Life-Oriented Behavioral Research for Urban Policy

Junyi Zhang
Editor

Life-Oriented Behavioral Research for Urban Policy

Springer

Editor
Junyi Zhang
Hiroshima University
Higashi-Hiroshima
Japan

ISBN 978-4-431-56470-6 ISBN 978-4-431-56472-0 (eBook)
DOI 10.1007/978-4-431-56472-0

Library of Congress Control Number: 2016955910

Printed on acid-free paper

This Springer imprint is published by Springer Nature
The registered company is Springer Japan KK
The registered company address is: Chiyoda First Bldg. East, 3-8-1 Nishi-Kanda, Chiyoda-ku, Tokyo 101-0065, Japan

Foreword I

Quality of life (QOL) is high in contemporary developed societies where people live longer and happier than ever in human history. One reason for this high OQL is in societal developments, such as greater wealth, better health care, and more safety. A related reason is greater individual choice, which means that more people can choose to live a life that fits them. These developments have created a demand for information about what determines OQL. Policymakers need information about the effects of their choices on the QOL of citizens, e.g., for deciding whether to invest in motorways or railways. Likewise, individual citizens need such information to help them make private choices, such as whether to buy a car or a train season ticket. The more we plan, the more information we need.

This need for information about effects that choices will have on QOL is met in several ways, by personal hearsay, listening to expert opinions, and discussions in the mass media. There is a growing stream of self-help advisory books on QOL, and the number and types of professional advisors available to us, e.g., policy consultants and lifestyle coaches, are growing. The information provided by such advisors depends very much on personal experience and conviction, but such professionals are drawing increasingly on empirical research. Much of that scientific knowledge has been gathered in the *Encyclopedia of Quality of Life and Well-Being Research..*

Scientific research on the effects of choices on QOL begins by looking for general patterns, such as whether life is typically better in small towns than in big cities. Several such common effects have been found in research on physical health, e.g., that smoking mostly works out to be bad for people's health and that eating an apple a day tends to keep people healthy. Yet research in subjective QOL has revealed few such common outcomes: typically it is found that effects of choice differ across persons and situations. This means that policymakers or individuals cannot make an informed choice using only some "rules of thumb" that apply always and everywhere. Contingencies must be taken into account; the trick is to find out what works for whom, when, and where.

These complexities have been acknowledged in the past, as I remember from the lectures on behavioral analysis in the 1960s delivered by my psychology professor, Rob Wentholt, who made me see that there are no iron laws and that mono-disciplinary thinking is unproductive. Yet acknowledging contingencies theoretically appears to be easier than applying this approach in empirical research. At that time samples were mostly too small to allow specification of sub-groups, statistical methods not sufficiently sensitive, and the body of research findings remained too small and scattered to allow for fruitful comparison across time and places. As a result most research on effects of choice has aimed at finding rules of thumb, often presented as "hypotheses" that x leads to y.

However, change is coming. Today an increasing number of researchers is delving into contingencies, not only because of theoretical enlightenment but also because easier questions have been settled and because advancements in research techniques allow us now to deal better with the more complex issues left. Today we have more and better data and are better able to exploit these data. This allows us to see choice and its consequences in a much wider context than before. In research on health and on family this approach is known as the "life course". In urban studies, this thinking has now crystallized into the "life-oriented approach" presented here.

This book marks one of the first steps, but certainly not the last, toward making better-supported decisions on issues that affect the quality of life at the level of populations, groups, and individuals.

Ruut Veenhoven
Emeritus Professor of Social Conditions
for Human Happiness,
Erasmus Happiness Economics Research
Organization EHERO
Erasmus University Rotterdam
Rotterdam
Netherlands
Director of the World Database of Happiness,
Founding Editor of the Journal of Happiness Studies
Rotterdam
Netherlands

Foreword II

Through a carefully curated selection of topics, Prof. Zhang and numerous colleagues have persuasively demonstrated the value of expanding our perspective beyond the single-domain focus that characterizes most social research, to investigate the interconnections among domains. The book offers tremendous breadth in the domains it examines and links, and presents a healthy mix of conceptual frameworks, methodological theory, and empirical application. This volume should be consulted by everyone who studies in any of these domains, and it is sure to prompt much-needed contemplation of inter-domain causes and effects, together with research and application collaborations across domains. The result will be greater understanding of the linkages between various realms of life and a new sensitivity to the impacts that trends, policies, constraints, and choices in one realm can have on other realms.

Patricia Lyon Mokhtarian
Professor of Civil
and Environmental Engineering
Georgia Institute of Technology
Atlanta
USA
Chair of International
Association for Travel Behaviour
Research (IATBR)
Former Professor
of Civil and Environmental Engineering,
University of California
Davis California
USA

Foreword III

I evaluate this book highly, because it has brought a new scientific method to policy making in town planning.

To improve the habitability of cities, policymakers should understand cause-and- effect relationships. There are good reasons for researchers to challenge decision- oriented studies on such relationships by examining actual situations. In the field of town planning, comparative case studies have been conducted to learn from their successes and failures. However, the definitions of success in these cases differ. In light of this situation, this book defines success as an improvement in quality of life (QOL). By revealing the relationships between QOL and various life choices, this book contributes to the establishment of effective policy. In addition, it seems reasonable to treat people's various life choices in an integrated manner because life choices are interrelated rather than independent. The content of this book is reliable and attractive because it has been constructed through discussions with many researchers at international conferences (especially the two international workshops that Prof. Zhang organized at the 14th International Conference on Travel Behaviour Research in July 2015 and the 95th Annual Meeting of Transportation Research Board in January 2016). This book also adds much more important information (e.g., women's labor participation, risky behaviors, mobility biographies and socialization, people's adaptation to natural disasters, and migration) than the Japanese edition, published by the Japan Society of Civil Engineers (JSCE) in March 2015 and edited by a research subcommittee led by Prof. Zhang.

Finally, I look forward to the day when effective innovative policies can be constructed based on findings from life-oriented behavior research that elucidates the relationship between diverse life choices and QOL.

Noboru Harata
Professor of the Department of Urban Engineering
Graduate School of Engineering,
The University of Tokyo
Tokyo
Japan

Preface

Policy makers in many sectors and researchers in many disciplines claim that their activities aim to improve people's quality of life (QOL). However, their claims are actually based on different "languages". Lack of a common "language" has hindered mutual understanding and meaningful collaboration between sectors and between disciplines. This consequently results in inefficient use of limited capital and waste of knowledge from various disciplines for urban policymaking. Motivated by such a troublesome situation, this book aims to present a new research stream, i.e., the life-oriented approach, as one of the "common languages" to facilitate the "talk" between different stakeholders for improving people's QOL. Even though various dialogues between different disciplines occur here and there, unfortunately, behavioral disciplines with truly interdisciplinary features could not be found in the literature for supporting urban policy decisions, which are usually associated with various life domains.

The life-oriented approach argues that people's various life choices, being attributable to QOL, are interrelated to one another. In other words, one life choice may not only result from other life choices but also affect other life choices. Such interdependencies are essential to understanding human decisions. For example, travel results from participation in various activities in different locations. Energy consumption also results from activity participation, and it occurs at home, at the office or school, or on the way from home to office or school, and so on. Health conditions are outcomes of not only lifestyles such as eating, drinking, sleeping, and physical exercises but also life choices such as residential location, daily travel behavior, and time-use behavior. Women's job participation is usually a result of considerations about family life arrangements (e.g., child care and education, care of parents, and other household affairs), a spouse's job, and the women's own life design. These life choices, among others, have been studied in various disciplines. There are various disciplines in favor of competition. The life-oriented approach puts more emphasis on collaborations in resolving various life issues than other approaches do.

I came up with the vague idea of the life-oriented approach in the very late 1990s when I started my consultant career in Tokyo, Japan. During that period, I witnessed how various civil services and policies had seriously suffered from bad collaborations across governmental sectors, and recognized that better jobs could be done under better collaborations across governmental sectors. Unfortunately, I could not find any truly interdisciplinary research field for supporting cross-sectoral policymaking.

Since 2002, when I joined my current workplace, I had been involved in two large-scale interdisciplinary research and education programs: (1) the 21st Century of Excellence (COE) Program "Social capacity development for environmental management and international cooperation" (April 2003–March 2008), supported by the Japan Society for the Promotion of Science (JSPS); and (2) the Global environmental leaders education program for designing a low-carbon society (July 2008–June 2012), supported by MEXT (Ministry of Education, Culture, Sports, Science and Technology) Special Coordination Funds for Promotion of Science and Technology, Japan. I worked together with researchers from disciplines such as economics, health science, environmental science, and education.

The above interdisciplinary research experiences further motivated me to meet the challenge of what I had not been able to do during my consultant period, i.e., studies on the life-oriented approach. In late 2009, I proposed a research project titled "Development of cross-sector urban planning and management methodologies by establishing a life-oriented approach" to the Japan Society for the Promotion of Science (JSPS) and successfully won a 4-year research "Grant-in-Aid for Scientific Research (A)" (April 2010–March 2014; No. 22246068). It was the first time that I formally used the name "life-oriented approach" in this project, for which I invited researchers in the fields of travel behavior, urban planning, transportation planning, environmental engineering, environmental economics, home economics, health science, architecture, sociopsychology, and related disciplines. Policies targeted in this project included low-carbon urban system design, mobility and social exclusion, urban tourism, promotion of healthy urban life, regeneration of central urban areas, and urban governance. After the above JSPS project, I won another JSPS Grant-in-Aid for Scientific Research (B) project titled "The progress of urbanization due to migrants from rural areas and its impacts on the low-carbon urban development under China's new urbanization policy (April 2014–March 2017; No. 26303003)" and a Grant-in-Aid for Scientific Research (A) project titled "Interdisciplinary research on policies promoting young people's migration to and permanent residence in local cities (April 2015–March 2019; No. 15H02271)", where the life-oriented approach is positioned as one of the core theoretical methodologies. Major research findings from these three JSPS projects are introduced in this book.

The life-oriented approach aims to evolve as a truly interdisciplinary behavioral discipline because it attempts to cover various life choices within the same research framework. In the writing of this book, I recommended that all authors focus more on literature review from the interdisciplinary perspective by selecting major references on life choices. I believe that readers can learn a lot not only about the life-oriented approach, but also about how to improve behavioral studies on the life choices of their interest from such interdisciplinary literature review. I am very proud of all the authors' excellent contributions to this book. My sincere thanks first go to all the authors of this book. This book would not have been published without the help of Springer staff and financial support by the Japan Society for the Promotion of Science (JSPS). I also deeply appreciate all my students involved in studies on the life-oriented approach and all members of the above three JSPS research projects. Finally, without the support and understanding of my wife Ziying Jiang and my daughter Xinyue Zhang (a second-year student at the Sauder School of Business at the University of British Columbia, Canada), I could not have devoted myself to this book, either.

Studies on the life-oriented approach are ongoing. Developing it as a truly interdisciplinary behavioral discipline needs more researchers' unremitting efforts. The door is always open. Welcome to this new academic continent.

San Francisco, USA Junyi Zhang
July 2016

Contents

Chapter 1
Life-Oriented Approach

Junyi Zhang

Abstract This chapter first emphasizes the importance of understanding human behavior for urban policymaking and discusses the motivations of proposing the core approach in this book, i.e., the life-oriented approach. Second, it describes the life-oriented approach, which argues that interdependencies are essential to understand various life choices. Third, this chapter summarizes the contents of each chapter included in this book.

Keywords Life-oriented approach · Cross-sectoral approach · Decision-making process of public policy · Human behavior · Quality of life · Interdependencies · Life choices · Inter-behavioral analysis

1.1 Introduction

Human activities have resulted in various changes to the land, water, and air as well as the society throughout several million years (Wolman 1993). Such changes involve many urban issues, such as urban sprawl, excessive land use, traffic congestion and accidents, housing issues, health issues, air pollution, and wastes. Currently, more than half of human beings are living in urban areas across the whole world. People pursue happiness. Many people believe that cities provide more opportunities to them for enjoying their life than rural areas do, and living in cities makes them experience a happier life. However, such belief is not always consistent with the reality in actual life. Accordingly, urban policies need to address the above issues for not only protecting natural environment, but also improving people's quality of life (QOL) (e.g., life satisfaction and happiness).

J. Zhang (✉)
Hiroshima University, Higashi-Hiroshima, Japan
e-mail: zjy@hiroshima-u.ac.jp; junyizh24@gmail.com

J. Zhang (ed.), *Life-Oriented Behavioral Research for Urban Policy*,
DOI 10.1007/978-4-431-56472-0_1

Various life choices (or consumption in life) affect the QOL, which has been investigated with respect to various life domains, such as residence, neighborhood, health, education, work, family life, leisure and recreation, finance, and travel behavior (e.g., Zhang and Xiong 2015). People usually perform different life choices under various constraints (e.g., money, time, and capability), and accordingly, they have to trade off between life choices, resulting in various interdependencies. In this sense, it is not desirable to incorporate different life choices separately in policymaking. Generally, the decision-making process of public policy consists of four stages: (1) agenda formation, (2) policy adoption, (3) policy implementation, and (4) policy review (Fawcett et al. 1988). No matter how important an issue related to a specific life choice may be, if its importance cannot not be recognized at the stage of agenda formation together with other issues, policies for resolving the issue cannot be made.

Urban policy decisions usually involve stakeholders from different vertically divided sectors. To date, criticisms of unsuccessful cross-sectoral policies have been directed at the lack of better institutional governance (e.g., Stead 2008; Cole et al. 2010). However, I would like to argue that the lack of interdisciplinary approaches, including the life-oriented approach proposed in this book, is more serious. As argued by Shafir (2013), the success or failure of public policy heavily depends on the understanding of human behavior. Policy resources are limited. Policy makers in different sectors need to know whether their sector-oriented policies improve a certain aspect of the QOL, but worsen other QOL aspects, if they do not collaborate with each other. In many case, collaboration between governmental sectors may generate synergic effects. Therefore, it is important for policy makers and other stakeholders to communicate with each other based on a common language.

As shown in the Shafir's (2013) book, economics, especially, behavioral economics has been the dominating discipline to provide behavioral foundation for public policy. Economics (or behavioral economics) can provide convincing behavioral evidence on the understanding of a single life choice. Unfortunately, it seems that interrelated life choices are not the interest of economists (or behavioral economists), or at least economists (or behavioral economists) have not made enough effort to develop frameworks for analysis of interrelated life choices.

Motivated by the above-mentioned practical issues and research gap in literature, this book presents the life-oriented approach, which is an interdisciplinary approach and expected to serve as a common language for supporting cross-sectoral policy decisions.

1.2 The Life-Oriented Approach

Needless to say, the life-oriented approach also argues that understanding human behavior is essential to urban policymaking. More importantly, it argues that people's decisions on various life choices are interdependent. Such interdependencies are essential to understand human behavior. A specific life choice may result from

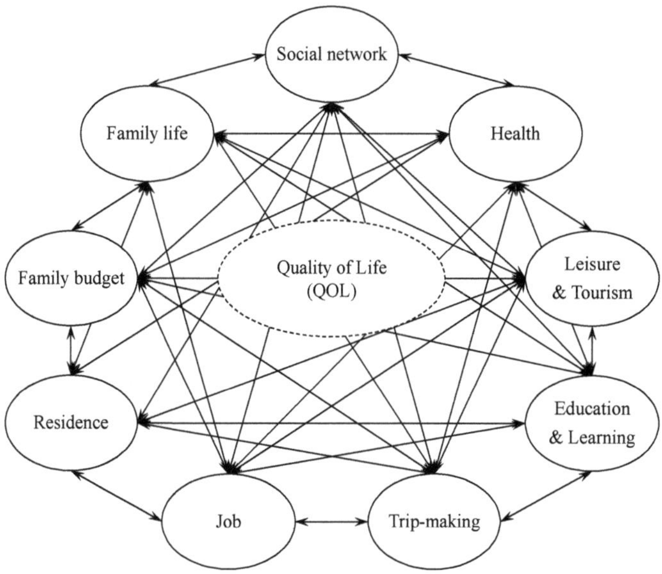

Fig. 1.1 An image of interdependencies across life choices

and/or affect other life choices. Figure 1.1 conceptually illustrates this argument. Note that the life domains shown are just some examples to classify the various life choices. As stated by Zhang (2015), there are various domain-generic and domain-specific reasons for such interdependencies. Improving the QOL, meeting various life needs, and sharing household resources (e.g., income, time, and living space) are some examples of common reasons across life domains. Health concerns are a part of domain-specific reasons why residential and travel behavior and health promotion behavior may be interrelated. Environmental concerns are another example of domain-specific reasons why residential and travel behavior and in-home energy consumption behavior may not be independent of each other. Various life choices also affect QOL. Better job may allow people to earn more money, which is essential to QOL. Good habits of performing physical exercise regularly and eating healthier foods usually result in good health conditions, which are a core element of health-related QOL. To many people, living in a good house is a symbol of social status, which is also indispensable for QOL. Especially, Chap. 2 of this book presents empirical evidence on interdependencies across life domains and effects of life choices on QOL. Interdependencies across life domains revealed in Chap. 2 can be illustrated in Fig. 1.2, showing an extremely complicated pattern of interdependencies. Readers can find more evidence from both literature review and empirical studies in other chapters.

Behaviorally, the ignorance of and inability to understand a specific life choice by considering the influence of other life choices may lead to a biased estimation of that specific life choice and behavioral changes in response to policies affecting

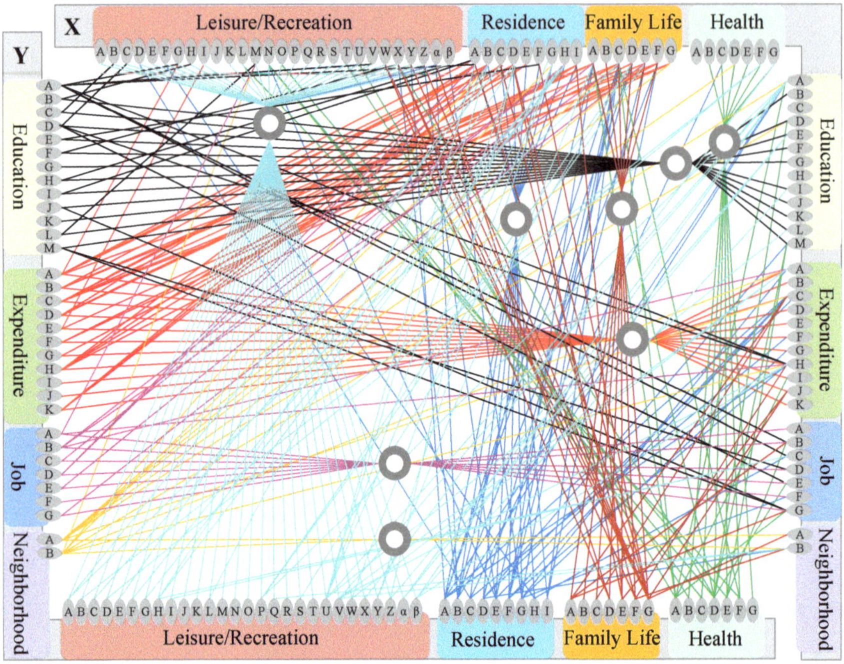

Fig. 1.2 Revealed relationships between 80+ life choice variables (Data collected in Japan in 2010)

it. In this sense, understanding of a specific life choice should not be constrained by the boundary of any single discipline. The ignorance of and inability to understand interdependent life choices may result in a failure of consensus building for policy decisions. Behavioral interdependencies between life choices suggest the necessity of cross-sectoral policies for QOL improvements. The life-oriented approach aims to serve as a common decision support method for various public policies and as a platform for negotiations across sectors and stakeholders.

1.3 Outlines of Chapters

This book consists of 18 chapters, including this chapter. Chapters 2–18 provide an extensive review of existing studies in various disciplines and present rich insights for future research.

First, Chap. 2 provides empirical evidence on the existence of interdependencies across an extensive set of life choice variables based on data from a cross-sectional survey, a panel survey, and a life history survey implemented in Japan in 2010 and 2014. It examines the interdependencies from both static and dynamic perspectives. It further investigates relationships between QOL and life choices.

Especially, evidence on cross-domain interdependencies and future expectations has long-lasting reference values.

Second, Chap. 3 focuses on the concept of lifestyle, which is usually defined by subjective factors (e.g., values and attitudes) and/or objective factors (including various life choices), and illustrates how this concept has been defined and analyzed in several major research disciplines. Related to the lifestyle, existing literature has often targeted ownership and usage of cars and various in-home appliances as well as residential behavior. In these two decades, information and communication technologies (ICTs) have become indispensable in many people's daily life and shaped their lifestyles in a different way from other technologies. In addition, many people prefer healthy lifestyles, in which not only daily activities but also non-daily activities (especially tourism) play important roles. With these considerations, Chap. 4 investigates car dependence in people's life, where new evidence on the decline in young people's car ownership and usage is presented based on a longitudinal dataset of household expenditure in Japan, together with descriptions about shared mobility, life-oriented studies, social exclusion, and behavioral changes. Chapter 5 examines ownership and usage of cars and various in-home appliances as well as residential location choices from the perspective of energy consumption, where an efficiency analysis is conducted for clarifying minimum energy consumption for a household, ABC factors (i.e., attitude, belief, and consciousness) and self-selection issues are emphasized, and an integrated dynamic energy consumption modeling system is introduced. Chapter 6 explores the association between ICT and people's life in terms of lifestyles, impacts of ICT on society and long-term decisions, urban form, travel behavior, shared mobility services, and the future of cities as well as autonomous vehicles (AVs). Chapter 7 describes health-oriented behavioral research by focusing on lifestyle habits, travel behavior (commuter paradox, active travel, etc.), park use, residential environments, and urban infrastructure, where health-related QOL is captured in terms of not only physical aspects, but also mental and social aspects; the famous stage of change model and the global movement of healthy cities are introduced. Chapter 8 treats life-oriented tourism behavior research by classifying tourism behavior into the following dimensions: information search and use, the social aspect, resources, the spatial aspect, activity participation and the temporal aspect. Literature review is given with respect to each dimension, followed by review about integrated tourism behavior models, relationship between tourism behavior and other life choices, tourism and quality of life, and determinants of tourism behavior. Importance of qualitative research in the future is emphasized.

Third, several typical behavioral issues related to urban policies are targeted in Chaps. 9–12. Chapter 9 deals with women's labor participation, where literature review is given with respect to women's labor participation associated with land use, transport, health, family, and leisure life as well as QOL, followed by a case study in Japan based on a recursive multiequation system. Focusing on the elderly mobility, Chap. 10 describes hierarchy of travel needs; discusses interdependencies between mobility and other life domains, mobility and well-being; argues the importance of measuring freedom to achieve and the components of mobility; and re-assesses policy goals on mobility of the elderly. Chapter 11 looks at risky behaviors in life, especially focusing on young people. It first describes risky behaviors in daily life and then review major theories (Heinrich's domino model, problem behavior theory, social development model for representing anti-social behavior, life history theory, lifetime utility theory). It further illustrates young people's risky driving by reviewing studies on driving tasks; risk homeostasis theory; applications of theory of planned behavior; influences of family, peers, and passengers on young people's risky driving behavior; avoidance driving; mood during driving and driving purpose; driving and nightlife; and self-driving cars and young people. Chapter 12 examines how people adapt their life to natural disasters by taking Bangladesh as a case study area. General literature review is given with respect to adaptation behaviors in terms of intercity travel and general life adaptations, followed by descriptions about a stated preference based case studies in the context of floods and cyclones.

Fourth, several major methodological issues related to life choices are explored, including general biographical research (Chap. 13), a new modeling method to represent various mobility decisions over the life course (Chap. 14), multi-dimensional household timing decisions in daily life (Chap. 15), theories of behavioral change (Chap. 16) and an application to explore migration in association with other life choices (Chap. 17). Concretely speaking, Chap. 13 describes the concept of mobility biographies (especially focusing on habits, domains of the life course, and transitions and key events in the life course), highlights mobility socialization and linked lives, argues that the importance of context, and discusses consequences for research. Chapter 14 supports the lifetime utility theory and applies the concept of multilinear utility to capture biographical interactions between residential, car ownership, household structure, and employment/education mobilities. An operational model is derived and its effectiveness is confirmed based on data from a life history survey collected in Japan in 2010. Chapter 15 deals with time use from the perspective of timing decisions, which have been an ill-defined issue in literature. It applied the concept of timing utility to represent household timing decision model with coupling constraints, first-order sequential correlations, nonnegative timing and sequencing constraints, where activities are distinguished between shared and nonshared activities and both observed and unobserved interdependencies are endogenously represented. Chapter 16 highlights life trajectories and choice models and especially describes promising individual-level modeling approaches for modeling lifecycle decisions and lifecycle driven behavioral changes, including discrete choice models with lifetime utility and social dynamics, attitudinal models, technology acceptance model, norm activation model, and value belief norm theory. Even though migration behavior is targeted, in fact, Chap. 17 presents an example how to capture behavioral changes across life domains. It argues that a behavioral change in one life domain may not only result from socio-psychological factors (e.g., behavioral intention, attitude, social norm, and perceived behavioral control) related to that domain, but also occur conditional on behavioral changes in other life domains.

Finally, Chap. 18 further discusses future research directions to promote the life-oriented approach for supporting various urban policies.

1.4 Summary

Urban policy serves for improving people's QOL. Both academic literature and actual policy practices suggest that such improvements rely heavily on better collaboration of different sectors. The life-oriented approach has various advantages for supporting urban policy over existing behaviorally oriented approaches. Such advantages are illustrated in each chapter. The life-oriented approach also has various unresolved research issues, which are discussed in each chapter as well. The life-oriented approach attempts to break the boundaries of various existing disciplines about human behavior research from a much broader perspective. The contents of the remaining chapters suggest that such cross-boundary efforts are not only important, but also feasible. Studies based on the life-oriented approach could be motivated by not only policy decisions, but also purely behavioral research. Policy makers may learn how to make cross-sectional policies by drawing on insights from such an interdisciplinary research, while researchers may learn how to resolve their single-discipline research issues by borrowing ideas from other disciplines in an integrated and consistent way.

This book introduces the life-oriented approach in a comprehensive and consistent way. It not only provides extensive literature review on interdependencies across various life choices in a variety of disciplines, but also presents new insights from new survey data based on new research methods. This book further illustrates inter-behavioral analysis frameworks with respect to various life domains based on case studies in different countries, along with a rich set of future research directions.

References

Cole R, Burke M, Leslie E, Donald M, Owen N (2010) Perceptions of representatives of public, private, and community sector institutions of the barriers and enablers for physically active transport. Transp Policy 17:496–504

Fawcett SB, Bernstein BS, Czyzewski MJ, Greene BF, Hannah GT, Iwata BA, Jason LA, Mathews RM, Morris EK, Otis-Wilborn A, Seekins T, Winett RA (1988) Behavior analysis and public policy. Behav Anal 11(1):11–25

Shafir E (2013) The behavioral foundations of public policy. Princeton University Press, Princeton

Stead D (2008) Institutional aspects of integrating transport, environment and health policies. Transp Policy 15:139–148

Wolman MG (1993) Population, land use, and environment: a long history. In: Jolly CL, Torrey BB (eds) Population and land use in developing countries. Committee on Population,

Commission on Behavioral and Social Sciences and Education, National Research Council. National Academies Press, Washington, DC
Zhang J (2015) The life-oriented approach and travel behavior research. A discussion paper for the workshop "Life-Oriented Approach for Transportation Studies" at the 14th international conference on travel behaviour research, Windsor, UK, July 19–23
Zhang J, Xiong Y (2015) Effects of multifaceted consumption on happiness in life: a case study in Japan based on an integrated approach. Int Rev Econ 62(2):143–162

Chapter 2
Empirical Evidence of Behavioral Interdependencies Across Life Choices

Yubing Xiong and Junyi Zhang

Abstract This chapter presents empirical evidence of behavioral interdependencies across more than 80 life choice variables, based on data collected from a cross-sectional survey, a panel survey, and a life history survey in Japan, respectively. Similar analyses are further conducted with respect to more than 20 indicators of life satisfaction and happiness, as a whole life and by life domain. Very complex patterns of cross-domain and within-domain interdependencies are revealed by using statistical modeling approaches. This is the first study in literature to clarify behavioral interdependencies across life choices from such a comprehensive way. Analyses also suggest a variety of research issues for promoting the life-oriented approach.

Keywords Life-oriented approach · Life choices · Life domain · Happiness · Life satisfaction · State dependence · Future expectation · Life history survey · Panel survey · Japan

2.1 Introduction

Many contemporary planning endeavors try to improve people's quality of life, and this goal has become central to the formulation of land use and transportation policies (Lotfi and Solaimani 2009). Quality of life (QOL) have been examined with respect to various life domains, such as residence (Heal and Chadsey-Rusch 1985; Wang and Li 2004; Cao 2016), social life (Honold et al. 2012; Delmelle

Y. Xiong (✉)
School of Transportation and Logistics, East China Jiao Tong University, Nanchang, China
e-mail: xiongmaozai1989@163.com

J. Zhang
Hiroshima University, Higashi-Hiroshima, Japan
e-mail: zjy@hiroshima-u.ac.jp; junyizh24@gmail.com

J. Zhang (ed.), *Life-Oriented Behavioral Research for Urban Policy*,
DOI 10.1007/978-4-431-56472-0_2

et al. 2013; Cambir and Vasile 2015; Lei et al. 2015), health (De Hollander and Staatsen 2003; Sturm and Cohen 2004; Curl et al. 2015; Tsai et al. 2016), education (Frisvold and Golberstein 2011; Winters 2011; González et al. 2016), employment (Huang and Sverke 2007; Zhao and Lu 2010; Tefft 2012), family life (Campbell 1976; Greenhaus et al. 2003; Huang and Sverke 2007), leisure and recreation (Leung and Lee 2005; Brajša-Žganec et al. 2011; Lin et al. 2013; Uysal et al. 2016), finance (Kaplan et al. 2008; Clark et al. 2008; Headey et al. 2008), and travel behavior (Abou-Zeid et al. 2012; Cao et al. 2013; Delmelle et al. 2013). Life choices in different life domains are usually made over different time scales and they are constrained by time and monetary considerations as well as by the various needs of households and their members. Therefore, changes in one of people's life choices may affect other choices. In other words, people's life choices are interdependent. Particularly over time, changes in residence/workplaces or vehicle ownership may have a significant impact on urban people's present/prospective life choices and QOL. Given these considerations, we can see that systematic investigations of various life choices, such as choice of residence and travel behavior, as well as QOL are important, especially from a dynamic and long-term viewpoint. However, many links between essential life choices and QOL embedded in land use and transportation planning are still unclear, because relevant studies are scarce in literature.

Links between transportation and QOL at the individual level have been recognized for several decades. Existing transportation studies have focused mainly on negative aspects of transportation, such as congestion, accidents, and air pollution. This is understandable because transportation policies, as one type of urban policy, must indicate how to mitigate the negative impacts of transportation externalities. In reality, however, travelers usually have both positive and negative feelings about travel activities (Zhang 2009; Ettema et al. 2010). Drivers stuck in traffic jams can experience stress and impatience, but multitasking during the use of transport systems allows people to make efficient use of time, which generates positive utility (Zhang 2009). Travel may also increase people's QOL because people's daily activities tend to be distributed across space, allowing them to strengthen social bonds and achieve personal goals (Ettema et al. 2010). Nordbakke and Schwanen (2013) found that having access to convenient transportation systems (e.g., living close to a public transit network) could generate feelings of freedom, competence, and belonging. A residence provides shelter, a fundamental human need, and people often need transportation to reach their home. Greater mobility (e.g., residential environment change) can also give people confidence and convince them that they are capable of realizing certain goals. Travel behavior is just a part of people's life choices. In this sense, travel behavior results from performing various human activities, as well as being a part of human mobility. People cannot survive without transportation; that is, transportation plays a vital role in meeting individuals' various needs (De Vos 2015).

This chapter has several purposes. First, using cross-sectional data, it: (1) statistically captures the interdependencies of life choices; and (2) clarifies the kinds of life choices, including residential choices and travel behavior, that affect people's

QOL and quantifies the effect sizes of these choices by controlling for the effects of land use attributes. Second, using midterm panel data, it: (1) examines the effects of the determinant factors of people's current life choices and QOL; and (2), illustrates the effects of changes in sociodemographics over time (individual attributes and changes of life events) on people's life choices and QOL. Third, from a long-term viewpoint, it: (1) clarifies biographical interdependences; and (2) demonstrates the changes in life choices and QOL in response to changes in people's life choices over the course of their lives.

2.2 Literature Review

2.2.1 Definition and Measurement of Quality of Life

Beginning in the 1960s, the question of quality of life (QOL) arose because the social costs of economic growth became more and more apparent to the public, especially environmental damage and the loss of future resources. Moreover, doubts grew about whether increasing the GDP would increase people's QOL (Tang 2007). Therefore, social scientists paid increasing attention to the QOL (Sirgy et al. 2000; George 2006), as did urban studies researchers (Khalil 2012; De Vos et al. 2013; Serag El Din et al. 2013). However, defining QOL is difficult, because it is a subjective experience that depends upon one's perceptions and feelings. There are over 100 definitions and models of QOL, but in recent years scholars have agreed that it is a multidimensional and interactive construct encompassing many aspects of people's lives and environments (Schalock 1996). Diener and Suh (1997) suggested that QOL is based on the experience of individuals. If a person experiences her/his life as good and desirable, it is assumed to be so, and factors such as feelings of joy, pleasure, contentment, and life satisfaction are paramount. Obviously, this definition of the QOL is most closely associated with the subjective well-being (SWB) tradition in the behavioral sciences. Andereck et al. (2007) and Uysal et al. (2012) have said that QOL refers to one's satisfaction with life and feelings of contentment or fulfillment with one's experiences in the world. It is concerned with how people view (or what they feel about) their lives. Similar situations and circumstances may be perceived differently by different people (Taylor and Bogdan 1990). QOL is a multifaceted and complicated concept. It is defined as a constellation of components that consists of three dimensions: positive, negative, and future expectations (Glatzer 2012). Future expectations are emphasized as a component of QOL because when someone experiences a bad situation, it matters whether that person is optimistic about the future or sees no way out.

To date, social indicators and subjective wellbeing (SWB) based approaches have been used to measure the QOL. Social indicators are societal measures that reflect people's objective circumstances in a given cultural or geographic unit. The hallmark of social indicators is that they are based on objective, quantitative statistics rather than on individuals' subjective perceptions of their social environment. Indicators such as infant mortality, doctors per capita, longevity, rape rates, homicide rates, and police per capita can be assessed to measure QOL. Nevertheless, objective indicators do not tell us how individuals perceive and experience their lives, whereas subjective evaluations define the experience of life more precisely. SWB refers to how people experience their whole lives, as well as specific life domains, and it includes both cognitive judgments and affective reactions (Diener 1984; Myers and Diener 1995). Concepts encompassed by SWB include positive and negative affects, happiness, and life satisfaction (Gilbert and Abdullah 2004). Happiness has been defined as transitory moods of "gaiety and elation" that people feel about their current state of affairs (Campbell 1976). Happiness is an affective mood or state (Bowling 1995), whereas life satisfaction refers to a cognitive sense of satisfaction with life (Kahn and Juster 2002; Diener 2000). Happiness occurs over shorter time frames and can be assessed via self-reported feelings or emotions during an interval or activity episode. Life satisfaction is a cognitive evaluation of a longer period of time (Diener and Suh 1997; Diener 2009). Both affect and judgments of satisfaction represent people's evaluations of their lives and circumstances.

More specifically, happiness has usually been measured with a question such as, "Taken all together, how happy would you say you are?" (Easterlin 2001; Veenhoven 2012). On a 10-point scale in which ten represents maximum happiness, one represents maximum unhappiness, and five represents neutrality, the median response was slightly over seven and the mean response not much lower (Myers and Diener 1996). As Veenhoven (2012) has noted, people may also derive happiness from a specific life domain (e.g., a happy marriage or a good job). Veenhoven (2012) found that there is only limited evidence about how different decisions affect happiness. He suggested that studies of the effects of time and monetary choices on happiness should be research priorities, and Zimmermann (2014) concurred. Dutt (2008) argued that happiness does not depend on consumption and income alone, but on many other things. People usually spend their income and time managing various types of life choices, such as education, housing, vehicles, tourism and leisure activities, and daily shopping. In addition, life satisfaction is a cognitive measure of QOL (Kahn and Juster 2002). It is widely accepted that life satisfaction can be measured saying, "Now I want to ask you about your life as a whole. How satisfied are you with your life as a whole these days?" This question from the 1976 national survey of the quality of American life (Campbell 1976) is typical of those that have been asked in many subsequent surveys. Typically, a five-point scale ranging from completely satisfied to completely dissatisfied is used. Measures of overall satisfaction with life allow respondents to weigh each life domain according to their own standards to form an evaluation of their satisfaction (Diener et al. 1985). Moreover, life satisfaction is jointly determined by context-specific factors in life domains. Some measures are simple summations or averages of domain-specific satisfaction scores, whereas others use weighting procedures in which responses to the direct questions about overall life satisfaction are dominant (Campbell 1976). Individuals judge different aspects of life more importantly than others and so it is important to understand which life domains contribute to life satisfaction. These questions depend upon the value an individual attaches to different experiences in life or the values they attach to various life domains (Sirgy 2010). However, how the domains interrelate, and which domains contribute most to overall life satisfaction, is unclear (Dolnicar et al. 2012).

2.2.2 Life Choices and Quality of Life

For individuals, the scientific understanding of quality of life (QOL) can guide important decisions in life, such as where and how to live and how to travel (Diener and Suh 1997). First, given the complex structural system of people's QOL, it is better to clarify how the life decisions made in different life domains affect people's QOL. Research from the life domain approach indicates that QOL is associated with various life domains, including residence, leisure and recreation, employment, health, social life, finance, education and learning, and family life (Knox 1975). The life domain approach maintains that satisfaction with each life domain determines overall well-being (Campbell 1976, 1981). These and other studies on life domain satisfaction suggest that satisfaction with health, family, and finance are the most important factors for overall life satisfaction (Cummins 1996; Salvatore and Munoz Sastre 2001; Van Praag et al. 2003). An earlier cross-sectional study by Cantril (1965) also indicates that economic factors, as well as health and family, rank highly among people's personal concerns. In an investigation of the livelihoods and well-being of low-income populations in Recife, Brazil, Maia et al. (2016) showed that the restricted mobility and activity patterns of citizens in these low-income communities influences or interacts with their QOL outcomes such as wealth, health, and well-being. Other research has confirmed that transportation planning and policy can play a role in enhancing people's future life chances. Specifically, with respect to the residential life domain, Wang and Li (2004) found that the residential satisfaction of young adults is influenced by individual local identity, financial capability, residence type, and an environment index based on comfort, convenience, and health. They also showed that housing ownership is central to residential satisfaction, based on a study in Beijing, China.

Cao (2016) adapted Campbell's model to examine the relationship between neighborhood characteristics and life satisfaction through perceptions and residential satisfaction and concluded that land use mix has both positive and negative impacts on life satisfaction, but the overall effect is insignificant. Both high density and poor street connectivity are detrimental to life satisfaction, but street connectivity is much more influential than density. To enhance life satisfaction, planners should limit neighborhoods with poor connectivity and implement strategies to promote positive responses to land use mix. As for the leisure or recreational domain, Brajša-Žganec et al. (2011) found that engaging in important leisure activities contributes to QOL, but the pattern of leisure activities varies somewhat by age and gender. Chen et al. (2016) examined the relationship between holiday recreational experiences and life satisfaction, as mediated by tourism satisfaction, for a sample of 777 respondents in the United States. They found that individuals who were able to control what they wanted to do, felt relaxed and detached from work, and had new and challenging experiences during a vacation were more likely to be satisfied with their holiday experiences and their lives in general. Uysal et al. (2016) made substantial contributions to the literature and provided guidance for future research on QOL and well-being in tourism. They pointed out that tourism experiences and activities have a significant effect on both tourists' overall life satisfaction and well-being of residents in tourist areas. That is, tourists' experiences and tourism activities tend to contribute to positive affect in a variety of life domains such as family life, social life, leisure life, cultural life, among others.

With respect to the financial domain, Clark et al. (2008) provided a good literature review of the effect of income on QOL, and they concluded that the relationship is generally positive. Headey et al. (2008) demonstrated that household income allocation is a stronger predictor of life satisfaction than household income alone. As for social life, Diener and Seligman (2002) found that social relationships are a major distinguishing factor in college students' happiness; the happiest students tend to have strong relationships with friends, family, and partners. Transportation-related social exclusion is increasingly recognized as having a significant impact upon QOL, especially for people who live in the rural areas (McDonagh 2006; Lamont et al. 2013). Cambir and Vasile (2015) described the state of art in the field of social inclusion in relation with the QOL and its material dimension and identified the main areas of Romania where national policies and strategies should be tailored to improve QOL. Lei et al. (2015) found that increased social participation among older adults in urban communities in China had a positive effect on various dimensions of health-related QOL. There is a need for policies that improve the integration of community-level public resources to encourage frequent social interaction among older adults and to promote health and social care as a whole.

Turning to family life, Campbell (1976) found that satisfaction with family life is a strong and significant predictor of overall QOL. With respect to employment, Zhao and Lu (2010) claimed that there is an urgent need to explore the determinants of workers' commuting time, as the reduced accessibility of jobs has had a serious negative effect on the quality of urban life, particularly in the megacities of China. Their analysis showed that the interaction of housing availability, the market system, and the *Hukou* system has a significant impact on individual commuting time, and by extension, on QOL. Alexopoulos et al. (2014) confirmed that higher levels of stress and longer work hours are related to job satisfaction and workers' QOL, although the magnitude of these associations varies depending upon age and gender. In the health domain, the role of the built environment in facilitating physical activity is well recognized. In a longitudinal study of "home zone" style changes designed to make residential streets more "livable" by reducing the dominance of vehicular traffic and creating shared spaces, Curl et al. (2015) examined broader self-reported behavioral (e.g., activity levels and perceptions), health, and quality of life outcomes. Among participants who were 65 or older, those in the intervention found it significantly easier to walk on the street near their home. Tsai et al. (2016) examined the cross-sectional and longitudinal association between sleep and health-related quality of life in pregnant women in Taiwan. They found that adequate sleep is essential for women at all stages of pregnancy and that improving the quantity and quality of nocturnal sleep in early gestation was especially important for an optimal health-related quality of life later in pregnancy. In the educational or learning domain, González et al. (2016) confirmed the motivational value and effectiveness of a gamification-training program that can prevent childhood obesity by using motor games and active videogames developed for overweight children aged 8–12. The outcomes included biometric variables, learning healthy habits, and experience with the intervention, and the results were highly satisfactory.

2.2.3 Behavioral Interdependencies of Life Choices

The interdependencies of life choices have not been satisfactorily explored, even though it is possible to identify studies that have examined several life choice variables. There is a large literature that investigates leisure related behavior and other life choices. Uysal et al. (2016) showed that tourists' experiences and tourism activities have positive effects in a variety of life domains, such as family life, social life, leisure life, and cultural life. Wilson et al. (2016) confirmed that participation in physical leisure activities, workload, and work environment all impact work-related fatigue. Tercan (2015) examined the relationship between leisure participation with one's family, family assessment, and life satisfaction among students at Akdeniz University and found that it is very important to understand students' family lives, as they develop leisure participation habits based on family life.

There is a great deal of literature on relationships between health-related behavior and other life choices. Fichera and Savage (2015) reported that there is a close relation between income and health improvement. They found that a 10 % increase in income is associated with a 0.02 (BMI: Body Mass Index) reduction in the number of illnesses in Tanzania. Based on a multilevel regression analysis of 1768 women living in the Paris metropolitan area, Vallée et al. (2010) discovered that the administrative characteristics of a neighborhood could promote or discourage the health-related behaviors of people whose daily activities are concentrated in the neighborhood. They confirmed the combined effects of activity space and neighborhood of residence on participation in preventive health-care activities.

Current theoretical models propose that work characteristics can influence health directly or indirectly via the work–family interface (Michel et al. 2009, 2011). Work–family conflict is a key construct that links the labor market and job quality to parents, family life, and children's home environments (Strazdins et al. 2013). For mothers and fathers, work–family conflict has been associated with poorer physical and mental health outcomes, poorer QOL, low job satisfaction and commitment, and high job turnover (Allen et al. 2000; Nomaguchi et al. 2005). Studies that have examined the early stages of the family life cycle have reported that work–family conflict is associated with poorer parental mental health and poorer parent–child interactions to a degree that measurably affects children's mental health (Cooklin et al. 2014, 2015a). Cooklin et al. (2015b) found that long and inflexible work hours, night shift work, job insecurity, a lack of autonomy, and more children in the household were associated with increased work–family conflict, and this was in turn associated with increased distress. In a survey of 3243 fathers of infants (aged 6–12 months) in Australia, job security, autonomy, and having a more prestigious occupation were positively associated with work–family enrichment and better mental health. With respect to social behavior and other life choices, Milner et al. (2016) reported that there is a strong direct effect of social support on mental health and that it differs between employed and unemployed persons. The availability of good social support buffers the mental health impact of unemployment considerably. Improvements in social support for the unemployed may reduce the mental health impacts of job loss. Given the well-established benefits of social support for mental health, studies have begun to explore how access to social support may be shaped by the residential context in which people live. Keene et al. (2013) used multilevel data from the Chicago Community Adult Health Survey to investigate the relationships between an individual's length of residence and measures of social integration, as well as the extent to which these relationships are moderated by neighborhood poverty. They found that the relationship between length of residence and some measures of social integration are stronger in poor neighborhoods than in ones that are more affluent. These findings suggest that long-term residence may contribute positively to well-being in low-income communities because residents have access to social resources that are likely to be health promoting. Most of the evidence indicates that various life choices are interdependent, and we need to understand the internal mechanism of interdependences to see how they contribute to QOL improvement.

2.2.4 Dynamics of Life Choices and Quality of Life

Transportation researchers have followed trends in other disciplines and started paying increased attention to subjectively experienced well-being and how this relates to travel behavior from a dynamic/life course perspective. It is well-known that travel behavior is both constrained and enabled by life events (Sharmeen et al. 2014; Oakil 2015), life cycle stages (Higgins et al. 1994; Lee and Goulias 2014), life course (Scheiner 2014; Schoendulet al. 2015), longer-term choices regarding lifestyle (Ritsema van Eck et al. 2005), residential location (Van Acker et al. 2010; van Acker 2015), and so on, and all of these aspects are closely related to well-being (De Vos et al. 2013). Many typical life events tend to cluster at certain stages in the life course, and they may have negative consequences for well-being if they do not occur at the usual age (McLanahan and Sorensen 1985). For instance, family formation (household structure change) usually occurs in young adulthood, whereas exit from the labor market is typically experienced towards the end of the life course. In a recent study, Powdthavee (2009) found that people who became severely disabled eventually returned to their pre-disability levels of satisfaction in various domains of life, with the exception of satisfaction with health and income, which remained significantly lower than before the onset of disability. Research by Plagnol and Scott (2011) offered further support for the idea that it is important for future research on QOL to take a life course perspective, as changes in the conceptualization of QOL may be linked to life course events. They found that entering a partnership and retirement have the largest effects on QOL. Sharmeen et al. (2014) found that in the year following the birth of a first child, travel behavior (such as car acquisition) and residential choices (such as living area) are independent. This means that policies aimed at reducing car use by changing housing situations may not be successful, as car ownership is affected by life choices other than changes in residential situation. In such cases, more detailed and longitudinal data are required. Scheiner (2014) noted that some key events, including the birth of a child, job participation, and changes in residential choices, have significant effects on travel mode choices. Abou-Zeid et al. (2012) reported that well-being is shaped by residential attributes and the dimensions of activities and trips, such as types of activities, duration of activities, persons with whom they are undertaken, and travel mode used. However, as Plagnol and Scott (2011) have said, we cannot completely rule out reverse causality, because it is possible people's QOL influences which events they experience. For instance, someone who believes in the importance of family is probably more likely to enter a long-term partnership and have children than someone who considers their career to be more important. Negative feelings such as stress can lead to immediate adjustments in people's activity and travel patterns and can have a spillover effect on subsequent travel behavior, as well as on choice of residential location. These reverse effects suggest that people may decide to change their residential location, dispose of or acquire vehicles, or reconfigure their mobility and activity patterns in order to improve their QOL. Hence, it is important to consider the multiple time scales implicated in the relationships between travel behavior, residential choices, and QOL, as QOL is temporally complex and has short-term and long-term dimensions.

2.3 Life-Oriented Behavioral Surveys: Cross-sectional, Panel, and Life History Surveys

In addition to long life expectancy (Coulmas et al. 2008), Japan is also known for its relatively traditional, rigid social structures with predetermined life courses and career paths (Sugimoto 2010), and especially the narrow wealth gap. These stable features suggest that an emphasis on the quality of life is more evident in Japan than in other societies (Inoguchi and Fujii 2009). Moreover, in order to capture the various behavioral interdependencies of life choices, especially from cross-sectional, dynamic, and long-term viewpoints, different time-series data sets are needed. Therefore, we conducted three Web-based surveys that covered all of the major cities in Japan, two life choice surveys in 2010 and 2014, and a life history survey in 2010.

2.3.1 The 2010 Web-Based Life Choice Survey

Considering the diversity and complexity of life choices, Zhang et al. (2011) conducted a Web-based life choice survey in Japan in January 2010 with the help of an Internet survey company that had more than 1.4 million registered panels at the time of survey. Respondents were randomly selected from the registered panels by considering the distributions of age, gender, and residential areas (here, referred to prefectures) across all of Japan. Zhang et al. (2011) argued that a Web-based survey is the most effective way to control the sample composition, which can be hard to achieve by other methods. However, we cannot deny that there are some sample selection biases. Nevertheless, considering that the Internet usage rate in Japan reached 75.5 % in 2010, the Internet might be an acceptable medium for conducting such a survey. A total of 2188 respondents participated in the survey, and 2178 provided valid answers for this study. The survey solicited very detailed information about individual's different life domains, including questions that asked about:

(1) Residence: location (zip code), length of stay, price (rental fee or purchase price), type, number of stories in the building, living area, number of rooms, distance to daily facilities, etc.
(2) Family budgets: income and expenditures.
(3) Health: subjective health condition, accidents and illnesses, amount of sleep, frequency and times of different types of physical exercise, and distance to places for physical exercise.
(4) Neighborhood: frequency of neighborhood communication and participation in community activities.
(5) Education and learning: academic degree, learning frequency and duration each time, distance, and major travel modes to different types of learning facilities.
(6) Job: location of workplace, commuting mode, job type, working days and hours per day, start and end time for a normal working day, paid holidays allowed and number of holidays actually taken, and number of years working.
(7) Family life: in-home and out-of-home time spent with family members on weekdays and weekends, frequency of communication with relatives, and care giving to preschool children and elderly or disabled family members.

(8) Leisure and recreation: discretionary time on weekdays and weekends, use of leisure time at different facilities (activity duration, frequency, distance to place, travel party (travel accompany during a trip such as relatives or friends), and major travel mode, tourism (domestic and overseas, frequency, travel party, and expenditure), and Internet usage (time and frequency).

A summary of the data characteristics is shown in Table 2.1. We expected decisions in the above domains to be interdependent. One can see that travel behavior such as possession of a driver's license, vehicle ownership (number and types of vehicles), and main travel mode are cross-domain behaviors. Furthermore, life satisfaction and happiness were also included to measure people's subjective QOL overall and in each domain, together with household attributes (numbers of preschool children, dependent students, and elderly members) and attributes of each

Table 2.1 Summary of characteristics of life choices survey data in 2010

Individual characteristics	Percentage	Individual characteristics	Percentage
Gender		*Household composition*	
Male	49.68	1 member	10.84
Female	50.32	2 members	28.83
Age		3 members	24.88
<15 years old	1.97	>3 members	35.45
15–17 years old	2.02	*Car ownership*	
18–34 years old	22.73	Have more than one car	26.91
35–64 years old	61.48	Have a private car	53.44
>64 years old	11.80	Have no car	19.65
Occupation		*Main travel mode*	
Employed	49.36	Cycling/walking	35.67
Part-time job	11.02	Public transit	23.51
Housewife	20.71	Car	36.64
Student	8.72	Others	4.18
Unemployed	10.19	*Health condition*	
Education level		Good	77.55
Having a bachelor degree	63.50	Not good	22.45
Having not a bachelor degree	36.50	*Life satisfaction*	
Marital status		Satisfied	57.07
Married	69.83	Neutral	32.87
Single	30.17	Dissatisfied	10.06
Household income		*Happiness*	
<2 million yen/year	7.76	9–10 point	13.22
2–6 million yen/year	46.46	6–8 point	51.56
>6 million yen/year	45.78	0–5 point	35.22

member (age, gender, marital status, relationship with household head, ownership of mobile phones, personal computer, etc.). For life satisfaction, respondents indicated on a 5-point scale how satisfied they were with their life as a whole and in each life domain (1 = very dissatisfied to 5 = very satisfied). For happiness, respondents indicated on a 11-point scale how happy they were currently (0 = very unhappy to 10 = very happy). For affective experience, the respondents assigned percentages to several moods (bad mood, low mood, pleasant mood, and very good mood) totaling to 100 % in each of the following domains: employment, social life, family life, and leisure and recreation. Based on these survey data, we found a bimodal distribution for happiness in Japan, with one peak at the center of the scale (5) and another at 7–8 (where 0 = very unhappy and 10 = very happy). The average happiness score was 6.37 (Fig. 2.1). The life satisfaction distribution is shown in Fig. 2.2.

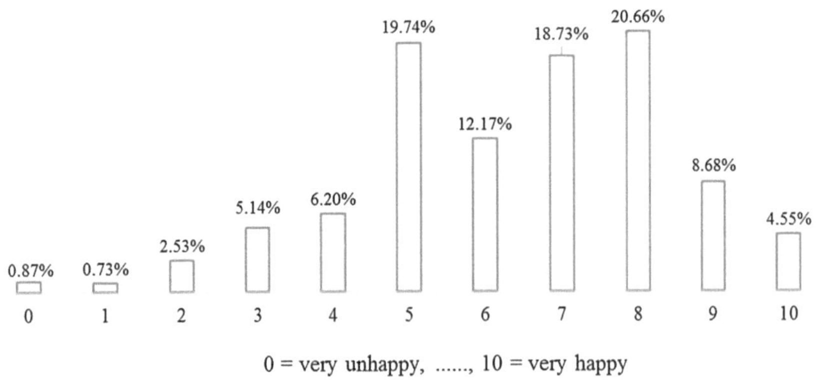

Fig. 2.1 Happiness scores

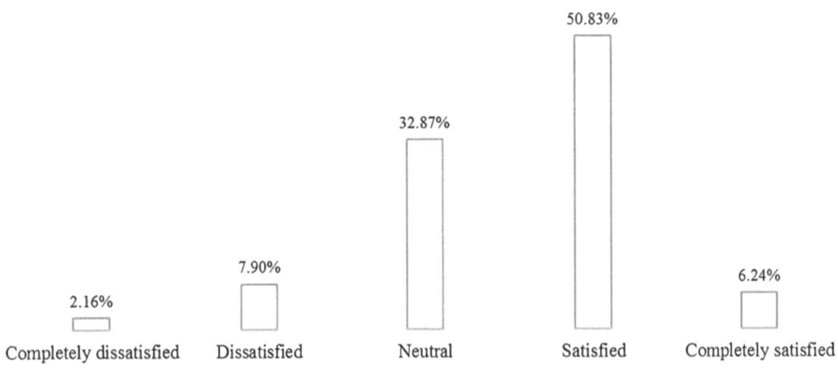

Fig. 2.2 Life satisfaction scores

2.3.2 The 2014 Web-Based Life Choice Survey

Zhang et al. (2014) conducted another life choice survey in January, 2014. Nine hundred respondents between 15 and 88 years old participated in the survey, and there were panel data for 422 participants who had responded to both the 2010 and the 2014 life choice surveys. The change rates for main life events and QOL indicators between 2010 and 2014 are shown in Fig. 2.3.

2.3.3 A Life History Survey

To disentangle behavioral interdependencies using a life course perspective, longitudinal data are required. Instead of a time-consuming panel survey, we used a retrospective approach that asked respondents to recall past mobility information. Using the same survey company mentioned above, this Internet-based life story survey was carried out in November 2010 in the major cities in Japan. Of the 6940 registered panels contacted, 1400 questionnaires were collected for which representative age, gender, and residential distributions across Japan are guaranteed. The response rate was 20.2 %. The survey focuses on four life events over the life course: residential mobility, household structure mobility, employment/education mobility, and car ownership mobility. Before answering detailed information about each type of mobility, respondents first indicated instances when their mobility changed, including the exact timing of relevant events (their age when the event occurred). To facilitate the reporting of detailed information, a simplified matrix showing these timings is presented in a separate window. Detailed information about each episode for each type of mobility is reported as follows:

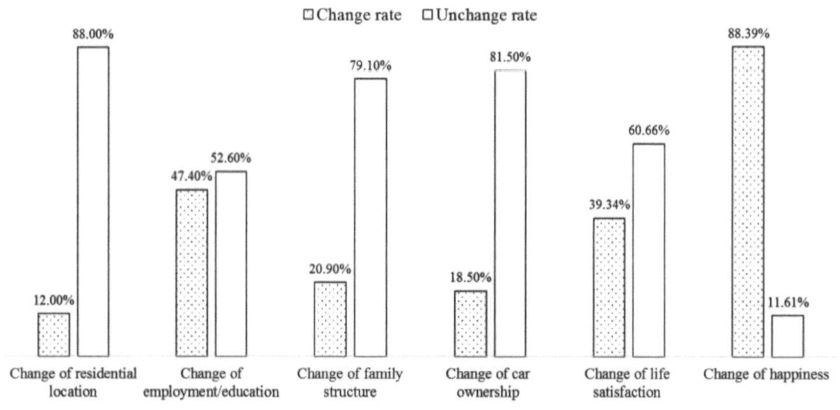

Fig. 2.3 The change rate of main life events based on panel data between 2010 and 2014

(1) Residential mobility: relocation place, income, residence property, and access (distance) to various facilities, including railways, bus stops, primary, junior, and high schools, hospitals, parks, supermarkets, and city hall, for each episode.
(2) Household structure mobility: household size, information about each household member for each episode, including age, gender, and relationship to householder.
(3) Employment/education mobility: job category, commute time to job/school, access to job/school, and travel mode for each episode.
(4) Car ownership mobility: number of cars, main user, car efficiency, purpose, and frequency of use for each episode.

In addition to the above information, QOL related variables (happiness and life satisfaction) were examined, and respondents were asked to report how confident they felt (11-point scale) about their answers to some major question items (e.g., access to facilities) with continuous values. Such confidence ratings can be used to reflect the reliability of the reported information as well as the quality of the retrospective survey. The data showed that the average confidence level varied from 7–9 across different cohorts (on the 11-point scale, 0 = not confident at all and 10 = completely confident), suggesting acceptable quality for the survey data. Figure 2.4 displays the mobility timing of residential location, car ownership,

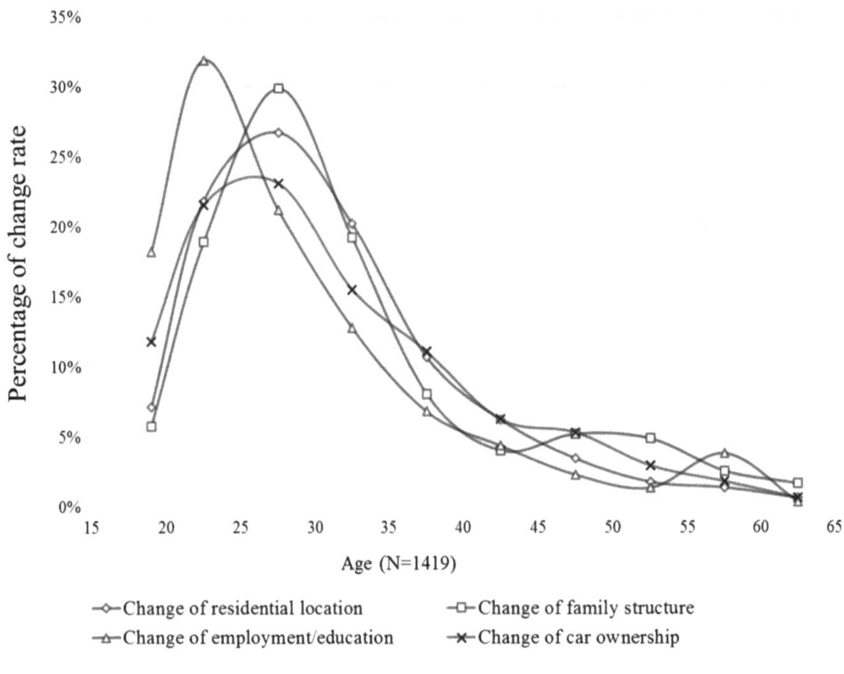

Fig. 2.4 Timing of mobilities in residential, household structure, employment/education, and car ownership

household structure, and employment/education over the life course in 5-year intervals. Obviously, there is a peak period of residential mobility between 20 and 35 years of age, and similar curves can be seen for the other three types of mobility.

2.4 Cross-sectional Analysis

2.4.1 Methodology

Considering the numerous life choice variables in this study, there are likely to be many correlations among them and more nonlinear relationships between these variables and QOL related variables, and these relationships must be treated properly. That is, a logical methodology will allow for consistent conclusions. Zhang (2014) has stated that there are interdependencies across the above eight life domains, and thus we must quantify such interdependencies in this analysis. To this end, we proposed an integrated approach employing a data mining method called Exhaustive Chi-squared Automatic Interaction Detector (CHAID) to clarify the kinds of life choice variables that have impacts on the target decisions (e.g., residence property, and QOL indicators). We also used a Bayesian Belief Network (BBN) approach to quantify the influence of the various variables. The results from the Exhaustive CHAID approach were used to build the network structure for the QOL indicators and life choices variables in the BBN approach.

2.4.1.1 Exhaustive CHAID Approach

Data mining is an analytical tool for exploring large datasets to identify consistent interdependencies among variables. CHAID, a decision tree technique based on adjusted significance testing, is one of the most popular methods used in science and business for prediction, classification, and detection (Kass 1980). It uses the available data to automatically build a series of "if–then" rules in the form of a decision tree. The tree begins with one root (parent) node for a target variable that contains all of the observations in the sample, and it grows to accommodate subgroups that are segmented based on predictors at various branch levels until the tree converges (based on stopping criteria). However, a CHAID analysis may not find the optimal split for a predictor variable. Exhaustive CHAID was developed to remedy this issue by continuing to merge categories of the predictor variables until only two super categories are left that have the strongest associations with the target variable. Thus, once a set of predictors is given for a target variable, the Exhaustive CHAID approach will automatically derive the best combination of predictors for the target variable. Thus, the arbitrary influences of analysts can be eliminated. However, the Exhaustive CHAID approach can only be used to clarify

Table 2.2 Explanatory variables

Land use attributes	**Employment domain**
Distance to railway station (km)	Occupation: officer; civil servant; merchant; part-time job; housewife; non-employee; others
Distance to bus stop (km)	
Distance to city hall (km)	Job type: technical professional; management; salesman; service staff; agriculture; others
Distance to community center (km)	
Distance to post office (km)	Commute mode[a]
Distance to hospital (km)	Working hours per day (paid)
Distance to supermarket (km)	Vacation actually taken (days/year)
Distance to Kindergarten (km)	Duration of tenure (years)
Distance to elementary school (km)	Monthly workdays (days)
Distance to secondary school (km)	**Health domain**
Distance to high school (km)	Sleep time
Distance to cinema/theatre (km)	Frequency of contact sports
Distance to sports facility (km)	Frequency of non-contact sports
Distance to park (km)	Frequency of gentle sports
Residence domain	Duration of contact sports (minutes)
Residence duration (years)	Duration of non-contact sports (minutes)
Living area (m^2)	Duration of gentle sports (minutes)
Housing type: attached house; terrace house; apartment; others	**Family life domain**
	Indoor time use on weekday
Number of stories of residential building	Outdoor time use on weekday
The floor where respondents lived	Indoor time use on non-weekday
Number of rooms	Outdoor time use on non-weekday
Residence property (own = 1; rent = 0)	Household composition
Main travel mode[a]	Frequency of having dinner with family
Vehicle ownership (number of vehicles)	Frequency of contact with relatives
Finance domain	**Leisure and recreation domain**
Household annual income: 1: < 1, 2: 1–2, 3: 2–3, 4: 3–4, 5: 4–5, 6: 5–6, 7: 6–7, 8: 7–8, 9: 8–9, 10: 9–10, 11:10–15, 12: > 15 million yen	Frequency of going to cinema and theatre
	Frequency of going to sports facilities
	Frequency of going to amusement parks
Percentage of food expenditure	Frequency of going to entertainment places
Percentage of housing expenditure	Frequency of going to racing facilities
Percentage of energy expenditure	Travel party[c] to cinema and theatre
Percentage of furniture expenditure	Travel party[c] to sports facilities
Percentage of clothes expenditure	Travel party[c] to amusement parks
Percentage of healthcare expenditure	Travel party[c] to entertainment places
Percentage of transport expenditure	Travel party[c] to racing facilities
Percentage of education expenditure	Travel mode to cinema and theatre[a]
Percentage of leisure expenditure	Travel mode to sports facilities[a]
Percentage of saving	Travel mode to amusement parks[a]
Percentage of other expenditure	Travel mode to entertainment places[a]
	Travel mode to racing facilities[a]
	Duration at cinema and theatre (minutes)
	Duration at sports facilities (minutes)
	Duration at amusement parks (minutes)
	Duration at entertainment places (minutes)
	Duration at racing facilities (minutes)
	Leisure frequency
	Tourism frequency
	Frequency of going home for a visit
	Leisure expenditure (yen/year)
	Tourism expenditure (yen/year)
	Expenditure on going home for a visit (yen/year)
	Internet usage frequency (use every day = 1,0)
	Internet usage time (minutes/day)

(continued)

Table 2.2 (continued)

Learning and education domain
Education level (bachelor = 1,0)
Frequency of language learning
Frequency of knowledge learning
Frequency of hobby learning
Frequency of job training
Duration of language learning (minutes)
Duration of knowledge learning (minutes)
Duration of hobby learning (minutes)
Duration of job training (minutes)
Travel mode for language learning[a]
Travel mode for knowledge learning[a]
Travel mode for hobby learning[a]
Travel mode for job training[a]
Neighborhood domain
Frequency of neighborhood communication[b]
Participation in community activities[b]

Note
[a]Travel mode or main travel mode or commute mode: car; walking; public transit; others
[b]Frequency of neighborhood communication/community activities: often; sometimes; rare
[c]Travel party: alone; family member; colleague/classmate; acquaintance; friend; others

effects of land use attributes. The results from Exhaustive CHAID are shown in Tables 2.3, 2.4, 2.5, 2.6, 2.7, 2.8 and 2.9, and the results of the BBN are shown in Tables 2.10 and 2.11. The BBN estimation (with predictors derived from the Exhaustive CHAID) shows the variance reduction (VR) calculated in parentheses after each predictor. Variance reduction is the expected reduction in the variance of a target node because of the introduction of an input node. In this sense, VR can be used to evaluate the degree of influence of each predictor on the target variable. In Tables 2.3, 2.4, 2.5, 2.6, 2.7, 2.8, 2.9, 2.10 and 2.11, the first column shows the indicators of various life choices, including travel behavior and residential choices, and the second and last columns show the predictors for each indicator. The value in parentheses after each target variable in Tables 2.3, 2.4, 2.5, 2.6, 2.7, 2.8, 2.9, 2.10 and 2.11 is the accuracy of the decision tree split, which ranged between 60 and 86 %, suggesting that the Exhaustive CHAID approach achieved acceptable accuracy. The classification accuracy of the BBN that was estimated using Netica software was evaluated based on standard scoring rules, including logarithmic loss, quadratic loss, and spherical payoff (Morgan et al. 1990). Spherical payoff values, the most useful index, vary from 0 to 1, with 1 indicating the best model performance. The logarithmic loss values are calculated using the natural log, between 0 and infinity (inclusive), where a smaller value suggests better performance. Quadratic loss values range from 0 to 2, with 0 being the best. For our model structure, the spherical payoff was 0.9091, the logarithmic loss was 0.53, and the quadratic loss was 0.6842. All of these values indicate that the BBN model performs well.

Given the results in Table 2.10, it is clear that income (i.e., household annual income) influences happiness, but this is only true with respect to happiness and

Table 2.3 Significant factors influencing the variables in residence life

Target variables	Predictors
Residence duration (82.6 %)	Percentage of housing expenditure, household annual income, distance to nearest park, duration at amusement park, distance to nearest hospital, percentage of furniture expenditure, household composition, frequency of going to cinema and theatre, percentage of education expenditure, residence property, distance to city hall
Living area (66.4 %)	Residence property, number of rooms, residence duration, frequency of neighbor communication, percentage of transport expenditure, house type, tourism expenditure, household composition, travel party to amusement park, percentage of clothes expenditure, main travel mode, job type, vehicle ownership, percentage of education expenditure, travel mode to entertainment places
Housing type (84.6 %)	Number of stories of residential building, residence property, number of rooms, living area, tourism frequency, distance to nearest kindergarten, travel mode for language learning, distance to nearest secondary school, travel party to cinema and theatre, duration of gentle sports, frequency of neighbor communication
Number of stories of residential building (91.70 %)	The floor lived, house type, distance to railway station, percentage of food expenditure, percentage of furniture expenditure, household annual income, percentage of transport expenditure, household composition, residence property, distance to supermarket, distance to city hall, distance to nearest elementary school
The floor where lived (71.90 %)	Number of stories of residential building, residence property, frequency of gentle sports, percentage of furniture expenditure, sleep time, residence duration, frequency of contact with relatives, frequency of neighbor communication, travel mode to entertainment places, distance to nearest kindergarten, travel party to cinema and theatre, frequency of going to sports facilities, travel mode to cinema and theatre, percentage of education expenditure, distance to city hall, distance to supermarket
Number of rooms (75.70 %)	Living area, outdoor time use on non-weekday, number of stories of residential building, education level, percentage of transport expenditure, residence duration, vehicle ownership, distance to supermarket, percentage of education expenditure, house type, frequency of contact with relatives, percentage of energy expenditure, household composition, frequency of neighbor communication

(continued)

Table 2.3 (continued)

Target variables	Predictors
Residence property (88.10 %)	House type, residence duration, living area, distance to railway station, number of rooms, number of stories of residential building, travel mode to amusement park, percentage of transport expenditure, distance to nearest elementary school
Main travel mode (70.90 %)	Commute mode, indoor time use on weekday, travel mode to sports facilities, vehicle ownership, frequency of having dinner with family, education level, occupation, travel mode to cinema and theatre, percentage of education expenditure, travel mode to entertainment places, household annual income
Vehicle ownership (62.20 %)	Household composition, main travel mode, house type, travel mode to amusement park, living area, percentage of furniture expenditure, percentage of saving, duration of tenure, household annual income, number of rooms, duration of non-contact sports, expenditure on going home for a visit, distance to nearest post office, frequency of neighbor communication, number of stories of residential building, percentage of transport expenditure

Note The value in the parenthesis after each target variable shows the accuracy of decision tree split based on the Exhaustive CHAID approach (100 % means a perfect representation)

the mildly pleasant mood produced by leisure activities. However, it was not the most influential factor. In the case of happiness, the variable with the greatest influence was the percentage of saving (i.e., income saved), with a VR of 30.80 %, which is about three times higher than that of income (VR = 10.76 %). As for the mildly pleasant mood produced by leisure activities, time spent at racing facilities was estimated to be the most influential factor (VR = 34.19 %), followed by income (VR = 24.19 %). For the land use attributes, distance to a park (7.93 %) played a dominant role in happiness. For the other life choice variables, only occupation and the length/frequency of job training were associated with several happiness indicators. Occupation was the most important variable in explaining all three types of mood assessed for working on the job. The length of job training influenced the mildly pleasant mood produced by leisure activities, and the frequency of job training influenced the good mood produced by leisure activities. However, both of these variables had less influence than did the consumption variables. For example, the VR values for the length and frequency of job training were 2.32 and 2.03 %, respectively, which is just 6.79 and 6.21 % of the VR values of the most influential factors.

Education-related life choice variables were associated only with being in a bad mood during one's job, family life, and neighborhood communication. The percentage of income spent on education and a person's education level were the top factors influencing bad moods during family life and neighborhood

Table 2.4 Significant factors influencing the variables in finance life

Dependent variables	Predictors
Household annual income (52.80 %)	Household composition, living area, number of rooms, percentage of saving, percentage of furniture expenditure, tourism expenditure, percentage of housing expenditure, residence duration, travel party to cinema and theatre, duration of tenure, distance to nearest kindergarten, distance to nearest post office, tourism frequency
Percentage of food expenditure (34.30 %)	Percentage of energy expenditure, percentage of saving, distance to nearest high school, living area, percentage of housing expenditure, distance to city hall, distance to railway station, percentage of clothes expenditure, percentage of leisure expenditure, frequency of neighbor communication, household annual income
Percentage of housing expenditure (28.20 %)	Percentage of transport expenditure, percentage of healthcare expenditure, residence property, vehicle ownership, percentage of furniture expenditure, distance to nearest supermarket, house type, frequency of contact with relatives, percentage of clothes expenditure, percentage of food expenditure, residence duration, percentage of saving, distance to nearest post office
Percentage of energy expenditure (45.60 %)	Percentage of transport expenditure, percentage of furniture expenditure, percentage of healthcare expenditure, house type, distance to railway station, duration of tenure, distance to supermarket, number of stories of residential building, percentage of leisure expenditure, household annual income, residence duration, percentage of housing expenditure
Percentage of furniture expenditure (54.40 %)	Percentage of clothes expenditure, percentage of transport expenditure, distance to nearest hospital, distance to nearest kindergarten, number of stories of residential building, percentage of energy expenditure, percentage of education expenditure, percentage of food expenditure, indoor time use on weekday, distance to nearest bus stop, the floor lived, percentage of leisure expenditure, residence property, residence duration, distance to nearest post office
Percentage of clothes expenditure (52.80 %)	Percentage of furniture expenditure, percentage of transport expenditure, distance to nearest hospital, vehicle ownership, distance to nearest secondary school, percentage of housing expenditure, percentage of healthcare expenditure, the floor lived, occupation, percentage of leisure expenditure, percentage of food expenditure, distance to nearest park, frequency of hobby learning, number of number of stories of residential building of residential building, percentage of energy expenditure, percentage of education expenditure

(continued)

Table 2.4 (continued)

Dependent variables	Predictors
Percentage of healthcare expenditure (42.30 %)	Percentage of transport expenditure, percentage of clothes expenditure, percentage of housing expenditure, vehicle ownership, percentage of food expenditure, indoor time use on non-weekday, household composition, percentage of education expenditure, leisure frequency
Percentage of transport expenditure (46.20 %)	Percentage of healthcare expenditure, percentage of energy expenditure, education level, percentage of clothes expenditure, percentage of education expenditure, travel party to cinema and theatre, percentage of furniture expenditure, frequency of contact with relatives, distance to nearest bus stop, distance to nearest park, frequency of neighbor communication, outdoor time use on non-weekday, distance to nearest high school, distance to nearest kindergarten
Percentage of education expenditure (49.70 %)	Percentage of transport expenditure, household composition, duration of hobby learning, residence duration, number of rooms, percentage of food expenditure, percentage of furniture expenditure, residence property, distance to nearest bus stop, frequency of neighbor communication
Percentage of leisure expenditure (43.70 %)	Percentage of transport expenditure, percentage of clothes expenditure, percentage of food expenditure, distance to nearest park, residence duration, distance to nearest kindergarten, percentage of education expenditure, distance to nearest bus stop, percentage of housing expenditure, residence property, commute mode
Percentage of saving (35.80 %)	Percentage of leisure expenditure, percentage of transport expenditure, percentage of housing expenditure, percentage of food expenditure, percentage of furniture expenditure, household annual income, house type

Note The value in the parenthesis after each target variable shows the accuracy of decision tree split based on the Exhaustive CHAID approach (100 % means a perfect representation)

communication, whereas education level was the third most influential variable on bad moods during one's job. Thus, in this study, education only contributed to negative affective experiences.

The residence-related life choice variables were found to influence eight happiness indicators, six of which were positive affects (a mildly pleasant mood during leisure activities and neighborhood communication, and a good mood during leisure activities, family life, one's job, and neighborhood communication) and two that were negative affects (a bad mood during one's job and neighborhood communication). Three residence-related life choice variables were influential: residence property, living area, and length of residence. Residence property and length of residence had mixed effects on affective experience—that is, they were associated with both positive and negative affects. In contrast, living area

Table 2.5 Significant factors influencing the variables in Education/Learning life

Dependent variables	Predictors
Education level (71.20 %)	Commute mode, household annual income, travel mode for hobby learning, established holiday, frequency of having dinner with family, occupation, number of rooms, job type, residence duration, frequency of contact with relatives, frequency of hobby learning, health condition, sleep time
Frequency of language learning (98.40 %)	Duration of language learning, frequency knowledge learning, percentage of healthcare expenditure, duration of job training, travel mode to racing facilities
Frequency knowledge learning (97.90 %)	Duration of knowledge learning, frequency of language learning, percentage of transport expenditure, travel mode to racing facilities, frequency of going to sports facilities, frequency of hobby learning, frequency of job training
Frequency of hobby learning (96.60 %)	Duration of hobby learning, frequency of job training, indoor time use on weekday, duration at amusement park, distance to city hall, working hours, frequency of neighbor communication
Frequency of job training (96.80 %)	Duration of job training, travel mode for job training, frequency of language learning, commute mode, education level, duration of non-contact sports, percentage of energy expenditure, frequency of hobby learning, sleep time, frequency of neighbor communication, health condition
Travel mode for language learning (92.70 %)	Travel mode for knowledge learning, frequency of language learning, distance to nearest bus stop, occupation, travel mode to cinema and theatre, duration of language learning
Travel mode for knowledge learning (91.60 %)	Travel mode for language learning, duration of knowledge learning, travel mode for hobby learning
Travel mode for hobby learning (86.00 %)	Travel mode for knowledge learning, duration of hobby learning, travel mode for job training, vehicle ownership, travel mode to cinema and theatre
Travel mode for job training (84.80 %)	Duration of job training, travel mode for knowledge learning, residence duration, duration of tenure, duration of gentle sports, main travel mode, commute mode
Duration of language learning (94.20 %)	Frequency of language learning, duration of knowledge learning, frequency of gentle sports, frequency of having dinner with family

(continued)

Table 2.5 (continued)

Dependent variables	Predictors
Duration of knowledge learning (92.60 %)	Frequency knowledge learning, duration of hobby learning, percentage of healthcare expenditure
Duration of hobby learning (83.20 %)	Frequency of hobby learning, duration of knowledge learning, travel mode for hobby learning, duration of job training, duration of contact sport, distance to nearest bus stop
Duration of job training (77.90 %)	Frequency of job training, travel mode for job training, duration of hobby learning, living area, household annual income, working hours, frequency knowledge learning, occupation, frequency of neighbor communication

Note The value in the parenthesis after each target variable shows the accuracy of decision tree split based on the Exhaustive CHAID approach (100 % means a perfect representation)

Table 2.6 Significant factors influencing the variables in employment life

Dependent variables	Predictors
Occupation (69.90 %)	Established holiday, workdays, frequency of contact with relatives, house type, living area, working hours, frequency of neighbor communication, education level, distance to nearest secondary school, duration of tenure
Job type (41.60 %)	Occupation, education level, household annual income, established holiday, expenditure on going home for a visit, travel party to amusement park, frequency of hobby learning, frequency of neighbor communication, commute mode
Commute mode (75.40 %)	Main travel mode, occupation, travel mode for job training, established holiday, distance to nearest park, household annual income
Duration of tenure (48.90 %)	Occupation, established holiday, distance to nearest hospital, household annual income, vacation actually taken
Monthly workdays (60.00 %)	Occupation, vacation actually taken, working hours, frequency of hobby learning, travel mode to cinema and theatre
Vacation actually taken (67.90 %)	Established holiday, workdays, frequency of going to cinema and theatre, household composition, residence property
Established holiday (73.20 %)	Vacation actually taken, occupation, distance to nearest elementary school, sleep time, frequency of going to entertainment places, duration of tenure, internet usage frequency, frequency of hobby learning
Working hours per day (51.10 %)	Occupation, workdays, frequency of having dinner with family

Note The value in the parenthesis after each target variable shows the accuracy of decision tree split based on the Exhaustive CHAID approach (100 % means a perfect representation)

Table 2.7 Significant factors influencing the variables in family and social life

Dependent variables	Predictors
Indoor time use on weekday (36.00 %)	Indoor time use on non-weekday, residence property, frequency of having dinner with family, frequency of neighbor communication, working hours, job type, vacation actually taken, outdoor time use on weekday, residence duration, occupation, sleep time, workdays
Outdoor time use on weekday (72.50 %)	Indoor time use on weekday, outdoor time use on non-weekday, travel mode to cinema and theatre, duration of tenure, frequency of neighbor communication, sleep time, indoor time use on non-weekday
Indoor time use on non-weekday (36.00 %)	Indoor time use on weekday, residence property, outdoor time use on non-weekday, education level, distance to nearest secondary school, commute mode, workdays, sleep time, frequency of neighbor communication, outdoor time use on weekday
Outdoor time use on non-weekday (46.30 %)	Indoor time use on non-weekday, outdoor time use on weekday, leisure frequency, duration at amusement park, residence duration, frequency of going to amusement park, percentage of housing expenditure
Frequency of having dinner with family (63.90 %)	Indoor time use on weekday, living area, main travel mode, established holiday, sleep time, frequency of contact with relatives, frequency of neighbor communication, house type, travel party to cinema and theatre, education level, number of rooms, vehicle ownership, travel party to sports facilities, number of stories of residential building, health condition
Household composition (51.4 %)	Indoor time use on non-weekday, residence property, health condition, percentage of education expenditure, vehicle ownership, frequency of neighbor communication, number of rooms
Frequency of contact with relatives (25.80 %)	Frequency of neighbor communication, travel mode to amusement park, living area, tourism frequency, commute mode, leisure frequency, number of rooms, frequency of going home for a visit, frequency of going to entertainment places, education level, frequency of going to amusement park, percentage of leisure expenditure, sleep time
Frequency of neighborhood communication (77.50 %)	Frequency of neighbor communication, distance to nearest high school, working hours, occupation, household composition, sleep time, percentage of saving, residence duration, commute mode, duration of non-contact sports, frequency of having dinner with family

(continued)

Table 2.7 (continued)

Dependent variables	Predictors
Participation in community activities (79.00 %)	Frequency of neighbor communication, residence property, duration at sports facilities, frequency knowledge learning, health condition, distance to supermarket, education level, distance to nearest hospital, frequency of contact with relatives, frequency of going to sports facilities, percentage of education expenditure, living area, household composition, percentage of energy expenditure, number of stories of residential building, travel party to amusement park

Note The value in the parenthesis after each target variable shows the accuracy of decision tree split based on the exhaustive CHAID approach (100 % means a perfect representation)

Table 2.8 Significant factors influencing the variables in health life

Target variables	Predictors
Sleep Time (61.20 %)	Working hours, occupation, commute mode, outdoor time use on weekday, frequency of hobby learning, frequency of gentle sports, internet usage frequency, education level
Frequency of contact sports (87.10 %)	Duration of contact sport, frequency of non-contact sports, commute mode, education level, frequency of neighbor communication
Frequency of non-contact sports (78.80 %)	Duration of non-contact sports, frequency of contact sports, frequency of going to amusement park, frequency of going to sports facilities, frequency of contact with relatives, frequency of gentle sports, frequency of job training
Frequency of gentle sports (62.60 %)	Duration of gentle sports, frequency of non-contact sports, percentage of transport expenditure, percentage of saving, duration of contact sport, sleep time, travel party to entertainment places, commute mode, percentage of housing expenditure
Duration of contact sport (87.60 %)	Frequency of contact sports, duration at sports facilities, duration at cinema and theatre, travel mode for job training
Duration of non-contact sports (81.70 %)	Frequency of non-contact sports, duration at sports facilities, duration at cinema and theatre
Duration of gentle sports (67.80 %)	Frequency of gentle sports, percentage of leisure expenditure, duration of non-contact sports, residence property, percentage of energy expenditure

Note The value in the parenthesis after each target variable shows the accuracy of decision tree split based on the exhaustive CHAID approach (100 % means a perfect representation)

Table 2.9 Significant factors influencing the variables in leisure/recreation life

Target variables	Predictors
Frequency of going to cinema and theatre (61.10 %)	Travel party to cinema and theatre, frequency of going to sports facilities, travel party to amusement park, travel mode to sports facilities, distance to nearest secondary school, frequency of neighbor communication, frequency of going to amusement park, travel mode to cinema and theatre, frequency of gentle sports, travel party to racing facilities, tourism expenditure
Frequency of going to sports facilities (75.80 %)	Duration at sports facilities, travel party to sports facilities, travel mode to amusement park, travel mode to amusement park, frequency of going to entertainment places, frequency of non-contact sports, duration of non-contact sports, frequency of going to amusement park
Frequency of going to amusement parks (61.80 %)	Duration at amusement park, travel party to amusement park, frequency of going to entertainment places, duration of knowledge learning, travel mode to cinema and theatre, number of rooms, frequency of going to cinema and theatre, frequency of gentle sports, travel mode to amusement park, travel mode to amusement park, frequency of neighbor communication
Frequency of going to entertainment places (72.50 %)	Duration at entertainment places, travel party to entertainment places, travel party to amusement park, frequency of going to sports facilities, frequency of having dinner with family, duration at amusement park, education level, leisure expenditure, duration of job training, frequency of going to amusement park, percentage of education expenditure
Frequency of going to racing facilities (93.60 %)	Duration at racing facilities, frequency of going to entertainment places, frequency of having dinner with family, travel mode to sports facilities
Travel mode to cinema and theatre (75.50 %)	Travel party to cinema and theatre, travel mode to entertainment places, travel mode to amusement park, residence property, frequency of neighbor communication, main travel mode, vehicle ownership, travel mode to sports facilities, frequency of hobby learning, frequency of going to cinema and theatre
Travel mode to sports facilities (82.70 %)	Duration at sports facilities, travel mode to racing facilities, travel mode to amusement park, travel party to amusement park, the floor lived, travel mode to cinema and theatre, main travel mode

(continued)

Table 2.9 (continued)

Target variables	Predictors
Travel mode to amusement parks (82.10 %)	Duration at amusement park, travel mode to entertainment places, distance to nearest secondary school, travel party to amusement park, travel party to sports facilities, duration at cinema and theatre, frequency of gentle sports, travel mode to sports facilities, travel mode to cinema and theatre, commute mode
Travel mode to entertainment places (82.50 %)	Travel party to entertainment places, travel mode to cinema and theatre, main travel mode, travel mode to amusement park, duration at entertainment places, travel mode to racing facilities, expenditure on going home for a visit
Travel mode to racing facilities (86.50 %)	Frequency of going to racing facilities, travel mode to sports facilities, travel mode to entertainment places, travel party to racing facilities, duration at sports facilities, frequency of neighbor communication
Duration at cinema and theatre (71.70 %)	Frequency of going to cinema and theatre, duration of non-contact sports, travel mode to cinema and theatre, travel party to cinema and theatre, duration at sports facilities, distance to railway station, distance to nearest elementary school, health condition, tourism expenditure
Duration at sports facilities (77.70 %)	Frequency of going to sports facilities, travel party to sports facilities, duration at cinema and theatre, travel mode to sports facilities, duration at entertainment places, vacation actually taken, duration at amusement park
Duration at amusement parks (76.70 %)	Travel mode to amusement park, frequency of going to amusement park, distance to city hall, frequency of going to cinema and theatre, travel party to sports facilities, residence duration, travel party to amusement park, duration at sports facilities, occupation, education level, percentage of education expenditure, travel mode to sports facilities
Duration at entertainment places (77.40 %)	Frequency of going to entertainment places, travel party to entertainment places, duration of gentle sports, travel mode to entertainment places, occupation, education level, percentage of transport expenditure
Duration at racing facilities (98.30 %)	Frequency of going to racing facilities, travel mode to racing facilities, duration at cinema and theatre, number of stories of residential building, distance to railway station, duration at entertainment places, frequency of neighbor communication

(continued)

Table 2.9 (continued)

Target variables	Predictors
Travel party to cinema and theatre (76.80 %)	Frequency of going to cinema and theatre, indoor time use on non-weekday, travel party to amusement park, living area, travel mode to cinema and theatre, duration of non-contact sports, frequency of hobby learning, travel party to entertainment places, outdoor time use on non-weekday, occupation
Travel party to sports facilities (80.70 %)	Frequency of going to sports facilities, travel party to racing facilities, duration at sports facilities, travel mode to sports facilities, frequency of having dinner with family, travel party to amusement park, percentage of transport expenditure, travel party to cinema and theatre
Travel party to amusement parks (81.60 %)	Frequency of going to amusement park, travel party to cinema and theatre, travel mode to cinema and theatre, travel party to racing facilities, travel mode to amusement park, frequency of going to entertainment places, indoor time use on weekday, travel mode to racing facilities, travel party to entertainment places, duration of tenure
Travel party to entertainment places (79.30 %)	Frequency of going to entertainment places, travel party to cinema and theatre, outdoor time use on non-weekday, travel party to amusement park, travel party to racing facilities, travel mode to entertainment places, duration at sports facilities, duration of gentle sports, duration at entertainment places
Travel party to racing facilities (93.20 %)	Frequency of going to racing facilities, travel party to entertainment places, travel party to sports facilities, duration at entertainment places, travel mode to sports facilities, frequency of hobby learning, travel mode to entertainment places, duration of knowledge learning, travel party to amusement park
Internet usage frequency (85.6 %)	Internet usage time, education level, outdoor time use on weekday, duration at amusement park, frequency of contact with relatives, percentage of transport expenditure, leisure frequency, frequency of hobby learning, frequency of going to entertainment places
Internet usage time (32.40 %)	Internet usage frequency, travel mode to entertainment places, health condition, education level, travel party to cinema and theatre, indoor time use on weekday, duration of job training, duration at cinema and theatre, percentage of education expenditure, frequency of neighbor communication, vehicle ownership, frequency of neighbor communication, frequency of contact with relatives, percentage of clothes expenditure, residence property

(continued)

Table 2.9 (continued)

Target variables	Predictors
Leisure frequency (37.50 %)	Tourism frequency, travel mode to amusement park, frequency of going to amusement park, duration of job training, percentage of leisure expenditure, travel mode to amusement park, indoor time use on non-weekday, outdoor time use on non-weekday, duration of non-contact sports, sleep time
Tourism frequency (61.60 %)	Tourism expenditure, occupation, frequency of having dinner with family, outdoor time use on weekday, frequency of hobby learning, frequency of job training, leisure frequency, percentage of furniture expenditure
Frequency of going home for a visit (70.30 %)	Expenditure on going home for a visit, number of stories of residential building, percentage of energy expenditure, occupation, distance to nearest elementary school, leisure frequency, residence property, sleep time, distance to nearest park
Leisure expenditure (78.40 %)	Tourism expenditure, duration at amusement park, percentage of leisure expenditure, frequency of contact with relatives, percentage of education expenditure, travel mode to amusement park, living area, travel party to sports facilities, household annual income, household composition, frequency of neighbor communication, outdoor time use on non-weekday, house type
Tourism expenditure (70.50 %)	Travel party to amusement park, education level, duration of knowledge learning, indoor time use on non-weekday, frequency of gentle sports, household annual income, frequency of contact with relatives, household composition, established holiday, sleep time, frequency of having dinner with family, travel party to cinema and theatre, frequency of going to amusement park
Expenditure on going home for a visit (68.50 %)	Residence duration, distance to city hall, distance to nearest park, percentage of saving, duration at amusement park, duration of gentle sports, distance to nearest elementary school, travel mode to amusement park, frequency of neighbor communication, education level, frequency of job training, occupation, frequency of contact with relatives, percentage of furniture expenditure, frequency of neighbor communication, sleep time

Note The value in the parenthesis after each target variable shows the accuracy of decision tree split based on the Exhaustive CHAID approach (100 % means a perfect representation)

Table 2.10 Significant factors influencing happiness

Target variables	Predictors
Happiness (79.2 %)	(1) Percentage of saving (30.80 %), (2) travel party to amusement parks (12.78 %), (3) household annual income (10.76 %), (4) tourism frequency (8.73 %), (5) distance to park (7.93 %), (6) duration of gentle sports (5.12 %), (7) frequency of contact with relatives (0.11 %), (8) frequency of neighborhood communication (0.07 %), (9) percentage of leisure expenditure (0.02 %)
Bad mood during leisure activities (71.3 %)	(1) Indoor time use on weekday (18.25 %), (2) frequency of contact with relatives (11.92 %), (3) percentage of leisure expenditure (10.61 %)
Mildly pleasant mood during leisure activities (69.4 %)	(1) Duration at racing facilities (34.19 %), (2) household annual income (24.19 %), (3) frequency of neighborhood communication (14.19 %), (4) main travel mode (11.76 %), (5) leisure expenditure (8.99 %), (6) residence property(7.93 %), (7) outdoor time use on holiday (5.701 %), (8) percentage of clothes expenditure (4.39 %), (9) duration of job training (2.32 %), (10) distance to bus stop (2.02 %)
Good mood during leisure activities (86.2 %)	(1) Duration at cinema and theatre (32.68 %), (2) percentage of transport expenditure (20.48 %), (3) residence property (10.40 %), (4) duration of language learning (8.30 %), (5) internet usage time (5.08 %), (6) frequency of job training (2.03 %)
Bad mood during family life (75.5 %)	(1) Percentage of education expenditure (4.32 %), (2) travel party to amusement parks (3.71 %), (3) percentage of transport expenditure (2.25 %), (4) percentage of food expenditure (1.16 %), (5) distance to city hall (1.08 %)
Mildly pleasant mood during family life (63.1 %)	(1) Indoor time use on holiday (12.75 %), (2) leisure expenditure (12.50 %), (3) duration of hobby learning (10.33 %), (4) distance to railway station (9.87 %), (5) frequency of contact with relatives (1.58 %), (6) duration of contact sports (1.03 %), (7) frequency of neighborhood communication (0.08 %), (8) duration at cinema and theatre (0.03 %)
Good mood during family life (66.3 %)	(1) Travel party to amusement parks (12.22 %), (2) tourism frequency (12.01 %), (3) percentage of healthcare expenditure (0.71 %), (4) indoor time use on holiday (0.10 %), (5) living area (0.004 %)
Bad mood during job (63.5 %)	(1) Occupation (8.20 %), (2) indoor time use on weekday (5.37 %), (3) education level (1.93 %), (4) vacation taken (1.13 %), (5) residence property (0.10 %), (6) distance to supermarket (0.08 %), (6) frequency of going to cinema and theatre (0.003 %)
Mildly pleasant mood during job (62.5 %)	(1) Occupation (7.60 %), (2) frequency of gentle sports (4.47 %), (3) duration at amusement parks (0.44 %), (4) percentage of others expenditure (0.23 %), (5) frequency of going to cinema and theatre (0.17 %), (6) frequency of neighborhood communication (0.14 %)
Good mood during job (61.1 %)	(1) Occupation (3.21 %), (2) distance to city hall (3.00 %), (3) distance to railway station (2.78 %), (4) frequency of going to cinema and theatre (2.60 %), (5) internet usage time (2.40 %), (6) residence duration (0.17 %), (7) vacation taken (0.14 %)

(continued)

Table 2.10 (continued)

Target variables	Predictors
Bad mood during social communication (63.3 %)	(1) Education level (30.34 %), (2) percentage of education expenditure (15.20 %), (3) outdoor time use on holiday (10.20 %), (4) travel party to cinema and theatre (9.19 %), (5) internet usage frequency (7.12 %), (6) internet usage time (2.32 %), (7) frequency of neighborhood communication (0.03 %), (8) residence duration (0.002 %)
Mildly pleasant mood during social communication (63.4 %)	(1) Frequency of neighborhood communication (18.98 %), (2) tourism frequency (9.37 %), (3) residence property (1.24 %), (4) percentage of food expenditure (1.06 %), (10) distance to bus stop (1.02 %)
Good mood during social communication (60.4 %)	(1) Frequency of neighborhood communication (21.28 %), (2) indoor time use on holiday (15.27 %), (3) frequency of going to entertainment places (3.03 %), (4) distance to high school (1.97 %), (5) frequency of gentle sports (1.02 %), (6) travel party to amusement parks (0.94 %), (7) travel party to entertainment places (0.02 %), (8) residence duration (0.009 %)

Note
The value in the parenthesis after each target variable shows the accuracy of decision tree split based on the Exhaustive CHAID approach, and the value in the parenthesis after each predictor is the variance reduction (VR) calculated from the BNN model

was associated only with a positive affect (being in a good mood in one's family life). Unfortunately, none of the residence-related variables influenced overall life happiness.

Happiness indicators were influenced by various other life choice variables. Regarding happiness as a whole, as mentioned above, the most influential life choice variable was the percentage of saving (VR = 30.80 %), whereas travel party to amusement parks was the next most influential variable (VR = 12.78 %), even stronger than income. In other words, investment in one's future is most important for enhancing people's current overall happiness level. For the four targeted life domains (jobs, family life, the neighborhood, and leisure and recreation), saving was less relevant for happiness. For experiences of a mildly pleasant mood during leisure activities, income was the second most influential factor, followed by the frequency of neighborhood communication.

Apart from income and the percentage of saving, happiness was clearly influenced by spending money to maintain an active lifestyle, including tourism and leisure activities, sports and entertainment, contact with relatives, and communication within the neighborhood. Active lifestyle was related to experiencing a positive affect in some life domains, but it was associated with a negative affect in others. Thus, the effects of active life related choices on happiness were mixed.

Table 2.11 Significant factors influencing life satisfaction

Dependent variables	Predictors
Life satisfaction (72.9 %)	(1) Vehicle ownership (28.5 %), (2) main travel mode (21.1 %), (3) occupation (19.13 %), (4) outdoor time use on non-weekday (12.56 %), (5) distance to bus stop (4.4 %), (6) commute mode (2.7 %), (7) frequency of going to cinema and theatre (1.92 %), (8) distance to railway station (0.9 %), (9) distance to sports facilities (0.551 %), (10) distance to city hall (0.49 %), (11) distance to park (0.389 %)
Satisfaction with residence (73.5 %)	(1) Main travel mode (33.3 %), (2) distance to kindergarten (11.8 %), (3) distance to secondary school (10.4 %), (4) vehicle ownership (11.03 %), (5) distance to station (1.27 %), (6) distance to bus stop (0.82 %), (7) travel mode to cinema and theatre (0.23 %), (8) internet usage time (0.21 %), (9) monthly workdays (0.18 %), (10) distance to city hall (0.08 %), (11) frequency of neighborhood communication (0.06 %)
Satisfaction with finance (68.9 %)	(1) Percentage of saving (30.9 %), (2) frequency of going to cinema and theatre (15.4 %), (3) vehicle ownership (9.74 %), (4) occupation (8.95 %), (5) main travel mode (2.11 %), (6) distance to railway station (1.83 %)
Satisfaction with health (75.6)	(1) Travel mode to sports facilities (23.8 %), (2) frequency to sports facilities (19.4 %), (3) commute mode (1.28 %), (4) occupation (1.02 %), (5) main travel mode (0.54 %)
Satisfaction with social (80.9 %)	(1) Frequency of neighborhood communication (28.1 %), (2) travel mode to park (23.6 %), (3) frequency to park (20.3 %), (4) travel mode to sports facilities (18.7 %), (5) distance to park (3.49 %), (6) distance to sports facilities (2.34 %), (7) occupation (1.12 %)
Satisfaction with education/learning (71.2 %)	(1) Outdoor time use on non-weekday (20.34 %), (2) distance to community center (10.44 %), (3) percentage of education expenditure (9.12 %), (4) monthly workdays (5.67 %), (5) distance to high school (3.12 %), (6) distance to kindergarten (1.63 %), (7) vehicle ownership (1.11 %)
Satisfaction with job (82.1 %)	(1) Vehicle ownership (10.4 %), (2) tourism frequency (7.61 %), (3) commute mode (5.59 %), (4) distance to station (4.32 %), (5) distance to bus stop (4.20 %), (6) job type (1.01 %)
Satisfaction with family life (82.3 %)	(1) Indoor time use on weekday (26.8 %), (2) main travel mode (12.90 %), (3) frequency of going to cinema and theatre (1.92 %), (4) vehicle ownership (0.78 %); (5) frequency to park (0.51 %), (6) frequency to sports center (0.045 %)
Satisfaction with leisure/recreation (65.3 %)	(1) Outdoor time use on non-weekday (30.3 %), (2) distance to park (15.04 %), (3) distance to station (12.52 %), (4) main travel mode (6.23 %), (5) distance to sports facilities (5.01 %), (6) frequency of contact with relatives (3.12 %), (7) frequency to park (0.51 %)

Note

The value in the parenthesis after each target variable shows the accuracy of decision tree split based on the Exhaustive CHAID approach, and the value in the parenthesis after each predictor is the variance reduction (VR) calculated from the BNN model

Of the 13 happiness indicators, the frequency of neighborhood communication influenced seven indicators (including positive and negative affective experiences), suggesting the importance of communicating with one's neighbors for happiness. The frequency of neighborhood communication had the greatest influence on experiences of positive moods (mildly pleasant and good moods) during neighborhood communication.

With respect to the influence of expenditures on happiness, besides bad and good moods during one's job and being in a good mood during neighborhood communication, expenditure variables influenced all the other happiness indicators, either negatively or positively. Leisure expenditure influenced happiness and the affective experience during leisure activities and family life, but with mixed effects. Transportation expenditure was associated not only with being in a good mood during leisure activities but also with being in a bad mood during family life. Food expenditure was related to both positive and negative affective experiences (good mood during neighborhood communication; bad mood during family life). Expenditure on clothes was only associated with positive affect (a mildly pleasant mood during leisure activities). Expenditure on health care was associated with being in a good mood during family life. Several of the expenditure variables were equally influential. The two most influential expenditure variables were the effect of the percentage of saving on overall life happiness, and the effect of the percentage of income spent on education on bad moods during family life. The next most influential expenditure variables were the effect of the percentage of income spent on leisure on bad moods during leisure activities, the effect of the percentage of income spent on transportation on good moods during leisure activities, and the effect of the percentage of income spent on education on bad moods during neighborhood communication. Tied for the third most influential expenditure variables were the effect of leisure expenditure on mildly pleasant moods during family life, and the effect of the percentage of income spent on health care on good moods during family life.

For the life choice variables, sports contributed to positive affects, whereas Internet usage and visiting amusement parks, cinemas, and the theater had mixed effects on affective experience. Indoor time use on a weekday was only related to two negative experiences: bad moods during leisure activities and during one's job. However, indoor time use during a holiday was associated with three types of positive affective experiences: mildly pleasant moods during family life, and good moods during family life, and neighborhood communication. Given that working hours and monthly working days did not significantly influence any of the 13 happiness indicators, whereas leisure- and tourism-related variables did, these results may imply that one's current work–life balance does not matter for happiness, but the use of one's free time outside of work definitely does.

Table 2.11 shows how QOL (in terms of life satisfaction) is affected by land use attributes, residential choices, travel behavior, and other life choices. First, land use attributes such as accessibility and travel behavior had a dominant role in life satisfaction. Specifically, vehicle ownership was the most influential factor (28.5 %), followed by main travel mode (21.1 %), and the distance to a railway station (0.9 %) also played a prominent role in life satisfaction. Second, the satisfaction with residence domain was mainly affected by main travel mode (33.3 %) and the distance to kindergarten (11.8 %). This reveals the strong association between closeness to childcare facilities and life satisfaction. Additionally, access to a railway station had a significant effect on satisfaction with finance, and access to a community center was important for the satisfaction with education and learning domain. This suggests that community centers (with museums, planetarium, and so on) in Japan are beneficial for those who would like to increase their knowledge, and that they generate greater enthusiasm for learning. Closeness to parks and railway stations have a positive influence on the life satisfaction in the leisure and recreation domain. This reveals that transit/leisure oriented environments are essential for participation in leisure activities.

2.4.3 Summary

This section of the chapter systematically examined various behavioral interdependencies across a broad set of life domains. Both the Exhaustive CHAID approach and the Bayesian Belief Network approach were shown to be the promising tools for quantifying the complex behavioral interdependencies between life choices and the quality of life. We used life choice survey data collected from residents in various Japanese cities in 2010. These data were originally collected for the life-oriented approach. The life-oriented analysis provides a foundation for this study. The findings are summarized below.

First, we confirmed that the life choices (decisions) that are relevant to various life domains are interdependent. For each life choice, the results showed other life choices as relevant predictors.

Second, we successfully captured the effects of different kinds of life choices on people's quality of life and quantified those effects. Some interesting findings include:

- Family life activities, leisure activities, and social activities are important for happiness and life satisfaction.
- Saving is the most important factor for enhancing people's happiness, whereas vehicle ownership is the primary factor for improving people's life satisfaction.
- Usage of one's free time outside of work increases happiness, but land use attributes and travel behavior play a vital role in life satisfaction.
- The effects of different types of expenditures and residence-related life choices on happiness and life satisfaction are mixed. However, most residence-related

and leisure-, social-, and family life-related life choice variables were related to positive affective experiences.

- Only the distance to the nearest park influenced people's happiness, whereas distance to bus stops, railway stations, sports facilities, and the city center influenced people's life satisfaction.

Finally, these results have valuable policy implications. We found that people who choose to live closer to the daily facilities of life (public railway stations, bus stops, city center, school, and so on) tend to have pleasant moods in each life domain. That is, geographic scales matter to levels of happiness and life satisfaction, reflecting the strong positive associations between: closeness to the city center and more employment opportunities; convenient transit and more trips; and closeness to school and higher education and enthusiasm for learning. People with more leisure activity opportunities have more positive social feelings and are more satisfied with most life domains.

2.5 Panel Analysis

2.5.1 Methodology

A Structural Equation Model (SEM) was developed for this study. Structural equation modeling is a very powerful tool and it is increasingly being used in travel behavior research (Golob 2003). A complete SEM consists of two components: the structural component and the measurement component. These components are defined by three sets of equations: structural equations, measurement equations for endogenous variables, and measurement equations for exogenous variables. This study includes both of the components and thus uses a full SEM model. Several measures are used to assess the goodness-of-fit of a SEM. However, in most cases, these measures do not agree (Fabrigar et al. 2010). Some take parsimony into account and others do not, and thus fit indices can be divided into general goodness of fit indices and parsimony fit indices. Roughly speaking, the first category of indices shows whether the model fits the data better than any other model. Parsimony fit indices address the possibility that the model may only be fitting the noise in the data and that it may not be representative of the wider population. Chi-square is an essential statistic to report, as are the Root Mean Square Error of Approximation (RMSEA) and the associated p-value (Hooper et al. 2008). Given the sensitivity of chi-square to model misspecification, the Standardized Root Mean square Residual (SRMR) is also reported. For a good fit, the value of SRMR should be less than 0.05, although values up to 0.08 are considered acceptable (Hooper et al. 2008). The RMSEA value should be less than 0.05 to indicate a good fit (Golob 2003). Given the complexity of the model for this study, we assessed the model fit of both of the aforementioned indices.

2.5.2 Model Estimation

2.5.2.1 Data

This analysis used data from a two-wave panel (2010 and 2014) Web-based survey with 422 respondents from major cities of different population sizes in Japan. The survey contained numerous life choice variables covering relevant travel behavior and eight life domains. The selected sociodemographic variables included personal and household characteristics, as shown in Table 2.12. The results indicate that males were slightly overrepresented in both samples, and most of the respondents were middle-aged, from 35 to 54 years old. In addition, the percentage of respondents with jobs, higher education degrees, and high household annual incomes increased, to varying degrees, from 2010 to 2014.

2.5.2.2 Conceptual Framework and Explanatory Variables

We used a structural equation model to represent the dynamics of life choices (including residential choices, and travel behavior) and QOL, after controlling for

Table 2.12 The sample characteristics of the two-wave panel survey data in 2010 and 2014

Variables (value)		Sample size: 422 persons	
		2010 (%)	2014 (%)
Gender	Male	56.64	56.64
	Female	43.36	43.36
Age	0–17	0.95	0.00
	18–34	18.72	10.90
	35–54	56.87	56.16
	55–64	10.66	15.17
	≥65	12.80	17.77
Education level	With bachelor degree or over	52.13	71.33
	No bachelor degree	47.87	28.67
Household annual income (Unit: million Yen)	Low (<200)	6.40	7.11
	Medium (200–599)	49.05	47.39
	High (≥600)	44.55	45.50
Employment status	With full/part-time job	69.67	71.56
	Housewife/students/no job	30.33	28.44
Household structure	Single	18.48	19.67
	Two members	27.01	26.54
	Three members	21.80	20.38
	Four members or more	32.69	33.41

the effects of changes in sociodemographics (in addition to age and gender, mainly the changes in key life events) over time. The proposed structural model takes state dependence of all life choices into account. Overall, we assumed that present residential choices, travel behavior, other life choices, and QOL are influenced by decisions made in the past. In particular, in addition to the effects of changes in sociodemographics over time, we assumed that current residential choices (travel behavior) are not only affected by previous corresponding residential choices but also by previous travel behavior and other life choices. We further assumed that other current life choices are not only influenced by current residential choices, travel behavior, and changes in sociodemographics but also by past residential choices, travel behavior, and other corresponding choices. Most importantly, we anticipated that the present QOL (and the effects of changes in sociodemographics produced by present and past life choices) would be simultaneously boosted by previous QOL. The conceptual framework is presented in Fig. 2.5.

This analysis contributes to the literature examining the dynamics of life choices, including residential choices and travel behavior, which are essential to the representation of higher overall QOL. Specifically, as time goes on, the current QOL is expected to be shaped by the past QOL. In this study, QOL was measured by life satisfaction and happiness, and thus it was essential that we obtain data for both constructs. Specifically, for life satisfaction, we asked respondents to use a 5-point scale (1 = very dissatisfied to 5 = very satisfied) to show how satisfied they were with life as a whole and with each life domain. For happiness, we asked respondents how happy they are currently, with response options ranging from 0 to 10 (0 = very unhappy to 10 = very happy). Thus, there were more than 140 variables in all. Zhang et al. (2014) provides details of data content. For the analysis, we constructed a structural equation model with latent variables to capture the complicated interdependencies between QOL, residential choices, and travel

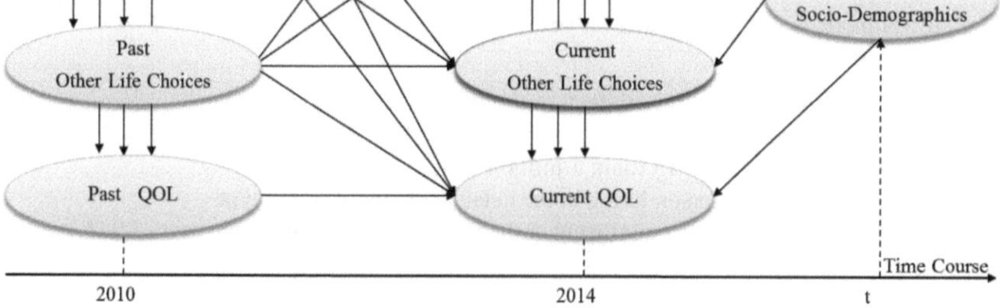

Fig. 2.5 The conceptual framework of panel data analysis between 2010 and 2014

behavior by explicitly incorporating the influence of other life choices over time. Based on the Chi-square test for life choice variables between 2010 and 2014, this analysis only used variables that differed significantly between 2010 and 2014 for the modeling. The Chi-square test results are shown in Table 2.13, and only statistically significant variables are presented and described.

Table 2.13 The Chi-square test results of the two-wave panel life choices variables in 2010 and 2014

Variables	Pearson Chi-square	Asymp. Sig. (2-sided)
Socio-demographics		
Education level (1: bachelor, 0: otherwise)	32.906	***
Employment status (1: employed, 0: otherwise[a])	0.365	**
Household annual income[b]	4.372	***
Household structure (number of family members)	4.968	***
Other life choices		
Percentage of household transport cost	18.254	**
Frequency of family meals weekly	36.772	***
Frequency of community activity participation	22.731	***
Time use in amusement park daily	12.787	**
Time use in doing gentle sports daily (e.g. golf)	16.823	**
Residential choices		
Distance from the city hall (city center) within 1 km (1: yes, 0: no)	1.639	*
Distance from nearest bus stop within 0.5 km (1: yes, 0: no)	2.511	**
Distance from nearest railway station within 1 km (1: yes, 0: no)	0.484	*
Residence duration (years you lived in the current house)	51.235	**
Residence type (living in the apartment = 1, 0[c])	0.801	*
Residence property (1: own, 0: otherwise)	1.708	**
Travel behavior		
Household vehicle ownership	3.484	**
Main travel mode is public transit (1: yes, 0: no)	1.914	**
Main travel mode is car (1: yes, 0: no)	0.324	*
Main travel mode is walking/cycling (1: yes, 0: no)	0.331	**

Note
[a]The value '0' refers to housewife, student, or the person without job
[b]Household annual income level: 1: < 1, 2: 1–2, 3: 2–3, 4: 3–4, 5: 4–5, 6: 5–6, 7: 6–7, 8: 7–8, 9: 8–9, 10: 9–10, 11:10–15, 12: > 15 (unit: 1 million Yen)
[c]The value '0' refers to the person living in the detached house or other types
*Significant at the 90 % level; **significant at the 95 % level; ***significant at the 99 % level

2.5.3 Dynamic Interdependencies of Life Choices

The maximum likelihood estimation procedure in the AMOS 20.0 software was used for the above structure equation model analysis. The estimated results are discussed in this section, including descriptions of the direct, indirect, and total effects of exogenous variables on endogenous variables. Table 2.14 shows the results of the interdependencies of sociodemographics, residential choices, travel behavior, other life choices, and quality of life (QOL) between 2010 and 2014. The goodness-of-fit measures reveal that the model is acceptable (GFI = 0.699, AGFI = 0.652, and RMSEA = 0.016). The parsimony indicator (PNFI = 0.556) also indicates that the models have modest applicability (Sharmeen et al. 2014). In Fig. 2.5, we assumed 29 direct effects among the latent variables, and 16 of the 29 direct effects were statistically significant. Corresponding to the insignificant direct effects, two indirect effects were significant. The estimated results consistently support our main assumed conceptual structure.

First, from a cross-sectional perspective, which offers insights into the direct and indirect effects on past QOL, the results indicate that past other life choices (−0.276) had a more prominent direct effect on QOL compared with past residential choices (0.158). Indirectly, the estimation indicated that past travel behavior (0.033) had a primary influence on past QOL, which suggests that the effect of travel behavior on QOL may be mediated by other life choices. This implies ignoring other life choices that are relevant to key life domains, such as health and leisure, and emphasizing that the straightforward impacts of transportation policies on QOL may not be fruitful, as QOL is affected by life choices other than changes in transportation situations. Second, from a longitudinal perspective, if we look at the significant direct and indirect effects over time, the results indicate that past QOL (0.826) has a substantial direct influence on current QOL, followed by past other life choices (−0.409), other current life choices (0.316), past travel behavior (−0.141), changes in sociodemographics (0.084), current residential choices (0.083), past residential choices (−0.045), and current travel behavior (0.031). There were also some statistically significant indirect effects, including for past residential choices (0.148) and past travel behavior (0.105). As these data show, past QOL contributes to current QOL, and they also show that other life choices play a prominent role in both past and current QOL. It may be that more and more residents are placing greater emphasis on leisure, social, family, and health oriented domains in order to enhance their overall QOL. The results show that life choices other than residential choices, travel behavior, and sociodemographics contribute to improvements in QOL over time. Thus, if we fail to examine life choices comprehensively and longitudinally, we may misunderstand how land use and transportation policies impact the QOL.

Table 2.14 Estimation results of cause-effect relationships based on structural equation model

Endogenous variables	Exogenous variables											
	Changes in socio-demographics			Past residential choices			Past travel behavior			Past other life choices		
	Direct effect	Indirect effect	Total effect	Direct effect	Indirect effect	Total effect	Direct effect	Indirect effect	Total effect	Direct effect	Indirect effect	Total effect
Latent variables												
Past travel behavior				−0.051		−0.051						
Past other life choices				−0.004	0.006*	0.002*	0.12*		0.12*			
Current residential choices	−0.271*		−0.271*	0.114*	−0.01	0.104*	0.039	0.055*	0.094*	0.403*	0.023	0.426*
Current travel behavior	0.1	0.015	0.115	0.029	−0.037	−0.008	0.534*	−0.009	0.525*	0.1	−0.016	0.084
Current other life choices	−0.088	0.042	−0.046	0.029	−0.012	0.018	0.036	−0.088	−0.051	0.98*	−0.063	0.917*
Past QOL				0.158*	−0.003	0.155*	0.044	0.033*	0.078*	−0.276*		−0.276*
Current QOL	0.084*	−0.034	0.05*	−0.045*	0.148*	0.104*	−0.141*	0.105*	−0.036*	−0.409*	0.1	−0.309*
Changes in socio-demographics												
Age in 2014	−0.186*		−0.186*									
Gender in 2014	0.031		0.031									

(continued)

Table 2.14 (continued)

Endogenous variables	Exogenous variables											
	Changes in socio-demographics			Past residential choices			Past travel behavior			Past other life choices		
	Direct effect	Indirect effect	Total effect	Direct effect	Indirect effect	Total effect	Direct effect	Indirect effect	Total effect	Direct effect	Indirect effect	Total effect
Changes of education level between 2010 and 2014 (Yes = 1, 0)	0.233*		0.233*									
Changes of household annual income between 2010 and 2014 (Yes = 1, 0)	0.717*		0.717*									
Changes of employment status between 2010 and 2014 (Yes = 1, 0)	0.207*		0.207*									

(continued)

Table 2.14 (continued)

Endogenous variables	Exogenous variables											
	Changes in socio-demographics			Past residential choices			Past travel behavior			Past other life choices		
	Direct effect	Indirect effect	Total effect	Direct effect	Indirect effect	Total effect	Direct effect	Indirect effect	Total effect	Direct effect	Indirect effect	Total effect
Changes of household structure between 2010 and 2014 (Yes = 1, 0)	0.61*		0.61*									
Past residential choices												
Distance from the City Hall (city center) within 1 km in 2010				0.165*		0.165*						
Distance from nearest Bus Stop within 0.5 km in 2010				0.698*		0.698*						
Distance from nearest Railway Station within 1 km in 2010				0.275*		0.275*						

(continued)

Table 2.14 (continued)

Endogenous variables	Exogenous variables											
	Changes in socio-demographics			Past residential choices			Past travel behavior			Past other life choices		
	Direct effect	Indirect effect	Total effect	Direct effect	Indirect effect	Total effect	Direct effect	Indirect effect	Total effect	Direct effect	Indirect effect	Total effect
Residence duration in 2010				0.024		0.024						
Residence type in 2010				0.718*		0.718*						
Tenure in 2010				0.767*		0.767*						
Past travel behavior												
Household vehicle ownership in 2010					−0.019	−0.019	0.382*		0.382*			
Main travel mode is walking/ cycling in 2010					0.047	0.047	-0.924*		−0.924*			
Main travel mode is public transit in 2010					−0.02	−0.02	−0.39*		−0.39*			

(continued)

Table 2.14 (continued)

Endogenous variables	Exogenous variables											
	Changes in socio-demographics			Past residential choices			Past travel behavior			Past other life choices		
	Direct effect	Indirect effect	Total effect	Direct effect	Indirect effect	Total effect	Direct effect	Indirect effect	Total effect	Direct effect	Indirect effect	Total effect
Main travel mode is car in 2010					−0.034	−0.034	0.678*		0.678*			
Past other life choices												
Percentage of household transport cost in 2010					−0.016*	−0.016*		0.009*	0.009*	−0.075*		-0.075*
Frequency of family meals weekly in 2010					0.015*	0.015*		−0.027	−0.027	0.221*		0.221*
Time use in amusement park daily in 2010					0.023*	0.023*		0.02	0.02	0.169*		0.169*
Time use in doing sports daily in 2010					0.036	0.036		−0.007*	−0.007*	0.058		0.058
Frequency of community activity participation in 2010					0.001*	0.001*		−0.091*	−0.091*	0.754*		0.754*

(continued)

Table 2.14 (continued)

Endogenous variables	Exogenous variables											
	Changes in socio-demographics			Past residential choices			Past travel behavior			Past other life choices		
	Direct effect	Indirect effect	Total effect	Direct effect	Indirect effect	Total effect	Direct effect	Indirect effect	Total effect	Direct effect	Indirect effect	Total effect
Current residential choices												
Distance from the city hall (city center) within 1 km in 2014		−0.068*	−0.068*		0.026*	0.026*		−0.024*	−0.024*		0.106*	0.106*
Distance from nearest bus stop within 0.5 km in 2014		−0.024*	−0.024*		0.009*	0.009*		−0.008*	−0.008*		0.038*	0.038*
Distance from nearest railway station within 1 km in 2014		−0.088*	−0.088*		0.034*	0.034*		−0.03*	−0.03*		0.138*	0.138*
Residence duration in 2014		0.12*	0.12*		−0.046	−0.046		0.042	0.042		0.188*	0.188*
Residence type in 2014		−0.191*	−0.191*		0.073*	0.073*		−0.066*	−0.066*		0.299*	0.299*

(continued)

Table 2.14 (continued)

Endogenous variables	Exogenous variables											
	Changes in socio-demographics			Past residential choices			Past travel behavior			Past other life choices		
	Direct effect	Indirect effect	Total effect	Direct effect	Indirect effect	Total effect	Direct effect	Indirect effect	Total effect	Direct effect	Indirect effect	Total effect
Tenure in 2014		0.188*	0.188*		−0.072	−0.072		0.065*	0.065*		0.295*	0.295*
Current travel behavior												
Household vehicle ownership in 2014		0.032	0.032		−0.002	−0.002		0.147*	0.147*		0.024	0.024
Main travel mode is car in 2014		0.071	0.071		−0.005	−0.005		0.325*	0.325*		0.052	0.052
Main travel mode is public transit in 2014		0.048	0.048		−0.003	−0.003		−0.221*	−0.221*		0.035	0.035
Main travel mode is walking/cycling in 2014		−0.107	−0.107		0.007	0.007		−0.488*	−0.488*		−0.078	−0.078
Current other life choices												

(continued)

Table 2.14 (continued)

Endogenous variables	Exogenous variables											
	Changes in socio-demographics			Past residential choices			Past travel behavior			Past other life choices		
	Direct effect	Indirect effect	Total effect	Direct effect	Indirect effect	Total effect	Direct effect	Indirect effect	Total effect	Direct effect	Indirect effect	Total effect
Percentage of household transport cost in 2014		0.005	0.005		−0.002	−0.002		0.005	0.005		−0.095*	−0.095*
Frequency of family meals weekly in 2014		0.004	0.004		−0.002	−0.002		0.005	0.005		−0.089	−0.089
Time Use in amusement park daily in 2014		0.009	0.009		−0.004	−0.004		0.01	0.01		0.186*	0.186*
Time Use in doing sports daily in 2014		0.007	0.007		−0.003	−0.003		0.02	0.02		0.239	0.239
Frequency of community activity participation in 2014		−0.04	−0.04		0.015	0.015		−0.045	−0.045		0.807*	0.807*
Past QOL												
Life satisfaction in 2010					0.128*	0.128*		0.064*	0.064*		−0.229*	−0.229*

(continued)

Table 2.14 (continued)

Endogenous variables	Exogenous variables														
	Current residential choices			Current travel behavior			Current other life choices			Past QOL			Current QOL		
	Direct effect	Indirect effect	Total effect	Direct effect	Indirect effect	Total effect	Direct effect	Indirect effect	Total effect	Direct effect	Indirect effect	Total effect	Direct effect	Indirect effect	Total effect
Changes of employment status between 2010 and 2014 (Yes = 1, 0)															
Changes of household structure between 2010 and 2014 (Yes = 1, 0)															
Past residential choices															
Distance from the City Hall (city center) within 1 km in 2010															
Distance from nearest Bus Stop within 0.5 km in 2010															
Distance from nearest Railway Station within 1 km in 2010															

(continued)

Table 2.14 (continued)

Endogenous variables	Exogenous variables														
	Current residential choices			Current travel behavior			Current other life choices			Past QOL			Current QOL		
	Direct effect	Indirect effect	Tctal effect	Direct effect	Indirect effect	Total effect	Direct effect	Indirect effect	Total effect	Direct effect	Indirect effect	Total effect	Direct effect	Indirect effect	Total effect
Residence duration in 2010															
Residence type in 2010															
Tenure in 2010															
Past travel behavior															
Household vehicle ownership in 2010															
Main travel mode is walking/cycling in 2010															
Main travel mode is public transit in 2010															
Main travel mode is car in 2010															
Past other life choices															

(continued)

Table 2.14 (continued)

Endogenous variables	Exogenous variables														
	Current residential choices			Current travel behavior			Current other life choices			Past QOL			Current QOL		
	Direct effect	Indirect effect	Total effect	Direct effect	Indirect effect	Total effect	Direct effect	Indirect effect	Total effect	Direct effect	Indirect effect	Total effect	Direct effect	Indirect effect	Total effect
Percentage of household transport cost in 2010															
Frequency of family meals weekly in 2010															
Time use in amusement park daily in 2010															
Time use in doing sports daily in 2010															
Frequency of community activity participation in 2010															
Current residential choices															
Distance from the city hall (city center) within 1 km in 2014	0.25*		0.25*												

(continued)

Table 2.14 (continued)

Endogenous variables	Exogenous variables														
	Current residential choices			Current travel behavior			Current other life choices			Past QOL			Current QOL		
	Direct effect	Indirect effect	Total effect	Direct effect	Indirect effect	Total effect	Direct effect	Indirect effect	Total effect	Direct effect	Indirect effect	Total effect	Direct effect	Indirect effect	Total effect
Distance from nearest bus stop within 0.5 km in 2014	0.09		0.09												
Distance from nearest railway station within 1 km in 2014	0.324*		0.324*												
Residence duration in 2014	0.442*		0.442*												
Residence type in 2014	0.703*		0.703*												
Tenure in 2014	0.692*		0.692*												
Current travel behavior															
Household vehicle ownership in 2014		−0.015	−0.015	0.281		0.281									
Main travel mode is car in 2014		−0.033	−0.033	0.619*		0.619*									

(continued)

Table 2.14 (continued)

Endogenous variables	Exogenous variables														
	Current residential choices			Current travel behavior			Current other life choices			Past QOL			Current QOL		
	Direct effect	Indirect effect	Total effect	Direct effect	Indirect effect	Total effect	Direct effect	Indirect effect	Total effect	Direct effect	Indirect effect	Total effect	Direct effect	Indirect effect	Total effect
Main travel mode is public transit in 2014		−0.023	−0.023	−0.421*		−0.421*									
Main travel mode is walking/cycling in 2014		0.05	0.05	−0.93*		−0.93*									
Current other life choices															
Percentage of household transport cost in 2014		0.015	0.015		−0.003	−0.003	−0.104		−0.104						
Frequency of family meals weekly in 2014		0.014	0.014		−0.003	−0.003	0.097*		0.097*						
Time Use in amusement park daily in 2014		0.029	0.029		−0.006	−0.006	0.202*		0.202*						
Time Use in doing sports daily in 2014		0.025	0.025		−0.002	−0.002	0.001*		0.001*						

(continued)

Table 2.14 (continued)

Endogenous variables	Exogenous variables														
	Current residential choices			Current travel behavior			Current other life choices			Past QOL			Current QOL		
	Direct effect	Indirect effect	Total effect	Direct effect	Indirect effect	Total effect	Direct effect	Indirect effect	Total effect	Direct effect	Indirect effect	Total effect	Direct effect	Indirect effect	Total effect
Frequency of community activity participation in 2014		−0.126	−0.126		0.026	0.026	0.88		0.88						
Past QOL															
Life satisfaction in 2010										0.828*		0.828*			
Happiness in 2010										0.791*		0.791*			
Current QOL															
Life satisfaction in 2014		0.027*	0.027*		−0.03*	−0.03*		0.238*	0.238*		0.624*	0.624*	0.753*		0.753*
Happiness in 2014		0.029*	0.029*		−0.032*	−0.032*		0.255*	0.255*		0.668*	0.668*	0.806*		0.806*

*significant at the 95 % level

2.5.3.1 Changes in Sociodemographics and QOL

Examining the six indicators of the latent variable changes in sociodemographics, the results indicate that changes in sociodemographics mainly occurred for life events change variables such as household annual income (0.717), followed by household structure (0.61), education level (0.233), and employment status (0.207), as well as a current individual attributes such as age (−0.186). The results for the total effects show that changes in sociodemographics had considerable influences on current residential choices (−0.271) and current QOL (0.05). Specifically, based on the positive signs of the changes in sociodemographics on current QOL and the above sample characteristics, the results show that QOL is enhanced when people increase their education, dedicate themselves to one career, and change their household annual income and household structure, which means that a QOL-oriented lifestyle may trigger life events. However, because of model limitations and the data used here, we cannot offer specific statements about how changes to household structure (such as having a baby) or changes in household annual income can improve QOL. The results also indicate that people who experienced changes in education level, household annual income, employment status, and household structure preferred to live in rental apartments close to the city center with good access to transit rather than own a detached house. This type of residential choice helps to improve QOL changing life events. However, this trend decreases with age. This implies that, to some extent, key life event changes can help explain improvements in QOL. Thus, life domains and life events should be considered together, which is consistent with Scheiner (2014).

2.5.3.2 Residential Choices and QOL

Examining the six indicators of past residential choices at a single point in time, the residential choices are featured by people's preferences for housing attributes and residential location/environment characteristics. As Chen et al. (2008) have noted, trade-offs between housing qualities and property, activity opportunities, and transportation accessibility have long been recognized as fundamental considerations in the decision to move and the selection of a residence. Residential property (0.767) was an important factor in people's residential choices, followed by residence type (0.718) (apartment or detached house), and location/environment characteristics, such as having the nearest bus stop within 0.5 km (0.698), the nearest railway station within 1 km (0.275) and the city center within 1 km (0.165). This implies that high-density, transit-oriented residential environments are critical factors in people's residential location choices. The findings above differ slightly from those in 2014. Similarly, the present respondents' residential choices were largely characterized by preferences for housing attributes relative to preferences for residential location/environment. However, residence type (0.703) played a dominant role in residential choices, in addition to residential property (0.692), length of residence (0.442), nearest railway station within 1 km (0.324), and distance to the city center within 1 km (0.25). In contrast, having the nearest bus stop within 0.5 km failed to influence residential choices. This implies that, compared with access to a bus stop, the current respondents cared more about access to railway stations.

If we examine the effects of the latent variable past residential choices, we can see that it has a significant direct effect on past QOL (0.158) and a significant indirect effect on past other life choices (0.006). With respect to the impact of residential choices on other life choices, the results indicate that living in one's own apartment, living close to the city center, railway stations, and bus stops, spending less on transportation, dining with family members more frequently, going to the amusement park, and greater participation in community activities had positive impacts on family life, leisure, and social life. These findings suggest that land use planning that emphasizes compactness and diversity enhances people's leisure and social and family lives, making residents more satisfied and happy. Thus, these findings also suggest that land use policies that try to improve QOL by changing housing situations or relocate residences may not be as beneficial to other life domains, such as leisure.

The latent variable current residential choices had a significant and direct effect on current QOL (0.083). Both in the past and currently, residents who live in a high-density or transit-oriented land use area, especially one with different kinds of facilities, feel more satisfied and are happier about their different life domains. Surprisingly, after controlling for the influence of other life choices over time, the consistent finding in the literature of an effect of residential choice on travel behavior was not observed in this study for past or current residential choices. This suggests that the influence of residential choices on travel behavior reported in the literature may be spurious because of the failure to control for other life choices. This re-confirms the importance of taking a life-oriented approach and suggests that more detailed and comprehensive research is required.

With respect to the impacts of past residential choices on current life choices and current QOL, we found that past residential choices had significant direct effects on current residential choices (0.114) and current QOL (0.045), and significant indirect effects on current QOL (0.303). Past residential choices did not have a significant effect on current travel behavior or other life choices. Considering the substantial total effect of past residential choices on current residential choices, we can surmise that as time passes, the respondents maintained their preferences for housing attributes and residential environments, possibly because of inertia. Most importantly, it is interesting to note that past residential choices exists the effect of future expectation on prospective QOL attainment. Having lived in high-density or transit-oriented land use areas in the past, residents still feel satisfied and happy in those same types of areas.

2.5.3.3 Travel Behavior and QOL

Of the four indicators of past travel behavior, main travel mode of walking/cycling (0.924) played a dominant role in characterizing the respondents' travel behavior, followed by main travel mode by car (0.678), main travel mode by public transit (0.39) and household vehicle ownership (0.382). These findings are similar to those for the present, but they are slightly different because of the trivial effects of current household vehicle ownership. We found that car acquisition played an important role in the respondents' past travel mode choices. If we examine all the impacts of past travel behavior, it only had significant effects on past other life choices (0.12) and past QOL (0.078); it did not have an effect on past residential choices. We found that the respondents who owned more vehicles and took more trips by car allocated more household income to transportation costs. In contrast, the respondents who walked/cycled more and who used public transit more were more likely to participate in more community activities and health oriented sports activities, which in turn improve their QOL. This is consistent with findings about current travel behavior that walking/cycling more and using public transit more (particularly, driving less) make residents happier and more satisfied.

Past travel behavior had a significant influence on current travel behavior (0.525), but less of an influence on current residential choices (0.094) and current QOL (−0.036). With respect to the effects of past travel behavior on current residential choices, we found that the respondents who preferred car use to public transit or active transportation (walking and cycling) were happier and more satisfied if they owned detached houses and lived far away from the city center in areas of dispersed land use patterns that are convenient for driving. On the other hand, the respondents who liked to walk/cycle and use public transit were more satisfied and happier if they lived in the high-density and transit-oriented neighborhoods, even when renting an apartment. We also found that self-selection helps explain QOL, which is consistent with Cao and Ettema's (2014) findings. Transportation policies that try to directly enhance QOL by reducing car use and promoting public transit and active transit may not be efficient, as QOL may be affected by life choices other than changes in transportation conditions. Again, further investigation is required.

2.5.3.4 Other Life Choices and QOL

The five indicators of past other life choices were family life, social life, health, leisure and recreation, and finance. The distinguishing characteristics of this latent variable were aspects of the social life domain, such as frequency of participation in community activities (0.754), which varied with the current other life choices, which was, in turn, primarily characterized by the leisure related domain and activities such as time spent in amusement parks (0.202). If we examine all of the effects of past other life choices, we see that it played a significant role in current other life choices (0.917), current residential choices (0.426), current QOL (−0.309), and past QOL (−0.276). With respect to the impact of past other life choices on current other life choices, we found that respondents who spent more time in social life, health-related, and leisure activities in the past were more likely to do the same in the future, just as they spent less money on transportation both in the past and present daily life, which may be because of inertia. As for the effect of past other life choices on current residential choices, we found that people who spent more time outdoor and less money on transportation in the past were more likely to move close to the city center and live in compact neighborhoods with accessible transit and a good walking environment. It may be that as time goes on, past life choices play a role in current life choices. Past other life choices also had an impact on the QOL indicators such that respondents who engaged in more social, leisure, and health-related activities in the past reported an improved current QOL. These results show that isolated land use and transport policies intended to improve people's QOL by changing housing situations and transportation conditions may not be effective, as QOL is broadly affected by other life choices rather than by changes in residential and travel factors.

2.5.4 Summary

Motivated by the variability of people's life choices over time, especially residential and employment changes, this section of the chapter examined changing life choices in the context of key life events. We examined changing life choices involving health, social life, education and learning, employment, family life, finance, and leisure and recreation domains jointly in order to shift the research focus from short-term behavioral analysis to midterm longitudinal analysis. We also extended the boundaries of the effects of changing life choices on QOL by incorporating the influence of key life events, which provides further insight into predicting people's prospective life decisions. To conduct this preliminary investigation of this complex system, we estimated a structural equation model based on panel data.

First, we examined a single point in time and found that other life choices have considerable effects on quality of life compared with the minor effects of residential choices and travel behavior. When examined over time, the results show that past and current other life choices played a dominant role in current quality of life relative to the slight influences of current and past residential choices, key life events, and the slight effect of current and past travel behavior. As such, ignoring other life choices that are relevant to people's key life domains (such as health and leisure) and key life events (such as changes in household structure) and only emphasizing the straightforward impacts of land use and transportation policies on quality of life may not be appropriate, because quality of life is greatly affected by other life choices—more so than by changes in residential and transportation situations. Second, we found that residents living in a high-density land use area (especially one with diverse facilities) or in a transit-oriented neighborhood feel more satisfied and happier with their lives. This finding indicates how land use patterns influence quality of life and provides insight into the worsening regional depopulation issue in Japan. Third, after controlling for the influence of other life choices over time, we failed to observe (both at a single point in time and over time) the consistently reported influence of residential choices on travel behavior. This suggests that the observed influence of residential choices on travel behavior in the literature may be spurious, possibly because previous research has not accounted for other life choices and key life events.

2.6 Life History Analysis

Once a transportation system is built or a land-use policy is carried out, it influences people's travel behavior and their lives for a long time. Therefore, it is important for policy makers to understand people's travel behavior decisions and their lives over a long period. However, little is known about the interdependencies of life domains, especially over the life course (i.e., biographical interdependencies). To address this gap, this section of the chapter aims to clarify the biographical interdependencies of households in relation to residential and car ownership biographies by explicitly incorporating the influence of household structure and employment/education biographies. Biography can be defined based on a general concept of mobility that indicates a change in a life domain. In November 2010, we conducted a Web-based life history survey, and 1000 households in major cities in Japan provided valid data. We performed aggregate and Exhaustive CHAID analyses, focusing on the occurrence times of mobilities in each biography.

Biography refers to the course of a person's life, and in this study it is defined as a series of mobilities in each life domain over the life course, whereas mobility indicates a change occurring in each domain. Mobility defined in this way is similar to the concept of a life event. Especially in the literature on residential and travel behaviors, such life events mainly refer to changes in jobs, workplaces, or household members (and/or their status), and they have been used as an explanatory variables for residential and travel behaviors. However, in this study, such life events are treated as dependent variables. For the above reasons, mobility is used instead of life event in this study. Four types of biographies that use the concept of mobility are defined as follows:

(1) Residential biography: a series of residential mobilities caused by relocation over the life course. Details from the survey: residential location, income, house property, access (which here refers to distance) to various facilities (including railway stations, bus stops, primary, junior and high schools, hospitals, parks, supermarkets, city hall) in each episode.
(2) Household structure biography: a series of mobilities in the status of household members. Details from the survey: household size, information about each household member in each episode (including age, gender, relationship with the respondent).
(3) Employment/education biography: a series of mobilities in one's job and/or school. Details from the survey: job category, commute time to job/school, access to job/school, travel mode in each episode.

(4) Car ownership biography: a series of mobilities of car ownership as a tool for travel. This is a specific type of travel biography (and refers to mobility biography in the general literature on transportation) that may include season passes or prepaid IC cards for public transportation systems, ownership of bicycles, and major travel modes in daily life. Details from the survey: number of cars, primary user, car efficiency, purpose, and frequency of use in each episode.

The results indicate obvious two-way cause–effect relationships over the life course between residential and car ownership biographies, which were further influenced by household structure and employment/education biographies. In particular, in both the short term and the long term, state dependence and future expectations within and across life domains were clarified. We found that household structure and employment/education biographies had a greater impact on residential biography than on car ownership biography. Although residential biography was found to be more influential on car ownership biography, the other two biographies also played an important role in explaining the car ownership mobility decision. All of these findings suggest the necessity of developing a unified framework of intra-domain and inter-domain biographical interdependence models with flexible structures that capture the influences of state dependence and future expectations over different time scales in the life course. The findings are summarized further below.

First, focusing on the occurrence times of mobilities in each biography, this study revealed obvious two-way cause–effect relationships between residential and car ownership biographies that were further influenced by household structure and employment/education biographies in a complex way. Therefore, the viewpoint that residential and travel behaviors should not be treated independently of other life domains in the life course was confirmed. This finding suggests that it is necessary to develop integrated models to jointly describe changes in the above four domains over the life course.

Second, substantial state dependence and future expectations were identified to explain the occurrence and nonoccurrence of residential relocation and car ownership mobilities. Both short-term and long-term state dependence and future expectations were clarified. These findings emphasize the need to develop a unified framework of dynamic models that incorporate higher-order state dependence and future expectations within and across domains over different time scales over the life course.

Third, household structure and employment/education mobilities were found to have a greater impact on residential mobility (relocation) than on car ownership mobility. Although residential mobility was found to have a greater impact on car ownership mobility, mobilities in the other two biographies also played an important role in explaining the car ownership mobility decision. These results call attention to the joint analysis of residential and car ownership mobilities by explicitly linking them to household structure and employment/education mobilities based on better behaviorally oriented approaches.

2.7 Conclusions

Using survey data from multiple points in time in several Japanese cities, this chapter presented empirical evidence of the behavioral interdependencies of life choices at a single point in time, over a midterm period, and from a life history viewpoint. Using several statistical methods, this study successfully captured the interrelationships between different life choices. In addition, we examined the value of a life-oriented approach (Zhang 2014, 2015) by incorporating various life choice interdependencies into the analyses. The findings suggest that it is necessary to describe the changes in life choices comprehensively, especially with respect to specific social issues.

First, we used cross-sectional data and an Exhaustive CHAID approach to identify predictors for life choices. In addition, we quantified the effects of life choices, including residential choices and travel behavior, on the quality of life (measured by happiness and life satisfaction indicators). We were able to identify which life choices affect people's life decisions and their quality of life.

Second, using a structural equation model based on midterm longitudinal data, we examined the changes in life choices after controlling for the effects of key life events over time. The results indicate that current life choices can be influenced by past life choices.

Third, from a life history viewpoint (using data from a Web-based retrospective life story survey in Japan), we made an additional attempt to represent biographical interdependencies among residential mobility, household structure mobility, employment/education mobility, and car ownership mobility. This analysis revealed obvious two-way cause–effect relationships between residential and car ownership biographies that were further influenced by household structure and employment/education biographies in a complex way. These results suggest that it is necessary to develop integrated models that jointly describe changes in these four domains over the life course.

Several important research issues should also be noted. First, the quality of life differs greatly at specific stages of the life course, especially in response to changes in residential location and employment. Additional longitudinal data should be collected and time series analyses should be conducted. Second, more advanced choice models should be built to jointly represent residential choices, travel behavior, and other life choices, as well as quality of life, in order to incorporate decision-making mechanisms into the analysis. Third, the effects of land use and transportation policies on the quality of life should be re-evaluated based on the conceptual framework proposed in this study and the future development of better choice models. Finally, to arrive at more comprehensive conclusions, more case studies should be conducted—not only in developed countries but also in developing countries, which are experiencing more dynamic changes economically, socially, and culturally.

References

Abou-Zeid M, Witter R, Bierlaire M, Kaufmann V, Ben-Akiva M (2012) Happiness travel mode switching: findings from a Swiss public transportation experiment. Transp Policy 19(1):93–104

Alexopoulos EC, Palatsidi V, Tigani X, Darviri C (2014) Exploring stress levels, job satisfaction, and quality of life in a sample of police officers in Greece. Saf Health Work 5(4):210–215

Allen TD, Herst DE, Bruck CS, Sutton M (2000) Consequences associated with work–to–family conflict: a review agenda for future research. J Occup Health Psychol 5(2):278

Andereck KL, Valentine KM, Vogt CA, Knopf RC (2007) A cross–cultural analysis of tourism and quality of life perceptions. J Sustain Tourism 15(5):483–502

Bowling A (1995) Measuring disease: a review of disease–specific quality of life measurement scales. Open University Press

Brajša-Žganec A, Merkaš M, Šverko I (2011) Quality of life and leisure activities: how do leisure activities contribute to subjective well–being? Soc Indic Res 102(1):81–91

Cambir A, Vasile V (2015) Material dimension of life quality social inclusion. Procedia Econ Finan 32:932–939

Campbell A (1976) Subjective measures of well–being. Am Psychol 31(2):117–124

Campbell A (1981) The sense of well–being in America: recent patterns and trends. McGraw-Hill

Cantril H (1965) The pattern of human concerns. Rutgers University Press, New Brunswick

Cao X (2016) How does neighborhood design affect life satisfaction? Evidence from twin cities. Travel Behav Soc 5:68–76

Cao X, Ettema D (2014) Satisfaction with travel and residential self-selection: how do preferences moderate the impact of the Hiawatha light rail transit line? J Transp Land Use 7(3):93–108

Cao X, Mokhtarian PL, Handy S (2013) Examining the impacts of residential self–selection on travel behavior: a focus on empirical findings. Transp Rev 29(3):359–395

Chen J, Chen C, Timmermans HJP (2008) Accessibility trade–offs in household residential location choice decisions. Transp Res Rec 2077(1):71–79

Chen CC, Huang WJ, Petrick JF (2016) Holiday recovery experiences tourism satisfaction life satisfaction–is there a relationship? Tour Manag 53:140–147

Clark AE, Frijters P, Shields MA (2008) Relative income, happiness, and utility: an explanation for the Easterlin paradox and other puzzles. J Econ Lit 46(1):95–144

Cooklin AR, Westrupp EM, Strazdins L, Giallo R, Martin A, Nicholson JM (2014) Fathers at work work–family conflict, work–family enrichment and parenting in an Australian cohort. J Family Issues. doi:10.1177/0192513X14553054

Cooklin AR, Westrupp EM, Strazdins L, Giallo R, Martin A, Nicholson JM (2015a) Mothers' work–family conflict and enrichment: associations with parenting quality and couple relationship. Child Care Health Dev 41(2):266–277

Cooklin AR, Giallo R, Strazdins L, Martin A, Leach LS, Nicholson JM (2015b) What matters for working fathers? Job characteristics work–family conflict enrichment fathers' postpartum mental health in an Australian cohort. Soc Sci Med 146:214–222

Coulmas F, Conrad H, Vogt G, Schad–Seifert A (2008) The demographic challenge: a handbook about Japan. Brill

Cummins RA (1996) The domains of life satisfaction: An attempt to order chaos. Soc Indic Res 38:303–328

Curl A, Thompson CW, Aspinall P (2015) The effectiveness of 'shared space' residential street interventions on self–reported activity levels and quality of life for older people. Landscape Urban Plann 139:117–125

De Holler AE, Staatsen BA (2003) Health environment and quality of life: An epidemiological perspective on urban development. Landscape Urban Plann 65(1):53–62

De Vos J (2015) The influence of land use and mobility policy on travel behavior: a comparative case study of Flanders and the Netherlands. J Transp Land Use 8(1):171–190

De Vos J, Schwanen T, van Acker V, Witlox F (2013) Travel subjective well–being: a focus on findings methods and future research needs. Transp Rev 33(4):421–442
Delmelle EC, Haslauer E, Prinz T (2013) Social satisfaction commuting neighborhoods. J Transp Geogr 30:110–116
Diener E (1984) Subjective well–being. Psychol Bull 95(3):542–575
Diener E (2000) Subjective well–being: the science of happiness and a proposal for a national index. Am Psychol 55(1):34–43
Diener E (2009) The science of well–being: the collected works of Ed Diener. Social indicators research series 37. Springer Science Business Media, Springer Netherlands
Diener E, Seligman ME (2002) Very happy people. Psychol Sci 13(1):81–84
Diener E, Suh E (1997) Measuring quality of life: economic social subjective indicators. Soc Indic Res 40(1–2):189–216
Diener ED, Emmons RA, Larsen RJ, Griffin S (1985) The satisfaction with life scale. J Pers Assess 49(1):71–75
Dolnicar S, Yanamram V, Cliff K (2012) The contribution of vacations to quality of life. Ann Tourism Res 39(1):59–83
Dutt AK (2008) The dependence effect consumption on happiness: Galbraith revisited. Rev Polit Econ 20(4):527–550
Easterlin RA (2001) Income and happiness: towards a unified theory. Econ J 111(473):465–484
El Din HS, Shalaby A, Farouh HE, Elariane SA (2013) Principles of urban quality of life for a neighborhood. HBRC J 9(1):86–92
Ettema D, Gärling T, Olsson LE, Friman M (2010) Out–of–home activities daily travel and subjective well–being. Transp Res Part A: Policy Pract 44(9):723–732
Fabrigar LR, Porter RD, Norris ME (2010) Some things you should know about structural equation modeling but never thought to ask. J Consum Psychol 20(2):221–225
Fichera E, Savage D (2015) Income and health in Tanzania: an instrumental variable approach. World Dev 66:500–515
Frisvold D, Golberstein E (2011) School quality and the education–health relationship: evidence from Blacks in segregated schools. J Health Econ 30(6):1232–1245
George L (2006) Perceived quality of life. In: Linstock R, George L (eds), Handbook of aging and the social sciences, The 6th Edition. Burlington, MA: Academic Press.
Gilbert D, Abdullah J (2004) Holiday taking and the sense of well–being. Ann Tourism Res 31(1):103–121
Glatzer W (2012) Cross–national comparisons of quality of life in developed nations including the impact of globalization. In: Land KC, Michalos AC, Sirgy MJ (eds) Handbook of social indicators and quality of life research. Springer, Netherlands, pp 381–398
Golob TF (2003) Structural equation modeling for travel behavior research. Transp Res Part B: Methodol 37(1):1–25
González CS, Gómez N, Navarro V, Cairós M, Quirce C, Toledo P, Marrero-Gordillo N (2016) Learning healthy lifestyles through active videogames motor games and the gamification of educational activities. Comput Hum Behav 55:529–551
Greenhaus JH, Collins KM, Shaw JD (2003) The relation between work–family balance and quality of life. J Vocat Behav 63(3):510–531
Headey B, Muffels R, Wooden M (2008) Money does not buy happiness: or does it? A reassessment based on the combined effects of wealth income and consumption. Soc Indic Res 87(1):65–82
Heal LW, Chadsey-Rusch J (1985) The lifestyle satisfaction scale: assessing individuals' satisfaction with residence, community setting, and associated services. Appl Res Mental Retard 6(4):475–490
Higgins C, Duxbury L, Lee C (1994) Impact of life–cycle stage and gender on the ability to balance work and family responsibilities. Fam Relat 43(2):144–150
Honold J, Beyer R, Lakes T, ver Meer E (2012) Multiple environmental burdens and neighborhood–related health of city residents. J Environ Psychol 32(4):305–317

Hooper D, Coughlan J, Mullen M (2008) Structural equation modelling: guidelines for determining model fit. Electron J Bus Res Methods 6(1):53–60

Huang Q, Sverke M (2007) Women's occupational career patterns over 27 years: relations to family of original life careers and wellness. J Vocat Behav 70(2):369–397

Inoguchi T, Fujii S (2009) The quality of life in Japan. Soc Indic Res 92(2):227–262

Janssens D, Wets G, Brijs T, Vanhoof K, Arentze T, Timmermans H (2006) Integrating Bayesian networks and decision trees in a sequential rule–based transportation model. Eur J Oper Res 175(1):16–34

Kahn RL, Juster FT (2002) Well-being: concepts and measures. J Soc Issues 58(4):627–644

Kaplan GA, Shema SJ, Leite CMA (2008) Socioeconomic determinants of psychological well–being: the role of income, income change and income sources during the course of 29 years. Ann Epidemiol 18(7):531–537

Kass G (1980) An exploratory technique for investigating large quantities of categorical data. Appl Stat 29(2):119–127

Keene D, Bader M, Ailshire J (2013) Length of residence and social integration: the contingent effects of neighborhood poverty. Health Place 21:171–178

Khalil HAEE (2012) Enhancing quality of life through strategic urban planning. Sustain Cities Soc 5:77–86

Knox PL (1975) Social well-being: a spatial perspective. Oxford University Press, Oxford

Lamont D, Kenyon S, Lyons G (2013) Dyslexia and mobility–related social exclusion: the role of travel information provision. J Transp Geogr 26:147–157

Lee JH, Goulias KG (2014) Examining differences and commonalities of life cycle stages indaily contacts and activity–travel time allocation. Compendium of papers CD-ROM, The93rd annual meeting of transportation research board. Washington, D.C., 12–16 Jan

Lei P, Xu L, Nwaru BI, Long Q, Wu Z (2015) Social networks and health-related quality of life among Chinese old adults in urban areas: results from 4th national household health survey. Public health 131:27–39

Leung L, Lee PS (2005) Multiple determinants of life quality: the roles of internet activities use of new media social support and leisure activities. Telematics Inform 22(3):161–180

Lin JH, Wong JY, Ho CH (2013) Promoting frontline employees' quality of life: Leisure benefit systems and work–to–leisure conflicts. Tour Manag 36:178–187

Lotfi S, Solaimani K (2009) An assessment of urban quality of life by using analytic hierarchy process approach (case study: comparative study of quality of life in the North of Iran). J Soc Sci 5(2):123–133

Maia ML, Lucas K, Marinho G, Santos E, de Lima JH (2016) Access to the Brazilian City—from the perspectives of low-income residents in Recife. J Transp Geogr (in press)

McDonagh J (2006) Transport policy instruments and transport–related social exclusion in rural Republic of Irel. J Transp Geogr 14(5):355–366

McLanahan SS, Sorensen AB (1985) Life course dynamics: trajectories and transitions 1968–1980. In Elder GH (ed) Life events and psychological well–being over the life course. Cornell University Press, Ithaca, pp 217–238

Michel JS, Mitchelson JK, Kotrba LM, LeBreton JM, Baltes BB (2009) A comparative test of work–family conflict models and critical examination of work–family linkages. J Vocat Behav 74(2):199–218

Michel JS, Kotrba LM, Mitchelson JK, Clark MA, Baltes BB (2011) Antecedents of work–family conflict: a meta–analytic review. J Organ Behav 32(5):689–725

Milner A, Krnjacki L, Butterworth P, LaMontagne AD (2016) The role of social support in protecting mental health when employed and unemployed: a longitudinal fixed–effects analysis using 12 annual waves of the HILDA cohort. Soc Sci Med 153:20–26

Mittal A (2007) Bayesian network technologies: applications and graphical models. IGI Global

Morgan MG, Henrion M, Small M (1990) Uncertainty: a guide to dealing with uncertainty in quantitative risk and policy analysis. Cambridge University Press, New York

Myers DG, Diener E (1995) Who is happy? Psychol Sci 6(1):10–19

Myers DG, Diener E (1996) The pursuit of happiness. Sci Am 274(5):70–72
Nomaguchi KM, Milkie MA, Bianchi SM (2005) Time strains and psychological well–being: do dual–earner mothers and fathers differ? J Fam Issues 26(6):756–792
Nordbakke S, Schwanen T (2013) Wellbeing and mobility: a theoretical framework and literature review focusing on older people. Mobilities 9(1):104–129
Oakil ATM (2015) Securing or sacrificing access to a car: Gender difference in the effects of life events. Travel Behav Soc 3:1–7
Plagnol AC, Scott J (2011) What matters for well–being: individual perceptions of quality of life before and after important life events. Appl Res Qual Life 6(2):115–137
Powdthavee N (2009) What happens to people before and after disability? Focusing effects lead effects and adaptation in different areas of life. Soc Sci Med 69(12):1834–1844
Ritsema van Eck J, Burghouwt G, Dijst M (2005) Lifestyles spatial configurations and quality of life in daily travel: an explorative simulation study. J Transp Geogr 13(2):123–134
Salvatore N, Munoz Sastre MT (2001) Appraisal of life; "area" versus "dimension" conceptualizations. Soc Indic Res 53(3):229–255
Schalock RL (1996) Reconsidering the conceptualization and measurement of quality of life. Qual Life 1(9):123–139
Scheiner J (2014) Gendered key events in the life course: effects on changes in travel mode choice over time. J Transp Geogr 37:47–60
Schoenduwe R, Mueller MG, Peters A, Lanzendorf M (2015) Analysing mobility biographies with the life course calendar: a retrospective survey methodology for longitudinal data collection. J Transp Geogr 42:98–109
Sharmeen F, Arentze T, Timmermans H (2014) An analysis of the dynamics of activity and travel needs in response to social network evolution and life–cycle events: a structural equation model. Transp Res Part A 59:159–171
Sirgy M (2010) Toward a quality–of–life theory of leisure travel satisfaction. J Travel Res 49:246–260
Sirgy M, Rahtz DR, Cicic M, Underwood R (2000) A method for assessing residents' satisfaction with community–based services: a quality–of–life perspective. Soc Indic Res 49(3):279–316
Strazdins L, OBrien LV, Lucas N, Rodgers B (2013) Combining work and family: rewards or risks or children's mental health? Soc Sci Med 87:99–107
Sturm R, Cohen DA (2004) Suburban sprawl and physical and mental health. Public Health 118(7):488–496
Sugimoto Y (2010) Introduction to Japanese society. Cambridge University Press
Takamiya M, Yamamoto K, Watanabe T (2010) Modeling and estimation of travel behaviors using Bayesian network. Intell Decis Technol 4(4):297–305
Tang TLP (2007) Income and quality of life: does the love of money make a difference? J Bus Ethics 72(4):375–393
Taylor SJ, Bogdan R (1990) Quality of life and the individual's perspective. In: Schalock RL (ed), Quality of life: perspectives and issues. American Association of Mental Retardation, Washington, pp 27–40
Tefft N (2012) Mental health and employment: the SAD story. Econ Human Biol 10(3):242–255
Tercan E (2015) An examination of leisure participation family assessment and life satisfaction in university students. Procedia-Soc Behav Sci 186:58–63
Tsai SY, Lee PL, Lin JW, Lee CN (2016) Cross–sectional and longitudinal associations between sleep and health–related quality of life in pregnant women: a prospective observational study. Int J Nurs Stud 56:45–53
Uysal M, Perdue R, Sirgy MJ (2012) Handbook of tourism and quality–of–life research: enhancing the lives of tourists and residents of host communities. Springer Science and Business Media
Uysal M, Sirgy MJ, Woo E, Kim HL (2016) Quality of life and well–being research in tourism. Tour Manag 53:244–261

Vallée J, Cadot E, Grillo F, Parizot I, Chauvin P (2010) The combined effects of activity space and neighbourhood of residence on participation in preventive health–care activities: the case of cervical screening in the Paris metropolitan area (France). Health Place 16(5):838–852

Van Acker V (2015) Defining, measuring, and using the lifestyle concept in modal choice research. Transp Res Rec 2495:74–82

Van Acker V, Van Wee B, Witlox F (2010) When transport geography meets social psychology: toward a conceptual model of travel behavior. Transp Rev 30(2):219–240

Van Praag BM, Frijters P, Ferrer-i-Carbonell A (2003) The anatomy of subjective well-being. J Econ Behav Organ 51(1):29–49

Veenhoven R (2012) Evidence based pursuit of happiness: what should we know, do we know and can we get to know? EHERO white paper Available: https://personal.eur.nl/veenhoven/Pub2010s/2012j-full.pdf. Accessed 1 Jul 2016

Verhoeven M (2010) Modelling life trajectories and mode choice using bayesian belief networks. Doctoral dissertation, Eindhoven University of Technology, The Netherlands

Verhoeven M, Arentze TA, Timmermans HJP, Van der Waerden PJHJ (2007) Examining temporal effects of lifecycle events on transport mode choice decision. Int J Urban Sci 11(1):1–13

Wang D, Li SM (2004) Housing preferences in a transitional housing system: the case of Beijing China. Environ Plann A 36(1):69–88

Wilson I, McDermott H, Munir F (2016) The role of working hours work environment and physical leisure activity on the need for recovery following a day's work among UK white–water raft guides: a within–subjects multilevel approach. Psychol Sport Exerc 23:123–131

Winters JV (2011) Human capital higher education institutions quality of life. Reg Sci Urban Econ 41(5):446–454

Zhang J (2009) Subjective well–being and activity–travel behavior analysis: applying day reconstruction method to explore affective experience during travel. In: Proceedings of the 14th international conference of Hong Kong Society for transportation studies, Hong Kong, 10–12 Dec, (2), pp 439–449 (Invited paper)

Zhang J (2014) Revisiting residential self–selection issues: a life–oriented approach. J Transp Land Use 7(3):29–45

Zhang J (2015) The life-oriented approach and travel behavior research. A discussion paper for the Workshop "life-oriented approach for transportation studies" at the 14th international conference on travel behaviour research, Windsor, UK, July 19–23

Zhang J, Tsuchiya Y, Fujiwara A, Chikaraishi M (2011) Citizens' life decisions and behavior survey: proposal and application to the evaluation of quality of life. In: Proceedings of infrastructure planning 43 (CD–ROM) (in Japanese)

Zhang J, Yu B, Chikaraishi M (2014) Interdependences between household residential and car ownership behavior: a life history analysis. J Transp Geogr 34:165–174

Zhao P, Lu B (2010) Exploring job accessibility in the transformation context: an institutionalist approach and its application in Beijing. J Transp Geogr 18(3):393–401

Zimmermann S (2014) The pursuit of subjective well–being through specific consumption choice. Available at SSRN: http://ssrn.com/abstract=2484660 or http://dx.doi.org/10.2139/ssrn.2484660

Chapter 3
Lifestyles and Life Choices

Veronique Van Acker

Abstract This chapter focuses on lifestyles and life choices. Although there is not a formally agreed definition of it, the 'lifestyle' concept—derived from sociology—might be useful in life choice studies. It highlights the importance of 'soft' factors next to the traditional 'hard' factors (e.g., demographic, socioeconomic and spatial characteristics) while explaining life choices. This chapter first provides a structured overview of the 'lifestyle' concept in terms of definitions and measurement methods. Two broad perspectives exists: (1) a mechanistic lifestyle approach considering a behavioral typology of activity and time use patterns, and (2) a sociographic lifestyle approach focusing on a behavioral orientations—values, attitudes and preferences—and a latent factor motivating behavior patterns. The second part of this chapter reviews how the 'lifestyle' concept has been used in life choice studies so far. It specifically focuses on applications in the research domains of demography and family studies, geography and urban studies, and transportation. Both perspectives are used interchangeably without little evaluation of the usefulness of various formal lifestyle classification systems. Moreover, most life choice studies consider 'lifestyles' as static and given, and not as something dynamic that might change over time. This calls for a more longitudinal perspective on the interaction between lifestyles and life choices. Other avenues for further research include the integration with a social network and a geographical perspective.

Keywords Lifestyles · Life choices · Mechanistic and sociographic approaches · Dynamics · Interactions · Sociology · Demography · Family studies · Geography · Urban studies · Transportation

V. Van Acker (✉)
LISER, Esch-sur-Alzette, Luxembourg
e-mail: veronique.vanacker@liser.lu

V. Van Acker
Ghent University, Department of Geography, Ghent, Belgium
veronique.vanacker@ugent.be

J. Zhang (ed.), *Life-Oriented Behavioral Research for Urban Policy*,
DOI 10.1007/978-4-431-56472-0_3

3.1 Introduction

Many studies relate particular life choices such as family formation, residential relocation or daily commuting to demographic, socio-economic and spatial factors only. Literature reviews such as Handy (2005), Ewing and Cervero (2010) on the interaction between residential location choices and daily travel choices summarize how various spatial variables such as density, diversity and design effect travel aspects such as modal choices and travel distances. These variables can objectively observed and measured, and are sometimes referred to as 'hard variables' (Sztompka 2000). However, different life choices can still be found within socioeconomic homogenous population groups (see, e.g., van Wee 2002; Mokhtarian and Cao 2008, for a reference to travel behaviour studies). Recently, some researchers have therefore argued in favour of including also more subjective explanations focusing on 'soft' variables such as individuals' attitudes, preferences, values and norms. Such soft variables are however not easily observed and measured by an outsider (Ross 1975; Sztompka 2000). This is where the 'lifestyle' concept is relevant. A variety of orientations towards family, work, leisure and consumption exists which might explain different life choices within population groups otherwise considered socioeconomically homogenous. The concept of 'lifestyle' thus adds a behavioural component to life choice models.

The first recorded use of the term 'lifestyle' is attributed to the psychologist Alfred Adler who used it in 1927 to describe the individual's unique, unconscious and repetitive way of responding to (or avoiding) the main tasks of living, i.e. friendship, love and work. It is reflected in the unity of thinking, feeling and acting. But despite its frequent and colloquial use since then, no formally stated agreed definition of the 'lifestyle' concept exists. Moreover, it is elaborated pragmatically rather than theoretically. Especially marketing studies (e.g., Mitchell 1983) use the 'lifestyle' concept in order to retrieve market sectors. These studies generally cluster analyse numerous data. Each cluster is then referred to as another lifestyle. Because results are data-dependent without a sound theoretical basis, each study 'finds' new lifestyles. This pragmatic approach is criticized by Sobel (1983) among others.

The remainder of this chapter is structured as follows. Despite the dominating pragmatic approach, some theoretical contributions have been made to the 'lifestyle' concept which are described in Sect. 3.2. Section 3.3 summarizes different methodologies to measure lifestyles. Against this theoretical and methodological background, the use of the 'lifestyle' concept in different life choice domains is discussed in Sect. 3.4. It examines the ways in which lifestyles influence the life choices of (i) family formation, (ii) residential location and migration, and (iii) traffic and travel behaviour. Finally, Sect. 3.5 presents some conclusions and possible future research directions.

3.2 The Concept of 'Lifestyle': Background and Definitions

A theoretical background of the 'lifestyle' concept can be found mainly in sociology by scholars such as Weber (1922), Bourdieu (1979), Ganzeboom (1988) and Schulze (1992). In sociology, social structure used to be explained in terms of *social class* measured by differences in education, profession and income. Such indicators clearly emphasize participation in labour force which seems adequate when describing the structure of an industrial society preoccupied with production. However, it has various disadvantages especially in modern societies which are more focussed on consumption rather than on production (Richter 2002). Social class structure was believed to be very stable throughout the years. However, in modern society changes can be noticed with respect to the use of free time, cultural behaviour and participation in society. For example, it no longer holds that employees and entrepreneurs vote conservative parties while workers vote socialist parties. During last decennia, prosperity increased resulting in increasing individualization and decreasing social control. Consequently, the social burden to behave uniformly according to social class membership disappeared, and traditional relations between behaviour and social class membership have broken down. Social structure is thus not as stable as it once was (Hradil 1987) and there is less uniformity of behaviour within social classes (Ferge 1972; Bootsma et al. 1993). Individuals nowadays not only behave according to their social class, but also to their personal lifestyles based on their values and interests in life. Consequently, a cultural and symbolic dimension needs to be added to the discussion on social structure (Helbrecht 1995).

Weber's *Wirtschaft und Gesellschaft* (Weber 1922) was one of the first sociological studies that contributed to the theoretical debate on lifestyles. Criticising Marx' class theory in which a person's behaviour is determined by his or her economic position (i.e., the possession of production means), Weber emphasized the importance of a cultural/symbolic and a political dimension. He argued that behaviour is not always based on what a person produces (i.e., economic dimension) but also on what he or she consumes (i.e., cultural/symbolic dimension). Through these consumption patterns, a person has a particular *social status*. According to Weber, social status refers to a group of people that shares the same prestige and who clarifies this prestige. Lifestyle is thus considered as a pattern of observable and expressive behaviours. Weber conceptualized lifestyles (or 'Lebensstil' in his work) through 'Lebensführung' (translated as life conduct) and 'Lebenschancen' (translated as life chances). 'Lebensführung' refers to choice and self-direction in a person's behaviour and 'Lebenschancen' refers to structural conditions that constrain these choices (e.g., economic conditions such as income and property but also social elements such as rights, norms and social relationships). Consequently, Weber recognized that people have choices in the lifestyles they adopt, but the actual realization of these choices is influenced by their life chances. Or in other words, lifestyle is the result of the interplay between choice and structure (Cockerham et al. 1993).

Following Weber, Bourdieu (1979) considered lifestyle as a pattern of behaviours indicating the social position of the individual. His work *La Distinction* is based on the analysis of consumption patterns in France. He combined socio-demographic data (e.g., education, profession, income) with information from thirty surveys on preferences and behaviours associated with lifestyle related subjects such as purchasing behaviour, holidays, car type, culinary preferences, fashion, cultural activities and taste. Based on this information, each individual occupies a position in a two-dimensional social space which is defined by the composition and the volume of capital. Within this two-dimensional space, traditional socio-demographic variables define the 'space of social position', whereas specific patterns of behaviour define the 'space of lifestyles'. Based on this, two hierarchies can be distinguished. One category reaches from the traditional lower status groups to the economic elites who pursue material welfare and obtain rather traditional aesthetic and moral beliefs. Another category reaches from the same lower status groups to cultural elites.

Ganzeboom (1988) builds on the work of Bourdieu in order to analyse lifestyles in the Netherlands. In his work, lifestyle is related (but not considered a synonym!) to the individual's socio-economic characteristics and also influenced by intermediate variables referring to opportunities and constraints offered by time budget, income, cognitive skills and status. Ganzeboom argues that lifestyles must not be considered as unambiguous types but rather as a continuum determined by three dimensions: an economic dimension, a cultural dimension, and a stage of life-dimension. The first two dimensions are clearly inspired by Bourdieu, but Ganzeboom considers economic and cultural capital as two separate dimensions instead of opposite extremes of one dimension. The third dimension originates from Bourdieu's 'space of social positions' which is based on traditional socio-economic variables.

Schulze's *Erlebnisgesellschaft* (experience society) (Schulze 1992) is another example of this postmodern approach. Moreover, he added a spatial dimension to the discussion on lifestyles. He observed that leisure consumption often occurs outside the home in specific places that attract a congenial group sharing similar lifestyles (e.g. cafes, shopping centres, football stadiums). Schulze refers to these specific sites as 'scenes': combinations of a congenial lifestyle group sharing similar leisure consumption behaviour. These scenes gain importance in a postmodern society at the expense of traditional urban living and working environments (van der Wouden and Kulberg 2002).

Without any intention of providing a comprehensive overview, this section illustrated how the theoretical discussion on lifestyle has evolved throughout the years. Two opposing views are apparent: Weber and Bourdieu who considered social class as an important determinant of lifestyles and thus a clear hierarchy of lifestyles, in contrast to Ganzeboom and Schulz who considered lifestyles as niches that are no longer in line with social classes in a postmodern society where old social structures are flattened (Tomlinson 1998). Nevertheless, they all agree on the communicative character of lifestyles and, therefore, a basic definition of the 'lifestyle' concept should at least refer to: "*The way by which the individual indicates his or her social position through specific patterns of behaviour, mainly in consumption and leisure behaviours*."

3.3 Measuring the 'Lifestyle' Concept

Defining the 'lifestyle' concept is one thing, measuring it is another one. Some empirical studies analyse what they would call lifestyles, but in fact combine various objective socio-economic and demographic characteristics of the individual and the household (e.g., Cooper et al. 2001; Hildebrand 2003 with applications in transportation research). Such studies are characterized by a *socio-economic and demographic approach* and rather measure stage of life or household composition than lifestyles. Statistical techniques such as cluster and factor analysis are frequently used to determine stage of life groups like youngsters, households with young children, single-parent families and the elderly. The advantage of this approach is that data on socio-economics and demographics are widely available. However, the theoretical discussion above illustrates that such characteristics do not necessarily reflect how people want to socially represent themselves towards other people. It is therefore questionable whether a socio-economic and demographic approach can be considered appropriate to measure lifestyles.

The theoretical discussion in Sect. 3.2 concluded with a basic definition of lifestyles as behavioural patterns, mainly in consumption and leisure, through which an individual elucidates his or her social position towards others. From this perspective, it makes sense to use data such as consumption behaviours, activity patterns and time-use. Lifestyle studies based on this type of data are using a *mechanistic lifestyle approach*. This approach considers the simplest content of the lifestyle concept: lifestyles as a way of living or as "*a condition of existence and a manner of being*" (Cathelat 1993, p. 97). The available data on (consumer) behaviours is often combined with socio-demographic data. The empirical analyses in Bourdieu's *La Distinction* can be considered as a good example. His two-dimensional social space is based on a correspondence analysis of socio-demographic data combined with information on consumption behaviour. The proximity of characteristics within this two-dimensional social space implies that these characteristics are often combined with one another.

But according to others, lifestyle includes more than observable patterns of behaviour. We behave in a particular way because we think in a particular way. Behaviour is thus related to personal thoughts, attitudes and preferences. No surprise that some lifestyle studies focus on such underlying opinions and motivations, including beliefs, interests and attitudes (Ganzeboom 1988), and use a *sociographic lifestyle approach*. Sociographic lifestyles studies aim at monitoring changes and trends in society by the analysis of changing individual and shared opinions and attitudes.

This contradiction between lifestyles as behaviours (or a way of acting) and attitudes (or a way of feeling and thinking) may confound our understanding of the 'lifestyle' concept. For that reason, Munters (1992) distinguished *lifestyles* from *lifestyle expressions*. He considered lifestyles as the individual's opinions and motivations, or orientations. Frequently studied lifestyle orientations relate to fields such as family-life, work-life, leisure, consumption and housing (Bootsma et al. 1993). Consequently, lifestyles are internal to the individual and are thus unobservable. A lifestyle, then, manifests itself in observable patterns of behaviour, or lifestyle expressions which is in line with the previously mentioned basic definition of lifestyles. In this way, observable patterns of behaviour (lifestyle expressions) are explained by underlying opinions and orientations (lifestyles). Two broad perspectives thus exist (for a more detailed overview, see Van Acker 2016):

1. lifestyles as a behavioural typology of activity and time use patterns (in accordance with 'lifestyle expressions' by Munters and the mechanistic lifestyle approach)
2. lifestyles as a behavioural orientation—values, attitudes and preferences—and a latent factor motivating behaviour patterns (in accordance with 'lifestyles' in its strict sense by Munters and the sociographic lifestyle approach).

3.4 Lifestyles and Life Choices

After having discussed different definitions and measurement methods, we now turn our attention to empirical studies that use the 'lifestyle' concept in relation to life choices. The 'lifestyle' concept is mainly used in research areas such as health sciences and medicines. Figure 3.1 is based on an ISI Web-of-Science literature search using 'lifestyle', 'life-style' and 'life style' as title words. This resulted in 15,768 articles that were then arranged by research area. It is striking how different disciplines of health sciences and medicines dominate Fig. 3.1. Many health studies relate diseases such as diabetes, obesity, cancer and depression to lifestyle activities such as diet, level of physical activity, substance abuse, social and personal interactions. From an empirical point of view, these studies clearly use a mechanistic lifestyle approach. But one cannot say that this focus on health-related lifestyle activities also highlights the communicative aspect of lifestyles. The individual's social position is not questioned through these health-related lifestyle activities. Consequently, such health studies use the 'lifestyle' concept rather pragmatically than theoretically.

The lifestyle concept is also used in research areas with a clear link to life choices, in particular in demography and family studies (e.g., family formation choices), geography and urban studies (e.g., residential location choices and the choice to migrate) and transportation (e.g., modal choices). The subsequent sections will summarize the main findings on lifestyles related to major life choices in each of these research areas. This literature review is based on the ISI Web-of-Science literature mentioned earlier. First, only articles with 'lifestyle', 'life-style'

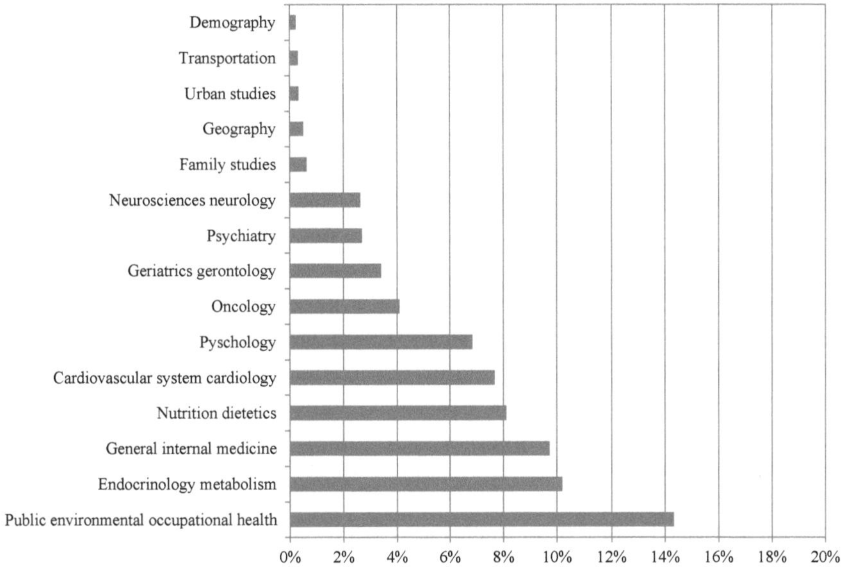

Fig. 3.1 Number of articles with 'lifestyle', 'life-style' or 'life style' in its title by research area. (% of 15,768 articles—search performed on May 17, 2016)

or 'lifestyle' in its title were selected. This resulted in a list of 15,768 articles. Second, articles were arranged by research area. Figure 3.1 summarizes the top 10 research areas using the 'lifestyle' concept (all in health sciences and medicines) as well as those research areas that are relevant to life choice research. Third, articles in those life choice related research areas were ranked according to relevance and finally reviewed. This chapter does not intend to provide a full comprehensive review of this body of work, but only highlights some examples and main findings related to various life choices.

3.4.1 Demography and Family Studies

One important topic in demographic and family studies is the study of life courses and within this the life choice of family formation. A traditional view on life courses considers a linear sequence of life stages divided from each other by clear life events. First graduating and finding a good job, then cohabiting before getting married and having children is still considered as the ideal life course and ideal path towards family formation, even today by many young adults (Elchardus and Smits 2005). But lifestyle features such as a family or career orientation, may explain why not everybody transitions from cohabitation into the first marriage at the same pace. Lois (2008) found that a family-oriented and religious lifestyle is positively linked to the probability of marriage, even after controlling for socioeconomic characteristics such as education or professional status. A career- and leisure-oriented lifestyles is negatively associated with marriage, but this can be partly explained by education, professional status and family formation. However, these associations between lifestyles and marriage can change all together depending on whether lifestyle features are shared between partners or not. The probability of marriage increases if both partners share the same career-oriented lifestyles, but it decreases if partner's family-oriented lifestyles are different. Divorce is another deviation from this ideal life course and family formation. Decurtins et al. (1997) studied the consequences of different lifestyles (in terms of a new partnership or not) for fathers after a divorce on the social network and health in comparison with married fathers. Based on interviews with divorced and married fathers in Zurich and Winterthur, Switzerland, they found that the social stress of divorced fathers with a new partner is similar to that of the other divorced fathers, but the social support they receive is higher and corresponds more to that of married fathers which then contributes to subjective well-being and satisfaction with the situation.

Most lifestyle-related demographic and family studies however question the traditional view on families and focus on more alternative forms of cohabitation, especially in developed countries. Such alternative forms received much social science attention in the 1960s and 1970s. It is however striking how some of these alternatives (e.g., cohabitation, stepfamilies) have become mainstream topics of scholarly research today, whereas the most extremes (e.g., swinging, group marriage, communes) have been largely ignored. Illustrative for this denial is how a journal such as *Alternative Life Styles: Changing Patterns in Marriage, Family, and Intimacy* founded in 1978 by Libby eventually changed its journal title in 1992 into *Journal of Family and Economic Issues* (Rubin 2001).

Many studies still start with married couples but then question traditional roles within the family. For example, an important increase in women entering the labour force can be noticed the last decades. This change has forced dual-income families to adopt new strategies with respect to combining work and family obligations (Paden and Buehler 1995), parenting (Jendrek 1993; Schneewind 1997) and commuting relationships (Anderson and Spruill 1993).

Combining work and family obligations might result in role overload and conflicts within the family. Paden and Buehler (1995) studied how married couples in a midsized Southeastern community in the U.S. cope with this problem and identified five coping mechanisms: planning, talking to others, withdrawing, cognitive restructuring and limiting job responsibilities. Coping mechanisms differed between spouses: planning and restructuring were significant buffering mechanisms for wives, restructuring and withdrawing for husbands. Direct effects of these coping mechanisms on well-being were minimal, but coping moderated several effects of role conflict and role overload on spouse's well-being. Seeking support through talking to others who can sympathise and provide a support system to relieve stress was found, surprisingly, to be an ineffective cooping mechanism. It exacerbated the relationship between husband's role overload and positive affect. Such a safety net is often offered by the grandparents who parent their grandchildren on a daily basis. Jendrek (1993) studied the effects of this parenting style on the lifestyles of the grandparents. The majority of grandparents reported an increase in the need to alter routines and plans, having more of a purpose for living and feeling more physically tired. But differences exists among grandparents, depending on the type of caregiving. Other couples remain childless voluntarily. Schneewind (1997) described profiles of voluntarily childless couples based on aspects such as personality, marital relations, parenting competence, family of origin relations, parenthood decision making but also lifestyles. No indications of a general anti-child orientation of these couples were found. Rather, it seems that their decision was based on an attitude of 'responsible non-parent-hood'. Whereas the previous studies focused on family obligations, Anderson and Spruill (1993) studied one specific coping mechanism related to work obligations in dual-income families. Most dual-income families are able to balance residential and job locations with each other so that the couple can live together at the same residence. But some couples cannot and eventually adopt a commuting relationship where both partners have separate residences in different cities and reunite regularly (e.g., in the weekends). Based on a sample of 39 couples throughout the U.S., Anderson and Spruill (1993) found that this non-traditional lifestyle is associated with a fairly traditional division of household labour, moderate levels of stress and an incomplete decision-making process.

Family studies also often question (the origins of) lifestyle homogamy in couple relationships. Some studies suggests that individuals choose a partner partly on the basis of similarity in terms of, for example, socio-economic background and leisure interests. Using data from the German Socieconomic Panel, Arranz Becker and Lois (2010) illustrate that alignment over time does indeed promote homogamy of leisure-related lifestyles in married and cohabiting couples. However, intermediate stages in the life course such as phases of active parenting and labour force participation tend to inhibit such alignment. Kalmijn and Bernasco (2001) reported similar results on the influence of life cycle factors for the Netherlands.

The research field also often refers to a wide array of modern factors that change the value orientation towards the family. Modern factors include external factors such as globalization (Okeke et al. 2011) and ICT use (Nwegbu and Echezona 2010; Ukwueze 2011) but also more personal factors such as migration of the family towards a new culture and value orientation towards the family and intergenerational differences in how to cope with this (Renzaho et al. 2011).

3.4.2 *Geography and Urban Studies*

The 'lifestyle' concept is applied in geography and urban studies with respect to two important life choices: residential location choices at a local scale and migration decisions at an international scale.

3.4.2.1 Residential Location Choice

Studies of residential location choice tend to focus on demographic and socio-economic factors only, but some argue that lifestyles are also relevant. Scheiner (2006) illustrates how lifestyles influence not only residential location choices but also activity spaces and modal choices. Using survey data from Cologne, Germany, he mainly used a sociographic lifestyle approach and defined lifestyles based on measures from four domains: leisure preferences, values and life aims, aesthetic taste and frequency of social contacts. Based on these four domains, he found that an out-of-home self-realisation lifestyle is associated with a positive location attitudes towards public transport and residential choices of good quality public transport locations. Residing in such high quality public transport locations eventually results in more public transport use and less car use. The same out-of-home self-realisation lifestyles was also found to be positively associated with a positive location attitude towards proximity of retail and services and residential choices with a high density of retail, service and leisure opportunities. However, not everybody agrees on the importance of lifestyles in residential location choices. Rossel and Hoelscher (2012), for example, found no important lifestyle influences using data from Leipzig, Germany. Household arrangements and economic resource endowments of persons were found much more important.

A remarkable part of the literature focuses on the very specific topic of gentrification or the inner-urban residential location choices of the upper-middle class. Brun and Fagnani (1994) pointed out how couples who live in the centre of Paris value traditional urban aspects such as proximity to shops, services and jobs. Moreover, those couples living in the centre are also very socially active and have a very 'open' lifestyle, despite the presence of children. Contrary to couples who choose to live in the suburbs and who have a much more family-oriented lifestyles. Similar results were found by McDowell (1997) who interviewed merchant bankers in the city of London. The majority of respondents argued that accessibility was a key factor in their decision to reside in inner London, especially as they worked long hours and did not want to lose free time in travel. A labour-oriented lifestyle clearly dominated their inner-city location choices. A few respondents lived outside London. For couples with children, their location outside London was clearly linked to a family-oriented lifestyle. Most of these people were satisfied with this, even if this means longer commuting times. Only a few were not. Totally different lifestyles were noticed among single people who choose to live outside London. Their choice was linked to particular hobbies involving for example sailing or riding, and thus a very specific active lifestyle.

The greater part of the literature focuses on residential location choice as a single event in someone's life course and respondents are often questioned which aspects determined that specific residential location choice. This suggests a state of 'topophilia', or that people have a rooted, static and stable set of relations with one specific residential location. However, Anderson and Erskine (2014) argue that this should be supplemented by 'tropophilia' or the love of mobility, change and transformation in the person-place relation. Some people—what they call 'lifestyle travellers—relocate often seeking dynamism, change and instability in their engagements with place. These relocations often cross borders. Therefore, it makes sense that the 'lifestyle' concept is used with respect to migration, a second topic in geography and urban studies.

3.4.2.2 Migration

In migration studies, the 'lifestyle' concept is used especially when referring to 'lifestyle mobilities'. Cohen et al. (2015) use the term 'lifestyle mobilities' to challenge discrete notions of travel, leisure and migration. Lifestyle mobilities are situated within the mobilities research, a contemporary paradigm in the social sciences (Sheller and Urry 2006). It considers physical and corporeal moving as an ongoing lifestyle choice linked to identity construction, meaning, belonging and place attachment. Such physical and corporeal moving ranges from daily travel trips to international migrations. Lifestyle mobilities are mainly studied in the latter context of international lifestyle migration, which is a rapidly growing worldwide phenomenon. For example, within Europe large numbers of northern Europeans are moving south in search of what they perceive as a better quality of life. This form of migration is typically considered as consumption-led, tourism-related and leisure-based (and not economic-led, labour-based or conflict-related). But recent studies also highlight the role of the local place in this type of migration process and the construction of individual and collective social identities (Benson 2011 for a sample of British residents in rural France; Torkington 2012 for a sample of British residents in the Algarve, Portugal; Huete et al. 2013 for lifestyle migrants in Alicante, Spain; Ono 2015 for a sample of Japanese retirees in Malaysia). Another type of international lifestyle migration is linked to very specific leisure activities such as 'action', 'alternative' or 'extreme' sports (e.g., snowboarding in Thorpe 2012; or rock climbing in Rickly 2016).

3.4.3 Transportation

3.4.3.1 Traffic Behaviour and Traffic Safety

Traffic behaviour and traffic safety is a first transportation research field that frequently refers to the concept of 'lifestyles'. Lifestyles are often used to explain risky driving behaviour, especially of young men (e.g., Gregersen and Berg 1994; Begg et al. 1999; Bina et al. 2006; Møller and Haustein 2013). A mechanistic lifestyle approach is frequently used. Lifestyles are often measured through a questionnaire in which respondents are asked to report their involvement in not only risky driving behaviours but also other health risk behaviours (such as drinking, drugs use, sleepiness, etc.) and leisure activities (such as sports, music, movies, reading, political engagement, religion, etc.).

Lifestyles related to religion/tradition (Gnardellis et al. 2008 for Greece) and culture (Chliaoutakis et al. 1999 for Greece; and 2005 for Crete) are often found to be negatively associated with the risk of causing car crashes, whereas the opposite holds for lifestyles dominated by aimless driving/cruising (Møller and Haustein 2013 for Denmark), antisocial behaviour (Bina et al. 2006 for Italy) and sports (Chliaoutakis et al. 1999, 2005). While in these studies 'lifestyles' are considered as important predictors of car crashes and injuries, in others its significance is rather limited. (e.g., Begg et al. 1999 for New Zealand).

3.4.3.2 Travel Behaviour

A second transportation research field that benefits from lifestyle-based insights is that of travel behaviour. The first explicit use of the word 'lifestyle' in travel behaviour research was at the end of the 1970s. Gillan and Wachs (1976) used it in relation to travel patterns of a very specific population group, namely the elderly. Wachs (1979, p. 21) stated: '*A particular combination of income, family status, educational attainment, residential density, and similar variables differentiates the patterns of living of those who share them from those who are represented by other ranges of the same variables*'. It is a clear example of the socio-economic and demographic lifestyle approach. The quote however does not highlight the communicative character of lifestyles. These early studies can, therefore, not be considered as representative of the theoretical perspective on 'lifestyles'.

Salomon and Ben-Akiva (1983, based on his PhD thesis in 1980) on the other hand used the 'lifestyle' concept in a sense much closer to its sociologic meaning. He defined lifestyles as '*the pattern of behaviour which conforms to the individual's orientation towards the three major roles: as a household member, a worker, and a consumer of leisure, and to the constrained resources available*' (Salomon 1980, p. 15). Alongside Salomon, the work by Kitamura (1988, republished in 2009) was also very influential in bringing this idea of lifestyles into travel behaviour research. Applications of 'lifestyles' in transportation research are since then mainly in activity-based travel modelling studies. By using the concept of 'lifestyle', activity-based studies seek to make a significant progress toward a more behavioural framework for simulating household travel behaviour (Krizek and Waddell 2002; Krizek 2006). Transport researchers are becoming aware that the utility maximization principle, which is widely used in transport economics and modelling, does not totally encompass the motivation of human behaviour (Talvitie 1997). Within this behavioural approach of travel behaviour, daily travel patterns are often considered within a hierarchical decision structure (e.g., Ben-Akiva 1973; Salomon 1980; Salomon and Ben-Akiva 1983). This hierarchy ranges from short-term decisions on daily activities and travel (such as activity type, activity duration, destination, route and mode choice), to mediate-term decisions on vehicle ownership, residential and workplace location, and long-term decisions on lifestyles (such as family formation, participation in labour force and orientation toward leisure). A significant challenge remains how to integrate these short- and long-term decisions (Glickman et al. 2015).

Various activity-based transport researchers have now tried to operationalize the 'lifestyle' concept quantitatively. A mechanistic lifestyle approach has frequently been applied using data on, for example, consumer expenditure (e.g., Deka 2015), time use (e.g., Fan and Khattak 2012) and/or activity behaviours (e.g., Lin et al. 2009). For example, Bagley and Mokhtarian (2002) used data from a 1993 survey carried out in five neighbourhoods in San Francisco. This survey included among others a list of more than 100 types of activities and interests. Respondents had to indicate what types of subjects they had read last month, how they spent their last weekend and what type of leisure activities they had conducted within the last year. These answers were factor analysed into eleven lifestyle factors such as culture lover, hobbyist and family-oriented. A more adventurous lifestyle appeared to be associated with longer travel distances by car. A similar survey was organized by Van Acker et al. (2011, 2014) in 2007 in Flanders. A low budget lifestyle was found to be related with less car use and more cycling, walking and public transport for leisure trips, whereas the opposite holds for an active family lifestyle.

Travel surveys also often collect data on attitudes and preferences. This allows the use of a sociographic lifestyle approach and to move towards the second perspective on lifestyles as a behavioural orientation. For example, Lanzendorf (2002) collected data from four neighbourhoods in Cologne, Germany, on leisure and mobility orientations. Applying factor and cluster analysis, he identified seven lifestyles (but used the word 'mobility styles' instead). He found that mobility styles significantly explained the decision to travel for various leisure purposes and distance travelled by car, while it was not a significant influence on modal choice. Contrary to Collantes and Mokhtarian (2007) who found similar effects on travel distances but also on modal choices. A 1998 survey in San Francisco included 18 attitudinal statements on work, family, money, status and time use. These statements were factor analysed, with four lifestyle factors emerging: frustrated, status seeker, workaholic and family-oriented. Family-oriented lifestyles as well as frustrated lifestyles were associated with less car use for short-distance trips. A family-oriented lifestyle was also found to be associated with fewer long-distance leisure trips. Furthermore, they found that workaholics travel significantly fewer short-distance as well as long-distance trips for leisure purposes.

Lifestyles might seem important correlates of travel behaviour at first sight, but some studies find very limited influences. Scheiner (2010), for example, found that the impact of lifestyles depends on trip purpose: it has a strong impact for leisure trips, but not so much on work and maintenance trips. Similarly, Van Acker (2016) illustrated how adding lifestyles increased the explained variances in models of modal choice for leisure trips, but other predictors such as driver licensing, car ownership and the built environment were more important.

3.5 Conclusions

This chapter illustrated how a lifestyle approach provides useful insights into life choices. Life choices are not simply made based on objective socio-economic and demographic characteristics such as income, prices, education and age, but are also related to subjective characteristics such as attitudes, status and preferences. This is where the 'lifestyle' concept becomes useful.

Despite its frequent and colloquial use, there is yet no agreement on the definition of the 'lifestyle' concept. Most empirical studies use the concept rather pragmatically, whereas this chapter also presented a theoretical overview of the 'lifestyle' concept. This eventually resulted in the formulation of a basic notion of 'lifestyles' as "*the way by which the individual indicates his or her social position through specific patterns of behaviour, mainly in consumption and leisure behaviours*". Such patterns of behaviour are actually 'lifestyle expressions' which are explained by underlying opinions and orientations, or 'lifestyles' in its strict sense. But the main argument is that lifestyles have a clear communicate character that highlights someone's social position towards others.

This theoretical overview indicated different dimensions of 'lifestyle', let only to measure as well. Two broad measurement perspectives were detected: (i) lifestyles as a behavioural typology of activity and time use patterns, and (ii) lifestyles as a behavioural orientation—values, attitudes and preferences—and a latent factor motivating behaviour patterns. These two perspectives are used interchangeably, also in life choice studies. This chapter referred to many examples and summarized main findings in demography and family studies, geography and urban studies, and transportation. Based on this, four avenues for further research on the lifestyle concept in life choice studies are identified:

- First, the two measurement perspectives are used interchangeably with little evaluation of which of the many formal classification systems are more useful. One exception in the research domain of transportation is Van Acker (2016) who compared a mechanistic with a sociographic lifestyle approach when studying modal choices for leisure trips in Flanders, Belgium. With respect to active travel (cycling and walking), no striking differences were found. But a mechanistic lifestyle approach seemed more appropriate with respect to the analysis of car use. This might suggest that car use is not as much associated with a value system (characteristic of the sociographic lifestyle approach) as active travel.
- Second, the discussion so far has mainly been about the question of how a specific lifestyle condition life choices of family formation, residential location, migration, and traffic and travel behaviour. Lifestyles are hereby considered as static and given. The reverse relationship of life choices enabling or constraining lifestyles is less well-studied. This reverse relationship then also raises the question how easily lifestyles can be changed under influence of particular life choices over the life course. Lifestyles must therefore be considered as dynamic rather than as static and given and which necessitates more longitudinal data.

- Third, there is not only a need for a more longitudinal perspective but also a social network perspective. Life choices not only depend on someone's personal lifestyle but also on the interaction with other people's lifestyle. For example, family and demography studies underline how decisions on family formation are influenced by the lifestyle of both partners. Marriage tend to be lower among people with a career-oriented lifestyle, but this no longer holds when both partners share the same career-oriented lifestyle (Lois 2008). This illustrates that a social network perspective on lifestyles is highly needed.
- Fourth, life choice studies in geography and urban form might suggest a process of spatial sorting of lifestyles in relation to residential location choices. Cultural and career-oriented lifestyles are often found in urban locations, traditional and family-oriented lifestyles in suburban locations. It might be useful to integrate the use of space and locations into the measurement of lifestyles (next to a behavioural typology of activity and time use patterns and behavioural orientations of values, attitudes and preferences).

References

Anderson EA, Spruill JW (1993) The dual–career commuter family—a life–style on the move. Marriage Fam Rev 19:131–147

Anderson J, Erskine K (2014) Tropophilia: a study of people place and lifestyle. Travel Mobilities 9:130–145

Arranz Becker O, Lois D (2010) Selection alignment and their interplay: origins of lifestyle homogamy in couple relationships. J Marriage Fam 72:1234–1248

Bagley MN, Mokhtarian PL (2002) The impact of residential neigborhood type in travel behavior: a structural equation modeling approach. Ann Reg Sci 36:279–297

Begg DJ, Langley JD, Williams SM (1999) A longitudinal study of lifestyle factors as predictors of injuries and crashes among young adults. Accid Anal Prev 31:1–11

Ben–Akiva M (1973) Structure of passenger travel demand models. Doctoral Dissertation, Department of Civil and Environmental Engineering, Massachusetts Institute of Technology, Cambridge

Benson M (2011) The movement beyond (lifestyle) migration: mobile practices and the constitution of a better way of life. Mobilities 6:221–235

Bina M, Graziano F, Bonino S (2006) Risky driving and lifestyles in adolescence. Accid Anal Prev 38:472–481

Bootsma H, Camstra R, de Feijter H, Mol A (1993) Leefstijl: Een dynamische levensorientatie (Lifestyle: a dynamic life orientiation). Rooilijn 26:32–37

Bourdieu P (1979) La Distinction Critique Sociale du Jugement. de Minuit, Paris

Brun J, Fagnani J (1994) Life–styles and locational choices—trade–offs and compromises: a case–study of middle–class couples living in the Ile–de–France region. Urban Stud 31:921–934

Cathelat B (1993) Socio–styles the new lifestyle classification system for identifying and targeting costumers and markets. Routledge, London

Chliaoutakis JE, Darviri C, Demakakos PT (1999) The impact of young drivers' lifestyle on their road traffic accident risk in greater Athens area. Accid Anal Prev 31:771–780

Chliaoutakis JE, Koukouli S, Lajunen T, Tzamalouka G (2005) Lifestyle traits as predictors of driving behaviour in urban areas of Greece. Transp Res Part F Traffic Psychol Behav 8:413–428

Cockerham WC, Abel T, Lüschen G (1993) Max Weber formal rationality and health lifestyles. Sociol Q 34:413–428
Cohen SA, Duncan T, Thulemark M (2015) Lifestyle mobilities: the crossroads of travel leisure and migration. Mobilities 10:155–172
Collantes GO, Mokhtarian PL (2007) Subjective assessments of personal mobility: what makes the difference between a little and a lot? Transp Policy 14:181–192
Cooper J, Ryley T, Smith A (2001) Contemporary lifestyles and the implications for sustainable development policy: lessons from the UK's most car dependent city. Belf Cities 18:103–113
Decurtins L, Niklowitz M, Meyer PC (1997) Life styles after the breakup consequences of different life styles for fathers after divorce on the social network and health in comparison with married fathers. Syst Fam 10:166–173
Deka D (2015) Relationship between households' housing and transportation expenditures examination from lifestyle perspective. Transp Res Rec J Transp Res Board 2531:26–35
Elchardus M, Smits W (2005) De levensloop van jongvolwassenen (The life course of adolescents). Research group TOR, Sociology Department, Free University Brussels, Brussels
Ewing R, Cervero R (2010) Travel and the built environment: a meta–analysis. J Am Plan Assoc 76:265–294
Fan YL, Khattak A (2012) Time use patterns lifestyles and sustainability of nonwork travel behavior. Int J Sustain Transp 6:26–47
Ferge S (1972) Social differentiation in leisure activity choices. In: Szalai A (ed) The use of time: daily activities of urban and suburban population in twelve countries. Mouton Den Haag, Netherlands, pp 213–227
Ganzeboom H (1988) Leefstijlen in Nederland: Een verkennende studie (Lifestyles in the Netherlands: an exploratory study). Sociaal Cultureel Planbureau Rijswijk
Gillan J, Wachs M (1976) Lifestyles and transportation needs of elderly in Los Angeles. Transportation 5:45–61
Glickman I, Ishaq R, Katoshevski-Cavari R, Shiftan Y (2015) Integrating activity–based travel–demand models with land–use and other long–term lifestyle decisions. J Transp Land Use 8:71–93
Gnardellis C, Tzamalouka G, Papadakaki M, Chliaoutakis JE (2008) An investigation of the effect of sleepiness drowsy driving and lifestyle on vehicle crashes. Transp Res Part F 11:270–281
Gregersen NP, Berg HY (1994) Life–style and accidents among young drivers. Accid Anal Prev 26:297–303
Handy S (2005) Critical assessment of the literature on the relationships among transportation, land use and physical activity. TRB special report 282 "Does the Built Environment Influence Physical Activity? Examining the Evidence"
Helbrecht I (1995) Differentiation of lifestyles: new challenges to social geography in urban research. Geographische Zeitschrift 83:222–237
Hildebrand ED (2003) Dimensions in elderly travel behaviour: a simplified activity–based model using lifestyle clusters. Transportation 30:285–306
Hradil S (1987) Sozialstrukturanalyse in einer fortgeschrittenen Gesellschaft. Leske and Budrich, Opladen
Huete R, Mantecon A, Estevez J (2013) Challenges in lifestyle migration research: reflections and findings about the Spanish crisis. Mobilities 8:331–348
Jendrek MP (1993) Grandparents who parent their grandchildren—effects on life–style. J Marriage Fam 55:609–621
Kalmijn M, Bernasco W (2001) Joint and separated lifestyles in couple relationships. J Marriage Fam 63:639–654
Kitamura R (2009) Life–style and travel demand. Transportation 36:679–710
Krizek K (2006) Lifestyles residential location decisions and pedestrian and transit activity. Transp Res Rec 1981:171–178
Krizek K, Waddell P (2002) Analysis of lifestyle choices—neighborhood type travel patterns and activity participation. Transp Res Rec 1807:119–128

Lanzendorf M (2002) Mobility styles and travel behaviour: an application of a lifestyle approach to leisure travel. Transp Res Rec 1807:163–173
Lin HZ, Lo HP, Chen XJ (2009) Lifestyle classifications with and without activity–travel patterns. Transp Res Part A 43:626–638
Lois D (2008) Influences of lifestyle features on the transition into first marriage. Zeitschrift für Familienforschung 20:11–33
McDowell LM (1997) The new service class: housing consumption and lifestyle among London bankers in the 1990s. Environ Plan A 29:2061–2078
Mitchell A (1983) The nine american lifestyles. Warner, New York
Mokhtarian PL, Cao XY (2008) Examining the impacts of residential self–selection on travel behaviour: a focus on methodologies. Transp Res B 42:204–228
Møller M, Haustein S (2013) Keep on cruising: changes in lifestyle and driving style among male drivers between the age of 18 and 23. Transp Res Part F 20:59–69
Munters QJ (1992) Bestaan leefstijlen (nog) wel? (Do lifestyles (still) exist?). Sociologische Gids 39:179–185
Nwegbu MU, Echezona RI (2010) Socio–cultural dimensions of ICT use among the youths and influences on family lifestyles. J Home Econ Res 12:138–147
Okeke EN, Ekomaru CI, Ihekoronye CN (2011) Globalization and changing patterns of family lifestyle: implication for home economics. J Home Econ Res 14:67–75
Ono M (2015) Commoditization of lifestyle migration: Japanese retirees in Malaysia. Mobilities 10:609–627
Paden SL, Buehler C (1995) Coping with the dual–income life–style. J Marriage Fam 57:101–110
Renzaho AMN, Green J, Mellor D, Swinburn B (2011) Parenting family functioning and lifestyle in a new culture: the case of African migrants in Melbourne, Victoria, Australia. Child Fam Soc Work 16:228–240
Richter R (2002) Lifestyle and social structure process of individualization in Eastern European countries. Revija za Sociologiju 33:169–180
Rickly JM (2016) Lifestyle mobilities: a politics of lifestyle rock climbing. Mobilities 11:243–263
Ross RB (1975) Measuring the influence of soft variables in travel behaviour. Traffic Q 29:333–346
Rossel J, Hoelscher M (2012) Life styles and residential choice. Kölner Zeitschrift für Soziologie und Sozialpsychologie 64:303–327
Rubin RH (2001) Alternative lifestyles revisited or whatever happened to swingers group marriages and communes? J Fam Issues 22:711–726
Salomon I (1980) Life style as a factor in explaining travel behavior. Doctoral Dissertation, Department of Civil Engineering, Massachusetts Institute of Technology
Salomon I, Ben-Akiva M (1983) The use of the life–style concept in travel demand models. Environ Plan A 15:623–638
Scheiner J (2006) Housing and action space: what role is played by lifestyle life situation and spatial structure. Geographische Zeitschrift 94:43–62
Scheiner J (2010) Social inequalities in travel behaviour: trip distances in the context of residential self–selection and lifestyles. J Transp Geogr 18:679–690
Schneewind KA (1997) Marriage yes children no—a lifestyle with a future? Syst Fam 10:160–165
Schulze G (1992) Die Erlebnisgesellschaft Kultursoziologie der Gegenwart. Campus Verlag, New York
Sheller M, Urry J (2006) The new mobilities paradigm. Environ Plan A 38:207–226
Sobel ME (1983) Lifestyle and social structure; concepts, definitions, analysis. Academic Press, New York
Sztompka P (2000) The turn toward soft variables in sociological theory. In: Sztompka P (ed) Trust: a sociological theory. Cambridge University Press, Cambridge, pp 1–17

Talvitie A (1997) Things planners believe in and things they deny. Transportation 24:1–31
Thorpe H (2012) Transnational mobilities in snowboarding culture: travel tourism and lifestyle migration. Mobilities 7:317–345
Tomlinson M (1998) Lifestyle and social class. Eur Sociol Rev 19:97–111
Torkington K (2012) Place and lifestyle migration: the discursive construction of 'glocal' place–identity. Mobilities 7:71–92
Ukwueze FN (2011) Influence of online communities on family lifestyles. J Home Econ Res 14:273–280
Van Acker V (2016) Lifestyle and modal choices: defining measuring and using the 'lifestyle' concept. Transp Res Rec 2495:74–82
Van Acker V, Mokhtarian PL, Witlox F (2011) Going soft: on how subjective variables explain modal choices for leisure travel. Eur J Transp Infrastruct Res 11:115–146
Van Acker V, Mokhtarian PL, Witlox F (2014) Car availability explained by the structural relationships between lifestyles residential location and underlying residential and travel attitudes. Transp Policy 35:88–99
Van der Wouden R, Kulberg J (2002) Stijloefeningen Leefstijlen in onderzoek en praktijk (Stylistic exercise lifestyles in research and practice). S and RO Stedenbouw and Ruimtelijke Ordening, 12–20
Van Wee B (2002) Land use and transport: research and policy challenges. J Transp Geogr 10:259–271
Wachs N (1979) Transportation for the elderly—changing lifestyles changing needs. University of California Press, Berkeley
Weber M (1922) Wirtschaft und Gesellschaft. Mohr, Tübingen

Chapter 4
The Car-Dependent Life

Junyi Zhang, Masashi Kuwano, Makoto Chikaraishi and Hajime Seya

Abstract This chapter focuses on car dependence in people's life. The authors first describe a new phenomenon about the decline in young people's car ownership and usage by providing additional facts and insights based on literature review and a case study in Japan. Especially, the case study in Japan uses data from a longitudinal national household expenditure survey and confirmed that car ownership and usage decisions in Japan are more or less associated with decisions about other household expenditures. Second, recent research on shared mobility is reviewed from the perspective of smart use of cars. Third, existing studies on cars from the life-oriented consideration are described by looking at shopping behavior (both store-shopping and online shopping) and general purchasing behavior as well as electric vehicle ownership and usage. As for electric vehicles, the influence of lifestyle is explored. Fourth, car ownership and usage for an inclusive society are discussed, where low-income persons, children, and the elderly are focused on. Fifth, behavioral changes toward less dependence on car from a long-term perspective are illustrated. Finally, discussions on car dependence from the life-oriented perspective are given.

Keywords Car dependency · Monetary expenditure · Lifestyles · Young people · Shared mobility · Behavioral change · Inclusive society · Travel time budget · Positive utility of travel time

---

J. Zhang (✉) · M. Chikaraishi
Hiroshima University, Higashi-Hiroshima, Japan
e-mail: zjy@hiroshima-u.ac.jp; junyizh24@gmail.com

M. Kuwano
Tottori University, Tottori, Japan

H. Seya
Kobe University, Kobe, Japan

J. Zhang (ed.), *Life-Oriented Behavioral Research for Urban Policy*,
DOI 10.1007/978-4-431-56472-0_4

4.1 Introduction

Since the Ford Model T was first produced in 1908, cars, and the huge investments across the world in highways, have changed human life remarkably. Cars have become an indispensable part of many people's lives because access to goods and services is much easier with a car than by other travel modes. Although cars were not invented to worsen people's lives and the environment, the excessive use of cars has surely caused troublesome traffic congestion and accidents, as well as air pollution, and these unintended consequences have diminished both people's lives and the environment. Various efforts have been made to address these problems, such as establishing public transportation systems (e.g., railways, subways, and buses), increasing transportation capacity, and constructing bypass roads to eliminate through traffic. Nevertheless, problems caused by automobile traffic have not been dramatically mitigated.

The average travel time for daily activities is about 60–80 min (e.g., Metz 2004; Van Wee et al. 2006; Vilhelmson 2007; Zumkeller 2009). Based on the Survey on Time Use and Leisure Activities conducted by the Ministry of General Affairs, we found that Japanese people's total travel time per day increased from less than 50 min in 1976 to more than 60 min in 2006, whereas travel time for the working population in Japan increased from more than 50 min in 1976 to more than 70 min in 2006. Travel time per day may vary across locations. According to the National Travel Survey of Japan conducted in 2010,[1] the national average travel time per day on weekdays was 65 min, with the highest value observed in the central cities of three major metropolitan areas (78 min) and the lowest value observed in smaller cities (48 min). In addition to longer travel times, drivers must park their cars somewhere for most of the day. In this sense, owning a car is costly and using it is not necessarily an efficient use of one's household budget. However, the number of private cars is predicted to grow from about 800 million in 2002 to more than 2 billion in 2030, a 250 % increase in less than 30 years (Sperling and Gordon 2009, as cited by Lucas et al. 2011). Considering that the world population is projected to reach 8.5 billion in 2030,[2] this means that one out of four persons will have a car in 2030. Both the number of private cars and the proportion of people who have cars are expected continue growing beyond 2030.

Car ownership has long been regarded as a good marker of material living standards (e.g., Smith et al. 1990; Gatersleben 2011; Delbosc 2012). This was true in the 20th century in developed countries, and now it is also true in developing countries. Based on an extensive review of studies included in the famous World Database of Happiness[3] [available at no cost on the Internet, also see Veenhoven (2014)], Veenhoven and his colleagues found that "car-ownership seems to boost

[1]http://www.mlit.go.jp/common/001032141.pdf (in Japanese) (Accessed February 25, 2016).

[2]http://esa.un.org/unpd/wpp/Download/Standard/Population/ (Accessed February 20, 2016).

[3]http://worlddatabaseofhappiness.eur.nl/ (Accessed February 21, 2016).

happiness" (Burger et al. 2015). Although having more cars (two or three cars) corresponds to increased happiness, when variability associated with income and other variables is controlled, this positive relationship disappears and even becomes negative. Owning an expensive car is associated with a happier life compared with owning a cheap one. Burger et al. (2015) further emphasized that the influence of cars on happiness may vary across persons and their life situations.

In recent years, some developed countries have observed a trend towards decreasing car ownership among young people (e.g., Metz 2010; Davis et al. 2012; Delbosc and Currie 2013; Goodwin and Van Dender 2013; Kuhnimhof et al. 2012, 2013).

Various factors derived from behavioral economics and social psychology theories have been identified in the literature as influencing car ownership and use, including past experience, peer pressure, intra-household interactions, materialism, affordability, and geographical/cultural characteristics (for a recent literature review of empirical findings, see Lucas et al. 2011). Jones (2011) reported that car dependence has been examined from various perspectives, such as the availability of other travel modes, the need to engage in activities that would be very difficult via other travel modes (e.g., carrying heavy goods, visiting multiple destinations in a single trip), lifestyle, self-esteem and identity, the liking of a car, limited mobility, convenience, and social exclusion.

In this chapter, we first focus on the recently identified decline in young people's car ownership and use by providing additional facts and insights based on a review of the literature and a case study in Japan (Sect. 4.2). Next, we review recent research on shared mobility (Sect. 4.3). Third, life-oriented studies on cars are briefly reviewed (Sect. 4.4). Fourth, car ownership and use for an inclusive society are discussed (Sect. 4.5). Fifth, behavioral changes toward less dependence on cars are described (Sect. 4.6). Finally, we discuss these issues from a life-oriented perspective in Sect. 4.7.

4.2 Young People's Decreasing Dependence on Cars: A New Phenomenon

4.2.1 General Observations

A decline in young people's car ownership has been observed in developed countries. Reasons for this trend have been discussed from a variety of perspectives, as summarized by Delbosc and Currie (2013) and Kuhnimhof et al. (2012):

(1) With the continuing economic slowdown, the motivation to purchase cars has decreased.

(2) Because of the diversification of values, interest in things other than cars has increased.

(3) With the spread of the Internet, it has become easier to communicate and interact with people without going out.
(4) There is an increased awareness of the disadvantages of owning and using cars, such as environmental problems and traffic accidents.

Related to some of these points, Delbosc and Currie (2014) collected data through an online "discussion forum" among 33, 17–23 year olds in Australia and found that having a car may be less symbolic of status and luxury and more symbolic of adulthood and maturity. Information communication technology was seen as a supplement to face-to-face contact, not a replacement for car travel. In addition, no one stated that environmental concerns shaped their travel choices.

Generally, car ownership is still growing in developing countries (OECD 2015). For example, in India, college students who believe that car use improves their social image and that car ownership contributes to happiness were more likely to own a car (Verma et al. 2015). This finding is understandable. The good news for the development of sustainable transportation in India is that college students who are satisfied with public bus systems were less likely to buy a car. Surprisingly, Verma et al. (2015) also found that male college students in India were less inclined to own a car in the near future than were their female counterparts.

The inefficiencies and costs associated with cars might be one reason why young people are less inclined to have cars. Delbosc and Currie (2013) examined cross-sectional and longitudinal studies in 14 developed countries to find the causes for the decline in young people's acquisition of driver's licenses, and they identified several factors, including changes in life stage and living arrangements, changes in motoring affordability, location and transportation, graduated driver licensing schemes, attitudinal influences, and the role of e-communication. They concluded that there were multiple causes rather than any single influence, even though evidence was weak and preliminary. They highlighted affordability and life stage factors as being most influential. Changing lifestyles might be another explanation for the decline in car usage among young people. Previously, owning a car was a symbol of social status for many people. Now, the symbolic value of car ownership seems less important for young people in some developed countries (Belgiawan et al. 2014). Many young people spend a lot of time on the Internet via computers, smartphones, and tablets. Spending time driving a car reduces opportunities to surf the Internet, which may be one more reason why some young people do not like to own cars. On a train or a bus, they can multitask (e.g., read, listen to music, and surf the Internet). There may be many other reasons related to life choices in other domains. First, both car users and non-car users may take advantage of public transport, which is sufficient to satisfy their mobility needs (Metz 2010; Kuhnimhof et al. 2012). Second, the structural relationships between income and car ownership and use have probably changed. Goodwin and Van Dender (2013) noted that "although the classic 'economic' factors are still seen to be important, without doubt, the nature of their importance seems to have changed, with a reduction over time of the size of some elasticities with respect to price and income, and more important through the medium of differential responses by population category and location." Unfortunately, most empirical studies that estimate elasticities have not considered population categories (e.g., Goodwin et al. 2004; Graham and Glaister 2004), and thus we need further empirical results to be able to draw sound conclusions.

4.2.2 Additional Observations in Japan

Some empirical studies of young people's car ownership and use have been done in Japan. Nishimura (2012) reported that, compared with their parents' generation, the current generation of young people does not really enjoy driving. A car tends to be regarded as a tool for moving around rather than as a status symbol. If this is true, young people who live near public transportation might be less likely to own and use cars. Fujioka et al. (2012) analyzed young women's travel behavior in Tokyo and found that married couples tend to use cars less, but this was not true for households with children. They concluded that the current urban structure in Tokyo may allow married couples to meet their activity needs without cars, whereas some activities for/with children may be impossible without cars. In discussing possible explanations for the rapid decline in the percentage of young men who are interested in cars (from 71 % in 2001 to 42 % in 2011), Yotsumoto (2012) cited cognitive dissonance theory. He argued that young men may unconsciously repress their desire to own a car for mainly financial reasons, but there is no clear evidence to support this explanation.

In this paper, we examine car ownership in Japan using micro data captured through the National Survey of Family Income and Expenditure for the years 1984, 1989, 1994, 1999, 2004, and 2009. Figures 4.1, 4.2 and 4.3 show changes in different population groups' car ownership by yearly income over time. Income

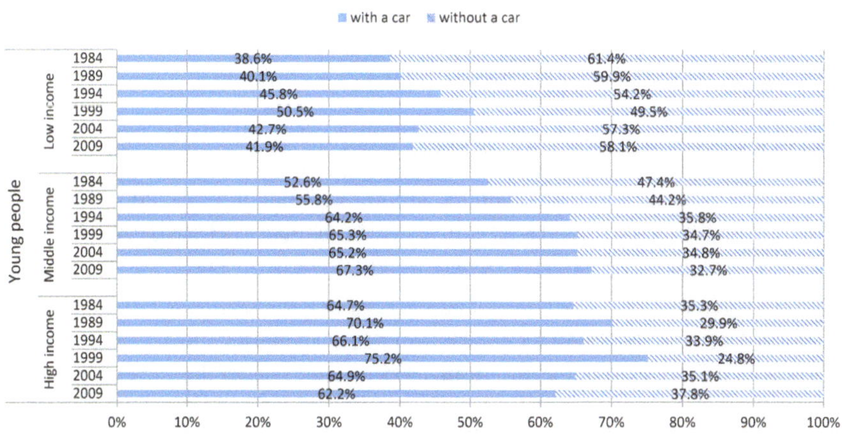

Fig. 4.1 Changes of young people' car ownership over time by income

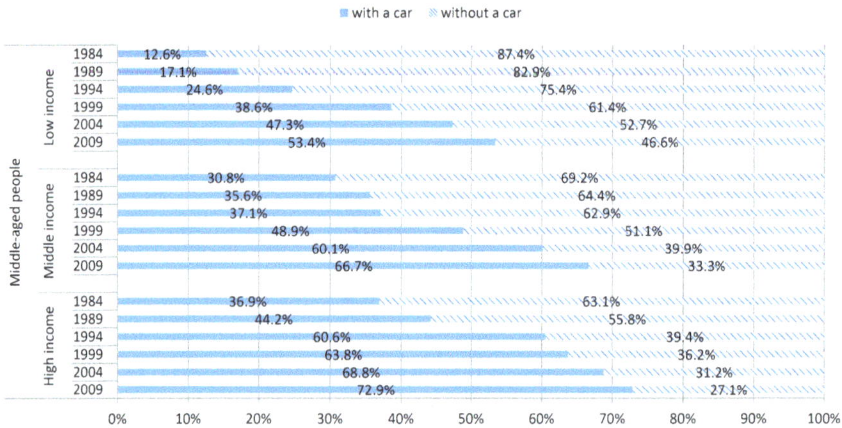

Fig. 4.2 Changes of middle-aged people' car ownership over time by income

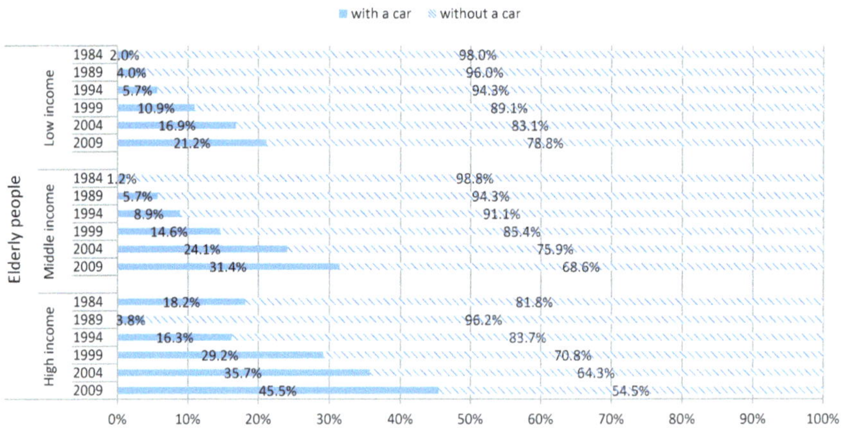

Fig. 4.3 Changes of elderly people' car ownership over time by income

groups were defined as Low income (<3 million yen), Middle income (3 million yen to 6 million yen), and High income (6 million yen +). Figures 4.4, 4.5 and 4.6 illustrate changes in the population groups' expenditures (including car usage costs) by income over time. These results are for one-person households. The findings displayed in these six figures can be summarized as follows:

- Irrespective of income, car ownership among middle-aged people (aged 35–64) and the elderly (aged 65+) showed a clearly increasing trend from 1984 to 2009. This was especially true from 1994 to 1999, when the increase was dramatic for middle-aged people. There was also an apparent trend for increasing car ownership among middle-income young people (aged 18–34), but the trend from 1994 to 2009 was not significant.

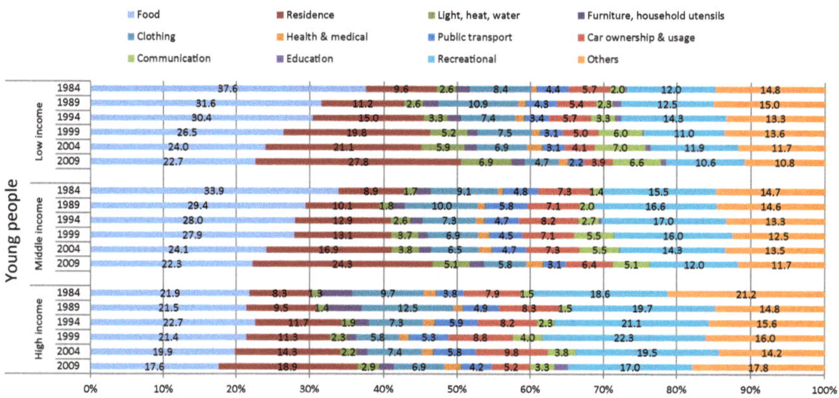

Fig. 4.4 Changes of young people' expenditure over time by income

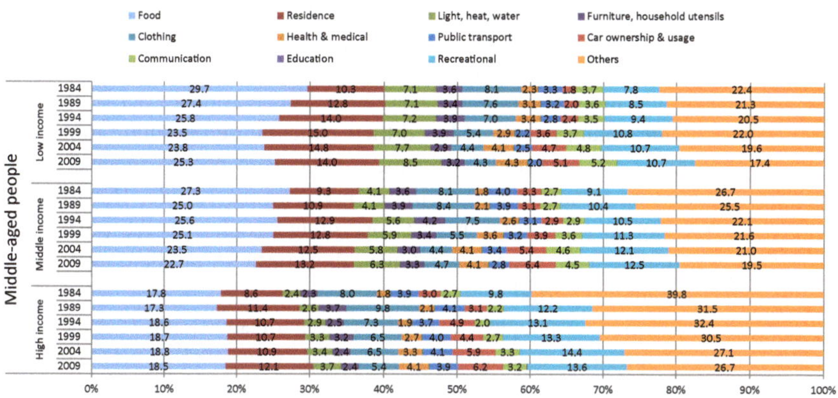

Fig. 4.5 Changes of middle-aged people' expenditure over time by income

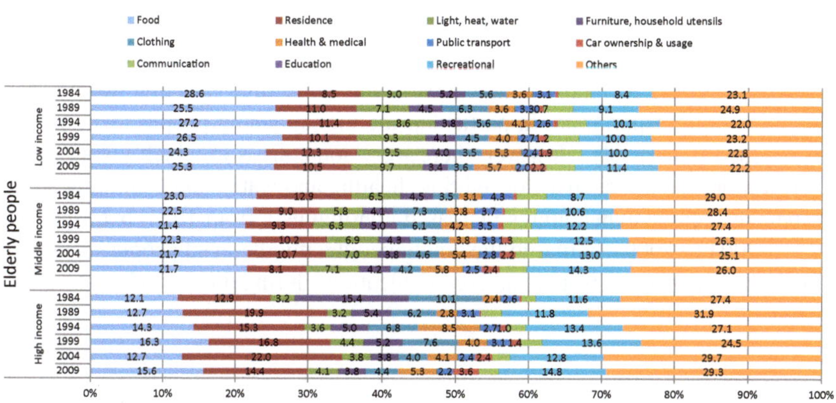

Fig. 4.6 Changes of elderly people' expenditure over time by income

- The low- and high-income young people increased their car ownership from 1984 to 1999. However, ownership dropped from 1999 to 2004, from 50.5 to 42.7 % for the low-income group (−7.8 points), and from 75.2 to 64.9 % for the high-income group (−10.3 points), which are dramatic changes relative to the drops that occurred between 2004 and 2009.
- As for expenditures,[4] the money young people spent on car use decreased for all of the income groups, from 5.7 % in 1994 to 3.9 % in 2009 for the low-income group, from 8.2 % in 1994 to 6.4 % in 2009 for the middle-income group, and from 9.8 % in 2004 to 5.2 % in 2009 for the high-income group. The decrease in the rate of car use expenditures was higher (−4.6 points) for the high-income group than for the others, but the decrease started earlier for the low- and middle-income groups than for the high-income group.
- Overall, the decrease in car ownership was greater than the decrease in car use.
- In contrast, middle-aged people and the elderly still showed increases, even in car use.
- With respect to expenditure on public transportation, low-income young people showed a continuous decrease from 4.4 % in 1984 to 2.2 % in 2009, whereas their middle-income counterparts' expenditure started to decrease in 1989, when their share of the total expenditures was 5.8 %, decreasing to 3.1 % in 2009. The high-income young people reduced their expenditure on public transportation from 2004. Low- and middle-income middle-aged people and the elderly showed decreasing trends similar to those of the young people. However, the decrease was not as substantial as that for young people. On the other hand, high-income middle-aged people maintained their ratio for public transit expenditures throughout this period.
- The low-income young people's expenditure on transportation (both car and public transit) decreased continuously from 10.1 % in 1984 to 6.1 % in 2009 (−4.0 points), whereas the decreases in transportation expenditure for middle- and high-income young people were somewhat less, from 12.1 % in 1984 to 9.5 % in 2009 (−2.6 points), and from 11.7 % in 1984 to 9.4 % in 2009 (−2.3 points), respectively.
- The changes in transportation expenditure listed above occurred in concert with changes in other expenditure. For example, young people spent less money on clothing and recreational activities at the same time that they were spending less on transportation. In particular, the money young people spent on food decreased remarkably. However, there were some areas in which young people spent more money, such as for lighting, heating and water, and communications. Their residential expenditures increased continuously from 1984, but especially from 2004 to 2009. Similar to the young people, middle-aged people spent more on lighting, heat and water, and communications during this period.

---

[4]Car purchase costs were excluded because, for each buyer, they only pertained to one year. Hence, car usage costs included the costs for gasoline and insurance, etc.

In a comparison of France, Germany, Great Britain, and the United States, Kuhnimhof et al. (2013) found that "even though all age classes have contributed to peak car, young adults stand out in this regard." However, our results clearly show the importance of considering income groups when conducting such analyses, and a similar finding has been reported for car use in France. Grimal et al. (2013) showed that diffusion of individual car use among low-income households was still ongoing in 2010, whereas it was ending for high-income households.

Owning a car is not like buying a bottle of water. Although both used and new cars are available, owning a car surely requires a lot of money. Spending on a car reduces the money that is available for other purposes, and thus it is natural to assume that people must make trade-offs when buying a car. People who want a car very much may work much harder to earn the money needed to buy a car rather than using that money for other purposes. Cermakova (2001) examined the influence of income differentiation on private consumption in the Czech Republic between 1988 and 1996 and found that increases in income differentiation led to increased spending on cars, houses, flats, and an overall growth of savings, but it also led to a decline in spending on food, clothing, and so on. Tsekeris (2012) found that spending on gasoline for private vehicles in Greek households was affected by spending on communications and tourism. However, the effects of car use on other expenditures were not analyzed. Using panel data from the Family Expenditure Surveys in the UK for 1982–1995, Dargay (2002) reported that rural households' car ownership was far less sensitive to motoring costs than was that of their urban counterparts. Dargay argued that increases in the costs of car transportation would pose a considerable economic burden for rural households. Using the Korea Household Expenditure Survey for the period between 1998 and 2007, Jung (2009) found that car ownership affected decisions on housing size. This indirectly indicates that spending on cars affects spending in other areas. Other relevant studies could not be found in literature. However, even these limited studies show that tradeoffs among expenditures are ignored by researchers.

Expenditure patterns displayed in Figs. 4.4, 4.5 and 4.6 should be interpreted carefully. Clearly, income seems to be an influential factor, but it is not the only important factor. Changes in lifestyle reflected in expenditure (or consumption) patterns should be examined more systematically. In other words, income itself is less important than how the income is spent. Expenditures are part of consumption in life (or life choices). One common goal of transportation policies and other public policies is the improvement of QOL (e.g., life satisfaction and happiness). Various life choices (or patterns of consumption) affect QOL. QOL has been investigated in various life domains, such as residence, neighborhood, health, education, work, family life, leisure and recreation, finances, and travel behavior. Using data collected in 2010 from 2178 respondents in various Japanese cities (including 77 consumption variables, 13 happiness indicators, and eight income-related variables), Zhang and Xiong (2015) found that income only influenced overall life happiness, but it was not the most influential factor. Saving was the most important variable with respect to overall life happiness. One's current work–life balance did not matter for happiness. Education-related consumption variables were only associated with negative affective experiences; surprisingly, they were unrelated to overall life happiness. The effects on happiness of expenditure- and residence-related consumption variables and of consumption choices related to an active lifestyle were mixed. Unexpectedly, none of the residence-related variables influenced overall life happiness. Communication with neighbors was important for positive affective experiences.

As Burger et al. (2015) have noted, people who have a car tend to be happier than people who do not have a car, even though owning a luxury car does not increase happiness beyond what people who own inexpensive cars report. If this is true for young people, the recent decreases in young people's car ownership should be regarded as a serious social issue. The availability of transportation to various facilities and locations is essential to one's life. Car users and people who use other travel means have different action spaces. Given these considerations, it might be important to investigate young people's car ownership behavior from the perspective of social exclusion (e.g., Stanley and Vella-Brodrick 2009; Stanley et al. 2011). On the other hand, decreasing car ownership is good for environmental sustainability. Policy makers are required to provide more support for public transportation to attractive and life-enhancing environments and opportunities. However, one critical question is whether, how, and to what extent car users can adapt to changing mobility and living environments, especially with respect to sustainable lifestyles. Related to this, it is worth exploring how the qualities of mobility environments oriented towards cars and public transportation differentially affect people's QOL via various life choices.

Because people have to spend a lot of money for a car, their ownership and usage decisions are more or less associated with decisions about other household expenditures, as evidenced in Figs. 4.4, 4.5 and 4.6. There are various studies of the relationships between residential behavior and vehicle ownership and use. Unfortunately, research on the influences of other life choices is very limited. For example, if a person's workplace is only accessible by car, he/she could not commute without a car. In this case, workplace location influences car ownership and use. Households with younger children may need a car to deliver and pick up their children, and such habitual use of a car may influence the children's future travel behavior, health behavior, and participation in various activities. These influences should be properly incorporated into the implementation of mobility management and into research on residential choices and activity-travel behavior.

4.3 Smart Use of Cars: Shared Mobility

Decreasing car ownership by young people is good news for the development of sustainable transportation, but it is not good news for the automobile industry. In fact, in recent years, many automobile makers have invested a lot of money to improve the design and functionality of cars to explicitly reflect young people's preferences in order to encourage them to continue the tradition of car ownership.

If people find that cars are not indispensable, the use of public transportation systems, cycling, or walking may increase, which should benefit their health. For people who must travel by car, car-sharing services are becoming more widely available. According to Kent and Dowling (2013), "small-scale car sharing already existed in the 1940s in Europe; however more successful programs were launched in Germany and Switzerland in the mid-1980s." Shaheen and Cohen (2013) reported that car sharing has expanded to approximately 1100 cities in 26 nations on five continents.

Mitropoulos and Prevedouros (2014) employed a life-cycle approach to explore sustainable transportation development and car-sharing systems. They compared six highway vehicles and modes: an internal combustion engine vehicle (ICEV), a hybrid electric vehicle (HEV), a car-sharing program with ICEVs, a car-sharing program with HEVs, a diesel bus, and a hybrid diesel electric bus. They found that including car sharing in the travel mix was the best option, and the most sustainable mode was car sharing with HEVs. Kent (2014) conducted a systematic review of the literature published from 2005 to 2013 and found that all of the studies reported reductions in vehicle ownership and use (distance traveled), increases in active transportation (walking and cycling), and increases in public transportation usage. All of these changes have potential health benefits.

Burkhardt and Millard-Ball (2006) found that most users of car sharing in North America were between 25 and 35 years old. Using data collected in Beijing and Shanghai, Shaheen and Martin (2010) found that younger and more educated residents were more interested in car sharing. Recognizing that car sharing was considered an exclusively middle-income, white, and young person phenomenon, Kim (2015) explored the possibilities for meeting the mobility demands of people in the marginalized neighborhoods of New York City. Kim found that it was feasible to expand the existing car sharing service boundaries to the outer boroughs as long as the affordability issues could be properly addressed, because car sharing in low-income neighborhoods did not differ from the typical car-sharing locations.

Given that most privately owned vehicles sit idle for more than 90 % of the day (Hampshire and Gaites 2011), customer to customer (C2C) car-sharing businesses have been started in the United States (e.g., RelayRides, Getaround), Japan (e.g., Anyca), China (e.g., Atzuche.com), and Singapore (iCarsclub) to help car owners rent their private cars to other drivers.[5] The C2C service [also called peer-to-peer (P2P) car sharing, see Hampshire and Gaites (2011), Craig Ballus-Armet et al. (2014)] allows vehicle owners to rent their personal vehicles to others in their surrounding area on a short-term basis. The rental rate (including driving insurance) is lower than conventional rental car services, car owners can decide what rate to charge, and they receive a much larger percentage of the rate than the company does. In a case study in Pittsburgh, PA, Hampshire and Gaites (2011) found that the market for P2P car sharing was economically viable, but uncertain and

[5]http://jp.techcrunch.com/2015/09/09/dena-lanched-anyca-c2c-car-sharing-service/ (in Japanese; Accessed December 13, 2015).

fragmented public policies and car insurance regimes threatened the growth of and investment in P2P car sharing. In California, Ballús-Armet et al. (2014) found very little awareness of P2P car sharing, and 25 % of those surveyed indicated that they would be willing to rent their personal vehicles through such a scheme. In contrast, more than 60 % of respondents without access to a vehicle would be willing to use P2P car sharing because of the convenience, availability, monetary savings, and expanded mobility. Chatterjee et al. (2013) found that car sharing attracted people who were already contemplating giving up their cars or who had been prompted by life events to consider giving up their cars. Schaefers (2013) identified four motivational patterns for car sharing: value seeking (e.g., saving money for other things, affordability, reasonable prices, free parking, and being able to go carless); convenience (e.g., saving time, flexibility, reduced responsibility, and a simple pricing scheme); lifestyle; and environmental concerns. The lifestyle motive, in particular, is affective rather than utilitarian. It is associated with a sense of belonging and a sense of community among car-sharing customers, and it is manifested by the desire to make a statement. Note that as early as the late 1990s, the use of a car-sharing service was regarded as indicative of a new lifestyle in literature (see Prettenthaler and Steininger 1999). Each of these four motives is associated with improving the users' quality of life.

Kent and Dowling (2013) discussed how to make car sharing successful based on the so-called "bundling of practices" related to transportation planning and road building, as well as those practices related to working, visiting, parenting, and consuming. Cars must be located within walking distance of work and home, but the time management of cars must also be efficient, reflecting the personal activity scheduling and competition for car use within the household. In fact, car-sharing users have been found to be more likely to plan their activity travel schedules (Chatterjee et al. 2013). In this sense, users' behaviors are also adaptive.

4.4 The Emergence of Life-Oriented Studies on Cars

In the field of transportation, the activity-based approach was developed to explain travel behavior (including car ownership and use) (e.g., Hensher and Stopper 1979; Jones 1990). Travel demand is thought to be derived from activity participation. Given that participating in daily activities is a part of people's lives, transportation research should focus more on such life perspectives.

For example, in the case of shopping by car, the activity "shopping" is the reason why a car was used, probably because the shopping center is only accessible by car. However, we might ask why the shopping trip was needed? If the shopper was buying items for a party, an activity that is important for maintaining his/her social network, then using the car to go shopping was, in fact, helping to maintain the shopper's social network. In addition, shopping requires both money and time (Zhang 2009). To save time, one might shop online rather than visit a store. Online shopping has become a routine behavior in people's daily lives and has certainly mitigated the constraints associated with inconvenient access to shopping facilities. Such a trend may influence people's residential location choices, ownership, and use of vehicles, and other travel-activity behaviors. Dennis et al. (2010) showed that young women prefer so-called social e-shopping to traditional e-shopping. In social e-shopping, shoppers are allowed to socialize and interact with each other. This implies that the act of shopping itself can be used to maintain social networks. Ahmed et al. (2007) conducted a survey on Malaysian students' visits to shopping malls and found that they visit a mall because of its interior design, accessibility of their favorite products, opportunities for socializing with friends, and the convenience of one-stop shopping. Erkip (2003) examined the role of the shopping mall in Turkey and found that shopping malls are regarded as emerging public spaces, which may also explain changes in urban lifestyle. Matthews et al. (2000) and Vanderbeck and Johnson (2000) pointed out that shopping malls are a convenient place to hang out, particularly for young people. Unfortunately, little research has been done, even with respect to joint analyses of time use and spending behavior. Because money and time are resource considerations for many other life choices, it is reasonable to assume that shopping behavior is associated with other life choices.

When we move from daily shopping to general purchasing behavior, more complicated behavioral issues need to be considered. General purchasing includes not only buying a bottle of juice that costs a few dollars; it also refers to also buying such things as a car that may cost tens of thousands of dollars or a house that may cost several hundred thousand dollars. We can expect that the more expensive a purchase is, the greater its influence on other life choices will be. People shop for reasons other than for buying goods. Given these considerations, we can identify two types of shopping: utilitarian and hedonic, where the former is for problem solving and the latter is for the affective experience or enjoyment of life (e.g., Babin et al. 1994; Babin and Darden 1995; Jones et al. 2006; Diep and Sweeney 2008). For instance, shopping by car may be more likely to improve a shopper's affective experience, which may be important for the shopper's quality of life.

Another example is the ownership and use of electric vehicles. Many studies have examined electric vehicles with respect to social cost analysis (Roosen et al. 2015; Nordelof et al. 2016), the spatial distribution of electric vehicle use (Chen et al. 2015), charging behavior (Davies and Kurani 2010; Sun et al. 2015), preferences and social psychological analyses (Caulfield et al. 2010; Hidrue et al. 2011; Woodjack et al. 2012; Axsen et al. 2013, 2015), charging infrastructure (Madina et al. 2016; Morrissey et al. 2016), and so on. It is true that limited driving ranges and long recharge times prevent many people purchasing electric vehicles (IEA 2011). However, the functionality, pleasures, problems, meanings, and values of vehicle purchases may unfold over time, in a process of lifestyle exploration and through which a new set of activities and values that outweigh the shortcomings might be discovered (Woodjack et al. 2012). Using the three-stage social process of science proposed by Nobel laureate Tim Hunt (discovery, translation, and application), Woodjack et al. (2012) maintained and empirically confirmed that drivers incorporate translated discoveries (e.g., evaluation of driving performance with members in their social networks) into their lifestyles, deepening their values and commitment. Woodjack et al. (2012) explored the influence of lifestyle from a social psychological perspective, but they did not examine the influences of activities via the use of electric vehicles. Axsen et al. (2013) examined the effects of lifestyle on consumer preference formation for pro-environmental technology via the use of electric vehicles. They investigated lifestyle through engagement in technology-oriented practices and pro-environmental practices, as well as overall lifestyle liminality (openness, flexibility, or transitionality). However, the limitations of the Woodjack et al. (2012) study also apply to those by Axsen et al. (2013, 2015). Thus, studies from a life-oriented perspective (i.e., that focus on various life choices) are scarce, with exceptions that examine lifestyle defined mainly by subjective factors. However, it is unclear how electric vehicles affect people's lives and how the ownership and use of electric vehicles are adaptive for people. In addition, the charging functions of electric vehicles can impact daily life. Electricity stored in the batteries of electric cars can be used for in-home purposes. For example, in Japan, the price of electricity is usually lower at night than it is in the daytime. Consuming electricity via batteries that were charged at night will save money, which can be used for other household needs. Interestingly, Yu et al. (2011, 2012, 2013a, b, c) conducted several studies investigating the interactions between in-home and out-of-home energy consumption. They treated vehicle use as out-of-home energy consumption, and residential location choices and time use behaviors were also incorporated. Such studies may provide a new way to look at the ownership and use of electric vehicles.

4.5 Car Ownership and Use for an Inclusive Society

If more people were to live close to railway stations or bus stops, the likelihood of car use might decrease significantly. However, in reality, partially because of higher land prices near railway stations and bus stops (e.g., Du and Mulley 2007; Medda 2012; Wang et al. 2015),[6] many low-income people have to live in areas with inconvenient access to the employment market and public transportation systems (e.g., Macintyre et al. 1993). This may indicate that if low-income people do not have access to a car, they will face various difficulties in their daily lives, including access to employment. For example, Ong (2002) found that, among welfare recipients in the Los Angeles metropolitan area, those with a car were more likely to be employed (by 9 %) than those without a car. Similarly, Cervero et al. (2002) found that once welfare recipients had access to a car, the likelihood of being employed increased remarkably, regardless of the distance to employment opportunities, suggesting that private mobility is more important than public

[6]Note that some studies show mixed effects of access to railway stations or bus stops based on land prices, such as Vessali (1996) and Debrezion et al. (2007).

mobility in helping inner-city residents find gainful employment and move off welfare. In fact, people in low-income households also prefer to live close to public transportation systems (e.g., Liao et al. 2015). For single mothers with no more than a high school education, Baum (2009) found that car ownership increases their employment. Thus, vehicles serve to reduce potential physical isolation from employment opportunities for transportation-poor populations. At the same time, these results also suggest that, as a matter of social policy, the preferences of people in low-income households should be reflected in the promotion of transit-oriented development. In related work, Gautier and Zenou (2010) found that car ownership was an important factor in the employment differences between ethnic minorities and white workers. They argued for the importance of better access to capital markets and better public transportation to reduce the differences in labor-market outcomes.

With respect to education, parents who are concerned about safety and security of their children's schooling tend to deliver children to and pick up them from school by car (e.g., Nasrudin and Nor 2013; Van Goeverden and de Boer 2013; Kelly and Fu 2014). This may also be true for people who live in areas with poor access to public transportation. As a result, the inability to own a car may keep children in these areas away from school. In Japan, it is common for children to attend cram schools to help them pursue studies at high-quality high schools and universities. Because cram schools are outside the public educational system, cram school hours often extend up to midnight. Therefore, most children are picked up and dropped off at cram schools by mothers who have exclusive use of a car (Japan Juku Association 2006). On the other hand, Delbosc and Vella-Brodrick (2015) suggested that having the freedom and means to go to work or school might give young people a sense of autonomy, which may lead to enhanced well-being. In contrast, Mackett (2002) argued that children who depend on cars might lose opportunities to gain independence from their parents, miss out on some social opportunities, and reduce their participation in physical activities. Long et al. (2015) confirmed that friends' car travel predicted high school students' car travel, suggesting the importance of social networks in explaining high school transportation choices. However, although living in the suburbs allows parents to raise their children in attractive natural environments, their concomitant dependence on cars may diminish their children's social skills and socialization opportunities (Andrews et al. 2014).

Providing the elderly with an accessible mobility environment is also essential to realizing an inclusive society. Based on a survey of 2500 Finnish citizens aged 65 and over from various areas, Siren and Hakamies-Blomqvist (2004) found that women, rural residents, the oldest elderly, and those without a driver license had reduced mobility. They concluded that access to a private car is crucial for elderly mobility. Focusing on social inequalities among disabled elderly men in Britain (3981 persons), Ramsay et al. (2008) observed that men who were not house or car owners were more likely than their house- and car-owning counterparts to experience functional limitations and disability in performing the activities of daily living, independent of behavioral risk factors, comorbidities, and social class. Distance traveled has been used as an indicator to measure people's quality of life. As reviewed by Mercado and Paez (2009), distance traveled decreases as age advances. Mercado and Paez (2009) found that, as car passengers, elderly women travel shorter distances than do men. In contrast, Van den Berg et al. (2011) showed that the average travel distance does not decrease as people get older. Considering that women live longer than men and that they have a greater tendency to give up driving (Rabbit et al. 1996; Blomqvist and Siren 2003), Mercado and Paez (2009) noted the importance of gender-sensitive transportation policies for the elderly. On the other hand, the elderly have more leisure time than their younger (working) counterparts and, potentially, they spend more time on social and leisure activities (Van den Berg et al. 2011). Gagliardi et al. (2007) compared the outdoor mobility and leisure activities of 3950 elderly persons in Germany, Finland, Hungary, The Netherlands, and Italy, and they found that "sports activities and hobbies were performed more often by younger men, by those with good physical functioning and by those who drove cars. Social activities were performed more by women and those who used public transport. Home activities were more frequently performed by those with low physical function and women." In fact, the proportion of active seniors is reported to have increased in various developed countries (Hjorthol et al. 2010). In an examination of the social activities of the elderly in the Netherlands, Van den Berg et al. (2011) reported that the elderly were just as mobile as their younger counterparts with respect to the number of social trips they made, but older seniors (75+) were less likely to use a bicycle than cars. Lord et al. (2011) conducted a qualitative longitudinal study and maintained that, even though elderly North Americans may show a trend towards increasing mobility, the immobility of the elderly is inevitable. Thus, they argued that built environment policies should be proposed that support the elderly mobility. For a more detailed discussion of elderly mobility, see Chikaraishi (2016).

4.6 Towards Reduced Dependence on Cars: A Long-Term Perspective on Behavioral Change

As Lucas et al. (2011) have argued, given the increasing world population and the trend towards total car ownership, it will be physically impracticable and unaffordable for nations to provide the necessary road infrastructure to support the current level of per capita car-based travel. Thus, it is important to reduce car dependence in our daily lives. Jones (2011) proposed four types of major policy options to reduce the need to travel and to increase the proportions of activities that can be performed in close proximity to home: (1) encouraging greater use of teleservices, (2) encouraging more mixed use and higher density developments, (3) encouraging more local sourcing of goods and services, and (4) improving local pedestrian networks. He also proposed four types of policies to promote accessible transportation environments that do not rely on cars: (1) car-restriction policies, (2) improvements to public transportation, (3) improved cycle facilities, and (4) more flexible land use provisions. In addition to the above measures/policies, Jones argued for policies that encourage people to modify their lifestyles, such as travel awareness campaigns (to raise awareness of the negative aspects of excessive car use), the provision of activity and travel information, and marketing campaigns (improving the image of non-car travel modes). However, the success of such policies relies on a better understanding of the behavioral changes needed to reduce car ownership and use toward a more sustainable lifestyle.

Based on a life history survey, Zhang et al. (2014) found that the relationship between car ownership behavior and residential relocation, household structure, and employment and education over the life course was extremely complex, in part because of both short-term and long-term state dependencies and future expectations within and across life domains. Such cross-domain dynamics make the representation of behavioral changes in car ownership and usage difficult. Thus, Zhang et al. (2016) extended the conventional theory of planned behavior to cover multiple life domains, and they empirically examined the ability of the new approach to capture the life-course dynamics of migration behaviors in relation to behavioral changes in jobs, dwellings, and childcare. The promotion of behavioral changes to reduce dependence on cars must take such a long-term perspective into account. Such considerations also emphasize the importance of lifestyle, which is usually formed over a long period. Interestingly, Hinde and Dixon (2005) argued that car-reliance (i.e., the trend that society systematically favors the automobile over other forms of mobility) not only results in physical inactivity but it also leads to a greater consumption of fast foods, both of which are not healthy.

Consistent with these considerations, Young and Caisey (2010) proposed a lifestyle approach to examine how to reduce car ownership and use by treating car ownership and use as the products of individual behaviors and lifestyle choices. Using a behavioral economics framework, they addressed behavioral changes by uncovering their underlying motivations, heuristics, and cognitive biases, and then they examined whether behavioral changes were sufficiently motivated based on social marketing theory. With respect to public health, Douglas et al. (2011) identified serious health issues related to private car use, including physical inactivity, obesity, death, and injury from crashes, cardiorespiratory disease from air pollution, noise, community severance, and climate change. They concluded that the public health community should strongly advocate for effective policies that reduce car use and increase active travel. Carse et al. (2013) noted the possibility of encouraging short-distance drivers to shift to cycling and walking in the cycle-friendly city of Cambridge, UK. With respect to lifestyle, Oakil et al. (2014) found strong relationships between car ownership changes and household formation and dissolution processes in the Netherlands. Specifically, they found that changing household car ownership level is affected by both past and future (anticipated) life cycle events such as residential relocation, changes in employment, and childbirth. Eakins (2015) showed that household composition is a strong and stable predictor of the level of car ownership over time. Using data from the first two waves (2009–2011) of the UK Household Longitudinal Study (UKHLS) (19,334 persons), Clark et al. (2016) found that changes in the composition of households and driving license availability were the strongest predictors of changes in car ownership, followed by employment status and income changes. Having children increased the probability of acquiring a car for non-car owners, and it increased the probability of eliminating a car for owners of two cars.

In examining these types of behavioral changes, we must also consider the influence of intra-household interactions on decisions about car ownership and use (Corfman and Gupta 1993; Zhang et al. 2002, 2005, 2009a; Ho and Mulley 2015; Kim and Parent 2016). The relative influences and roles of different household members in negotiations and joint decisions depend upon the nature of intra-household interactions. In addition, the intergenerational transfer of vehicle preferences should be addressed. For example, Hjorthol and Fyhri (2009) showed that greater dependence on cars in childhood contributed to greater dependence on cars in adulthood because of parental influences. In addition, social conformity effects (Ajzen 1985), such as following the opinions of others and conforming to the behaviors of friends, acquaintances, and public opinion, influence behavioral changes associated with car ownership and use (Kuwano et al. 2013).

4.7 Discussion: A Life-Oriented Perspective

Car ownership and usage change over time, and this involves a complicated decision-making process. Cars have become an indispensable part of many people's lives, even though car owners usually park their cars for most of the day. Various studies have shown that owning and using a car are motivated not only by its utilitarian functions, but also by its affective functions. Here, we would like to argue for the importance of life-related factors in examinations of car ownership and use, as well as relevant behavioral changes. Zhang (2014, 2015) has proposed the life-oriented approach, which argues that people's life choices in various domains (e.g., residence, neighborhood, health, education, work, and family life, leisure and recreation, finances, and travel behavior) are interdependent. For instance, various life decisions associated with the quality of life influence travel behavior, but they are also influenced by travel behavior, which means that travel behavior also impacts the quality of life. In other words, travel (including travel by car) is not just a burden; it is also an indispensable part of life. The activity-based approach has been well developed in the field of transportation (e.g., Hensher and Stopper 1979; Jones 1990). However, given the breadth of its scope, the life-oriented approach could be developed to include the activity-based approach as a special case. In fact, transportation research from such a life perspective has begun. Some people own cars just for fun, but many other people own and use cars to meet various needs in life (not just for fun) that are associated with various life choices. In other words, car ownership and usage are derived from other (non-travel) life choices, just as the life-oriented approach suggests. The limited literature on associations between other life choices and car ownership and usage is discussed below.

4.7.1 Travel Time Budgets and the Positive Utility of Travel Time

The notion that the average travel time per day remains constant (at least at the aggregate level: 60–90 min) has been discussed since the early 1970s, when Szalai (1972) and Zahavi (1973) published their seminal papers on the concept of travel time budgets (Zahavi and Ryan 1980; Lyons and Urry 2005). Although there have been many proponents of this concept, the notion remains subject to much debate (e.g., Lyons and Urry 2005; Chikaraishi et al. 2011). Hojer and Mattsson (2000) summarized three theoretical explanations proposed by Vilhelmson (1990): biological programming, utility maximization, and social routine. Unfortunately, a consensus on this issue has not been reached in literature. The life-oriented approach (Zhang 2014, 2015) argues that travel is both influenced by and influences various life decisions that are closely related to the quality of life. With respect to the notion of constant travel time, the life-oriented approach suggests that this concept should be examined by considering everyday life, which is consistent with Vilhelmson's (1990) third explanation, "social routine." In other words, everyday life is full of settled routines, of which travel is a part, and it is allocated its share of time among all other routines (Hojer and Mattsson 2000; as cited by Lyons and Urry 2005). It is worth exploring how travel by car and travel by other means fare in this debate. For example, using a car allows a person to participate in nighttime activities that are not accessible by public transportation. It would be interesting to know how such differences contribute to total travel time. Unfortunately, nighttime travel by car has rarely been studied. The biological programming explanation is consistent with the role of human habits in travel as being part of the human evolutionary process, and the utility maximization explanation argues that travel has both positive and negative effects on activities: there are positive effects because travel allows access to activities, and there are negative effects because of conflicts between time allocated to travel versus other activities. In partial agreement with this argument, Mokhtarian and Salomon (2001) suggested that positive utility is gained from the activities conducted at the destination, activities that can be conducted while travelling, and/or the activity of travelling itself. For example, Redmond and Mokhtarian (2001) reported that the ideal commuting time for 1300 commuters in the San Francisco Bay Area in 1998 was about 16 min, on average. Based on data from a 2008 survey of 547 public transportation commuters in Hiroshima City, Japan (Zhang et al. 2009b), we also found that many commuters' ideal travel time is not zero.

These brief examples of research from the life-oriented approach support the value of this approach to better understand travel time use and its impact on urban and transportation policies.

4.7.2 Life Connected by Cars

Considering the many urban problems in cities across the world, such as traffic congestion, accidents, air pollution, and damage to natural resources, population size must surely be a major factor. In fact, even the location and distribution of populations are problematic. For example, Cooper et al. (2001) argued that, "the rise in demand for car travel is fueled more by the increased spatial separation of homes and workplaces, shops and schools than by any rise in trip making." In particular, the mismatch between the locations of jobs and housing has been largely due to market failures and ineffective governmental interventions. On the other hand, people spend time in various activities, some of which are mandatory and repeated on a daily basis, such as work and schooling, and others of which are selective. The efficient use of limited amounts of time obviously requires reductions in travel time. Thus, the balance between jobs and housing location becomes important. Such a balance can be achieved via compact city developments that allow people to participate in daily activities within a much smaller area than do car-dependent urban developments. However, some reasons for the mismatch between job and housing locations could be related to housing preferences. For example, some people may not want to spend the additional money on housing needed to live closer to work, either because of budget constraints or because they think it is not worth the expense considering their lifestyle. If someone really enjoys driving, he/she might decide to work at a place that is easily reached by car. Other people may want to live close to their workplace, but they do not out of consideration for other members of the household, such as living near their children's study activities and the homemaker's daily activities. Other reasons for the imbalance between housing and workplace locations are related to workplaces themselves. For example, areas with automobile and chemical factories are clearly not suitable as residential areas, which forces employees to suffer longer commutes than they might have if they worked elsewhere. If a workplace is located in an area that is only accessible by car, employees must commute by car. In such a case, the workplace determines car use. In addition to the jobs–housing location balance, other life domains may affect car ownership/use behaviors, as explained in Sect. 4.6.

Thus, car ownership and usage seem to be associated with job, residence, household composition, and other factors that should be examined over the life course (e.g., Zhang et al. 2014). Residential behavior and travel behavior have been often studied together, and residential self-selection is regarded as a core behavioral phenomenon. The dominant argument states that residential self-selection has two sources: attitudes and sociodemographic traits. Zhang et al. (2014)

have argued that life choices must be included in this two-source framework as an additional set of decision variables, which would require reviewing the existing studies on employment, family budgets, health, neighborhoods, education and learning, family life, leisure and recreation, and empirical evidence from case studies in Japan. Similar arguments might be applicable to car ownership and usage, which is worth exploring in future.

References

Ahmed ZU, Ghingold M, Dahari Z (2007) Malaysian shopping mall behavior: an exploratory study. Asia Pacific J Mark Logistics 19:331–348

Ajzen I (1985) From intentions to actions: a theory of planned behavior. In: Kuhi J, Beckmann J (eds) Action-control: from cognition to behavior. Springer, New York, pp 11–39

Andrews FJ, Rich S, Stockdale R, Shelley J (2014) Parents' experiences of raising pre-school aged children in an outer-Melbourne growth corridor. Health Place 27:220–228

Axsen J, Bailey J, Castro MA (2015) Preference and lifestyle heterogeneity among potential plug-in electric vehicle buyers. Energy Econ 50:190–201

Axsen J, Orlebar C, Skippon S (2013) Social influence and consumer preference formation for pro-environmental technology: the case of a UK workplace electric-vehicle study. Ecol Econ 95:96–107

Babin BJ, Darden WR (1995) Consumer self-regulation in a retail environment. J Retail 71(1):7–70

Babin BJ, Darden WR, Griffin M (1994) Work and/or fun: measuring hedonic and utilitarian shopping value. J Consum Res 20(4):644–656

Ballús-Armet I, Shaheen SA, Clonts K, Weinzimmer D (2014) Peer-to-peer carsharing exploring public perception and market characteristics in the San Francisco Bay Area. Calif Transp Res Rec 2416:27–36

Baum CL (2009) The effects of vehicle ownership on employment. J Urban Econ 66(3):151–163

Belgiawan PF, Schmöcker JD, Abou-Zeid M, Walker J, Lee TC, Ettema D, Fujii S (2014) Car ownership motivations among undergraduate students in China, Indonesia, Japan, Lebanon, Netherlands, Taiwan, and USA. Transportation 41(6):1227–1244

Blomqvist LH, Siren A (2003) Deconstructing a gender difference: driving cessation and personal driving history of older women. J Safety Res 34:383–388

Burger M, Chiperi F, Kang X, Veenhoven R (2015) Consumption and happiness: a review of research. In: The keynote paper for the workshop "Life-Oriented Approach for Transportation Studies" at the 14th International conference on travel behaviour research. Windsor, UK, July 19–23 (to be published in the Conference Proceedings as a book)

Burkhardt J, Millard-Ball A (2006) Who's attracted to car-sharing? Transp Res Rec 1986:98–105

Carse A, Goodman A, Mackett RL, Panter J, Ogilvie D (2013) The factors influencing car use in a cycle-friendly city: the case of Cambridge. J Transp Geogr 28(100):67–74

Caulfield B, Farrell S, McMahon B (2010) Examining individuals preferences for hybrid electric and alternatively fueled vehicles. Transp Policy 17:381–387

Cermakova J (2001) The influence of income differentiation on the structure of household expenditures. Czech J Econ Finance (Finance A Uver) 51(1):33–45

Cervero R, Sandoval OS, Landis J (2002) Transportation as a stimulus of welfare-to-work: private versus public mobility. J Plann Educ Res 22(1):50–63

Chatterjee K, Andrews G, Ricci M, Parkhurst G (2013) Qualitative insights into the effect on travel behavior of joining a carshare. Transp Res Rec 2359:76–84

Chen TD, Wang Y, Kockelman KM (2015) Where are the electric vehicles? A spatial model for vehicle-choice count data. J Transp Geogr 43:181–188

Chikaraishi M (2016) Mobility of the elderly. In: Zhang J (ed) Life-oriented behavioral research for urban policy. Springer, Heidelberg (Chapter 10)

Chikaraishi M, Fujiwara A, Zhang J, Axhausen KW, Zumkeller D (2011) Changes in variations of travel time expenditure: some methodological considerations and empirical results from German mobility panel. Transp Res Rec 2230:121–131

Clark B, Chatterjee K, Melia S (2016) Changes in level of household car ownership: the role of life events and spatial context. Transportation 43(4):565–599

Cooper J, Ryley T, Smyth A (2001) Contemporary lifestyles and the implications for sustainable development policy: lessons from the UK's most car dependent city, Belfast. Cities 18(2):103–113

Corfman KP, Gupta S (1993) Mathematical models of group choice and negotiations. In: Eliashberg J, Lilien GL (eds) Handbooks in operations research and management science, vol 5: Marketing. North-Holland, Amsterdam, pp 83–142

Dargay J (2002) Determinants of car ownership in rural and urban areas: a pseudo-panel analysis. Transp Res Part E 38(5):351–366

Davies J, Kurani KS (2010) Recharging behavior of households' plug-in hybrid electric vehicles observed variation in use of conversions of 5-kw-h blended plug-in hybrid electric vehicle. Transp Res Rec 2191:75–83

Davis B, Dutzik T, Baxandall P (2012) Transportation and the new generation: why young people are driving less and what it means for transportation policy. Frontier Group—US PIRG Education Fund

Debrezion G, Pels E, Rietveld P (2007) The impact of railway stations on residential and commercial property value: a meta-analysis. J Real Estate Finance Econ 35(2):161–180

Delbosc A (2012) The role of well-being in transport policy. Transp Policy 23:25–33

Delbosc A, Currie G (2013) Causes of youth licensing decline: a synthesis of evidence. Transp Rev 33:271–290

Delbosc A, Currie G (2014) Using discussion forums to explore attitudes toward cars and licensing among young, Australians. Transp Policy 31:27–34

Delbosc A, Vella-Brodrick D (2015) The role of transport in supporting the autonomy of young adults. Transp Res Part F 33:97–105

Dennis C, Morgan A, Wright LT, Jayawardhena C (2010) The influences of social e-shopping in enhancing young women's online shopping behavior. J Customer Behav 9:151–174

Diep VCS, Sweeney JC (2008) Shopping trip value: do stores and products matter? J Retail Consum Serv 15:399–409

Douglas MJ, Watkins SJ, Gorman DR, Higgins M (2011) Are cars the new tobacco? J Public Health 33(2):160–169

Du H, Mulley C (2007) The short-term land value impacts of urban rail transit: quantitative evidence from Sunderland, UK. Land Use Policy 24(1):223–233

Eakins J (2015) Household car ownership in Ireland across time: an analysis of the effects of expansion and contraction in the Irish economy. Int J Transp Econ 42(3):315–342

Erkip F (2003) The shopping mall as an emergent public space in Turkey. Environ Plann A 35:1073–1094

Fujioka K, Ishigami T, Takahashi K (2012) Macro-analysis of travel behavior of youth in the Tokyo Metropolitan Area, with a focus on the life stages of women. IATSS Rev 37(2):31–38

Gagliardi C, Spazzafumo L, Marcellini F, Mollenkopf H, Ruoppila I, Tacken M, Szémann Z (2007) The outdoor mobility and leisure activities of older people in five European countries. Ageing Soc 27:683–700

Gatersleben B (2011) The car as a material possession: exploring the link between materialism and car ownership and use. In: Lucas C, Blumemberg E, Weinberger R (eds) Auto motives: understanding car use behaviours. Emerald, Bingley, pp 137–148

Gautier PA, Zenou Y (2010) Car ownership and the labor market of ethnic minorities. J Urban Econ 67(3):392–403

Goodwin P, Dargay J, Hanly M (2004) Elasticities of road traffic and fuel consumption with respect to price and income: a review. Transp Rev 24(3):275–292

Goodwin P, Van Dender K (2013) 'Peak car'—themes and issues. Transp Rev 33:243–254

Graham DJ, Glaister S (2004) Road traffic demand elasticity estimates: a review. Transp Rev 24:261–274

Grimal R, Collet R, Madre JL (2013) Is the stagnation of individual car travel a general phenomenon in France? A time-series analysis by zone of residence and standard of living. Transp Rev 33(3):291–309

Hampshire RC, Gaites C (2011) Peer-to-peer carsharing market analysis and potential growth. Transp Res Rec 2217:119–126

Hensher DA, Stopher PR (1979) Behavioral travel demand modelling. Croom Helm, London

Hidrue MK, Parsons GR, Kempton W, Gardner MP (2011) Willingness to pay for electric vehicles and their attributes. Resour Energy Econ 33:686–705

Hinde S, Dixon J (2005) Changing the obesogenic environment: insights from a cultural economy of car reliance. Transp Res Part D: Transp Environ 10:31–53

Hjorthol R, Fyhri A (2009) Do organized leisure activities for children encourage car-use? Transp Res Part A 43(2):209–218

Hjorthol RJ, Levin L, Siren A (2010) Mobility in different generations of older persons: the development of daily travel in different cohorts in Denmark, Norway and Sweden. J Transp Geogr 18:624–633

Ho C, Mulley C (2015) Intra-household interactions in transport research: a review. Transp Rev 35(1):33–55

Hojer M, Mattsson LG (2000) Determinism and backcasting in future studies. Futures 2:613–634

IEA (International Energy Agency) (2011) Technology roadmap: electric and plug-in hybrid electric vehicles (EV/PHEV). Available: http://www.ieaorg/publications/freepublications/publication/EV_PHEV_Roadmappdf. Accessed 25 Feb 2016

Japan Juku Association (2006) Safety guidelines for children to attend cram school. Available: http://www.jjaorjp/children/data/0603gl-allpdf. Accessed 25 Feb 2016 (in Japanese)

Jones P (1990) Development in dynamic and activity-based approaches to travel analysis. Gower, Aldcrshot

Jones P (2011) Conceptualising car 'dependence' In: Lucas C, Blumemberg E, Weinberger R (eds) Auto motives: understanding car use behaviours. Emerald, Bingley, pp 39–61

Jones MA, Reynolds KE, Arnold MJ (2006) Hedonic and utilitarian shopping value: investigating differential effects on retail outcomes. J Bus Res 59(9):974–981

Jung KO (2009) A study of the decision of an individual household on the housing size using Korea expenditure survey data. J Korean Public Policy 11(2):29–151

Kelly JA, Fu M (2014) Sustainable school commuting—understanding choices and identifying opportunities: a case study in Dublin, Ireland. J Transp Geogr 34:221–230

Kent JL (2014) Carsharing as active transport: what are the potential health benefits? J Transp Health 1(1):54–62

Kent JL, Dowling R (2013) Puncturing automobility? Carsharing practices. J Transp Geogr 32:86 92

Kim K (2015) Can carsharing meet the mobility needs for the low-income neighborhoods? Lessons from carsharing usage patterns in New York City. Transp Res Part A 77:249–260

Kim C, Parent O (2016) Modeling individual travel behaviors based on intra-household interactions. Reg Sci Urban Econ 57:1–11

Kuhnimhof T, Armoogum J, Buehler R, Dargay J, Denstadli JM, Yamamoto T (2012) Men shape a downward trend in car use among young adults—evidence from six industrialized countries. Transp Rev 32:761–779

Kuhnimhof T, Zumkeller D, Chlond B (2013) Who made peak car, and how? A breakdown of trends over four decades in four countries. Transp Rev 33:325–342

Kuwano M, Tsukai M, Matsubara T (2013) The influence of social conformity in promoting electric vehicle sales. In: Roorda MJ, Miller EJ (eds) Travel behaviour research: current foundations, future prospects. Lulu Press, Toronto, pp 369–386

Liao FH, Farber S, Ewing R (2015) Compact development and preference heterogeneity in residential location choice behaviour: a latent class analysis. Urban Stud 52(2):314–337
Long J, Harre N, Atkinson QD (2015) Social clustering in high school transport choices. J Environ Psychol 41:155–165
Lord S, Despres C, Ramadier T (2011) When mobility makes sense: a qualitative and longitudinal study of the daily mobility of the elderly. J Environ Psychol 31(1):52–61
Lucas C, Blumemberg E, Weinberger R (2011) Auto motives: understanding car use behaviours. Emerald, Bingley
Lyons G, Urry J (2005) Travel time use in the information age. Transp Res Part A 39:257–276
Macintyre S, Maciver S, Sooman A (1993) Area, class and health: should we be focusing on places or people? J Soc Policy 22:213–234
Mackett R (2002) Increasing car dependency of children: should we be worried? In: Proceedings of the Institution of Civil Engineers—Municipal Engineer, vol 151, no 1, pp 29–38
Madina C, Zamora I, Zabala E (2016) Methodology for assessing electric vehicle charging infrastructure business models. Energy Policy 89:284–293
Matthews H, Taylor M, Percy-Smith B, Limb M (2000) The unacceptable Flaneur: the shopping mall as a teenage hangout. Childhood 7:279–294
Medda F (2012) Land value capture finance for transport accessibility: a review. J Transp Geogr 25:154–161
Mercado R, Paez A (2009) Determinants of distance traveled with a focus on the elderly: a multilevel analysis in the Hamilton CMA, Canada. J Transp Geogr 17(1):65–76
Metz D (2004) Travel time constraints in transport policy. In: Proceedings of the Institution of Civil Engineers—Transport, vol 157, no 2, pp 99–105
Metz D (2010) Saturation of demand for daily travel. Transp Rev 30:659–674
Mitropoulos LK, Prevedouros PD (2014) Multicriterion sustainability assessment in transportation: private cars, carsharing, and transit buses. Transp Res Rec 2403:52–61
Mokhtarian PL, Salomon I (2001) How derived is the demand for travel? Some conceptual and measurement considerations. Transp Res A 35:695–719
Morrissey P, Weldon P, O'Mahony M (2016) Future standard and fast charging infrastructure planning: an analysis of electric vehicle charging behavior. Energy Policy 89:257–270
Nasrudin N, Nor ARM (2013) Travelling to school: transportation selection by parents and awareness towards sustainable transportation. Procedia Environ Sci 17:392–400
Nishimura H (2012) Sociological perspectives on youth and automobiles with special reference to contemporary Japan. IATSS Rev 37(2):21–30
Nordelof A, Messagie M, Tillman AM, Soderman ML, Van Mierlo J (2016) Environmental impacts of hybrid, plug-in hybrid, and battery electric vehicles-what can we learn from life cycle assessment? Int J Life Cycle Assess 21(1):134–135
Oakil ATM, Ettema D, Arentze T, Timmermans HJP (2014) Changing household car ownership level and life cycle events: an action in anticipation or an action on occurrence. Transportation 41(4):889–904
OECD (2015) ITF Transport Outlook 2015. OECD publishing, Paris
Ong PM (2002) Car ownership and welfare-to-work. J Policy Anal Manage 21(2):239–252
Prettenthaler FE, Steininger KW (1999) From ownership to service use lifestyle: the potential of car sharing. Ecol Econ 28:443–453
Rabbit P, Carmichael A, Jones S, Holland C (1996) When and why older drivers give up driving. AA Foundation for Road Safety Research, Manchester, UK
Ramsay SE, Whincup PH, Morris RW, Lennon LT, Wannamethee SG (2008) Extent of social inequalities in disability in the elderly: results from a population-based study of British men. Ann Epidemiol 18(12):896–903
Redmond LS, Mokhtarian PL (2001) The positive utility of the commute: modeling ideal commute time and relative desired commute amount. Transportation 28:179–205
Roosen J, Marneffe W, Vereeck L (2015) A review of comparative vehicle cost analysis. Transp Rev 35(6):720–748

Schaefers T (2013) Exploring carsharing usage motives: a hierarchical means-end chain analysis. Transp Res Part A 47:69–77

Shaheen SA, Cohen AP (2013) Carsharing and personal vehicle services: worldwide market developments and emerging trends. Int J Sustain Transp 7(1):5–34

Shaheen SA, Martin E (2010) Demand for carsharing systems in Beijing, China: an exploratory study. Int J Sustain Transp 4(1):41–55

Siren A, Hakamies-Blomqvist L (2004) Private car as the grand equaliser? Demographic factors and mobility in Finnish men and women aged 65+. Transp Res Part F 7(2):107–118

Smith GD, Shipley MJ, Rose G (1990) Magnitude and causes of socioeconomic differentials in mortality: further evidence from the Whitehall Study. J Epidemiol Community Health 44(4):265–270

Sperling D, Gordon D (2009) Two billion cars: driving towards sustainability. Oxford University Press, Oxford

Stanley JR (2011) Social exclusion. In: Currie G (ed) New perspectives and methods in transport and social exclusion research. Emerald, Bingley, pp 27–43

Stanley JR, Vella-Brodrick D (2009) The usefulness of social exclusion to inform social policy in transport. Transp Policy 16(3):90–96

Sun XH, Yamamoto T, Morikawa T (2015) Charge timing choice behavior of battery electric vehicle users. Transp Res Part D 37:97–107

Szalai A (1972) The use of time: daily activities of urban and suburban populations in twelve Countries. Mouton Publications, The Hague

Tsekeris T (2012) Disaggregate analysis of gasoline consumption demand of Greek households. Inzinerine Ekonomika-Engineering Econ 23(1):41–49

Van den Berg P, Arentze T, Timmermans H (2011) Estimating social travel demand of senior citizens in the Netherlands. J Transp Geogr 19(2):323–331

Van Goeverden CD, de Boer E (2013) School travel behaviour in the Netherlands and Flanders. Transp Policy 26:73–84

Van Wee B, Rietveld P, Meurs H (2006) Is average daily travel time expenditure constant? In search of explanations for an increase in average travel time. J Transp Geogr 14:109–122

Vanderbeck RM, Johnson J, James H (2000) "That's the only place where you can hang out": urban young people and the space of the mall. Urban Geogr 21:5–25

Veenhoven R (2014) World database of happiness: archive of research findings on subjective enjoyment of life Erasmus University Rotterdam (Available at: http://worlddatabaseofhappiness.eur.nl)

Verma M, Malayath M, Verma A (2015) Analysis of aspiration for owning a car among youths in a city of a developing country, India. In: Proceedings of the Third Conference of Transportation Research Group of India (3rd CTRG), Kolkata, India, December 17–20 (CD-ROM)

Vessali KV (1996) Land use impacts of rapid transit: a review of the empirical literature. Berkeley Plann J 11(1):71–105

Vilhelmson B (1990) Vår dagliga rörlighet—om resandets utveckling, fördelning och gränser TFB-rapport 1990:16 Stockholm: Transportforskningsberedningen, 1990

Vilhelmson B (2007) The use of the car—Mobility dependencies of urban everyday life. In: Garling T, Steg L (eds) Threats from car traffic to the quality of urban life: problems, causes, and solutions. Elsevier, Oxford, pp 145–164

Wang Y, Potoglou D, Orford S, Gong Y (2015) Bus stop, property price and land value tax: a multilevel hedonic analysis with quantile calibration. Land Use Policy 42:381–391

Woodjack J, Dahlia G, Andy L, Thomas ST, Gil T, Michael AN (2012) Consumer perceptions and use of driving distance of electric vehicles: Changes over time through lifestyle learning process. Transp Res Rec 2287:1–8

Yotsumoto M (2012) Loss of interest among youth toward automobiles: analysis of the present state and the possibility of a break through. IATSS Rev 37(2):39–47

Young S, Caisey V (2010) Mind shift, mode shift: a lifestyle approach to reducing car ownership and use based on behavioural economics and social marketing. Perspect Public Health 130(3):36–142
Yu B, Zhang J, Fujiwara A (2011) Representing in-home and out-of-home energy consumption behavior in Beijing. Energy Policy 39(7):4168–4177
Yu B, Zhang J, Fujiwara A (2012) Analysis of the residential location choice and household energy consumption behavior by incorporating multiple self-selection effects. Energy Policy 46:319–334
Yu B, Zhang J, Fujiwara A (2013a) Evaluating the direct and indirect rebound effects in household energy consumption behavior: a case study of Beijing. Energy Policy 57(C):441–453
Yu B, Zhang J, Fujiwara A (2013b) A household time-use and energy-consumption model with multiple behavioral interactions and zero consumption. Environ Plann B Plann Des 40(2):330–349
Yu B, Zhang J, Fujiwara A (2013c) Rebound effects caused by the improvement of vehicle energy efficiency: an analysis based on a SP-off-RP survey. Transp Res Part D Transp Environ 24:62–68
Zahavi Y (1973) The TT-relationship: a unified approach to transportation planning. Traffic Eng Control 15N(n/5):205–212
Zahavi Y, Ryan JM (1980) Stability of travel components over time. Transp Res Rec 750:19–26
Zhang J (2009) A model of pedestrian time and monetary consumption behavior at city center. In: Timmermans HJP (ed) Pedestrian behaviour: models, data collection and applications. Emerald, Bingley, pp 157–193
Zhang J (2014) Revisiting the residential self-selection issues: a life-oriented approach. J Land Use Transp 7(3):29–45
Zhang J (2015) The life-oriented approach and travel behavior research. In: A discussion paper for the Workshop "Life-Oriented Approach for Transportation Studies" at the 14th international conference on travel behaviour research. Windsor, UK, July 19–23
Zhang J, Xiong Y (2015) Effects of multifaceted consumption on happiness in life: a case study in Japan based on an integrated approach. Int Rev Econ 62:143–162
Zhang J, Timmermans HJP, Borgers A (2002) A utility-maximizing model of household time use for independent, shared and allocated activities incorporating group decision mechanisms. Transp Res Rec 1807:1–8
Zhang J, Timmermans HJP, Borgers A (2005) A model of household task allocation and time use. Transp Res Part B 39:81–95
Zhang J, Kuwano M, Lee BJ, Fujiwara A (2009a) Modeling household discrete choice behavior incorporating heterogeneous group decision-making mechanisms. Transp Res Part B 43:230–250
Zhang J, Uno M, Fujiwara A (2009b) Cause-effect structure analysis of influential factors related to affective experience of using transit systems based on day reconstruction method. In: Proceedings of Infrastructure Planning, 39 (CD-ROM) (in Japanese)
Zhang J, Yu B, Chikaraishi M (2014) Interdependences between household residential and car ownership behavior: a life history analysis. J Transp Geogr 34:165–174
Zhang J, Xiong Y, Jiang Y, Tanaka N, Ohmori N, Taniguchi A (2016) Behavioral changes in migration associated with jobs, residences, and family life. In: Zhang J (ed) Life-oriented behavioral research for urban policy, Chapter 17. Springer, Heidelberg
Zumkeller D (2009) The dynamics of change—latest results from the German mobility panel. In: Paper presented at the 12th international conference on travel behaviour research. Jaipur, India, December 13–18 (CD-ROM)

Chapter 5
Household Energy Consumption Behavior

Biying Yu and Junyi Zhang

Abstract This chapter deals with not only household car ownership and usage, but also ownership and usage of in-home electric and electronic appliances from the perspective of energy consumption. Household energy consumption is an outcome of a series of life choices including end-use ownership, end-use efficiency, end-use usage, time use, expenditure allocation, residential location choice, employment choice, and household structure decisions. It is related to all life domains and also has externalities such as impacts on health. Life-oriented methodology that considers the potential interactions between household energy consumption and other life choices would be more appropriate to investigate this issue. To that end, this chapter sheds light on three fundamental questions related to household energy consumption: (1) How much is the minimum energy demand for households in the context of their life choices? (2) How do factors of attitude, belief and consciousness work on residential choice and household energy consumption? (3) How can household energy demand be actively managed by designing life choice-oriented interdisciplinary policies? In this chapter, the externality of household energy use on health is discussed as well.

Keywords In-home and out-of-home energy consumption · Integrated behavior model · Energy demand management system · Waste energy · Re-bound effects · Self-selection effects · Health

B. Yu (✉)
Beijing Institute of Technology, Beijing, China
e-mail: yubiying_bj@bit.edu.cn

J. Zhang
Hiroshima University, Higashi-Hiroshima, China
e-mail: zjy@hiroshima-u.ac.jp; junyizh24@gmail.com

J. Zhang (ed.), *Life-Oriented Behavioral Research for Urban Policy*,
DOI 10.1007/978-4-431-56472-0_5

5.1 Background

In recent years, great progress has been made to slow down and stop the pace of climate change. Indeed, good signs have been seen that economic growth and energy-related emissions, which have historically moved synchronously, are starting to decouple. The energy intensity of the global economy continued to decline in 2014 despite economic growth of over 3 %. However, increasing effort is still needed if we are aiming to limit the rise in global mean temperature to 2 °C (IEA 2015). To that end, efforts to develop cleaner and more efficient energy technologies should be further enhanced. Globally, the industrial final energy consumption fell by 4 % from 1973 to 2011 (Fig. 5.1). In addition, residential consumption accounted for about a quarter of global total final consumption. This share has remained stable over the last 35 years and is likely to remain more or less the same in the future in spite of technology change (IEA 2014), probably because of the contribution from the developing countries, whose shares are continuing to increase due to the unsaturation of domestic end uses as well as poor living conditions. For the transport sector, the total final energy consumption increased from 23 % in 1973 to 27 % in 2011(IEA 2014), suggesting that energy savings from new efficient technologies are likely to be offset by increasing demand for transport.

Based on these statistics, it is not difficult to realize that, in contrast to industrial and service sectors, residential and private transport energy consumption requires more active controls in addition to technology improvement, because they are associated with the way individuals and households use energy to heat, cool, and light their homes, run an increasing number of electric appliances, and drive their cars. All forms of consumption are a result of life choices (e.g., end-use ownership, efficiency choice, end-use usage, time allocation, expenditure allocation, residential location choice, and job choice) and can be a form of self-expression (Hubacek et al. 2009; Schaffrin and Reibling 2015; Wei et al. 2007).

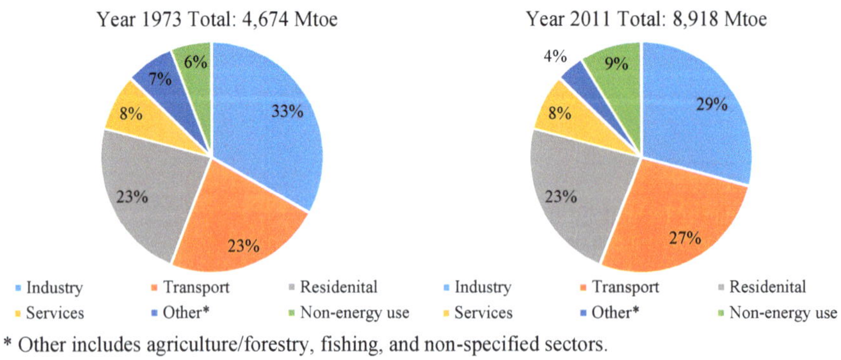

Fig. 5.1 Shares of sectors in total final consumption for the world (1973 and 2011) (IEA 2014)

In other words, determining how to achieve sustainability in these two sectors relies to a large extent on household/individual daily behavior in all life domains, which might be quite different across the population, making it more difficult to control through regulation than other energy-consuming sectors. The incentives for bundling residential consumption and private transport consumption together as household consumption have been demonstrated repeatedly in the literature (Yu et al. 2011, 2012, 2013a, b, c). Therefore, this chapter will depart from the context of a comprehensive household sector by including both residential and private transport sectors.

5.2 Energy Consumption, Life Choices, Quality of Life, and Environmental Consequences

Motivated or restrained by attitude, belief, and consciousness (ABC) factors, as well as sociodemographic and economic factors, people make a series of interrelated choices about their employment, residence, and family composition, which may further influence their other life choices, such as daily activities and monetary consumption. These life choices are further attributable to people's quality of life (Veenhoven 2014; Zhang and Xiong 2015). It is worth noting that self-selection effects (Cao et al. 2009; Mokhtarian and Cao 2008; Van Wee 2009) might exist between these choices (Zhang 2014). To support daily activities, households/individuals need to purchase the necessary goods and end uses (end-use ownership choice) with appropriate technologies (technology choice), and decide how long and how often to use them (end-use usage). In turn, this causes additional expenditure on goods, appliances, and/or vehicles. The activity pattern of a household/individual relates to the main driving forces of direct residential and passenger transport energy consumption, namely the duration of use of energy-consuming appliances, the number of trips taken to support daily activities, the mode of travel, and the timing of travel (Ellegård and Palm 2011; Widén et al. 2009). On the other hand, expenditure on goods and end uses will induce energy consumption during the life cycle of industrial production for materials or services (Bin and Dowlatabadi 2005; Wei et al. 2007). Consequently, the choices of activity pattern and expenditure may be further linked to energy consumption. In other words, household energy consumption is a result of all the aforementioned life choices, as shown in Fig. 5.2, and changing any one of them may have derivative effects on the others. Using data from 198 countries for the period 1990–2009, Al-mulali (2016) found that "energy consumption improves the life quality of 70 % of the countries despite their different incomes. ... the life quality indicators also increase energy consumption, a phenomenon that appears to be true in 65 % of the countries." Thus, energy consumption and quality of life are interrelated.

The world still depends on fossil fuels that represent 81 % of total energy consumption (Al-Mulali 2016). The OECD extensively examined environmental pressure from households from the perspectives of waste generation and recycling, personal transport choice, residential energy demand, environmentally responsible food choice, and residential water use (OECD 2008). It is predicted that environmental pressure from households will significantly increase by 2030: total residential energy use in OECD countries will increase by an average of 1.4 % per year from 2003 to 2030 and non-OECD residential energy use will be nearly 30 % higher than the OECD total in 2030 (Ferrara and Serret 2008). Zaman et al. (2016) confirmed the relationships between energy, environment, health, and wealth in BRICS countries (Brazil, Russia, India, China, and South Africa) over the period 1975–2013, and suggested that a carbon-free economy should be the priority for the green growth agenda that helps prevent environmental health hazards. More evidence of the negative effects of energy consumption on public health is seen in Wang (2010). On the other hand, Ellegård and Palm (2011) argued that policies reducing environmental loads from households must relate to and rely on individuals' daily choices and household routines, i.e., what they do in their everyday lives.

Under the full picture in Fig. 5.2, this chapter sheds light on three fundamental questions related to household energy consumption. (1) How much is the

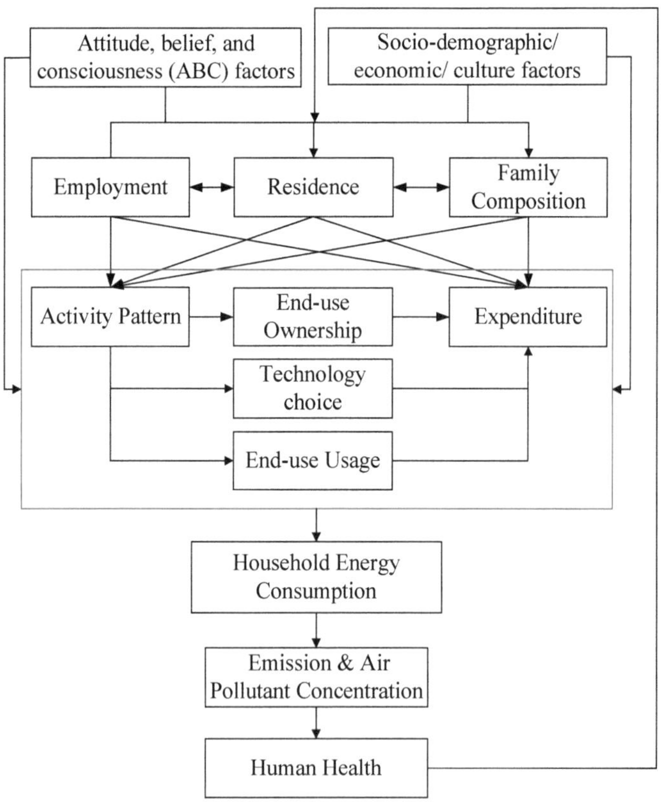

Fig. 5.2 Life choices and environmental consequences

minimum energy demand for households in the context of their life choices? (2) How do the ABC factors work on residential choice and household energy consumption? (3) How can household energy demand be actively managed by designing life choice-oriented interdisciplinary policies? As an extension, the externality of household energy use on health will be discussed through a review.

5.3 Household Energy Consumption, How Much Can Be Cut Down?

5.3.1 Behavioral Mechanism

Energy is an indispensable resource for household production and is consumed in meeting different needs in daily life (e.g., eating, showering, cooling and heating, entertainment, working, and so on). Energy consumption for meeting basic needs is not the same as that for meeting higher-order needs. The energy consumption for basic needs may not be significantly different between households if household composition and other attributes are the same, and there is probably no potential to cut down this part of consumption by external policies because the minimum quality of life should be ensured for each household. However, for higher-order needs, energy consumption across households with the same composition and attributes could differ significantly. Only for these needs might "unnecessary" consumption exist and be able to be reduced by policy instruments, along with the constraints of basic needs (Baxter et al. 1986; Schaffrin and Reibling 2015). The question of energy consumption for human basic needs immediately raises the issue of a minimum threshold energy budget; i.e., one above which human basic needs can reasonably be met. Filippini and Hunt (2012) estimated the underlying efficiency of residential energy consumption for each US state; substantial variation of efficiency was found between different states, suggesting that the phenomenon of "waste energy" is quite prevalent. Chung (2011) reviewed dozens of articles related to the benchmarking of buildings in light of energy-use performance (i.e., the lowest energy-use buildings), and the main methodologies [including Ordinary Least Squares (OLS), Stochastic Frontier Analysis (SFA), and Data Envelopment Analysis (DEA)] for dealing with energy efficiency were summarized and compared.

5.3.2 Case Study: Does "Waste Energy" Exist or Not?

In this section, based on an empirical study in the context of Beijing, we give an example of how to address the questions concerning whether "waste energy" exists or not and how much household energy consumption can be cut down. Stochastic frontier analysis (SFA) (Fernández et al. 2005) is applied to identify the end uses showing inefficient consumption in households, as well as the lower bound of energy expenditure (minimum expenditure) for these end uses in each household. The data employed here are obtained from a household energy consumption survey conducted in Beijing in 2010 (Yu et al. 2015).

To analyze the inefficiency of end uses, the single-output nature SFA analysis with frontier cost function is conducted for each end use. It is unlikely that all households operate at the frontier with minimum consumption, and failure to attain the cost frontier implies the existence of consumption inefficiency. The part of consumption excluding the inefficient consumption equals the part for basic needs. The mathematical expression is denoted as:

$$\ln Y_{ij} = \beta \ln X_{ij} + u_{ij} + v_{ij}, \quad u_i \geq 0 \quad (i = 1, 2, \ldots, N \quad \text{and} \quad j = 1, 2, \ldots, 9) \tag{5.1}$$

where i is household, j is end use, and X_{ij} is a group of variables representing the household/individual heterogeneity; the first error term u_{ij} is a one-sided nonnegative disturbance reflecting the inefficiency of end use j in household i, $u_{ij} \sim idN^{+}(0, \sigma_u^2)$; the second error term v_{ij} is a two-sided disturbance capturing the effect of measurement error and random factors, $v_{ij} \sim iidN(0, \sigma_v^2)$.

Inefficiency is indexed by the ratio of the actual costs (the actual energy expenditure) to the lowest cost level (the minimum energy expenditure):

$$\text{Inefficiency}_{ij} = \frac{\left(Y_{ij} \middle| u_{ij}, X_{ij}\right)}{\left(Y_{ij} \middle| u_{ij} = 0, X_{ij}\right)} = \frac{\beta \ln X_{ij} + u_{ij}}{\beta \ln X_{ij}} \geq 1 \tag{5.2}$$

The variables used to describe the cross-sectional heterogeneity in SFA are listed in Table 5.1. In total, nine durable end uses are targeted: refrigerators, electric fans, air conditioners (AC), gas showers, washing machines, TVs, PCs, microwave ovens, and private cars. The results in Table 5.2 and Fig. 5.3 show that for these nine end uses, only for the usage of refrigerators, washing machines, microwave ovens, and cars is there significant inefficient consumption. The inefficiency level of the domestic end uses (i.e., refrigerators, washing machines, and microwave ovens) ranges from 1 to 5, and almost 80 % of the sample is below 3. By contrast, the inefficiency level of cars is much wider (i.e., 1–19), indicating a

Table 5.1 Variables in the stochastic frontier analysis (SFA)

Variable		Description
Y_{ij}		Energy consumption per person on end use j in household i
x_{ijm} ($m = 1$–7)	x_{ij1}	Household annual income level
	x_{ij2}	Household size
	x_{ij3}	Accessibility to the nearest bus stop/MRT station
	x_{ij4}	Accessibility to the nearest supermarket
	x_{ij5}	Energy intensity of the end use
	x_{ij6}	Accessibility to the nearest shopping mall
	x_{ij7}	Accessibility to the nearest park
$\ln(x_{ijm}) * \ln(x_{ijn})$		($m, n = 1$–$7, n \geq m$) interacted terms between each two of the above seven x variables

Table 5.2 Estimation results of SFA model

	Refrigerator	Fan	AC	Shower	Washer	TV	PC	Microwave oven	Car
$\ln x_1$	0.032	0.234	−0.035	−0.545	***−0.867***	−0.510	***1.335***	0.413	−0.119
$\ln x_2$	−0.163	***−2.579***	***−0.722***	0.773	−0.709	***−1.439***	***−1.167***	−1.650	−1.783
$\ln x_3$	0.336	−0.134	−0.011	0.251	−0.451	***−1.421***	0.783	0.239	***3.382***
$\ln x_4$	0.214	0.551	0.296	0.579	***1.739***	−0.144	−0.851	1.734	***3.717***
$\ln x_5$	***−0.634***	***0.824***	***1.232***	0.905	0.409	***3.587***	***7.093***	0.732	1.654
$\ln x_6$	***−0.621***	0.991	−0.470	***−1.627***	−0.417	−0.651	−0.441	***4.065***	***−3.382***
$\ln x_7$	0.146	***−1.421***	***−0.969***	−0.387	−0.458	0.699	0.516	***−5.659***	***−2.456***
$\ln x_1 \ln x_1$	0.044	***−0.248***	−0.022	−0.056	***0.379***	−0.034	−0.059	−0.154	0.114
$\ln x_1 \ln x_2$	−0.007	−0.126	***−0.240***	0.264	−0.007	***0.321***	0.068	***0.479***	−0.233
$\ln x_1 \ln x_3$	***0.114***	−0.183	0.102	***0.276***	0.046	−0.171	0.026	0.238	***−0.372***
$\ln x_1 \ln x_4$	***−0.169***	−0.026	***−0.276***	***−0.518***	***−0.545***	***0.240***	−0.180	−0.008	***−0.787***
$\ln x_1 \ln x_5$	0.017	−0.024	***0.486***	0.002	0.034	−0.009	***−0.171***	−0.058	0.102
$\ln x_1 \ln x_6$	0.089	0.078	***0.313***	***0.369***	0.112	−0.013	−0.110	−0.396	***0.641***
$\ln x_1 \ln x_7$	−0.055	0.217	0.111	0.285	***0.313***	0.120	0.029	***0.370***	***0.372***
$\ln x_2 \ln x_2$	0.014	***0.321***	***0.280***	−0.042	−0.169	0.076	***0.209***	−0.210	0.023
$\ln x_2 \ln x_3$	***0.139***	−0.203	−0.044	0.291	−0.033	0.137	***−0.391***	0.476	−0.078
$\ln x_2 \ln x_4$	0.008	−0.087	−0.040	−0.297	0.152	0.030	0.086	−0.464	0.019
$\ln x_2 \ln x_5$	***0.139***	***0.286***	***−0.854***	***−0.569***	−0.008	0.066	−0.040	0.103	0.780
$\ln x_2 \ln x_6$	−0.033	***0.600***	−0.049	0.171	0.105	0.178	0.221	0.131	0.175
$\ln x_2 \ln x_7$	0.029	0.018	***0.310***	***−0.422***	0.115	***−0.312***	−0.195	−0.161	***−0.450***
$\ln x_3 \ln x_3$	−0.069	−0.173	−0.137	***0.332***	−0.129	***0.203***	0.108	−0.310	−0.124
$\ln x_3 \ln x_4$	0.042	0.283	−0.239	***−0.477***	0.156	−0.025	***−0.277***	−0.288	0.279
$\ln x_3 \ln x_5$	***0.089***	−0.039	0.200	−0.321	0.078	***0.212***	***−0.175***	−0.260	***−0.875***
$\ln x_3 \ln x_6$	−0.019	−0.214	0.154	0.041	0.154	0.065	***0.620***	***0.760***	***−0.488***

(continued)

Table 5.2 (continued)

	Refrigerator	Fan	AC	Shower	Washer	TV	PC	Microwave oven	Car
ln x_3 ln x_7	0.031	***0.700***	0.104	−0.123	−0.042	−0.002	−0.160	0.405	***−0.480***
ln x_4 ln x_4	0.068	***−0.462***	0.123	0.229	***−0.299***	−0.202	0.029	0.303	−0.160
ln x_4 ln x_5	−0.016	0.065	***−0.488***	−0.037	***−0.164***	0.009	***0.289***	−0.141	***−0.989***
ln x_4 ln x_6	***−0.154***	0.226	−0.293	−0.155	0.020	***0.365***	***−0.356***	−0.062	***−0.559***
ln x_4 ln x_7	−0.069	−0.305	0.214	***0.456***	−0.281	***−0.302***	−0.053	−0.349	0.264
ln x_5 ln x_5	***−0.099***	0.008	−0.017	0.039	***0.057***	***−0.254***	***−0.601***	−0.007	−0.570
ln x_5 ln x_6	***−0.063***	***−0.267***	−0.064	***0.625***	−0.058	0.184	0.063	***−0.566***	0.907
ln x_5 ln x_7	0.003	0.175	***0.330***	0.030	−0.029	−0.089	−0.090	***0.895***	***0.974***
ln x_6 ln x_6	***0.152***	−0.076	***0.395***	0.147	***0.299***	***−0.303***	−0.027	***0.432***	***0.933***
ln x_6 ln x_7	0.086	***−0.481***	−0.273	−0.159	0.002	−0.097	−0.073	−0.360	−0.422
ln x_7 ln x_7	***−0.107***	***0.414***	***0.299***	0.164	0.149	***0.195***	0.140	−0.079	***0.492***
Intercept	***4.829***	0.314	***5.914***	***3.360***	0.538	***−6.024***	***−15.02***	−3.278	***3.982***
Lambda	***1.608***	0.732	1.272	1.437	***1.453***	0.029	0.031	***0.991***	***2.630***
Sigma2	0.288	0.707	0.873	0.866	0.905	0.375	0.604	1.633	0.961
R-square	0.726	0.816	0.622	0.651	0.737	0.994	0.996	0.846	0.873

Note Lambda = σ_u/σ_v, Sigma2 = $\sigma_u^2 + \sigma_v^2$. Bold and italic numbers mean significant at the 90 % level

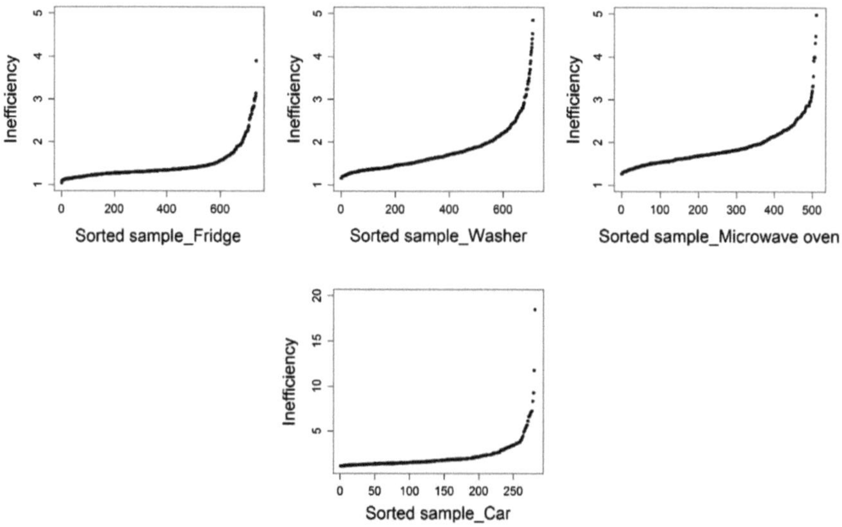

Fig. 5.3 Inefficiency level of the end uses (Yu et al. 2015)

substantial variance. It can be inferred that energy consumption for cars might be easier to control and the extent for reduction will also be broader than domestic end uses when the relevant policies [e.g., integrating persuasive technology with energy delegates (IPTED) (Emeakaroha et al. 2014), rumor propagation (Han et al. 2014), and eco-feedback systems (Jain et al. 2013)] are carried out. The minimum expenditure or the lower bound ($\underline{y}_{ij} = \beta \ln X_{ij}$) of the end-use usage in each household can be further calculated and this limit is supposed to change with household/individual characteristics in future years.

5.3.3 Summary

The findings on inefficient consumption and the minimum threshold for households are enlightening because they contribute to target setting and the effectiveness of the climate policies that encourage the proenvironmental behavior of households. The results in the Beijing case study show that the demand for the service of electric fans, ACs, gas showers, washing machines, TVs, and PCs is to meet basic life needs, implying that the energy consumption on these five end uses is difficult to cut down by policies other than technology improvement. For the four end uses with inefficient consumption, it should be noted that irrespective of the policies carried out, there is always a maximum bound for energy saving.

Furthermore, considering life needs may change with the progress through life stages; decision-making patterns may or may not be transferred from one stage to the next stage(s). This issue should be investigated using panel approaches to capture the dynamic change of consumption for basic needs.

5.4 ABC Factors and Household Energy Consumption

5.4.1 Behavioral Mechanism

In relation to the need for energy in life, in addition to objective factors such as income and household composition, subjective factors such as attitude, belief, and consciousness (ABC) of different life activities may play a role in understanding household energy consumption behavior. The question whether environmental attitudes, beliefs, and consciousness result in proenvironmental behaviors with regard to energy conservation has been extensively studied (Abrahamse et al. 2005; Ohler and Billger 2014; Ozaki and Sevastyanova 2011). A growing body of research indicates that many people and households engage in proenvironmental actions (e.g., recycle their waste or sort garbage themselves (Czajkowski et al. 2014), and buy organic food or efficient appliances (Steg et al. 2014) with the consideration of benefiting other people, future generations, and the environment, even though these actions may be costly. These proenvironmental actions accordingly induce energy savings or emission reductions (Bolderdijk et al. 2013; Gadenne et al. 2011; Martinsson et al. 2011; Sapci and Considine 2014; Yu et al. 2011). Even though the targeted areas, the analysis methods, and the survey data used in these studies are quite varied, similar relationships between these psychological factors and energy consumption are identified. Consequently, it is plausible that changing such unobserved factors, e.g., ABC factors, by informational or educational campaigns could be an alternative means to reduce energy use for a proportion of households.

On the other hand, the subjective factors are usually the inherent characteristics of people, implying that they may impact two or multiple life choices and activities: extroverts may enjoy staying out and socializing more with others (less in-home energy use); car addicts may buy a car and become a heavier car user (more fuel consumption); workaholics may spend most of their time working and less time on other activities (more consumption on work-related activities); proenvironmentalists may buy high-efficiency appliances and take public transport (less energy consumption); and so on. Indeed, all of these subjective factors are related to household energy consumption behavior, suggesting that household energy consumption should be analyzed jointly with other life choices.

5.4.2 Case Study: Self-selection Effects Between Residential Location Choice and Household Energy Consumption Behavior

Residential location choice has a long-term influence on household energy consumption behavior, referring to end-use ownership and usage. Brand et al. (2013) found that urban/rural status, home-to-work distance, home-to-retail distance, and home location had a significant influence on energy consumption and carbon dioxide emissions from motorized passenger travel in the UK. Nässén (2014) and Rahut et al. (2014) identified different domestic energy consumption patterns for rural and urban households in Sweden and Bhutan, respectively. In addition to the above causal effect from the residential environment (RE) characteristics to household energy consumption behavior, many researchers argue that there are other noncausal associations between these two dimensions derived from intervening variables that cause both. This relationship is called the "self-selection effect" (Mokhtarian and Cao 2008; Yu et al. 2012). Statistically, self-selection arises in any situation in which individuals select themselves into a group. The self-selection effect might come from ABC factors (Ohler and Billger 2014; Ozaki and Sevastyanova 2011), social factors such as lifestyle and life stage (Lutzenhiser 1993; Weber and Perrels 2000), and cultural factors (Abrahamse et al. 2005; Lutzenhiser 1992) among others. It is further argued that the self-selection effect might vary with life domains. For example, households that do not like cooking may choose to reside in a neighborhood with good catering facilities (e.g., restaurants and/or supermarkets), consequently, with fewer cooking-related end uses; households with a preference for driving may prefer to live in suburban areas to satisfy their desire to drive. Obviously, these two effects are distinct. This section introduces a case study that sheds light on household energy consumption behavior by incorporating multiple self-selection effects.

To that end, an integrated model, termed a mixed multinomial logit–multiple discrete-continuous extreme value (MNL–MDCEV) model, is built. This model covers residential location choice, end-use (including in-home appliances and out-of-home cars) ownership, and usage behavior, by considering a comprehensive set of RE and sociodemographic variables, as well as multiple self-selection effects. Bearing in mind the focus of this section, we only discuss the results related to the effect of unobserved factors (e.g., ABC factors) that cause self-selection effects on household energy consumption behavior; other results and conclusions can be found in Yu et al. (2012).

The MNL–MDCEV model includes the unobserved factors associated with both residential choice and household energy consumption behavior, which are regarded as the cause of multiple self-selection effects. To represent the sample heterogeneity, these factors are assumed to follow a normal distribution and Table 5.3 lists the estimation results of the mean and standard deviation for each end use. Based on the means, it was found that there is a significant unobserved component simultaneously affecting residential location choice and the ownership and usage of all end uses, indicating a correlation between long-term residential location choice behavior and medium/short-term household energy consumption behavior. In addition, the self-selection effects differ across end uses, verifying the need to incorporate multiple self-selection effects into the integrated model. Specifically, for in-home end uses (i.e., refrigerator, AC, electric shower, washing machine, TV, and PC), the positive self-selection effect indicates that some unobserved factors make households select themselves to a particular neighborhood and be more likely to own and spend more money on these end uses. For electric fan, gas shower, microwave oven, and car, the negative sign means that

Table 5.3 Unobserved factors related to self-selection effects

Unobserved factors	Fridge	Fan	AC	Electric shower	Gas shower	Clothes washer	TV	PC	Microwave oven	Car
Mean	6.663	−30.112	39.05	2.840	−2.637	8.764	8.189	5.608	−5.603	−9.826
s.d.	2.844	3.968	3.798	2.461	5.098	2.333	2.218	1.984	3.886	4.023

certain unobserved factors make households select themselves to some other particular neighborhood and be less likely to own these end uses or spend less money on them. For the standard deviations, it is confirmed that the multiple self-selection effects on the residential choice and energy consumption behavior of refrigerator, AC, electric shower, washing machine, TV, PC, and car vary significantly between households. Furthermore, these heterogeneous self-selection effects are more obvious for the ownership and usage of electric shower and car. This also supports the rationality of accommodating end-use-specific self-selection effects instead of using a common effect for all end uses. Although based on the model results, we cannot clarify what the self-selection effect exactly is or how to change it; however, after controlling for the self-selection effect in the model, the relatively true effect from residential environment variables can be captured, leading to less biased evaluation of land-use policy for household energy consumption.

To identify how much various factors influence household energy consumption behavior, we calculate the contribution ratio by each factor. For ease of interpretation, the total effects from three groups of variables are compared: household attributes (including household income, household size, presence of children and elders, number of workers and education level), residential environment attributes (including the CBD, suburban area, number of shopping malls, supermarkets, recreational facilities, restaurants, parks, bus lines and train lines in the neighborhood), unobserved factors only related to household energy consumption behavior, and unobserved factors associated with self-selection effects. It can be seen in Fig. 5.4 that different attributes have their own leading domain. Household and

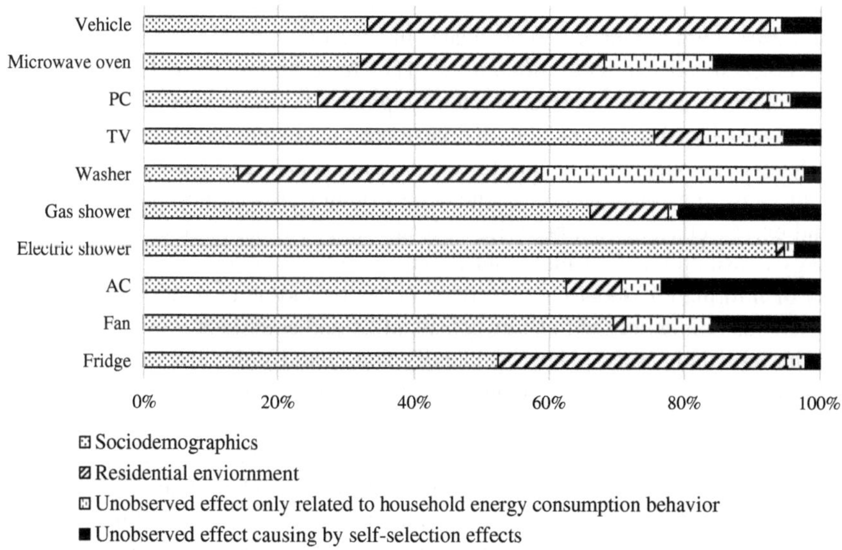

Fig. 5.4 Contribution of different attributes on household energy consumption behavior for end uses

individual attributes dominate for the energy consumption behavior of refrigerator, electric fan, AC, electric shower, gas shower, and TV. For washing machine, PC, microwave oven, and car, residential environment attributes play a more important role in explaining ownership and usage behavior. The contribution of unobserved factors varies greatly with end uses, ranging from 5 to 41 %, among which the portion causing self-selection effects varies from 2 to 24 %, suggesting a significant contribution that cannot be neglected when modeling the interaction between residential choice and household energy consumption behavior.

5.4.3 Summary

This section emphasizes the importance of considering the unobserved factors that influence household energy consumption behavior. The significant unobserved factors associated with the self-selection effects in the case study suggest that residential environment attributes are not completely exogenous in household energy consumption behavior. In other words, the effect of land-use policy on household energy use would be incorrectly estimated due to the existence of self-selection effects. This is an example showing the interaction between different life choices (i.e., residential location choice and household energy consumption decision choices) triggered by the subjective factors. As noted above, ABC factors are usually the inherent characteristics of people, meaning that besides the residential domain, there might be some other life domains interacting with household energy consumption due to ABC factors. Future analysis could start from this notion. In addition, in the case study, the self-selection effect was found to vary between 2 and 24 % with end uses. This validates the need to consider end-use-specific or life-choice-specific self-selection effects. The above finding strongly suggests that when planners attempt to develop interdisciplinary policy to save energy, in addition to the objective factors (e.g., RE attributes, sociodemographics, and housing attributes), the subjective factors (e.g., the ABC, social, and cultural factors) that might cause the self-selection phenomenon should also be introduced to understand energy consumption behavior. It is also implied that to conserve household energy consumption, it is important to introduce "soft policy", such as the provision of information about energy-saving behavior and an evaluation platform for households to monitor their energy consumption and emissions.

The remaining issue is how to identify and quantify the exact effect of ABC factors to determine the appropriate policies. Some researchers ask about people's environmental awareness or willingness to pay for environmentally improving measures (Tsushima et al. 2015; Wang et al. 2015); however, it is argued that those households that have positive environmental concerns and attitudes do not always consume less energy or do not recognize the relevance of energy savings (Gaspar and Antunes 2011; Holden and Linnerud 2010). Such inconsistencies should be taken into account. Panel surveys or field experiments might produce better data and the multilevel model could be an alternative method to stratify ABC factors.

5.5 Interdisciplinary Policy Scheme

5.5.1 Behavioral Mechanism

To achieve sustainable energy demand management, it is important to design a proper policy scheme to combine the effects of new technology, awareness campaigns, social norms, city structure, and comparative information (Khansari et al. 2014); in other words, a series of interdisciplinary countermeasures should be designed and carried out at the same time or successively put into practice. Accordingly, evaluating the collective effect of these countermeasures on household energy demand via an examination of the behavior change becomes the crucial challenge. Gomi et al. (2011) highlighted three types of relationships between policies: (1) policies that have an accelerating effect on other policies; (2) policies that are the prerequisite policies for others; and (3) policies that are parallel policies. However, in reality, there might also be a hindering effect between different policies, perhaps due to the inappropriate time sequence of the policies. For example, if the measures for improving people's environmental awareness are implemented in advance of a rebate program, one of the interactions between these two policies could be that more people utilize the rebate, while another result could be that because consumers have already contributed to energy savings by altering their lifestyle as their incremental awareness increases, they are hindered from participating in the rebate program, and vice versa. In this case, the rebate policies that are supposed to increase technology efficiency will not work as expected. This behavior could also occur between social-norm-related policies and technology improvements. Sometimes such hindering effects are not easily perceived, resulting in the failure of the planned policies. Therefore, when the interdisciplinary policies are implemented together, the overall effect should not be calculated as the sum of the effects of every single policy; instead, the system that can reflect the policy interactions from the consumers' behavioral perspective is required. To date, few attempts have been made to systematically couple these insights into a quantitative framework. As a result, a serious methodological gap exists between the perceived importance of closing the loop from the energy demand side and quantitative modeling frameworks or even policy scheme analysis.

5.5.2 Case Study: A Dynamic Active Energy Demand Management System

This section outlines a trial analysis to address the methodological gap noted above by extending the analysis in Sects. 5.3 and 5.4 to a simulated dynamic active energy demand management system (DAEDMS), which evaluates the collective effects of a set of nonprice policies, including urban planning, soft policies for improving household/individual unobserved factors (such as ABC factors), technology improvement/rebate programs, market end-use diffusion control, and social norms, on changing household behavior (i.e., end-use ownership, technology efficiency choice, and end-use usage) and the accompanying energy consumption in the residential and private transport sectors. The timing effect of each policy is also considered in DAEDMS, on the one hand to account for the interactions between the policies, and on the other hand to show the possible pathways to achieve the target. To present the implementation of DAEDMS, Beijing is taken as an example. The core model structure in DAEDMS builds on the methodology (i.e., the logit and resource allocation model) proposed in Yu et al. (2013a) and the estimation results related to self-selection effects in Yu et al. (2012). DAEDMS includes six modules, of which four modules directly act on the static policy variables (the technology improvement/rebate module, the soft policy for the ABC change module, the land-use change module, and the sociodemographic/economic factor (SDEF) change module); the other two modules play the role of introducing the dynamic change due to the market and other households (the market diffusion change module and the neighborhood social interaction module). Compared with the existing top-down and bottom-up energy system models (Fortes et al. 2014), such as decision analysis-based energy modeling (Wang and Poh 2014) and the demand side management system in the power sector (Jalali and Kazemi 2015), DAEDMS is focused on the energy demand side in both residential and private transport sectors, but with much more detailed and in-depth description of the behavioral mechanisms for household energy consumption, especially the interaction between residential energy consumption behavior and travel behavior, the rebound effects when the technology improves, the self-selection effects when the residential environment changes, the ownership change when the end-use penetration increases in the market, and the inefficient consumption and minimum service demand when considering the social influence. Furthermore, the interactions between policies within one scheme caused by the timing effect are explicitly incorporated in DAEDMS.

(1) *Referring aspects in the simulation*

In the simulated DAEDMS, the base year is 2010 and the future five years of 2011–2015 are targeted. Although the period can be easily extended, a short-term projection assuming similar economic and societal environment in the future is recommended because the adopted model estimation result is based on cross-sectional data. The following aspects in DAEDMS are addressed:

1. the natural change of the sociodemographic and socioeconomic characteristics (e.g., income, retirement with age increase, and the presence of children younger than 12 years) in the future year;
2. the influence of technology improvement or the rebate policy that causes the end-use efficiency changes;
3. the influence of soft policy (e.g., proenvironmental education);
4. the influence of the urban planning policy that changes the number of surrounding facilities;

5. the influence from the change of the market diffusion rate of the end uses;
6. the influence of social norms due to the households living in the same neighborhood;
7. the inefficiency level of the end uses and the minimum energy required for each end use.

(2) *Embedded model for predicting the future end-use consumption in DAEDMS*

DAEDMS is developed to evaluate the collective effect of the policy scheme on changing household energy consumption in the future. To that end, the logit and resource allocation model (Logit & RA) is embedded in DAEDMS to predict the end-use energy consumption every time certain policies occur. This model is derived from the combination of the model structure in Yu et al. (2013a) and model results in Yu et al. (2012). Based on the results of the mixed MNL–MDCEV model in Table 5.3, the unobserved factors associated with self-selection effects are extracted. By including these factors and household socioeconomic characteristics as well as residential environment attributes and technology efficiency collected from the household survey into the Logit & RA model and estimating it, the model coefficients used for dynamic simulation are finally obtained. In this way, we can describe how urban planning, soft policy, and technology improvement affect household energy consumption behavior in the same model structure, while dealing with both rebound effects and self-selection effects.

(3) *Interface and flowchart of DAEDMS*

A visual user interface was designed for DAEDMS (Fig. 5.5), in which the parameters for controlling policy interventions in the simulation program can be set externally based on the survey data or assumptions. The parameters shown in the interface are regarded as the policy parameters. In addition, policy makers can select the years to implement different types of policies to find the potential pathways to achieve energy conservation. If certain policies are not included in the policy scheme, then 0 is input to the corresponding option box for the policy year.

Households first access the four parallel modules (the technology improvement/rebate module, the soft policy for the ABC change module, the land-use change module, and the SDEF change module) to update their technology efficiency, unobserved factors related to ABC, residential environment, and SDEF; next, the market diffusion change module is accessed to ensure that the end-use ownership keeps pace with the whole market; finally, the social interaction module is accessed to indicate the interaction with other households. The concrete flowchart and interpretation of each module can be found in Yu et al. (2015).

In DAEDMS, we set the policy year option for technology improvement, soft policy, and urban planning policy; regarding the influence of the market and the social network, we assume that it always exists. The time step is set as one year, meaning that household energy expenditure will be re-estimated every year. However, it is easy to shorten the time step to one month or one day, and the continuous implementation of a policy (i.e., more than one year) can be easily

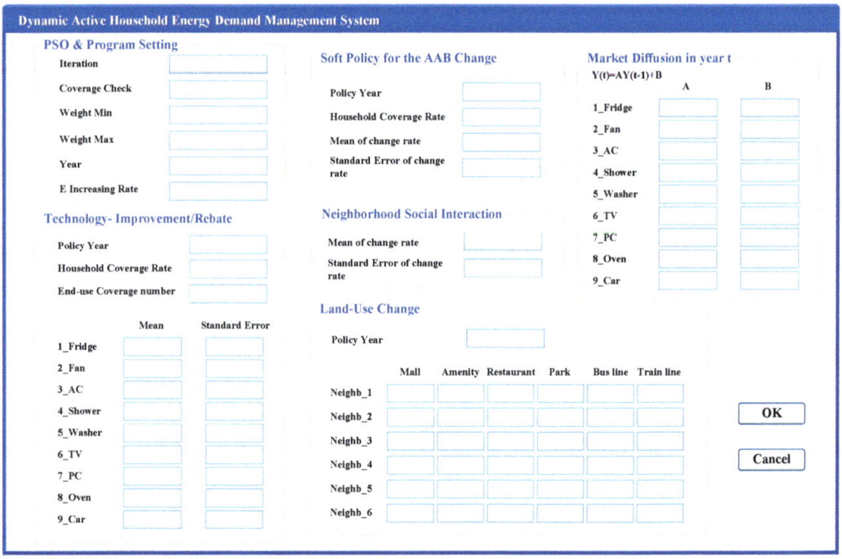

Fig. 5.5 DAEDMS interface (Yu et al. 2015). *Note* The base year is 2010, the 1st policy year is 2011, the 2nd year is 2012, and the 5th year is 2015

implemented in this program. Here, we only provide an example of how to manipulate such an integrative policy analysis system for household energy consumption behavior.

(4) *Simulation results on policy effects*

Because of the lack of data, several assumptions have been made in the simulation process, which results in less reliable estimation of the policy effects. Nevertheless, the main focus of this study is to demonstrate how to evaluate quantitatively the overall effect of this policy scheme on household energy consumption behavior rather than proposing effective countermeasures for policy makers.

Regarding the outputs, the simulated DAEDMS produces the annual energy expenditure and consumption for each end use in every household in the targeted period (2011–2015 in this empirical analysis). In addition, the effects of policy schemes (or scenarios) composed of a single policy or multiple policies can be examined for any predefined execution time for the relevant policies. To evaluate the overall effect of policy schemes and to examine the timing effect, the policy scenario in the empirical analysis refers to the scheme including all of the DAEDMS policies with predefined policy years, and the scenario with only the influence of the market diffusion rate and social interaction is set as the reference scenario.

With the increasingly saturated diffusion of end uses in the market and the influence of the social network, the annual growth rate of household energy consumption decreases significantly in the reference scenario. This result suggests

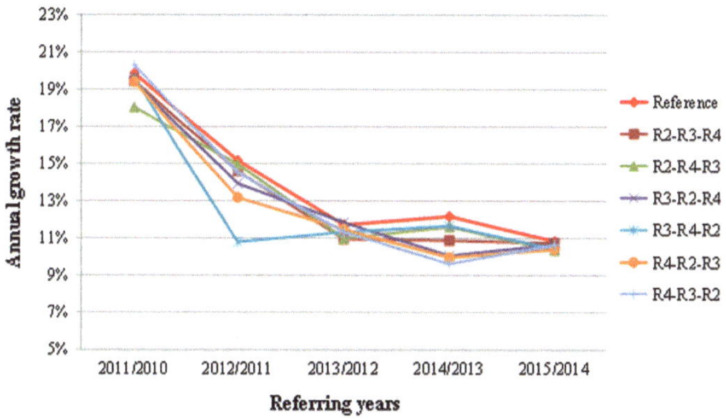

Fig. 5.6 Annual growth rates of policy scenarios. *Note* R2-S3-L4 is used to index the policy scenario, which means that the technology improvement/rebate is performed in the second year (2012), the soft policy in the third year (2013), and the land-use policy in the fourth year (2014). The same meanings are retained for the other scenarios

the effectiveness of market regulation and social interaction-oriented policies for reducing household energy use. Compared with the reference scenario, the lines of all of the policy scenarios are under the reference line (Fig. 5.6), and the predicted energy consumption at the end of 2015 will be reduced by 2–12 % (Fig. 5.7), meaning that the other three policies (i.e., rebate program, soft policy, and land-use policy) effectively achieve further energy conservation in the household sector. Nevertheless, these results reveal the variant efficacy of the same policy scheme, but with different execution timings. In other words, the interactions between policies caused by sequential implementation exist and are nonnegligible for evaluating the genuine collective effect of the policies within the same scheme.

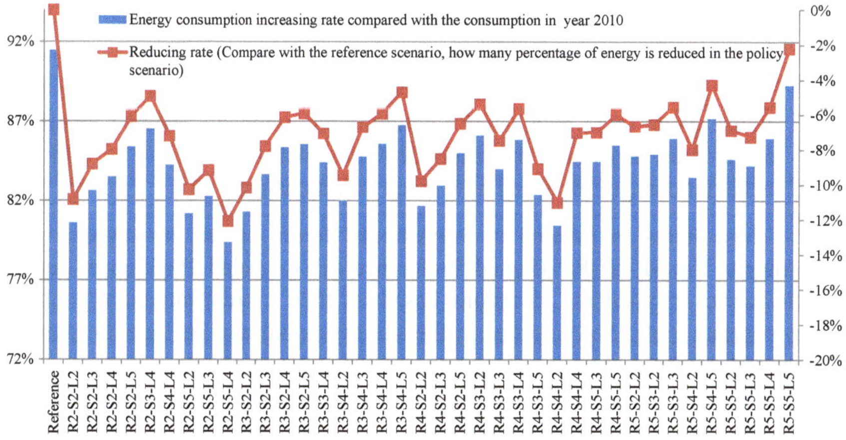

Fig. 5.7 Annual growth rates of policy scenarios

particles. Inhaled particle count is positively associated with proximity to motorized traffic. Despite the promotion of green travel modes worldwide, concerns about health risk should be always kept in mind; e.g., the supplementary policies that would locate bicycle lanes a safe distance away from motorized traffic should be considered together.

Because household energy consumption behavior and lifestyle contribute to both indoor and outdoor air pollution, health considerations influence the development of environmental policies aimed at reducing these adverse health impacts, such as building and construction codes that define the amount of ventilation in industrial and domestic kitchens, ventilation in commuter modes, reduction of emissions from key transport modes, and urban planning (Delgado-Saborit 2012).

5.7 Conclusion

Household energy consumption is an outcome of a series of life choices including end-use ownership, end-use efficiency, end-use usage, time use, expenditure allocation, residential location choice, employment choice, and household structure decisions. It is related to all life domains and also has externalities such as impacts on health. Life-oriented methodology that considers the potential interactions between household energy consumption and other life choices would be more appropriate for investigation of this issue. However, developing a systematic framework that includes as many life domains as possible without overcomplicating the analysis is the most challenging step. Although the methodology for dealing with self-selection effects is one alternative, a structure that can portray the direct relationship is to be preferred. A comprehensive demand management system that can cover multiple life domains is one such framework.

As emphasized in this chapter, household energy consumption is composed of basic-needs consumption and higher-order-needs consumption. Policy makers need to be aware of those policies that target both basic and higher-order needs and those that are only effective for higher-order consumption. In this way, they have a general idea of the maximum influence of the proposed policies, and can then set a reasonable and feasible target. Figure 5.8 provides a guide to how the policies work for household consumption. For technology improvement, land-use policy, and lifestyle-related policy (e.g., telecommuting and ICT promotion), they may affect household energy use from basic needs to higher-order needs, because they are likely to change people's life needs. Technology improvement is a little different from other two types of policies, because it may have no influence at all on people's lives if households simply maintain their original life without any changes. However, we should always be aware of rebound effects. Therefore, it is suggested that it is better to package technology improvement with additional policies (e.g., well-designed price/tax policies) that can contain the potential rebound effects. The self-selection phenomenon was expounded in Sect. 5.4; when implementing land-use policies, some soft policies (e.g., education, information

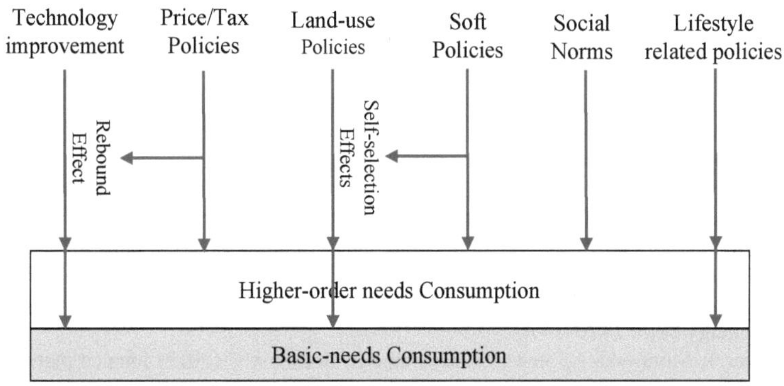

Fig. 5.8 Instructions on the policy performance

provision, and feedback) for improving household/individual ABC factors can be carried out simultaneously to diminish the negative effect and enhance the positive effect caused by self-selection. Price/tax policies, soft policies, and social norms can only have an effect on the consumption of higher-order needs. Hence, if they are likely candidates, their effectiveness should be evaluated under the constraint of minimum consumption for basic needs. In Sect. 5.5, we provided an example of the estimation of the collective effect of a group of interdisciplinary policies by considering basic-needs consumption and the applicability of a number of policies. As an initial trial, the structure is relatively simple; a more sophisticated policy assessment system, building on the viewpoints emphasized here, and a richer dataset are encouraged as the next step.

Given the apparent cause-effect relationship between lifestyle, household energy consumption, air pollution, and health, the issue concerning how a comprehensive framework should be built to unite all these domains is a challenge for the future. Existing methodologies include the residential energy demand model, the traffic model, emission inventory construction, the air quality model, the technology choice model, the lifestyle method, health impact assessment, sociological and psychological methods, all of which are relevant, suggesting that an interdisciplinary analysis is imperative.

References

Abrahamse W, Steg L, Vlek C, Rothengatter T (2005) A review of intervention studies aimed at household energy conservation. J Env Psychol 25(3):273–291

Al-mulali U (2016) Exploring the bi-directional long run relationship between energy consumption and life quality. Renew Sustain Energy Rev 54:824–837

Baxter LW, Feldman SL, Schinnar AP, Wirtshafter RM (1986) An efficiency analysis of household energy use. Energy Econ 8(2):62–73

Bin S, Dowlatabadi H (2005) Consumer lifestyle approach to US energy use and the related CO2 emissions. Energy Policy 33(2):197–208

Bolderdijk JW, Steg L, Geller ES, Lehman P, Postmes T (2013) Comparing the effectiveness of monetary versus moral motives in environmental campaigning. Nat Climate Change 3(4):413–416

Brand C, Goodman A, Rutter H, Song Y, Ogilvie D (2013) Associations of individual household and environmental characteristics with carbon dioxide emissions from motorised passenger travel. Appl Energy 104:158–169

Bruce N, Perez-Padilla R, Albalak R (2000) Indoor air pollution in developing countries: a major environmental and public health challenge. Bull World Health Organ 78(9):1078–1092

Cao XJ, Mokhtarian PL, Handy SL (2009) The relationship between the built environment and nonwork travel: a case study of Northern California. Transp Res Part A 43(5):548–559

Chung W (2011) Review of building energy-use performance benchmarking methodologies. Appl Energy 88(5):1470–1479

Cole-Hunter T, Morawska L, Stewart I, Jayaratne R, Solomon C (2012) Inhaled particle counts on bicycle commute routes of low and high proximity to motorised traffic. Atmos Environ 61:197–203

Czajkowski M, Kądziela T, Hanley N (2014) We want to sort! Assessing households' preferences for sorting waste. Resour Energy Econ 36(1):290–306

Delgado-Saborit JM (2012) Use of real-time sensors to characterise human exposures to combustion related pollutants. J Environ Monit 14(7):1824–1837

Ellegård K, Palm J (2011) Visualizing energy consumption activities as a tool for making everyday life more sustainable. Appl Energy 88(5):1920–1926

Emeakaroha A, Ang CS, Yan Y, Hopthrow T (2014) Integrating persuasive technology with energy delegates for energy conservation and carbon emission reduction in a university campus. Energy 76:357–374

Fernández C, Koop G, Steel MF (2005) Alternative efficiency measures for multiple-output production. J Econometrics 126(2):411–444

Ferrara I, Serret Y (2008) Household behaviour and the environment reviewing the evidence. Organization for Economic Cooperation and Development, Paris France, pp 153–180

Filippini M, Hunt LC (2012) US residential energy demand and energy efficiency: a stochastic demand frontier approach. Energy Econ 34(5):1484–1491

Fortes P, Pereira R, Pereira A, Seixas J (2014) Integrated technological-economic modeling platform for energy and climate policy analysis. Energy 73:716–730

Gadenne D, Sharma B, Kerr D, Smith T (2011) The influence of consumers' environmental beliefs and attitudes on energy saving behaviours. Energy Policy 39(12):7684–7694

Gaspar R, Antunes D (2011) Energy efficiency and appliance purchases in Europe: consumer profiles and choice determinants. Energy Policy 39(11):7335–7346

Gomi K, Ochi Y, Matsuoka Y (2011) A systematic quantitative backcasting on low-carbon society policy in case of Kyoto city. Technol Forecast Soc Chang 78(5):852–871

Han S, Zhuang F, He Q, Shi Z, Ao X (2014) Energy model for rumor propagation on social networks. Physica A 394:99–109

Holden E, Linnerud K (2010) Environmental attitudes and household consumption: an ambiguous relationship. Int J Sustain Dev 13(3):217–231

Hubacek K, Guan D, Barrett J, Wiedmann T (2009) Environmental implications of urbanization and lifestyle change in China: ecological and water footprints. J Clean Prod 17(14):1241–1248

IEA (2014) Energy efficiency indicators: fundamentals on statistics international energy agency, Paris. https://www.iea.org/publications/freepublications/publication/IEA_EnergyEfficiencyIndicatorsFundamentalsonStatistics.pdf

IEA (2015) World energy outlook special report 2015: energy and climate change international energy agency, Paris. https://www.iea.org/publications/freepublications/publication/WEO2015SpecialReportonEnergyandClimateChange.pdf

Jain RK, Gulbinas R, Taylor JE, Culligan PJ (2013) Can social influence drive energy savings? Detecting the impact of social influence on the energy consumption behavior of networked users exposed to normative eco-feedback. Energy Build 66:119–127

Jalali MM, Kazemi A (2015) Demand side management in a smart grid with multiple electricity suppliers. Energy 81:766–776

Khansari N, Mostashari A, Mansouri M (2014) Conceptual modeling of the impact of smart cities on household energy consumption. Procedia Comput Sci 28:81–86

Lutzenhiser L (1992) A cultural model of household energy consumption. Energy 17(1):47–60

Lutzenhiser L (1993) Social and behavioral aspects of energy use. Annu Rev Energy Env 18(1):247–289

Martinsson J, Lundqvist LJ, Sundström A (2011) Energy saving in Swedish households The (relative) importance of environmental attitudes. Energy Policy 39(9):5182–5191

Mokhtarian PL, Cao X (2008) Examining the impacts of residential self-selection on travel behavior: a focus on methodologies. Transp Res Part B Methodol 42(3):204–228

Nässén J (2014) Determinants of greenhouse gas emissions from Swedish private consumption: time-series and cross-sectional analyses. Energy 66:98–106

OECD (2008) Household behaviour and the environment: reviewing the evidence, OECD. https://www.oecd.org/environment/consumption-innovation/42183878.pdf

Ohler AM, Billger SM (2014) Does environmental concern change the tragedy of the commons? Factors affecting energy saving behaviors and electricity usage. Ecol Econ 107:1–12

Ozaki R, Sevastyanova K (2011) Going hybrid: an analysis of consumer purchase motivations. Energy Policy 39(5):2217–2227

Rahut DB, Das S, De Groote H, Behera B (2014) Determinants of household energy use in Bhutan. Energy 69:661–672

Sapci O, Considine T (2014) The link between environmental attitudes and energy consumption behavior. J Behav Experimental Econ 52:29–34

Schaffrin A, Reibling N (2015) Household energy and climate mitigation policies: investigating energy practices in the housing sector. Energy Policy 77:1–10

Steg L, Bolderdijk JW, Keizer K, Perlaviciute G (2014) An integrated framework for encouraging pro-environmental behaviour: the role of values situational factors and goals. J Env Psychol 38:104–115

Steinle S, Reis S, Sabel CE, Semple S, Twigg MM, Braban CF, Leeson SR, Heal MR, Harrison D, Lin C, Wu H (2015) Personal exposure monitoring of PM25 in indoor and outdoor micro-environments. Sci Total Environ 508:383–394

Tsushima S, Tanabe Si, Utsumi K (2015) Workers' awareness and indoor environmental quality in electricity-saving offices. Build Environ 88:10–19

Van Wee B (2009) Self-selection: a key to a better understanding of location choices travel behaviour and transport externalities? Transp Rev 29(3):279–292

Veenhoven R (2014) Findings on happiness and consumption. World Database of Happiness Erasmus, University Rotterdam. http://worlddatabaseofhappinesseur.nl/hap_cor/desc_topicphp?tid=6265. Assessed Mar 2016

Wang Y (2010) The analysis of the impacts of energy consumption on environment and public health in China. Energy 35(11):4473 4479

Wang Q, Poh KL (2014) A survey of integrated decision analysis in energy and environmental modeling. Energy 77:691–702

Wang Y, Sun M, Yang X, Yuan X (2015) Public awareness and willingness to pay for tackling smog pollution in China: a case study. J Clean Prod 112(2):1627–1634

Weber C, Perrels A (2000) Modelling lifestyle effects on energy demand and related emissions. Energy Policy 28(8):549–566

Wei YM, Liu LC, Fan Y, Wu G (2007) The impact of lifestyle on energy use and CO_2 emission: an empirical analysis of China's residents. Energy Policy 35(1):247–257

WHO (2013) Indoor air quality guidelines: household fuel combustion. World Health Organization. http://www.who.int/indoorair/guidelines/hhfc/en/

Widén J, Lundh M, Vassileva I, Dahlquist E, Ellegård K, Wäckelgård E (2009) Constructing load profiles for household electricity and hot water from time-use data—Modelling approach and validation. Energy Build 41(7):753–768

Yu B, Zhang J, Fujiwara A (2011) Representing in-home and out-of-home energy consumption behavior in Beijing. Energy Policy 39(7):4168–4177

Yu B, Zhang J, Fujiwara A (2012) Analysis of the residential location choice and household energy consumption behavior by incorporating multiple self-selection effects. Energy Policy 46:319–334

Yu B, Zhang J, Fujiwara A (2013a) Evaluating the direct and indirect rebound effects in household energy consumption behavior: a case study of Beijing. Energy Policy 57(C):441–453

Yu B, Zhang J, Fujiwara A (2013b) A household time-use and energy-consumption model with multiple behavioral interactions and zero consumption. Environ Plann B 40(2):330–349

Yu B, Zhang J, Fujiwara A (2013c) Rebound effects caused by the improvement of vehicle energy efficiency: an analysis based on a SP-off-RP survey. Transp Res Part D 24:62–68

Yu B, Tian Y, Zhang J (2015) A dynamic active energy demand management system for evaluating the effect of policy scheme on household energy consumption behavior. Energy 91:491–506

Zaman K, Bin Abdullah A, Khan A, Bin Mohd Nasir MR, Hamzah TAAT, Hussain S (2016) Dynamic linkages among energy consumption environment health and wealth in BRICS countries: green growth key to sustainable development. Renew Sustain Energy Rev 56:1263–1271

Zhang J (2014) Revisiting residential self-selection issues: a life-oriented approach. J Transp Land Use 7(3):29–45

Zhang K, Batterman SA (2009) Time allocation shifts and pollutant exposure due to traffic congestion: an analysis using the national human activity pattern survey. Sci Total Environ 407(21):5493–5500

Zhang J, Xiong Y (2015) Effects of multifaceted consumption on happiness in life: a case study in Japan based on an integrated approach. Int Rev Econ 62(2):143–162

Chapter 6
ICT-Dependent Life and Its Impacts on Mobility

Giovanni Circella

Abstract The rapid development of information and communication technology (ICT) is revolutionizing people's lives in many ways. Among their numerous impacts, ICT solutions allow for more flexibility in individuals' schedules, and provide new alternatives for the organization of work, social and recreational activities. Several types of relationships are possible between the adoption of ICT and travel behavior, leading to the eventual *complementarity with*, *substitution of*, *modification of*, or *neutrality with* travel. Modern technologies play an important role in affecting individuals' long- and medium-term decisions as well as numerous daily choices. The application of information and communication technologies is also behind the introduction of new shared mobility services that were barely imaginable only a few years ago. These services expand the set of travel options available to individuals. The effects of the availability and adoption of these technologies on individual behaviors are still largely unclear. They will likely cause long-lasting impacts on travel patterns, vehicle ownership, and life organization.

Keywords Information and communication technology · Lifestyles · Mobility · Travel behavior · Shared mobility services · Complementarity · Substitution · Modification · Neutrality · Urban form · Connected and autonomous vehicles

---

G. Circella (✉)
School of Civil and Environmental Engineering, Georgia Institute of Technology, Atlanta, GA, USA
e-mail: giovanni.circella@ce.gatech.edu

G. Circella
Institute of Transportation Studies, University of California, Davis, USA

J. Zhang (ed.), *Life-Oriented Behavioral Research for Urban Policy*,
DOI 10.1007/978-4-431-56472-0_6

6.1 ICT and Modern Lifestyles

Information and communications technology (ICT) applications are quickly changing the way we live, work, socialize and travel, to a degree that would have been barely imaginable only a few years ago. The readers simply need to look around themselves to see tangible examples of how modern technologies affect their lives and contribute to modifying their habits. ICT applications are nowadays an intrinsic part of daily activities and of most tools of common use, to the point that it is often difficult to identify and separate their presence from the activities and tools themselves. Over the course of the last few decades, technology has allowed for a number of revolutionary transformations spanning several different areas. Not only it has led to a complete transformation of many traditional activities, e.g. through the automation of the most tiring, boring or unpleasant tasks in one's life (such as washing the dishes, or doing laundry). It has improved individuals' quality of life through providing the ability to precisely organize production processes and maintenance tasks, e.g. finely controlling heating or air conditioning in most people' houses, or remotely controlling most household or office appliances. Probably even more revolutionary, technology has improved communications, in the work environment as well as for personal and social purposes, and it has given access to a variety of sources of information and entertainment, e.g. through the continuous improvement in the quality and availability of appliances and services, and the access to a broad selection of contents, which are increasingly available through online streaming. The most recent frontier in the application of modern communication and information technologies allows the integration of various technologies that were initially developed in different fields as independent, standalone applications. All these changes have considerably simplified one's life through a combination of effects.[1] For example, one can nowadays perform a number of activities remotely, from investing in the stock market to controlling the temperature of their home and optimizing its energy consumption based on their real-time schedule (and any fine adjustments to it), through a smartphone app, independently from where they are. They can perform these activities while they ride in a taxi or a car provided by some *ride-sourcing* services such as Uber or Lyft, on the way to dinner (which they have also booked through a dedicated app on their mobile device). They contemporaneously maintain real-time communications with the friends they are supposed to meet for dinner through some instant messaging services, and micromanage the details of their appointment (place to meet and time of arrival), minimizing the waiting time, and accommodating any eventual disruptions (e.g. due to travel delays, etc.). Such types of behavior are becoming increasingly common at least for the majority of

[1]Technology can also make someone's life more complicated, due to the need to learn how to use new technologies and services, the increased number of available activities and services, and the related burden on one's time.

"tech-savvy" users, for whom it is even difficult to imagine a time in which technology did not permeate society as it currently does.

The increased computational power and miniaturization of modern computer processors, the development and application of increasingly cheap and reliable sensors, the adoption of global positioning system (GPS) geolocation technologies, and the access to powerful and reliable communication networks have forever transformed society. They have enabled us to live in a way that would have been barely imaginable to previous generations. The continuous developments in the field of *domotics* are further modifying individuals' life: the path towards a *smart home* paves the way to a future in which common household appliances make large use of automation and electronic technologies, and are increasingly connected through fast and reliable communication technologies. Similarly, technological development is deeply changing the *work* environment. It is also rapidly transforming the features of most vehicles, in a continuous race to improve travel safety, security, comfort and ability to carry out many activities in a variety of conditions. The ubiquitous presence of information and communications technologies has revolutionized individuals' behavior through the ability (and related expectations) to be continuously connected to others.[2]

ICT applications considerably reshape the relationships with time and space. As they simplify the execution of many tasks, they make it easy to engage in additional activities in the same unit of time. Similarly, they often reduce the friction of distance, making travel easier, and letting information and news circulate over long distances in shorter (or almost no) time. The increased presence of ICT devices and services also expands the set of known and available choices in most decision processes, and it increases the amount of related accessible information. Thus, technology enables individuals to access options that would have otherwise been unavailable, or too difficult (and expensive) to access, or of which they would have ignored the existence, if modern information and communication technologies did not exist.

The adoption of ICT solutions is modifying individual lifestyles through several subtle modifications to the organization of work and leisure activities, and the social habits of individuals. Larger effects are associated with specific segments of the population, such as younger and better-educated individuals, and those that live in central regions and cities, who have access to more options, i.e. they are exposed to a larger number of technological innovations.

The effects of the adoption of ICT on individual choices and mobility patterns are not fully understood, and still largely unclear. Numerous studies have investigated the impact of ICT on lifestyles and mobility. Early studies shared an optimistic view that most ICT applications would have contributed to enriching one's life, while at the same time they would have reduced total travel, thus bringing

[2]In this chapter, I generically refer to "others" as either other people (e.g. family members, friends, co-workers) or things (e.g. cell phones, TVs and other home appliances, personal vehicles, office and work networks).

some environmental benefits through the substitution of physical travel with technological alternatives. The reality is, however, more complex: ICT certainly contributes to increasing the amount of options available to users when they perform many activities, and has significantly changed the quality and nature of many of these options, allowing the physical replacement of travel with technological alternatives. It also enables a considerable amount of additional activities, and opportunities to engage in them, which did not exist in the past.[3] This also includes the increased need to travel.

6.2 Impact of ICT on Society

The adoption of modern information and communication technologies is generating sizable impacts on many components of modern life. It contributes to changing the organization of the work environment, including office and retail space, and affects the organization of cities and regions and the logistics of good distribution. In addition, communication technologies are reshaping many aspects of individuals' lives, including the way they interact in real time, and access information through new media.

During the last few years, in particular, *online social networks* have acquired an important role in society. The quick growth in the popularity of services such as Facebook, Twitter, and LinkedIn, which have become a popular presence with a user base that includes millions of individuals in every world region, has contributed to restructuring time use and interpersonal relationships, and has affected countless daily choices that people make. The ability to be constantly "connected" (and the related expectation to do so) is revolutionizing many familiar aspects of social and economic life, with impacts on the mobility of people and goods that are still often unclear. ICTs, and social networks in particular, are also reshaping many aspects of political and social life, often modifying the language of the political debate, and increasing the opportunities, and interest, for civic engagement of some groups, e.g. younger adults, who are heavier users of these technologies. Telecommunications increase the coverage and the speed with which news reaches voters and the general public audience. They have changed the political agenda of parties and leaders, and the way they communicate. Online social media, in particular, with their continuous stream of news, the easy sharing of comments and videos, and the amplification of public excitement, disappointment, disapproval and blame, have already established an important role in political processes. Understanding the specific role of these technologies and services, and their outcomes, is not easy, as it comprises a complex pattern of direct and indirect effects. Among the more direct, and visible, effects, is the rise of grassroots movements

[3]This fact, per se, could be interpreted as a positive contribution to the quality of life of most individuals that have access to these modern solutions.

and the emergence of candidates and leaders who share a stronger engagement with the masses of active social media users, and directly use these technologies to spread their message and increase their consensus. Telecommunications and social media also have a more subtle effect, modifying the political agenda of many parties and candidates, as an effect of the feedback obtained from online platforms, organized groups and the general public.[4]

Finally, ICTs affect the political process and public decision-making in a more indirect way, for example, through their effects on the outcomes of general and local elections, with the prevailing of certain candidates and parties who are more able to adjust to social media and are more at ease in communicating their message through these communication channels. This in turn affects the political agenda of governments, for example, in terms of foreign policies, immigration, and infrastructure investments. In the transportation sector, it has important consequences in terms of the delicate (and/or more polarizing) decisions related e.g. to the funding of public transportation, and the delivery of important infrastructure such as high-speed rail systems, or mass transportation in metropolitan areas, vs. the prioritization of road infrastructure investments.

Similar changes are happening in the economy, with ICT playing an important role in assisting and promoting economic development. In almost every field of the economy, those businesses that have easily adjusted to a modern internet-based reality, and were more able to harvest the many opportunities enabled by modern ICTs, have reinforced their presence in the market, while other players have gone out of business or are slowly disappearing. Further, the equilibrium among the various sectors of the economy has changed as a result of the development of modern information and communication technologies, and the production and distribution of related products and services. More traditional economic fields have been shrinking: they have heavily modified the nature of their production, or have increasingly relocated to other regions or countries, where the lower labor costs still make their activity economically sustainable.[5] This has led to the rise of entirely new sectors in the economy, e.g. companies specialized in IT hardware and software, smartphone apps, and the production of internet and other media content. It has also contributed to reshaping the physical patterns of development,

---

[4]An important role in any political campaign is nowadays played by experts in public relations, as well as polling and online media consultants, who explore the trends in the electoral basis, and analyze the popularity of the political message. They recommend ways in which a candidate should address specific topics, or should communicate (keeping in high consideration the messages received from the political base and general audience) through popular online social networks such as Facebook and Twitter.

[5]Also in the case of delocalization to remote regions or foreign countries, as discussed in more details in the following sections, ICTs play a central role in allowing firms to maintain communications among the members of a geographically distributed partnership, and between the central offices located in major cities and the remote production centers housed in the other regions (or countries) where labor (and other production) costs are lower.

with the impressive growth of some cities and regions and the decline of more traditional industrial centers.[6]

As one of the effects of the adoption of technological solutions, including computers, smartphones, other technological devices and internet-based services, modern lifestyles in the first part of the 21st century considerably rely on the provision of efficient and reliable high-speed transmission and digital networks (Audirac 2005; Tranos et al. 2013). These often provide a way to circumvent the lack of physical accessibility in those locations that are not easy to reach by traditional transportation modes, or because of physical limitations of an individual. The massive adoption of modern technologies, smartphones and online services generates a new type of *virtual accessibility*. The few places that are left outside of this network and communication grid (e.g. because of topography, or the high investments to connect them) become less desirable, and disadvantaged, in a world that is dominated by fast and reliable communications. This factor also opens additional business opportunities, aimed at overcoming these limitations, through providing increased access to WiFi and cellular networks in areas that are not reached by other technological networks (landline phones, cable connections), or when traveling (e.g. on planes, trains or buses).

6.3 Impact of ICT on Long-Term Decisions

At the time this book was printed, the access to online social media and communication technology played an important role in shaping the response to emergencies and humanitarian crisis in areas that are torn by civil war, political turmoil and instability. The recent flow of refugees escaping from the war zone in the Middle East and trying to reach Europe (and, to a less visible scale, any migration flows in other parts of the world) has been considerably shaped by the rise of social media, and the access to online information and wireless communications, as an important characteristic of this massive international migration. Probably for the first time in history, wireless communications and real-time information provided by other friends and members of an online network of contacts have been guiding thousands of refugees through their journey, crossing entire regions on foot, or by other informal transportation options. Modern migrants rely on cell phones, instant-messaging apps, and online mapping services to navigate themselves through a complex pattern of topographic, natural and political difficulties. Similarly, the response from many governments, informing the refugees and migrants about the policies that are available to them (or that sometimes are

[6]An emblematic sign of the changes in economic activity associated with the rise of modern technologies is signaled by the rise of San Francisco and the Silicon Valley as one of the main cores of innovation and production of advanced hi-tech services and products, with the contemporaneous decline of Detroit, the former capital of the U.S. auto industry.

designed to keep them away), has been largely organized, and communicated to the public, through online social media, further affecting the migration flows and the movements of masses of refugees in search for freedom and a shelter from persecution and war.

Even in times of peace, and during more conventional migration processes, ICT plays an important role in affecting relocation patterns and decisions on where to live. Migration decisions are usually well-informed rational choices among economic opportunities at various locations (Yankow 2003), which are affected by interpersonal networks, environmental considerations and the available information about the destination options. In the era of massive access to the internet and widespread adoption of ICT devices, modern technologies play an important role in all major phases of the migration process (Villhelmson and Thulin 2013; Dekker et al. 2015). They act as an enabler or *catalyst*, reinforcing the propensity to migrate of an individual, or stimulating the desire in making such long-term and life changing decisions in other individuals, through the increased access to information (*augmented awareness*) and increased knowledge, as well as through affecting personal tastes and decisions with multiple composite impacts (Stevenson 2009; Villhelmson and Thulin 2013).

The widespread adoption of mobile phones, email messages, instant messaging, live chat, and online social networks enables a socially and spatially extended network of friends, family, acquaintances, and colleagues, which reinforces organizational and interpersonal ties, connects local labor markets, and channels immigrants to particular destinations and into particular occupations. These tools help nourish old ties between immigrants and their places of origin, and develop new ties in their new places. They also support temporary migration decisions (e.g., for education or temporary employment), in particular among the most dynamic segments of the population, and increase the level of satisfaction among such *connected migrants* (Komito 2011).

ICTs also affect other important individuals' long-term decisions, as in the case of residential location, through affecting both the decision *process*, i.e. the way in which an individual accesses information and makes a decision, and the *outcome*, i.e. the actual location or housing unit where an individual (or household) decides to relocate. ICT also increases the flexibility in the choice of the place where to relocate, e.g. through the increased adoption of telecommuting and other remote connectivity-based options (e.g. e-shopping), which can reduce the friction of distance, and eventually allow some individuals to relocate further away from the places where they need to commute or travel for other purposes. This process increases the ability to accommodate household members' needs, while fulfilling their preferences, for example, for larger, cheaper, or simply different lots or housing units, or their desire to be located near vibrant parts of a city/region or other amenities (Mokhtarian et al. 2004; Nijkamp and Salomon 1989).

6.4 ICT and Urban Form

The adoption of modern information and communication technologies is leading to the gradual modification of a number of relationships behind the current spatial form of cities. It affects the organization of productive activities, and modifies the distance constraints that limit the mobility of people and goods. Historically, technology has contributed to the process of *time-space convergence*, allowing for the contraction of the average travel times to reach a destination (Janelle and Gillespie 2004). It has also expanded the number of destinations that can be reached in a certain unit of time. More recently, ICT has contributed to further relaxing the space-time constraints, through the ability of telecommunications to (at least partially) compensate for physical distance. Physical proximity is thus a less binding constraint for the location of residences and activities at a time "when dominant forces such as globalization and telecommunications seem to signal that place and the details of the local no longer matter" (Sassen 2000, p. 144). The impact of ICT on urban geography has led some to even hypothesize the "end of geography" (O'Brien 1992), and the "death of distance" (Craincross 2001).

Quantifying the effects of ICT on urban geography is not easy: modern telecommunication services can help firms and residences move to places where land is cheaper or where amenities are more attractive, and this may lead to a decrease in urban density, although the effects could vary significantly by region, and with the *scale* of the local economies and local conditions (Nijkamp and Salomon 1989). This would cause negative environmental effects of travel behavior, as lower-density development is usually associated with greater distances traveled, and a reduction in urban density leads to higher reliance on private vehicles (Ewing and Cervero 2010).

One effect of ICT on work organization is associated with the ability for firms to change their structure, in particular moving production activities and back offices farther away from the central business district to locations where land (and/or labor) is cheaper. Only higher-paying and white-collar jobs, management activities and the front offices that need closer interactions with customers remain in central locations. The adoption of modern and reliable telecommunication services allows firms to maintain regular communications and coordination of activities among the central offices and the production sites (and back offices) that relocate to more distant locations. Further, by loosening the effects of distance, ICT can support the rise of spatially distributed work teams and enable larger spatial separation between the manufacturing sites and the end use of goods.

The advent of information and communication technologies is also deeply revolutionizing the relationship of individuals with shopping and, to a wider extent, the entire organization of retail activities. Online shopping already accounts for a sizable percentage of total sales, and its importance continues to increase steadily every year. In the US, the total volume of e-shopping sales has increased from $138 billion in 2007 to $305 billion in 2014. The recent introduction of smartphone apps and additional user-friendly solutions for e-shopping that provide users with increased opportunities to access online retailers and obtain the purchased items in a fast and convenient way is contributing to further boosting sales and the total volume of business for this economic sector.

The rise of internet shopping has also brought important changes in the organization of traditional retail. On one hand, hybrid forms of "bricks and clicks" stores have emerged, in order to integrate internet sales in the business of more traditional retailers.[7] Further, the advent of internet shopping has deeply modified the nature, and organization, of retail itself. The adoption of technological solutions has modified the nature of many products, as in the case of the dematerialization of books, CDs, and DVDs, which have been gradually replaced by their digital alternative, and by the introduction of online streaming. For other products and services, the large adoption of internet services has deeply changed the channel through which these goods and services are purchased, as in the case of airline tickets, or banking and insurance services, for which the internet has largely replaced purchases made over the phone, or in person at traditional stores and offices. The introduction of modern information and communication technologies has also contributed to reshaping the structure of many physical stores, which have increasingly evolved into entertainment centers that include restaurants, cafes, space for cultural attractions and social gathering, etc., and thus provide additional services that are less amenable to substitution, and thus less subject to the competition of internet shopping.

Through all the changes discussed above, ICTs contribute to changing the urban form, through a process that according to many authors may contribute to further increasing the decentralization of cities, due to the reduction in the importance of physical proximity, and the increase in the importance of technological substitutes. In addition, the application of ICT is transforming the organization of many activities in cities through a number of additional effects, which modify the number of alternatives available to individuals, as well as the characteristics of transportation options, and the way to organize personal schedules. The following sections discuss in more details the changes that ICT brings to daily choices and many individual decisions related to transportation.

6.5 ICT and Mobility

Understanding the impact of information and communication technologies on transportation is not easy. ICTs include numerous and diverse applications: in this chapter, I primarily refer to goods and services involved in the production, collection, storage, analysis and/or transmission of information in electronic form,

[7]To date, all large retailers, and many smaller companies, have an internet presence, which compete with giant online retailers, such as Amazon.com, and e-shopping portals, such as E-bay.com, among others.

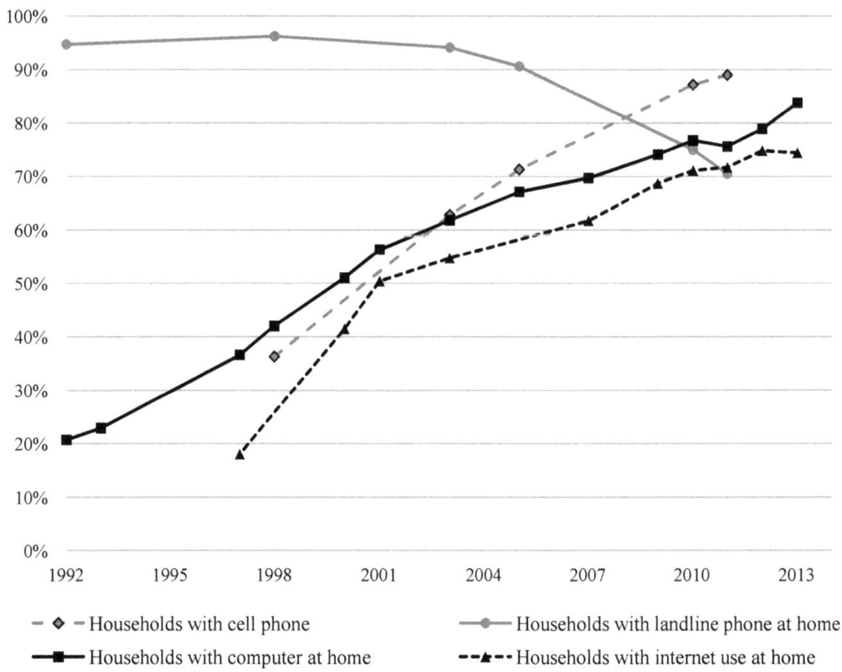

Fig. 6.1 Percentage of U.S. households using various types of technologies at home: 1990 to 2013 (*Source* Modified from Circella and Mokhtarian, forthcoming. Data from the U.S. Census Bureau)

whether ranging from end-user applications such as smartphones, tablets and computers to network-services that are used to exchange communication and information among users (and/or things, or businesses). The adoption of modern forms of information and communication technologies has experienced a rapid increase during the last few years. In general, more advanced technologies have quickly conquered a large number of users, sometimes substituting for the use of older-generation technologies (as in the case of the use of landline vs. mobile cell phones among US households, shown in Fig. 6.1).

To date, smartphones and internet connections have become a common presence in the life of most American households. The same happens in other developed and (increasingly so) developing countries. The latter, in particular, have experienced a rapid growth in the adoption of some types of technology, e.g. mobile phones and more recently smartphones, which have helped them fill a gap in the availability of communication technologies. In all geographical contexts, the adoption of communication technologies has contributed to reshaping daily habits, the participation in activities and individual lifestyles, in particular through the increased access to multiple services and the easy share of information with others. Overall, technology has increased the flexibility with which many activities can be carried out.

The adoption of modern information and communication technologies can lead to a complex pattern of eventually counteracting effects on transportation. The replacement of travel with ICT alternatives has long been seen as a promising solution to many societal problems, including traffic congestion, air pollution, greenhouse gas emissions, the reduced economic opportunities for the mobility-limited, and the need to improve individuals' work-life balance (Salomon 1998; Mokhtarian et al. 2005). ICTs certainly replace a lot of travel, but they can also generate additional travel as well. ICTs modify an individual's time-space constraints, and affect the participation in activities and travel behavior in a number

Table 6.1 Impacts of ICT on travel

Neutrality	Complementarity	Substitution
Not all ICT-based activities reduce travel: 1. Not all activities have an ICT counterpart 2. Even when an ICT alternative exists, it might not be practically feasible 3. Even when feasible, ICT might be not a desirable substitute 4. Travel carries a positive utility per se, not just as a means to access places 5. Not all uses of ICT constitute a replacement for travel	ICT actively increases travel: 6. ICT saves time and/or money for other activities, some of which involve travel 7. ICT permits travel to be sold more cheaply 8. ICT increases the efficiency of transportation (and its attractiveness) 9. Personal ICT increases the productivity and enjoyment of travel (thus it decreases its disutility) 10. ICT directly stimulates travel, through its ability to stimulate communications and transactions 11. ICT enables new travel options (e.g. shared mobility services, or connected and autonomous vehicles) which might induce additional travel demand 12. ICT is an engine driving the globalization of commerce 13. ICT facilitates shifts to more decentralized and lower-density land use patterns	ICT activities may reduce travel: 14. ICT may directly substitute for making a trip 15. ICT activities consume time and/or money that could be spent on travel 16. When travel becomes costly, difficult or dangerous, ICT substitution increases 17. ICT can make shared means of transportation more attractive 18. ICT can reduce unnecessary travel (e.g. browsing items online, and reducing trips to stores)

Source Created by the author, based on Mokhtarian (2009)
Note In addition to the effects listed above, ICT might modify the characteristics of existing travel (*modification*), e.g. affecting the choice of a trip destination, or mode choice, or causing the replacement of a trip made for one purpose (e.g. fewer commute trips due to the adoption of telecommuting) with trips made for other purposes (e.g. trips to meet a new client that was acquired through the use of ICT)

of ways (Schwanen and Kwan 2008; Circella and Mokhtarian, forthcoming): they relax some constraints, while imposing some new ones.

Mokhtarian (2009) discusses several ways in which ICTs affect mobility. Depending on the situation, ICTs can have no relevant effect on travel (*neutrality*), generate new travel (*complementarity*), modify the characteristics of travel that would have happened anyway (*modification*), or reduce travel (*substitution*). Table 6.1 summarizes numerous ways in which ICT affects travel.

The overall impacts of ICT on travel depend on a number of local conditions, and can involve a complex combination of several of the (often counteracting) effects listed in Table 6.1. At the disaggregate level, various forms of ICTs are responsible for different effects on individual choices. The following section discusses some of the likely impacts of ICTs on the everyday choices related to the participation in activities and travel.

6.6 ICT and Individual Travel Behavior

Information and communication technologies have brought a number of modifications to individual behaviors, through their revolutionary impacts on the way individuals work, socialize and travel. The previous sections have already discussed how ICTs have an important impact on work organization and the office environment, the shopping experience and retail organization, and more in general how they contribute to reshaping the relationships with space and time, increasing the opportunities for extended forms of team work and social networking opportunities also over long distances. ICTs reduce (though do not eliminate) the physical constraints of distance, reducing the importance of proximity to the work place, and central parts of cities, or to the other members of one's social network. Further, they increase the ability to remain in contact with a geographically-dispersed network of contacts, and increase the ability to access (and exchange) information at distance, thus affecting migration and relocation processes. Further, they increase the flexibility in the choice of residential location of individuals and households. As discussed in the next section of this chapter, modern information and communication technologies have given rise to a number of new mobility services and solutions that reduce the reliance on private vehicle ownership, and might affect medium-term choices such as a household's decision on the number of vehicles to own. In addition, ICTs affect a number of additional choices that individuals make on a daily basis, and affect individual' lifestyles and participation in activities. In particular, the adoption of ICT can have a number of effects on various components of travel-related decision processes.

Specifically for *business travel*, ICT has long been attributed a role in replacing some portion of business-related travel, due to the adoption of virtual alternatives (e.g. teleconferencing). Certainly, ICT does substitute for some portion of business and work-related trips, while at the same time it generates additional opportunities and needs for travel (for the reasons reported in Table 6.1). In particular, travel substitution with ICT alternatives becomes particularly attractive (and allows individuals and businesses to maintain contact with clients and other peers) also at times in which travel becomes particularly dangerous, difficult or impossible. Business travel has continued to grow in recently years, and will likely continue to grow during a time in which the world becomes increasingly globalized, and the adoption of technology and the movement of goods and people become easier and cheaper: business people travel ever farther and more frequently to develop new clients and serve existing ones (Mokhtarian 2009). The increased adoption of technology is causing several modifications in the nature and characteristics of business travel, though. A number of scholars have commented, for example, on how teleconferencing, and ICT in general, substitutes for some types of face-to-face interaction, e.g. replacing intra-company business trips. However, it does not substantially reduce and often stimulates a growth in other types of trips, e.g. meetings with new clients located in more remote locations that have been acquired through the use of ICT (Denstadli et al. 2012; Circella and Mokhtarian, forthcoming).

With regards to *commuting*, ICT solutions (predominantly, the ability to telecommute) have the potential to significantly affect individuals' commuting patterns. Several studies have investigated the impact of telecommuting on travel: telecommuting offers increased flexibility in the organization of individuals' activities, as well as increased flexibility in the choice of residential location, with larger opportunities to accommodate the needs of the partner, children and other household members. The literature has long debated on the dominant impact of telecommuting on the amount of travel, depending on the different types of telecommuters, e.g. *substituters* (who replace an entire commute trip with working remotely from home or another location), *complementers* (who work at home in addition to the regular hours worked in the office or other work location), *remote back-office workers*, etc. Accordingly, telecommuting can generate a complex mix of multifaceted effects on travel. It provides the ability to replace a work trip with working remotely, but also increases the flexibility in the choice of home locations farther away from work and central locations of a city, which might generate longer (even if less frequent) commuting trips. It also enables telecommuters to engage in additional home-based travel for other purposes during a day (Mokhtarian and Tal 2013; Circella and Mokhtarian, forthcoming). To date, the evidence indicates that telecommuting tends to reduce total travel, even if by a small degree (Choo and Mokhtarian 2005; Helminen and Ristimäki 2007), while it generates additional effects in terms of changes in travel mode, route, and departure time of trips (Downs 2005).

ICT certainly affects the generation and characteristics of *leisure trips*, and the participation in many social activities. Early research in this field suggested that ICT might substitute for some leisure trips, through consuming time and resources that would have been otherwise devoted to the participation in social activities and physical travel. However, the majority of recent research supports the opposite conclusion: the adoption of modern communication technologies and online social networks tends to increase the number of choice options for leisure activities available to an individual, the motivation to participate in them, and the opportunities for travel. Overall, a greater adoption of internet-based activities is usually associated with more time spent with friends and acquaintances, thus complementing the amount of total travel and not reducing it (Robinson and Martin 2010). Online social networks and improved mobile telecommunications also affect how leisure activities, and trips, are organized. They allow micro-coordination of time and location for social gatherings and last-minute schedule adjustments. Thus, they make it easier to engage in trips that otherwise would have not been made (Circella and Mokhtarian, forthcoming), and influence trip objectives and purposes, mode choice, origins and destinations, and the specific route that is chosen for a trip (Kellerman 2009).

As Mokhtarian and Tal (2013, p. 250) point out, "the same types of roles of ICT generally apply across destination, mode, and route choices": ICT can serve as inspiration, information provider, explanatory variable, and/or as one of the alternatives. ICT also influences decisions related to the time and duration of activities, through the related mechanisms of fragmentation and multitasking (Circella and Mokhtarian, forthcoming):

- *Destination choice*: ICT provides an important channel for acquiring information about potential destinations of a trip. It affects individuals' choices through the increased awareness about the available destinations, it makes it possible to compare the information on a variety of candidate destinations for a given activity (e.g., eating out) and it provides information about how to reach these destinations, contact the vendor/service provider, and make instant reservations. Further, ICT provides access to travel information to reach a destination, making it possible to make adjustments before and during a trip, also as an effect of the reaction to temporary conditions (e.g. traffic congestion, temporary street closures) and coordination with other members of one's social network. ICT also provides a number of opportunities to affect travelers' choices through the availability of internet-based and location-based marketing, online reviews of commercial facilities and companies, instant-sharing of videos and photos, and GPS-enabled location and navigation services.
- *Mode choice*: ICT can make the choice of specific modes more convenient and appealing to travelers, e.g. through the access to information on traffic conditions, and travel time and costs for each specific mode through smartphone apps and advanced traveler information systems. For example, the availability of real-time accurate information on waiting time and expected in-vehicle time at public transportation stops or before the beginning of a trip can make traveling by transit more appealing (Watkins et al. 2011). ICT also affects the subjective evaluation and rating of different travel modes, making some transportation modes (e.g. cycling) more popular among the members of some specific groups of users, or in certain segments of the population that are more exposed to peers' influence or targeted campaigns. It can also provide specific benefits associated with the adoption of specific travel solutions, as in the case of the ability to work productively using ICT devices while riding transit. The possibility to increase the *utility* (or reduce the *disutility*) of travel time might

significantly enhance travelers' experience and become a factor in the choice of the travel mode to use for a trip. Thus, travelers might be willing to travel by public transportation even at the expense of longer total travel time, if they can make positive use of their time while traveling or while waiting at a terminal (Malokin et al. 2015; Dong et al. 2015). Finally, ICT offers increased opportunity for the adoption of new technology-based transportation solutions and travel modes, as in the case of new shared-mobility and ride-matching services, contributing to shifting modal distribution in particular among those individuals, such as younger adults, who are more familiar with these technologies (Circella et al. 2016).

- *Route Choice*: ICTs, and advanced traveler information systems, have a strong role in affecting route choice before and during a trip, and in prompting a route change, for example, in case of heavy traffic congestion or temporary road closures. They might also serve an inspirational role, affecting the selection of the travel route, for example in the case of scenic routes, or historical or cultural interests. Finally, ICT can affect the trip experience of passengers, for example through entertainment systems that deflect attention from the unpleasantness of an unappealing route.
- *Fragmentation of activities*: ICT promotes the blurring of space-time boundaries between and among activities associated with home, work, shopping, and entertainment, and an increased fragmentation of activities in time and space (Couclelis 2004; Hubers et al. 2008). Increased fragmentation usually implies a shorter duration of the fragments of time dedicated to the activities, but a higher number of activities (e.g. increased opportunities to communicate with a larger network of peers through instant messaging), which may generate a larger number of trips, for those activities that cannot be carried out "virtually". Further, a number of additional technological solutions, from the "nanny-cam" and medical-alert systems to daily blogs and frequent tweets, help reassure a traveler that all is well at home and conversely (White and White 2007). At the margin, this process supports travel that might otherwise have been suppressed in favor of staying home (Mascheroni 2007, Circella and Mokhtarian, forthcoming), and modifies the characteristics of those trips that would have been made even if ICTs were not available.

6.7 Shared Mobility Services

Technological innovations have also allowed the growth of new mobility services that are quickly reshaping the transportation sector. The massive adoption of ICT combined with the continuously increasing number of smartphone applications provides a great opportunity for users to access transportation services long imagined but never deployed on a large scale. These services, which combine the benefits of modern communication technologies with the principles of the sharing economy, provide access to a number of mobility options without bearing the costs of owning a vehicle. They can affect key factors affecting travel decisions including travel cost, convenience and security (Taylor et al. 2015). Over longer horizons, the adoption of these services can affect the level of auto ownership of a household, and impact daily schedules, lifestyles, and even residential location. Modern shared mobility services range from *car-sharing* services, including fleet-based round-trip or one-way services (such as Zipcar or Car2Go, in the U.S. market) and peer-to-peer services (such as Turo), to *ridesharing* services, including dynamic *carpooling* (such as Carma, among others) and on-demand ride services (also known as *ridesourcing* or *transportation network companies*, or TNCs, such as Uber and Lyft), and *bike-sharing* services.

The range and availability of shared-mobility services is continuous evolving, and new services and related smartphone apps are introduced almost on a daily basis. Hallock and Inglis (2015) found that 19 of 70 U.S. major cities already have access to nearly all new mobility options included in their review. In addition, 35 other cities have access to most emerging transportation options (but not all), leaving only 16 cities where few technology-enabled transportation options are available. Although the share of total trips made with new shared-mobility services is still rather small, the foreseeable increase in the popularity of these services is expected to cause large effects on future passenger travel. According to the Special Report 319 from the U.S. Transportation Research Board (Taylor et al. 2015), numerous social and environmental effects may derive from the adoption of these services, depending on the regulations and policies that are enacted.

There is no doubt about the potential revolutionary effect that these new mobility services can have on travel behavior. The new services expand the set of choices available to travelers, and can affect key travel-related decisions and the way individuals evaluate factors such as travel cost, convenience and security (Taylor et al. 2015). The effects of emerging transportation and shared mobility services may significantly vary based on the characteristics of each type of service, the local context in which the service is provided, the characteristics of the different groups of users, and the eventual behaviors observed among different subsets of the population. New shared-mobility services may expand the set of choices available to users. They provide a valid alternative to the use of private cars, and may contribute to reducing car ownership and VMT, or stimulate additional demand for trips that would have not been made if these services were not available. Under some circumstances, they can boost transit ridership by better serving the first and last mile, improving the experience of riding transit services (Hallock and Inglis 2015; Shaheen et al. 2015; Taylor et al. 2015), or providing the availability of a ride home outside the hours of operation of public transit or at a time in which traveling by transit and/or walking to/from the transit stops may be considered unsafe (Circella et al. 2016).

The adoption of new shared-mobility services may vary significantly among members of different segments of the population. Not surprisingly, young adults (also known as *millennials*) are reported to be the most frequent users of these emerging transportation options. According to a 2013 study commissioned by Zipcar, millennials are more willing than older peers to use technology-enabled

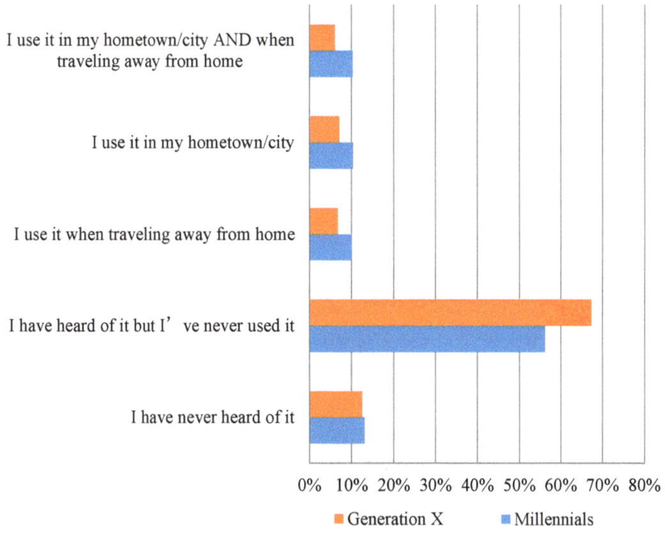

Fig. 6.2 Familiarity and usage of on-demand ride services (e.g. Uber, Lyft) among young adults ("millennials", age 18–34) and middle-age adults (members of the Generation X, age 35–50) in California (*Source* Circella et al. 2016)

transportation options. In a recent statewide study in California, Circella et al. (2016) found that millennials were consistently more likely to report higher awareness, adoption and frequency of use of all shared mobility services controlled in the study, including fleet-based car-sharing, peer-to-peer car-sharing, bike-sharing, dynamic ridesharing, and on-demand ride services (see Fig. 6.2), if compared to the members of the older Generation X that live in the same regions. Similarly, in a survey of bikesharing users in Washington D.C., Buck et al. (2013) showed that more than half of the annual members of the bikesharing program are in the age group between 25 and 34. In another study, Rayle et al. (2014) showed that the majority of the users of on-demand ride services are young and highly educated people.

Millennials are found to be heavy users of these services, possibly due to the familiarity with technological solutions in general, or because of their residential location, and the availability of new mobility options: millennials seem to be more interested in living in central, urban areas and more open to adopting alternative means of transportation. The two factors combined would mean that not only do millennials have higher accessibility to new mobility options, but when exposed to them they are also more inclined to adopt them. Overall, though, the user base of new shared-mobility services seems to be continuously growing among all age groups.

Carsharing encompasses some of the most well-known technology-enabled transportation services, which can be provided through a variety of business and operational models. While fleet-based carsharing services have achieved rather large popularity in the denser areas of major US and international cities, peer-to-peer carsharing is emerging as an important alternative because of its capability to expand the benefits of carsharing to the suburbs and to rural areas. In these areas, the lack of critical mass associated with the lower urban densities, the high proportion of home-based trips, and the higher auto-ownership rates, makes fleet-based carsharing unprofitable. Carsharing can potentially affect vehicle ownership and mode use, and influence travel behavior in a number of ways. It allows individuals to access a vehicle when needed without bearing the associated fixed costs (e.g. cost of insurance, maintenance, and long-term parking). While this effect can contribute to increasing car use among those individuals that do not feel the need to (or cannot afford to) own a car (or travel far away from the place where their personal vehicle is located), it also contributes to reducing the importance of car ownership among other users, i.e. those that already own one or more vehicles. Thus, carsharing can contribute to reducing vehicle ownership, allowing at least a portion of their users to get rid of one (or all) of their vehicles. Cervero and Tsai (2004) found that 30 % of the members of car-sharing programs were willing to sell one or more of their vehicles, while other members postponed the purchase of an additional vehicle after using carsharing services for about two years. More recently, Mishra et al. (2015) found that vehicle holding among the members of urban carsharing programs is lower by about 10–14 %, while the proportion of transit, biking and walking trips are all higher. However, the behavior of early adopters of these services may not be typical of later entrants to the car-sharing market. In another study, Martin and Shaheen (2011) surveyed members of car-sharing programs in the United States and Canada, and concluded that adding another vehicle to the fleet of shared cars would replace 9–13 privately-owned vehicles among members of car-sharing services, which might contribute to a 27–43 % reduction in vehicle miles traveled (VMT). Chatterjee et al. (2013) suggested that carsharing could enhance the access to the other modes and as a result enrich multimodality.

Bikesharing programs are becoming an increasingly popular presence in many American cities. Bikesharing provides users with on-demand access to bicycles for short-distance trips that seem too long for walking. Like carsharing, bikesharing is offered in various operational and business models, including dock-based bikesharing programs (by far the most common model of bikesharing services in large urban areas), dockless or GPS-based systems, and peer-to-peer bikesharing services. Bikesharing programs have been found to reduce driving and taxi use in almost every city in which they are available. In addition, while in small cities bikesharing tends to increase transit use through better serving the first and last mile, in large cities bikesharing may reduce transit ridership through providing a faster and cheaper travel option for many trips (Shaheen et al. 2014). Similarly, bikesharing programs may increase transit use for those living in the urban periphery, where access to public transportation by walk is limited, and decrease transit use for individuals in the urban core (Martin and Shaheen 2014).

Unlike other emerging transportation services, *ridesharing/carpooling* has always been a travel option available to travelers. Thus, the introduction of modern smartphone-based ridesharing apps has not introduced a new service or travel mode, but rather it has modified the qualities of an existing option. It changed the way travelers can match their travel needs, by helping them find other peers with whom to share a ride. Technological advances have revolutionized traditional ridesharing/carpooling by easily matching riders with drivers in real-time, or on a very short notice. Compared to traditional ridesharing, dynamic ridesharing has higher flexibility, which can improve accountability and reliability of the ridesharing services and can expand its potential markets, even for occasional non-work trips.

One of the most controversial and rapidly growing forms of shared mobility services include *on-demand ride services*, also known as *ridesourcing* or *transportation network companies* (*TNCs*), such as Uber and Lyft in the U.S. market. On-demand ride services primarily resemble taxi services, in that they connect travelers requesting a ride with the pool of drivers through a smartphone application. On-demand ride services are different from dynamic ridesharing because drivers who participate in dynamic ridesharing programs only offer rides to other travelers on the route, including small deviations from it, on which the drivers intended to travel for their own needs. The growth of TNCs has been very rapid, but the information on the effect that these services have on the use of other modes is limited. Not surprisingly, respondents who live in central urban areas (where distances are shorter, parking is more scarce, and these services are more easily available) are found to use on-demand ride services more frequently than users in more suburban or rural areas. As it is common with many technological innovations, several researchers have reported that early adopters and frequent users of these services mainly include higher-educated young adults (Rayle et al. 2014). As these services become increasingly common, future adoption rates and overall impacts on the use of other modes will depend on a number of factors, including the perceived convenience of using these services, for various categories of travelers, and whether current users will continue to use these services with the same frequency as they transition in their stages of life and move to other residential locations. It is currently difficult to ascertain how riders change their behaviors with regard to the use of other transportation modes as a result of the adoption of TNCs (Taylor et al. 2015). For example, in a recent study about millennials' mobility in California, Circella et al. (2016) found that a larger proportion of millennials (compared to the members of Generation X) reported that the overall effect of their last trip with an on-demand ride service company such as Uber or Lyft was to substitute for a trip for which they would have otherwise walked or biked. Instead, a relatively larger proportion of members of the previous Generation X reported that their Uber/Lyft trip replaced a trip that they would have made by car (Fig. 6.3).

It is reasonable to expect that shared-mobility services influence travel demand and mode choice, with their effects varying with the local context, the characteristics of the users, the land use features and the transportation alternatives that are available in each area. Newer services that allow multiple users to share a ride in the same vehicle are also being introduced in many regions: if this type of service became dominant in the field of on-demand ride services, a reduction in

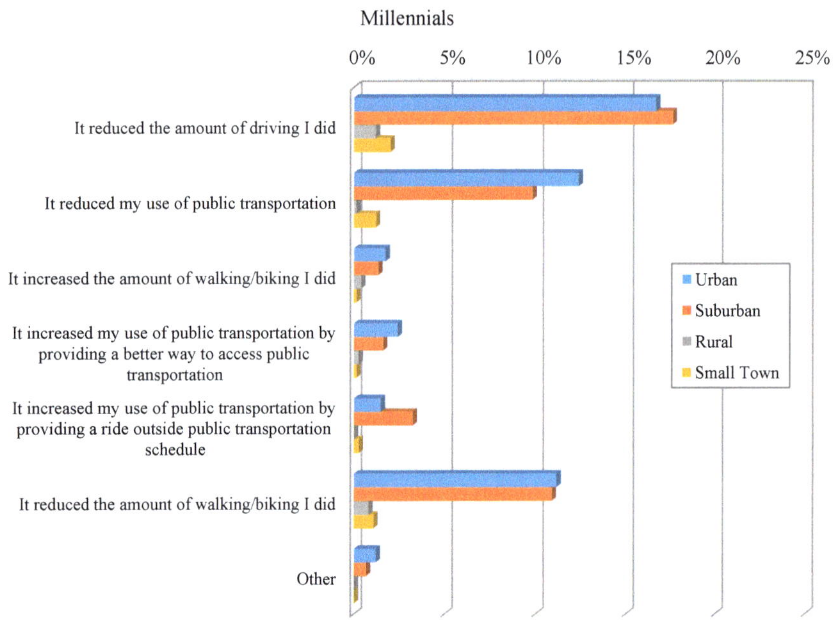

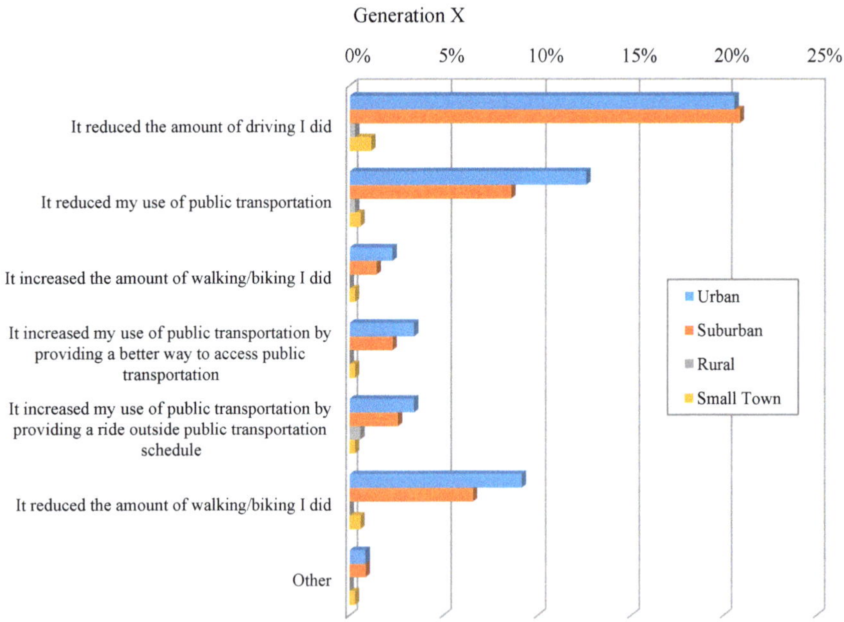

Fig. 6.3 Impact of the last trip made with Uber or Lyft on the use of other means of transportation, among young adults ("millennials", 18–34) and middle-age adults (members of the Generation X, 35–50) in California (*Source* Circella et al. 2016)

total travel could result (Taylor et al. 2015). Certainly, these emerging transportation services have the potential to change the relationships of individuals with auto ownership, and they may eventually reduce the importance of owning a private vehicle, in favor of having access to transportation options when and where needed. ICT can play an important role in making this cultural transition become reality.

6.8 ICT and the Future of Cities

Modern technologies are quickly revolutionizing the way we work, live, socialize and travel. This has forever changed the lifestyles of most individuals, and their organization of activities. The adoption of modern information and communication technologies is also contributing to reshaping cities through the reduction in the importance of physical proximity, and the increased flexibility in location choices and adoption of virtual alternatives. Modern technologies have also given rise to new technology-based services, and have helped apply the principles of the sharing economy revolutionizing several economic fields (e.g. hospitality industry) and bringing innovation to transportation through the introduction of new shared-mobility services. All these changes contribute to changing individual behaviors, preferences and habits, through a complex combination of often counteracting effects associated with the adoption of technology.

Understanding the impact that ICT will continue to have on cities is not easy: ICT is already contributing to reshaping the form of cities, eventually increasing the level of decentralization through the increased reliance on modern telecommunications. This effect, to some extent, seems to be counterbalanced by other trends happening in society. For example, at the same time in which ICTs become ubiquitously common, the process of urban decentralization is slowing down, thanks to the resurgence of downtown and other central areas of cities, and the increased demand for housing units that are located close to the most vibrant and accessible parts of cities in the United States and other developed countries (Wachs 2013). Additional changes in the form of cities will continue to happen in future years, as new technologies hit the market, and contribute to reshaping the life of millions of individuals, e.g. through the organization of *smart cities*, and the increased availability of technology-based services to a larger pool of individuals. In this continuously-changing scenario, planners and policy-makers are called to provide answers to new emerging issues associated with the *digital divide* and *social equity*, the access to new technology-based services, and the eventual gap suffered by those users who, due to personal disabilities, lack of education or economic resources, might not have sufficient access to the ICT devices and services that are quickly becoming part of the new standards of living.

In the field of transportation, additional changes will be associated with the introduction of additional transportation services. Shared-mobility services, including car-sharing, bike-sharing, and on-demand ride services such as Uber and Lyft, have already revolutionized transportation. They contribute to reducing the dependence on auto ownership in denser urban areas, potentially shifting the importance from ownership to access to transportation options.

In the future, even larger changes will be associated with the introduction of new revolutionary technologies, and in particular with the advent of connected and autonomous vehicles (AVs). The automobile industry has already made significant strides in automating driving: many current car models include features like cruise control, parking assist and other assistive technologies which are all components of what will be needed in the future for full automation of cars. Still, the mass deployment of full self-driving automation (Level 4, according to the classification of the U.S. Department of Transportation's National Highway Traffic Safety Administration) on public roads will require several more years, due to a combination of engineering, economic, and regulatory factors.

Assuming that these technologies will prove to be fully successful and become available to the mass market, subject to regulatory approval and/or any restrictions from federal, state and local agencies, AVs have the potential to dramatically change future travel patterns and individual behaviors. Among other effects, they may lead to safer roads, reduced congestion, increased network capacity, improved travel comfort, and reduced parking requirements. Connected and autonomous vehicles may provide mobility for those too young to drive, the elderly and the disabled. AVs will likely reduce the fatigue associated with driving, and increase the ability to perform activities while traveling. They will further change the way individuals organize their schedule and activity participation, and the concept of travel as a transition between different activities conducted at the origin and destination of a trip. They are expected to increase the utility of using a car, as travelers can combine the scheduling flexibility of being a driver with the comfort of riding as a passenger. Thus, AVs are likely to lower the value of travel time for car users, and affect mode choice by favoring the adoption of private vehicles for a larger number of trips at the expenses of other travel modes (Malokin et al. 2015). The adoption of AVs will likely result in higher per-capita VMT due to latent demand, and the increased utility of using a car: the increased mobility among the elderly and others, as well as lower travel efforts and congestion delays, will almost certainly lead to large increases in car travel, unless demand-management strategies are thoughtfully implemented (Fagnant and Kockelman 2015).

However, the overall effects of AVs on passenger travel will largely depend on the policies and regulations that are implemented, including, but not limited to, eventual restrictions in some portions of the road network (e.g. city centers and local roads), regulations for specific categories of users (e.g. unaccompanied minors), ownership models (e.g. personal autonomous vehicles vs. shared autonomous vehicles), traffic regulations and parking requirements (e.g. whether empty vehicles will be allowed to travel back home or will need to be parked at the final destination of a trip). Further, the use of AVs might be integrated in other transportation services: TNCs such as Uber and Lyft are already evaluating the future integration of fully autonomous vehicles into their fleets, thus revolutionizing on-demand ride services through the use of driverless shared vehicles. To date, it is still unclear when fully autonomous vehicles will become commercially available, and how quickly consumers will adopt them. Some studies predict that AVs will be an accepted technology by 2030 (or even earlier) and dominate personal transportation by 2050 (Greenblatt and Shaheen 2015). Overall, more research is needed in order to better understand the impacts of AVs on future travel, and the way the introduction of this revolutionary technology will modify the future of cities, and our life.

Acknowledgments I am deeply grateful for the support and great contributions to the content of this chapter that I received from Patricia L. Mokhtarian and Farzad Alemi.

References

Audirac I (2005) Information technology and urban form, challenges to smart growth. Int Reg Sci Rev 28(2):119–145

Buck D, Buehler R, Happ P, Rawls B, Chung P, Borecki N (2013) Are bikeshare users different from regular cyclists? A first look at short-term users, annual members, and area cyclists in the Washington, DC, region. Transp Res Rec 2387:112–119

Cairncross F (2001) The death of distance: how the communications revolution is changing our lives. Harvard Business School Press

Cervero R, Tsai Y (2004) City CarShare in San Francisco, California: second-year travel demand and car ownership impacts. Transp Res Rec 1887:117–127

Chatterjee K, Andrews G, Ricci M, Parkhurst G (2013) Qualitative insights into the effect on travel behavior of joining a carshare. Transp Res Rec 2359:76–84

Choo S, Mokhtarian PL (2005) Do telecommunications affect passenger travel or vice versa? Structural equation models of aggregate US time series data using composite indexes. Transp Res Rec 1926(1):224–232

Circella G, Fulton L, Alemi F, Berliner RM, Tiedeman K, Mokhtarian PL, Handy S (2016) What affects millennials mobility? Part I: investigating the role of environmental concerns, lifestyles, mobility-related attitudes and adoption of technology of young adults in California. National Center for Sustainable Transportation, May 2016

Circella G, Mokhtarian PL (forthcoming) Impact of information communication technology on transportation. In: Hanson S, Giuliano G (eds) Geography of Urban Transportation. The Guilford Press, New York

Couclelis H (2004) Pizza over the Internet: e-commerce, the fragmentation of activity and the tyranny of the region. Entrepreneurship Reg Dev 16(1):41–54

Dekker R, Engbersen G, Faber M (2015) The use of online media in migration networks. Population Space Place 22(6):539–551

Denstadli JM, Julsrud TE, Hjorthol RJ (2012) Videoconferencing as a mode of communication: a comparative study of the use of videoconferencing and face-to-face meetings. J Bus Tech Commun 26(1):65–91

Dong Z, Mokhtarian PL, Circella G, Allison JR (2015) The estimation of changes in rail ridership through an onboard survey: did free Wi-Fi make a difference to Amtrak's Capitol Corridor service? Transportation 42(1):123–142

Downs A (2005) Still stuck in traffic: coping with peak-hour traffic congestion. Brookings Institution Press

Ewing R, Cervero R (2010) Travel and the built environment: a meta-analysis. J Am Plann Assoc 76(3):265–294

Fagnant DJ, Kockelman K (2015) Preparing a nation for autonomous vehicles: opportunities, barriers and policy recommendations. Transp Res Part A 77:167–181

Greenblatt JB, Shaheen S (2015) Automated vehicles, on-demand mobility, and environmental impacts. Current Sustain/Renew Energy Rep 2(3):74–81
Hallock L, Inglis J (2015) The innovative transportation index: the cities where new technologies and tools can reduce your need to own a car. Frontier Group. U.S. PIEG Education Fund, February 2015
Helminen V, Ristimäki M (2007) Relationships between commuting distance, frequency and telework in Finland. J Transp Geogr 15(5):331–342
Hubers C, Schwanen T, Dijst M (2008) ICT and temporal fragmentation of activities: an analytical framework and initial empirical findings. Tijdschrift voor economische en sociale geografie 99(5):528–546
Janelle DG, Gillespie A (2004) Space-time constructs for linking information and communication technologies with issues in sustainable transportation. Transp Rev 24(6):665–677
Kellerman A (2009) The end of spatial reorganization? Urban landscapes of personal mobilities in the information age. J Urban Technol 16(1):47–61
Komito L (2011) Social media and migration: virtual community 2.0. J Am Soc Inform Sci Technol 62(6):1075–1086
Malokin A, Circella G, Mokhtarian PL (2015) How do activities conducted while commuting influence mode choice? Testing public transportation advantage and autonomous vehicle scenarios. Compendium of Papers CD-ROM, the 94th Annual Meeting of the Transportation Research Board, Washington, D.C., January 11–15
Martin E, Shaheen S (2011) The impact of carsharing on public transit and non-motorized travel: an exploration of North American carsharing survey data. Energies 4(11):2094–2114
Martin EW, Shaheen SA (2014) Evaluating public transit modal shift dynamics in response to bikesharing: a tale of two US cities. J Transp Geogr 41:315–324
Mascheroni G (2007) Global nomads' network and mobile sociality: exploring new media uses on the move. Inf Community Soc 10(4):527–546
Mishra GS, Clewlow RR, Mokhtarian PL, Widaman KF (2015) The effect of carsharing on vehicle holdings and travel behavior: a propensity score and causal mediation analysis of the San Francisco Bay Area. Res Transp Econ 52:46–55
Mokhtarian PL (2009) If telecommunication is such a good substitute for travel, why does congestion continue to get worse? Transp Lett 1(1):1–17
Mokhtarian PL, Collantes GO, Gertz C (2004) Telecommuting, residential location, and commute-distance traveled: evidence from State of California employees. Environ Plann A 36:1877–1897
Mokhtarian PL, Salomon I, Choo S (2005) Measuring the measurable: why can't we agree on the number of telecommuters in the US? Qual Quant 39(4):423–452
Mokhtarian PL, Tal G (2013) Impacts of ICT on travel behavior: a tapestry of relationships. In: Rodrigue J-P, Notteboom T, Shaw J (eds) The sage handbook of transport studies. Sage Publications, London, pp 241–260
Nijkamp P, Salomon I (1989) Future spatial impacts of telecommunications. Transp Plann Technol 13(4):275–287
O'Brien R (1992) Global financial integration: the end of geography. Council on Foreign Relations Press
Rayle L, Shaheen S, Chan N, Dai D, Cervero R (2014) App-based, on-demand ride services: comparing taxi and ridesourcing trips and user characteristics in San Francisco. University of California Transportation Center UCTC-FR-2014-08, University of California, Berkeley
Robinson JP, Martin S (2010) IT use and declining social capital? More cold water from the General Social Survey (GSS) and the American Time-Use Survey (ATUS). Soc Sci Comput Rev 28(1):45–63
Salomon I (1998) Technological change and social forecasting: the case of telecommuting as a travel substitute. Transp Res Part C 6(1):17–45
Sassen S (2000) New frontiers facing urban sociology at the Millennium. Br J Soc 51(1):143–159

Schwanen T, Kwan M-P (2008) The Internet, mobile phone and space-time constraints. Geoforum 39(3):1362–1377

Shaheen S, Chan AN, Bansal A, Cohen A (2015) Shared mobility: a sustainability and technology workshop: definition, industry development and early understanding. University of California, Berkeley

Shaheen SA, Martin EW, Cohen AP, Chan ND, Pogodzinsk M (2014) Public bikesharing in North America during a period of rapid expansion: understanding business models, industry trends & user impacts. MTI Report 12–29

Stevenson B (2009) The Internet and Job Search. NBER Chapters, 67–86

Taylor B, Chin R, Melanie C, Dill J, Hoel L, Manville M, Polzin S (2015) Special report 319: between public and private mobility: examining the rise of technology-enabled transportation services. Transportation Research Board: Committee for Review of Innovative Urban Mobility Services

Tranos E, Reggiani A, Nijkamp P (2013) Accessibility of cities in the digital economy. Cities 30:59–67

Vilhelmson B, Thulin E (2013) Does the Internet encourage people to move? Investigating Swedish young adults' internal migration experiences and plans. Geoforum 47:209–216

Wachs M (2013) Turning cities inside out: transportation and the resurgence of downtowns in North America. Transportation 40(6):1159–1172

Watkins KE, Ferris B, Borning A, Rutherford GS, Layton D (2011) Where is my bus? Impact of mobile real-time information on the perceived and actual wait time of transit riders. Transp Res Part A 45(8):839–848

White NR, White PB (2007) Home and away: tourists in a connected world. Ann Tourism Res 34(1):88–104

Yankow JJ (2003) Migration, job change, and wage growth: A new perspective on the pecuniary return to geographic mobility. J Reg Sci 43(3):483–516

Chapter 7
Health-Related Life Choices

David Pérez Barbosa and Junyi Zhang

Abstract Health has been of growing interest for professionals in a variety of disciplines, including engineers and urban planners among many others. Urban and transport policies may be interlinked with health at many levels, directly or indirectly, because connections between life choices and health may be bidirectional. A healthy life means a balanced condition of not only physical health, but also mental and social health. However, existing studies have mainly focused on the physical health and ignored the mental and social aspects in people's health-related quality of life (QOL). Therefore, this chapter makes a review of health behavior and health-related QOL with respect to health lifestyle habits, health promotion activities, active and non-active travel behavior (active travel refers to walking, bicycling and partially refers to use of transit systems), park usage, residential environment, and urban infrastructure. Lifestyle habits are reviewed by focusing on smoking, alcohol drinking, eating, sleeping, social contacts, and commuting, etc. Various future research issues are finally discussed.

Keywords Physical health · Mental health · Social health · Lifestyle habits · Stage of change model · Commuter paradox · Active travel · Residential environment · Infrastructure · Healthy city

7.1 Introduction

The World Health Organization defines health as "a state of complete physical, mental and social well-being and not merely the absence of disease or infirmity" (WHO 1948). Other conceptualizations of health include other aspects of life,

D.P. Barbosa (✉) · J. Zhang
Hiroshima University, Higashi-Hiroshima, Japan
e-mail: dapbarbosa@gmail.com

J. Zhang
e-mail: zjy@hiroshima-u.ac.jp; junyizh24@gmail.com

J. Zhang (ed.), *Life-Oriented Behavioral Research for Urban Policy*,
DOI 10.1007/978-4-431-56472-0_7

such as "being able to move about freely, enjoy food and sex, feel good, remember things, have family and friends" (Breslow 1999; Goetzel 2009).

We need to understand and examine in more detail the forms in which the health of city dwellers is linked to our environments and the life choices we are able to make within our environments. Decisions about how spaces are used and developed for residential, industrial, retail, and other facilities have impacts on the health of the people who live, work, and play within these spaces.

Spatial planning is generally considered to have positive influences on human health when facilities such as gardens or urban parks are available and measures to address overcrowding, improve sanitation, standardize and regulate construction, and control traffic have been implemented (Croucher et al. 2012). The decisions that are made about the spaces where we live and move certainly have some influence on health. However, as individuals we also make decisions about where we live and how we live (lifestyle habits), and these decisions have consequences for our health-related quality of life.

In previous studies, we observed how health-related QOL is influenced by lifestyle habits and how these in turn might be influenced by the residential environment for some groups of people, depending upon their travel behavior characteristics (Perez Barbosa et al. 2016). Lifestyle habits are influenced by the family environment and knowledge of good lifestyle habits, which usually form over a long period. It is necessary to understand how decisions about lifestyle behaviors, such as working hours and intensity, physical exercise, sleep, relaxation, recreation and leisure, communication with others (i.e., spending time with family, friends, neighbors, etc.), and use of active travel modes (walking, bicycling, and transit systems) affect health in different ways. Depending upon the importance people attach to certain life activities, they might have no motivation to change their attitude towards a healthy life (Zhang 2015).

Individual health behaviors and lifestyles are mediated by a range of external factors, including social and community influences, living and working conditions, and general socioeconomic and cultural conditions, as well as built and natural environmental conditions (Croucher et al. 2012). The life-oriented approach argues that people's decisions in various life domains (e.g., residence, neighborhood, health, education, work, family life, leisure and recreation, finances, and travel behavior) are not independent of each other and that an understanding of life choices should not be constrained by the boundary of any single discipline (Zhang 2015).

7.2 Health and Lifestyle Habits

Zeratsky (2014) mentions several of the most important habits of healthy people, including physical activity, strength and flexibility, adequate sleep, adequate portion size, contact with family and friends, preventive healthcare screenings, and addressing addictive behaviors. The importance of other habits in the spiritual sphere is usually underestimated, such as the effects of forgiveness, laughter, peace of mind, and gratitude for a good health, and there is relatively little information on these habits in the health-related scientific literature.

Exercise and physical activity are considered to be intrinsically good, and they can offer additional benefits as well, such as having fun, unwinding, being outdoors, and social interaction. Someone who finds an enjoyable physical activity and practices it every day has a better chance of feeling happy.

Generally, at least 30 min of physical activity a day is considered an acceptable, healthy activity level. More exercise or higher intensity activities are recommended for alternative purposes, such as losing weight or increasing one's fitness level.

The goal of 30 min of activity can be easily met by incorporating easy physical activities in people's daily routines, such as using stairs, walking, standing, and stretching. The use of a pedometer or other activity monitor can help people monitor their activity, and this option is available in many smartphones.

Socially, much can be done to promote physical activity. Finding a workout partner or taking fitness classes at local parks, schools, or gyms, or joining a jogging group, etc. can be very supportive and help people achieve their physical activity goals.

Apart from exercising regularly, public health officials and health care providers have stressed the critical importance of adherence to a healthy lifestyle, which includes a diet high in fruit and vegetables, avoiding or quitting smoking, and consuming alcohol in moderation (Matheson et al. 2012). These lifestyle habits are considered essential to any efforts to reduce premature morbidity and mortality.

The National Health and Nutrition Examination Survey (NHANES) III is a nationally representative survey in the United States. It has a complex sampling design that allows for weighted population estimates of the noninstitutionalized U.S. population (Matheson et al. 2012). Below, we briefly mention each of the healthy lifestyle habits.

Smoking

Smoking status was determined by self-report of current cigarette, pipe, and cigar smoking (Matheson et al. 2012).

Alcohol consumption

According to the USDA Dietary Guidelines for Americans (2005), the limits for moderate consumption of alcohol are of up to one drink per day for women and up to two drinks per day for men. As for the beneficial effects of moderate alcohol consumption, the USDA says:

> Moderate alcohol consumption may have beneficial health effects in some individuals. In middle-aged and older adults, a daily intake of one to two alcoholic beverages per day is associated with the lowest all-cause mortality. More specifically, compared to non-drinkers, adults who consume one to two alcoholic beverages a day appear to have a lower risk of coronary heart disease.

Apart from those benefits, the negative health effects of alcohol consumption that the USDA highlights include alteration in judgment, risk of dependency or addiction, and liver, pancreas, heart, and brain damage. Among other important hazards are the risks of motor vehicle accidents, other injuries, high blood pressure, stroke, violence, some types of cancer, and suicide.

Diet

The healthy eating index dataset, which contains data on the number of servings of food consumed by survey participants, indicates an intake of at least five servings of fruit and vegetables a day (Matheson et al. 2012). Consumption of fruit and vegetables is thought to protect against cancer and cardiovascular disease, and increasing this type of eating is a central objective of health promotion programs worldwide (Steptoe et al. 2003). Fruit and vegetable consumption is often found to be inversely related to socioeconomic position, and increasing the consumption of fruit and vegetables among low-income populations is recommended, as it may help to redress socioeconomic inequalities in health (UK Department of Health). The departments of health services in the United Kingdom (Public Health England) and the United States (U.S. Department of Health and Human Services) have established "five a day" programs to improve access to, and increase the consumption of, fruit and vegetables (Centers for Disease Control and Prevention, 2005). Five a day programs that target people of all ages in schools, the community, industries, restaurants, churches, and work sites, etc. can be used effectively to promote access to fruit and vegetables.

Physical activity

In some studies, level of physical activity is determined by the frequency of participation in leisure-time physical activities in the previous month (Matheson et al. 2012). Examples of these activities include walking, jogging or running, riding a bicycle or exercise bicycle, swimming, aerobic exercise, aerobic dancing, regular dancing, calisthenics, gardening or yard work, weightlifting, and other similar activities. All of these activities are listed in a *Compendium of Physical Activities*, which includes 605 different physical activities with a coding scheme that classifies physical activities by rate of energy expenditure (Ainsworth et al. 2000).

The amount of physical activity that is desirable for an individual varies among studies. Matheson et al. (2012) divided participants into two frequency groups based on whether they exercised more than 12 times a month (0–12 and >12 times per month), a threshold that was consistent with national recommendations at the time the NHANES III was conducted.

In the United States, the recommendations for dietary energy intake make use of the Estimated Energy Requirement (EER) as a key indicator, referring to calories needed for a healthy individual to maintain his or her own weight (Grosvenor and Smolin 2012). EER takes into account gender, age, height, weight, and activity intensity, etc. People can be classified into the following types based on the EER (Smolin and Grosvenor 2005).

- Sedentary type: This type refers to a person who does not participate in any activity beyond those activities required for a daily independent living, which may include—without being limited to—tasks such as gardening, walking from/to the bus, household tasks such as vacuuming or mopping, loading and unloading the car. In addition, it is assumed that people spend approximately 2.5 h per day in these types of activities.
- Low active type: A person belonging to this type participates in vigorous physical activities (e.g., aerobics, soccer, tennis, swimming, fast bicycling, fast walking, or jogging) for 15–30 min per day or moderate activities (yoga, calisthenics, golf, slow swimming, skating, or cycling leisurely) for 30–60 min per day. For example, a 70 kg adult would need to expend energy equivalent to walking 3.5 km (at 4.8–6.4 kph) in addition to the energy required for daily living activities.
- Active type: A person in this type spends 30–60 min per day in vigorous physical activities or more than 60 min per day in moderate physical activities. For example, a 70 kg adult would need to expend for walking 11 km (at 4.8–6.4 kph) in addition to the energy required for daily living activities.
- Very active type: A person in this type engages in vigorous physical activities for 1.00–1.75 h per day or in moderate activities for more than 2.00–2.50 h per day. For example, a 70 kg adult would need to expend for walking 27 km (at 4.8–6.4 kph) in addition to the energy required for daily living activities.

In the United States, it has been recommended that all citizens engage in at least 30 min of moderate-intensity activity five or more days per week, or at least 20 min of vigorous-intensity activity at least three days per week (U.S. Department of Health and Human Services 2000). These recommendations are mainly based on the benefits of regular physical activity to reduce the risks of coronary heart disease, hypertension, obesity, diabetes, osteoporosis, and mental health disorders, regardless of age. Other authors classify respondents as active if they engage in moderate intensity activity for at least half an hour a day, or at least three weekly sessions of 20 min (or more) of vigorous activity (Jimmy and Martin 2005).

The recommendation to adopt active travel (cycling and walking) as a way to exercise 30 min a day is generally encouraged by governments and institutions worldwide. Among the health benefits of daily active travel are reduced risks of coronary heart disease, non-insulin-dependent diabetes, obesity, hypertension, and colon and breast cancer. Daily active travel could also help to: maintain bone mass and protect against osteoporosis; improve balance, coordination, mobility, strength, and endurance; increase self-esteem; reduce levels of mild to moderate hypertension; and promote overall psychological well-being (WHO 2010).

The importance of adopting habits that support good health is frequently underestimated. Good sleep (regular sleep cycles and getting enough sleep), stress management, appropriate use of pharmaceuticals, access to sunlight, exercising one's mind, spiritual practices (thoughts of gratitude, meditation, appreciation, forgiveness, turning negative thoughts into positive thoughts, and becoming a more giving person, etc.), and social habits (socializing with friends, expressing positive emotions, and avoiding toxic relationships) are some habits with implications for individual and public health that should be researched in more depth.

In addition, there is still a great deal of uncertainty about how lifestyle interacts with commonly used control variables such as socioeconomic indicators or marriage (Matheson et al. 2012). Other weaknesses of the methodologies used to research lifestyles include the limited accountability for changes in lifestyle habits over time, an overreliance on the accuracy of self-reports of healthy habits, and the frequent inability to prove causation from associations between health habits and desired outcomes such as decreased mortality.

An interesting case study can be found on Okinawa Island, Japan, which is in a region that has one of the longest life expectancies in the world (81.2 years) and the lowest rates of heart disease, cancer, and stroke. These benefits can be attributed to several factors, including eating only until one is 80 % full (*Hara Hachi Bu* in Japanese), healthy and active lifestyles, low-stress environments, and a moderate diet high in soy, vegetables, and fish and low in salt and alcohol. The Okinawan Centenarian Study, which began in 1976, is an ongoing research effort to identify genetic, dietary, and lifestyle factors that contribute to healthy aging in Okinawa (Smolin and Grosvenor 2005).

At the other extreme, some studies estimate that in the United States as many as 250,000 deaths (or 12 % of the yearly mortality rate) can be attributed to physical inactivity (Brownson et al. 2007). Given the tremendous benefits of a healthy lifestyle, policies and programs that encourage adherence to healthy lifestyles should be encouraged, both locally and at the national level. In addition, Matheson et al. (2012) found that there is an evident association between healthy lifestyle habits and decreased mortality risk, regardless of baseline BMI.

The importance of regular counseling about the lifestyle adjustments needed to adopt a healthy lifestyle cannot be overstated. This is not just important for obese or overweight people, as the lack of time spent counseling patients to adopt healthy lifestyles has been raised as a general concern, and research suggests that the failure to counsel people about healthy behaviors is common. This lack of emphasis on counseling is particularly troubling because counseling has been shown to be effective in decreasing smoking, increasing fruit and vegetable consumption, moderating alcohol consumption, and increasing the frequency of exercise (Matheson et al. 2012).

Future projects to develop and disseminate physical activity counseling schemes should encourage different groups of physicians to discuss physical activity with their patients and provide them with assessment tools that yield more accurate measures of their physical activities (Jimmy and Martin 2005).

The awareness that physical inactivity is a key public health issue is growing and bringing more attention to epidemics such as obesity. At the same time, researchers are increasingly acknowledging that primary care physicians have a key role to play in the health of the population (Eakin et al. 2004).

7.2.1 Stage of Change Model

People vary in their readiness to make healthy changes such as eating more fruit and vegetables, stopping smoking, or increasing leisure time physical activity. Steptoe et al. (2003) have suggested that the most suitable methods of encouraging and sustaining behavior changes have five stages:

- Precontemplation—The person does not intend to change his/her behavior in the foreseeable future (for example, the person was not thinking of eating more fruit and vegetables).
- Contemplation—The person is aware of the problem and is seriously thinking about changing but has not yet made a commitment to take action and is not confident of being able to sustain a change in behavior (for example, the person was thinking about eating more fruit and vegetables, but either he/she was not intending to do so in the next month or he/she was not confident of being able to stick to the plan).
- Preparation—The person is seriously planning to take action in the next month and is confident of success (for example, the person was thinking about eating more fruit and vegetables and was confident that he/she could do so in the next month).
- Action—The person successfully modified his/her behavior within the past six months.
- Maintenance—The person has maintained the behavior change for at least six months.

Future work should investigate methods for improving the initiation and sustained delivery of physical activity counseling in primary care, as well as the impact of improving links between primary care and community support for physical activity (Eakin et al. 2004). Such counseling need not be limited to physical activity, as it would be appropriate for primary care providers to counsel people about modifying any number of health-related behaviors, including smoking, physical activity, and diet (Sciamanna et al. 2004).

On the other hand, the poor dissemination of evaluation research and policy advocacy is onc of thc factors limiting the impact of evidence-based physical activity interventions on public health. There is a need to collaborate with policy experts from other fields to improve the interdisciplinary science base for diffusion and dissemination (Owen et al. 2006). Although existing health promotion diffusion and dissemination models are valuable, they are limited because they do not provide sufficient guidance for dissemination (Owen et al. 2006).

Although diffusion and dissemination research is needed to inform public health practice, policies that support the adoption of evidence-based physical activity interventions will be required to ensure sustained success. Policies can enhance both the supply and demand of evidence-based interventions, but different policies will be needed in various settings and for different target populations.

To meet the challenges of diffusion and dissemination of evidence-based interventions, physical activity researchers and service providers will not only need to increase their own knowledge and skills but they will also have to develop partnerships with experts in business, policy, and advocacy (Owen et al. 2006).

7.2.2 Health and Health Promotion Activities

Health promotion has been defined as "the science and art of helping people change their lifestyle." From this, we can derive that lifestyle changes can be facilitated through a combination of efforts to enhance awareness, change behavior, and create environments that support good health practices (Goetzel 2009).

A recent report by the City of London Corporation (2014) is pertinent to the four lifestyle habits discussed earlier, as it discusses evidence for the short-term effectiveness of interventions in the following areas:

Physical activity

There is a strong body of evidence that community-wide campaigns are effective in increasing levels of physical activity, as indicated by an increase in the percentage of people engaging in physical activity, energy expenditure, or other measures of physical activity (Kahn et al. 2002).

Among the most recommended initiatives by the City of London Corporation (2014) were prompts to increase stair use, pedometer programs, Internet-based approaches (such as online walking or cycling challenges), access to places and opportunities for physical activity, education, employee and peer counseling/support, multicomponent interventions combining nutrition and physical activity, and programs matching individuals to their stage of behavioral readiness. The positive reaction of patients and physicians alike showed that this primary care scheme on based physical activity was not only feasible but also appreciated by all of the people involved (Jimmy and Martin 2005).

Nutrition

This involves multicomponent interventions that include physical activity, nutrition strategies (such as nutrition education, dietary prescription, behavioral skills development, and training to control adult obesity), enhanced access to and availability of nutritious foods (especially fruit and vegetables), and the promotion of healthy foods at point-of-purchase. Steptoe et al. (2003) showed that brief counseling carried out by primary care nurses led to marked increases in reported fruit and vegetable consumption in an ethnically mixed sample. They also observed that individual counseling in primary care may be an effective means of increasing consumption in less affluent adults, and so targeting low-income groups may help redress social inequalities in health. In addition, behaviorally oriented methods allowed for greater changes than just nutrition counseling alone.

Tobacco control

This involves interventions directed towards individual smokers to increase the likelihood that they will quit smoking, and tobacco policies and bans to decrease cigarette consumption at work and to prevent nonsmoking employees from being exposed to tobacco smoke. Incentives and competitions can be effective, but only when combined with additional support, such as client education, smoking cessation groups, and telephone cessation support.

Alcohol

This involves brief interventions to encourage employees to consider their alcohol intake and contemplate changes, interventions included in health and lifestyle checks, psychosocial skills training, and peer referral (in which a colleague or peer recommends an intervention for someone).

Some people argue that preventive measures do not save money when compared with the cost of treating the disease because the screening costs for healthy people far outweigh treatment costs for the few who develop the disease. However, we can change this debate from a "saving money" perspective (through prevention or treatment) to a "cost-benefit" perspective, which encourages the discovery of the most cost-effective ways to improve health (Goetzel 2009).

7.2.3 Counseling Programs

It is important to note that health is not merely the absence of disease and that health promotion is not the same as disease prevention. Goetzel (2009) categorizes prevention as primary, secondary, and tertiary. Secondary prevention measures are directed at people who are at high risk of contracting diseases but who might not yet be sick, whereas tertiary prevention is comparable to disease management.

Primary prevention, which emphasizes disease avoidance and the promotion of good health practices, is the most pertinent prevention category for discussions about health promotion. Primary prevention involves things such as obtaining proper immunizations, managing one's weight, being physically active, eating a healthy diet, not smoking, drinking moderate amounts of alcohol, getting enough rest, surrounding oneself with family and friends, driving safely, managing stress, and, in general, living what most would agree is a healthy lifestyle.

Most of these behaviors can be adopted without the services of medical personnel, and they can reduce the likelihood of chronic and debilitating diseases and their concomitant costs. Proper advice from a clinician with follow-up counseling can encourage older, primary care patients to take up moderate-intensity physical activity. Pinto et al. (2005) found that extended counseling about physical activity led to a significant improvement in motivational readiness for more frequent exercise. For instance, extended telephone counseling has proved to be a highly effective complement to physician advice. This additional support may be especially important to help reduce sedentary behavior among older adults.

In the United States, there is increasing acknowledgment of the need to more aggressively promote the goals of Healthy People 2000 and to offset the cross-sectional declines in physical activity and health outcomes associated with age (Caspersen et al. 2000). The Healthy People 2000 program has several objectives for leisure-time physical activity and fitness, and it provides a useful framework for assessing the physical activity of adolescents and adults. Men have been reported to have somewhat better patterns of physical activity, but they have a greater drop off in activity with increasing age than do women. The availability of physical activity facilities and programs in workplaces should be increased, and preretirement counseling about exercise should be provided.

With respect to the promotion of physical activity, the Centers for Disease Control and Prevention (a U.S. Department of Health and Human Services agency) recommends the expansion of intramural and extramural offerings (indoor or protected locations should be encouraged to provide safe places for walking in any weather, for example), the encouragement of community-based programs, facilities, and sports participation, the marketing of existing programs to increase levels of participation, and the incorporation of physical activity into people's daily lives (Caspersen et al. 2000).

Kahn et al. (2002) noted the importance of providing information to change knowledge about the benefits of physical activity, increase awareness of community opportunities for increasing physical activity, explain methods for overcoming barriers and negative attitudes about physical activity, and increase participation in community-based activities. They reviewed interventions such as (1) "point-of-decision" prompts to encourage the use of stairs rather than elevators or escalators, (2) community-wide education campaigns, (3) mass media campaigns, and (4) classroom-based health education focused on information provision and skills related to decision making. Both community settings and healthcare settings are important locations for the dissemination of evidence-based programs and policies (Rabin et al. 2006).

Family-based interventions attempt to change health behavior through the use of techniques that increase the support of family members for behavioral change. The family is a major influence on children through the modeling of health behaviors and, thus, it is an appropriate target for intervention. Many disease risk factors, both behavioral and physiological, are associated with families. Moreover, a supportive social environment has been shown to increase the maintenance of behavioral change (Kahn et al. 2002).

These interventions target factors in the social environment and interpersonal and behavioral patterns that are likely to influence physical activity behaviors. Programs should include joint or separate educational sessions about health, goal setting, problem solving, and family behavioral management, and they will often incorporate some physical activities (Kahn et al. 2002).

In the United States, estimates indicate that only 9 % of health-related research funding focuses on prevention research, and within this body of inquiry, less than 10 % of prevention research involves dissemination research (Brownson et al. 2007). Given this sparse attention to dissemination research, the necessity for studies that provide more information about the impacts of prevention and dissemination as well as their manifestation into public health action becomes evident.

7.2.4 Avoiding Long Commutes

The negative health effects of long commutes have been widely discussed, and there are things employers can do to reduce the negative consequences of long commutes.

Many employers have considered reevaluating their options for helping workers manage those effects, particularly in light of the costs associated with reduced well-being. For instance, the costs of short-term and long-term sickness absence in the workplace have been estimated in the order of hundreds of billions of pounds in the United Kingdom (Black 2008; City of London Corporation 2014). Alternatives such as telecommuting can help to balance the physical and emotional toll of long commutes and it might even outweigh the social benefits of having employees together in the workplace.

From the perspective of employees, the reduction in commuting expenses could contribute to a greater peace of mind and reduced levels of worry (Crabtree 2010). Employees with long work hours or long commuting times may experience more difficulty in accessing health professionals (e.g., doctors, psychologists, and therapists) and health services, which might put an additional detriment to an eventually deteriorated health condition produced by the inconvenience of excessively long commutes. Surprisingly, Huinink and Feldhaus (2012) even revealed a negative correlation between long-distance commuting and female fertility. Furthermore, since unemployment can bring adverse health effects for different segments of population that include healthy people of working age, disabled people, and social security beneficiaries, etc., worklessness can be clearly associated with poorer well-being (Waddell and Burton 2006).

Assuming that this definition of "work" can be extended to the human and social interactions that are originated at the workplace, policies oriented to avoid commutes might be counterproductive for the health-related QOL. In Sweden, it is found that commuting by car is significantly associated with low social participation and low general trust compared with active commuting, and that only long-duration public commuters show similar levels of low social participation and trust (Mattisson et al. 2015). Further studies should be conducted in a variety of locations, in order to understand which circumstances of travel mode choice, travel time, and built environment and so on can significantly affect the health-related QOL, as well as to which extent they can affect it, in a comprehensive way.

7.2.5 Alliance for Healthy Cities

The Alliance for Healthy Cities is an international network intended to protect and enhance the health of city dwellers. The Healthy Cities approach is based on the concept that the social, economic, and physical environments are the key to the health of city dwellers.

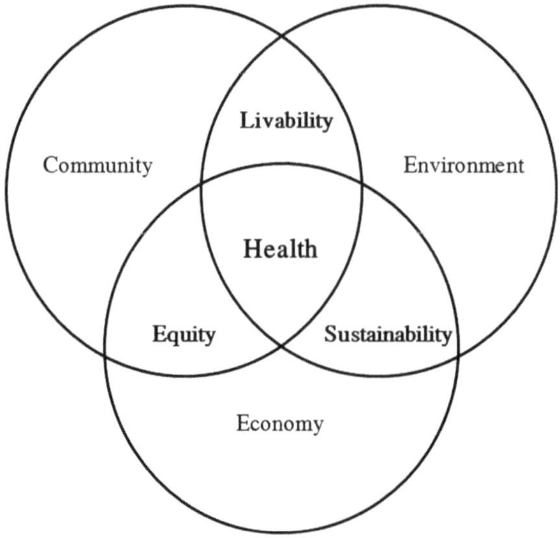

Fig. 7.1 Healthy cities model [adapted from Hancock (1993) and WHO (2011)]

"A healthy city is one that is continually creating and improving those physical and social environments and expanding those community resources which enable people to mutually support each other in performing all the functions of life and in developing to their maximum potential" (Hancock and Duhl 1998).[1]

Key features of a Healthy Cities project include high political commitment; inter-sectoral collaboration; community participation; the integration of activities in elemental settings; the development of a city health profile and a local action plan; periodic monitoring and evaluation; participatory research and analyses; information sharing; the involvement of the media; the incorporation of views from all groups within the community; mechanisms for sustainability; linkage with community development and human development; and national and international networking (Dora 2013; Dora et al. 2015).

The original intersectoral nature of Healthy Cities remains essential and leads to co-benefits for different sectors, as can be illustrated through Hancock's model (see Fig. 7.1), which focuses on human health and development (WHO 2011):

- The community needs to be convivial, with its members living harmoniously together, building social support systems and participating fully in the life of the community. The built environment needs to be livable, designed to maintain cordial relationships and to sustain a viable human presence. The community also needs to be equitable, where members are treated with fairness and justice, their basic needs are met, and equal opportunity exists for all.

[1]http://www.alliance-healthycities.com/htmls/resources/index_resources.html (Accessed May 1, 2016).

- The economy needs to be adequately prosperous, generating enough wealth to enable all of its members to achieve a satisfactory level of health. This economic wealth must be socially equitable, with wealth distributed fairly within the community. The economy also must be environmentally sustainable so that economic activity does not deplete renewable resources by using them beyond a sustainable level.
- The environment must be viable for humans, which requires a suitable range of temperature and solar radiation, clean air and water, and plants and animals to provide food. The environment must be sustainable over the long term so that the great web of life in all its richness and diversity is maintained. The environment must be livable, considered in terms of not only the natural environment but also the built environment.

The principal elements of a healthy cities project include health advocacy, intersectoral coordination, community participation, vision development, political commitment, and a setting approach (schools, markets, workplaces, and communities). More specifically, the essential features of a Healthy Cities project (WHO 2000) are:

- Improved health and quality of life for all citizens or people in the city, and a future vision of the city that respects the social and cultural values of the communities and which is developed by consensus.
- Encouragement of participatory planning for health.
- Priorities for project activities that are based on considerations that include the following two types of assessments of needs: (a) relationships between living conditions and health status, as determined by epidemiological analysis and/or the assessment of public health professionals; and (b) perceptions of the community on priority health and quality of life issues.
- Priority project activities that are undertaken by multidisciplinary teams that include substantial community participation.

Similarly, for the evaluation of health outcomes, the Healthy Cities project proposes some medium-term indicators (WHO 2000):

- Health literacy (encompassing health-related knowledge, attitudes, behavioral intentions, and interpersonal skills).
- Social action and influence (including community participation, community empowerment, social norms, and public opinion).
- Healthy public policy and organizational practices (including policy statements, legislation, regulation, resource allocation, and organizational practices).
- Healthy lifestyles (tobacco use, physical activity, food choices, etc.).
- Healthy environments (particularly a safe physical environment and supportive economic and social conditions).
- Effective health services (provision of preventive services and access to appropriate health services).

7.2.6 Additional Remarks

Freudenberg (2000) argues that the interactions between process and outcome in health promotion interventions are often complex and understudied. In urban communities, population diversity, difficulties in enlisting the participation of distrustful or disadvantaged residents or overburdened organizations, and the effect of multiple other influences on urban life make it especially difficult to attribute changes in population health status to specific interventions. A related problem is that most urban neighborhoods have many interventions in place simultaneously, with little effort to understand their cumulative impact or their synergistic interactions.

In fact, public health workers can help to forge an expanded practice of health promotion that contributes to healthier cities. Creating healthier cities requires locating health promotion interventions in a wide array of settings, enlisting more neighborhood residents and institutions to implement programs, and defining health in broader ways (Freudenberg 2000). In light of these considerations, places such as cultural centers, churches, sports facilities, housing projects, public transportation vehicles, and shops and supermarkets, play an important role and can become effective means to achieve healthier cities by supporting actions that include access to quality primary care, increasing health knowledge and social support, improving urban physical environments, and creating supportive social environments.

7.3 Health and Travel Behavior

It has been widely reported that long commutes can have very negative consequences for human health. Researchers have associated long commutes with obesity (Gies 2006), back and neck pain, cardiovascular disease, arthritis, asthma, headaches, divorce, self-reported stress, loneliness, and insomnia. Thus, high impedance commuting can easily lead to adverse effects on blood pressure, mood, frustration tolerance, illness occurrences, work absences, job stability, and overall life satisfaction (Novaco et al. 1991).

Given these implications of commuting, many people find it unpleasant and stressful. The challenges of driving and parking, the potential for unintentional injuries, and the hardships and inconveniences of vehicle maintenance and purchase (perceived traffic stress) have been associated with lower general health status and depression (Gee and Takeuchi 2004). Such findings suggest that commuting is particularly unpleasant, and it may be one of people's least favorite common activities. In a comparison between workers with very long commutes (more than 90 min) and those with very short commutes (approximately 10 min), Lowrey (2011) found that the former group felt less rested and experienced less enjoyment.

In addition, long commuting times are one of the most robust predictors of social isolation. For instance, Putnam (2000) found that every 10 min spent commuting is associated with 10 % fewer "social connections." Because social connections tend to make us feel happy and fulfilled, such findings become very important if we consider that the drive times for urban sprawl commuters are three to four times as long as those for individuals who live in well-planned, dense communities (OCFP 2005).

Commuting makes drivers less healthy and less fit, and they have less time for such activities as fixing meals at home, exercising, spending time with family and friends, and sleeping. The source of the unhappiness, then, is not so much commuting per se, but the time that commuting takes from other activities (Paumgarten 2007).

Additionally, for car commuters, the lack of social contact increases the bad effects for mental or social health. As an example of this, we have road rage, which refers to the sudden violent anger that the actions of one driver can provoke in another driver. Road rage can lead to disputes between drivers that can eventually become violent and involve people who are not usually violent. This type of behavior may be facilitated by the perceived absence of other people when we are in a car, because people behave differently outside of the bounds of social contact. Thus, social contact is very important, as it promotes the perception of fellowship with others, which can be a means of social control and regulation (Paumgarten 2007).

The benefits of social contact can be obtained through public transit, such as commuting by train. In addition, commuting by public transit offers the benefits of multitasking, which may add utility value to a commuting trip. On a train, one can sleep, read, send e-mails, play cards, or any of the many things smartphones allow. These new possibilities for improving the well-being of passengers should be considered in future urban transportation policies.

7.3.1 The Commuter Paradox

Bruno Frey and Alois Stutzer, economists at the University of Zurich, released a study called, "Stress That Doesn't Pay: The Commuting Paradox" (Stutzer and Frey 2008).

The commuting paradox refers to the notion that many people who are supposedly rational (according to classical economic theory, at least) commute to work, even though it makes them miserable. In the final accounting, they are not adequately compensated. They have to trade off social and immaterial goods such as sleep, exercise, and fun, which are undervalued, for material goods such as money, a house, or prestige, which have been overvalued. In the end, people with longer commuting times systematically report lower subjective well-being.

For many people, commuting involves stress with no pay off. The balance between, and nature of, rational choice and constrained choices must be carefully considered when we discuss residential location choice, travel mode choice, and other related life choices. From this perspective, it is necessary to understand in more detail the implications that commuting has for people's lives in order to gain valuable insights into the institutional and behavioral restrictions to compensation. Moreover, it may help commuters to increase their individual well-being, which should be directly reflected in their overall health.

Putnam (2000) states the following idea: we can imagine a triangle with points that represent the places for sleeping, working, and shopping (see Fig. 7.2). The sides of the triangle can vary from very short (a five-minute walk from one point to the next) to very long (an hour or two travelling each side, as in many U.S. cities). The smaller the triangle, the happier the human will be, as long as there is social interaction to be had. With smaller triangles (with mixed-use zoning and mixed-income dwellings), people would not have to travel so far to go to work or to buy what they need (Paumgarten 2007). In addition, social capital would be strengthened by short commutes.

In smaller triangles, people would be more likely to use active travel modes, whereas in larger triangles, people must necessarily use cars and other motorized means of travel to reach its corners. Once again, the overdependence on motorized transportation may have adverse health effects (Lopez-Zetina et al. 2006). More time spent commuting is associated with less time spent exercising, preparing food, and sleeping (Christian 2009).

Very often, commuting is delayed by traffic congestion. The loss of time in traffic congestion frequently leaves people overwhelmed by time demands, health impairments, psychological adjustments, decreased work performance, and a reduced overall satisfaction with life (OCFP 2005). Thus, traffic congestion easily becomes aversive and frustrating, as it elevates arousal levels, elicits a negative affect, and produces stress, all of which are relevant to choices of travel mode, residential location, and job location (Novaco et al. 1990).

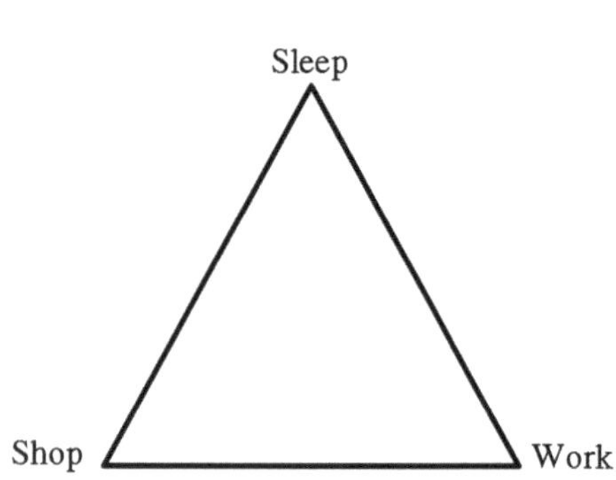

Fig. 7.2 Putnam's triangle

7.3.2 Active Travel and Health

Although there is evidence that people are more physically active in walkable neighborhoods, the evidence is mixed as to whether there is also a positive association with other health indicators, such as BMI or rates of depression (Croucher et al. 2012).

It has been suggested that commuting by walking, bicycling, public transit, or carpooling can actually improve mental health and counteract the negative effects of using motor vehicles. The positive effects increase significantly with walkable, mixed-use neighborhood designs that encourage the development of social capital through enhanced levels of community and social engagement (OCFP 2005).

However, the effects of active travel might be counterproductive as well. For example, walking to promote a healthy lifestyle is less attractive in suburban or semirural neighborhoods, which often lack sidewalks or trails. Unfortunately, often the healthy and harmful features of environments go unnoticed (Rainham et al. 2010).

In previous studies, we found that the effects of residential environments on active travel behavior are mixed and limited, depending upon who is travelling. The active travel behavior of citizens in Japan had no direct effects on health-related quality of life, and so conceptualizations of both travel behavior and health-related quality of life need to be examined in future studies to understand the nature of these associations (Perez Barbosa et al. 2016). However, it is often the interplay between people and place that ultimately influences healthy behaviors and health-related quality of life, and thus it should always be considered by practitioners.

7.4 Health and Park Use

According to the APA (2003), cities can use parks to improve public health in different ways, including contact with nature, opportunities for physical activity to help increase fitness and reduce obesity, and by mitigating the impacts of climate change and air and water pollution. Park characteristics such as size, accessibility, availability, and the quality of amenities influence park use. Because parks vary in size, shape, quality, and character, they can satisfy a broad spectrum of opportunities for contact with the natural world at various levels (Maller et al. 2009).

In addition, different kinds of parks may offer different health benefits, from small neighborhood parks, which may contribute to social interaction and physical activity, to larger parks that can perform important ecological functions and provide citizens with more intense and beneficial contacts with nature (APA 2003). Access to large, attractive, public open spaces has been associated with increased walking (Cohen et al. 2007).

Parks play a critical role in facilitating physical activity in minority communities, not only by providing facilities and scheduled, supervised activities but also by providing destinations to which people can walk—even though they may be sedentary after arriving there. Based on these findings, Cohen et al. (2007) have suggested that communities should be designed so that everyone has a park within a mile of their residence. In addition, special groups such as seniors may need special programs or incentives to use park facilities.

Park facilities and services have individual, social, economic, and environmental benefits. Some of these benefits affect entire communities, not just the park users (Bedimo-Rung et al. 2005). Some of the most relevant benefits include:

- Physical health benefits: There is strong evidence that when people have access to parks, they are more likely to exercise, which can reduce obesity and its associated problems and costs (Gies 2006). In many cases, people who live closer to parks exercise more often than people who live greater distances far from green spaces. In general, there is enough evidence to support the idea that parks improve health and vigor and extend life expectancy (Maller et al. 2009).
- Mental health benefits: From nearby natural environments, people get "feelings of open space," "change of scenery," and a "place to escape," etc. A park can be a great source of pleasure for residents who live nearby. Lower levels of anxiety, sadness, stress, and depression and the restorative effects of nature can be counted among the psychological (mental) health benefits of parks (Bedimo-Rung et al. 2005). Benefits associated with reducing problems related to Attention Deficit Disorder and the development of children's brains have also been investigated (Isenberg and Quisenberry 2002; Gies 2006).
- Social benefits: Parks may facilitate social interactions that are critical to maintaining community cohesion, pride, and social capital. In a park, people can develop social ties, be influenced by the healthy behavior of others, increase their social capital (relationships among people that facilitate productive activity), and be more easily integrated in their social environment. Park settings in which there are more trees and vegetation appear to inhibit crime, aggression, and violence while promoting social interaction among individuals (Bedimo-Rung et al. 2005). Consequently, if the parks are in bad condition (crowded, dangerous, and noisy), the formation of neighborhood social ties will be severely restricted, with the subsequent negative consequences for social health.

Parks and nature are currently undervalued as a means of improving and maintaining health. Although most people are aware of the health benefits of sports and recreation activities, the range of other health and well-being benefits from contact with nature are virtually unknown. In addition to their contribution to public health and well-being through ecosystem services, parks also contribute to health and well-being by providing settings for community engagement (Maller et al. 2009).

The lack of park spaces can hinder human health. There is evidence that when people cannot reach parks, they often go without exercise (Gies 2006). The idea that isolation from the natural world may be harmful to health is not limited to scientists and researchers; it is also seen in the choices of everyday people (Maller et al. 2009).

Baum (1999) argues that healthy communities should provide varied opportunities for their citizens to meet and interact in both formal and informal settings. Recent research indicates that parks make a key contribution to meeting this requirement (e.g., Krenichyn 2006). However, it has been asserted that, if not well-maintained and used, parks that form boundaries between neighborhoods of different cultural, ethnic, and socioeconomic characteristics can become "green walls" that divide communities rather than be places of community interaction (Solecki and Welch 1995; Maller et al. 2009).

For low-income segments of the population, the importance of well-maintained parks and green spaces for health is especially relevant. For instance, parks offer low-income people who cannot afford gym memberships a place to exercise. This is an excellent way to reduce social inequities. In many U.S. cities, for example, there is a notable paucity of parks in poor communities. More generally, there are correlations between poverty, minority status, obesity, ill health, and neighborhood factors that discourage exercise, including the absence of parks and recreation facilities (Gies 2006).

Parks can also stand as very strong symbols of change that people make in their own lives to improve their personal condition and their environment. The involvement of communities in the planning stages of parks gives people a sense of ownership, it brings people together to create the best possible environment they can imagine, and it also creates a sense of success that is very positive for individuals and communities in a neighborhood. Therefore, it is always important to consult the community about the types of parks people would be most likely use and how they would be used.

In fact, parks are ideal catalysts for the integration of environment, society, and health (which have been demonstrated to be inextricably linked) because they promote an ecological approach to human health and well-being based on contact with nature (Maller et al. 2009). Parks contribute to physical, mental, and social health in many ways that still need to be more fully investigated from a multidisciplinary approach, including considerations of the heterogeneity in people's ages, health needs, social and economic backgrounds, physical activity preferences, and attitudes toward nature, etc.

Despite the existence of a large body of evidence suggesting the positive effects of urban green spaces, Lee and Maheswaran (2011) found that although many studies tried to assess links between urban green spaces and health benefits, the results were "weak, inconsistent, and occasionally contradictory." This absence of significant associations may be attributable to the hidden or included effects of density and accessibility, as well as differential effects for separate population groups, depending upon the urban features analyzed in those studies (Melis et al. 2015). Therefore, more detailed studies are required to bring more clarity to these apparently contradictory issues.

7.5 Health and Residential Environments

It is easy to find support for the idea that the health can be strongly influenced by the residential environment, in both positive and negative ways. In fact, we found that the residential environment may have both direct and indirect effects on health-related quality of life, where the indirect effects were observed via lifestyle habits and active travel. However, self-reported health indicators may not be sufficient to capture the impacts of repeated daily travel on health. In addition, although residential environments influence active travel, the effects are limited and mixed, with different influences on certain groups depending upon their lifestyles (Perez Barbosa et al. 2016).

Conventional approaches to delineating boundaries effectively negate the concept of dynamic populations in residential environments. Sometimes for urban dwellers, using a single address or residential boundary to identify the primary place where health behaviors or outcomes occur may not provide an accurate view of the impact of the environment (Rainham et al. 2010).

Apart from the built infrastructure, assessments of successful residential environments must consider the concept of social capital. Social capital can be defined as the social, political, and economic networks and interactions that inspire trust and reciprocity among citizens, leading to common good and mutual obligation (Putnam 2000). If people can connect with others in their area, share a sense of belonging in their neighborhood, and find enough time for recreation, voluntary activities, civic engagement, and self-care, then that area has very good signs of social capital. A positive association has been demonstrated between social relationships and health, and the higher the quality and quantity of these relationships, the greater the health benefits can be (Frumkin 2003).

7.5.1 Natural Environment and Health

There has been a considerably growing body of evidence highlighting the beneficial aspects of natural environments for humans. Kuo and Sullivan (2001) found that residents living in “greener” surroundings reported lower levels of fear, fewer incivilities, less aggressive and violent behavior, a stronger sense of community, better relationships with neighbors, and less heated domestic conflicts. Berry et al. (2015) found that visual exposure to natural environments is associated to less impulsive decision-making processes by individuals. Impulsivity in decision making sometimes leads to poor human decisions that have implications that underlie many environmental issues, individual and societal dilemmas such as drug addiction and obesity. The exposure to natural environments is further beneficial to mental health because it can be associated with lower levels of stress, depression, anxiety, and improved cognition and memory abilities (Pearson and Craig 2014). Furthermore, active lifestyles can be encouraged among the population via use of transport mode and participation in leisure activities (Calogiuri and Chroni 2014). However, Pearson and Craig (2014) argue that much of the existing evidence on the effects of natural environments on human health are based on a too simplistic "natural" and "built" environment dichotomy, letting other relevant aspects poorly represented, such as people's attitudes and beliefs toward health and the environment and their interactions with behavioral responses.

Currently, more than half of the world population are living in cities where they are spending less time exposed to natural environments as a direct consequence. Therefore, it is important for spatial planning policy makers to put the development of green space in a more central position for improving the health situation of urban residents (Maas et al. 2006). Pearson and Craig (2014) highlight the need for empirical research that finds more in detail which properties and which forms of interactions with the natural environment are most likely to lead to mental health benefits.

The WHO has recommended for adults of any age that 'muscle-strengthening activities should be done involving major muscle groups on two or more days a week'. Therefore, interventions should pay more attention to promote physical activities with greater potential for muscle conditioning through whole-body involvement, given their great potential contribution to improve cardiorespiratory and muscular fitness, bone health, as well as to reduce the risk of non-communicable diseases and depression (WHO 2010; Calogiuri and Chroni 2014). The above existing studies suggest that the mere existence of green and natural spaces might not be enough to encourage physical activities if underlying beliefs, possible barriers to physical activity practices and preferred environmental characteristics are not correctly understood. In this sense, any interventions should act at a multilevel scale that includes not only infrastructural interventions but also social campaigns inducing the necessary behavioral changes in the population, such as promoting visits to natural environments, programming activities that encourage social interactions in the natural environments, providing information about the health benefits of physical activities, and paying attention to maintaining a good quality in the natural environments in terms of safety, accessibility, and aesthetics (Calogiuri and Chroni 2014).

7.5.2 Negative Impacts of Urban Sprawl

One the assumptions about the prevalence of car commuting is that many people move to the suburbs to escape the "ills of the city." Part of the motivation to move out of the city can be to be closer to the country air, have a bigger yard for children to play, or to get away from the noise and bustle of the city. Although suburban life has some benefits, as discussed previously, there is a growing body of evidence suggesting that there are significant public health costs of dispersed urban development, often called "urban sprawl" (OCFP 2005).

Urban sprawl can seriously disturb the natural environment, including negatively affecting biodiversity. Thus, people who leave urban areas to find a greater connection with nature in the sprawling suburbs may be disappointed. In spread-out communities, homes are usually far away from schools, workplaces, stores, and services, forcing people to drive virtually everywhere. More time driving means less time with family and friends, less time for oneself, and less time to engage in community activities (Putnam 2000). In addition, the psychological impact of traffic fatalities associated with urban sprawl can be very serious.

Thus, urban sprawl negatively affects well-being by eroding social capital, increasing the social stratification of communities, robbing people of all ages of the opportunity to have a balanced, healthy lifestyle, degrading the surrounding natural environment, and increasing the stress of commuting, which affects both mental and physical health. Jones (2014) maintains that the built environment affects mental health through the stress produced by car commuting, the limits to social interaction (isolation), and the exacerbation of mental disorders. A 2004 study by the RAND Corporation think tank found that living in a high sprawl area has the equivalent health effect of aging four years, in part because of the higher incidence of health problems such as diabetes, breathing difficulties, migraine headaches, and high blood pressure (Gies 2006).

The most obvious mechanism through which a sprawling environment affects health is by limiting opportunities for physical activity through its infrastructure. In addition, sprawl appears to have a disproportionate impact on the physical health of the elderly and possibly the poor, making them much more vulnerable to the known negative effects of sprawl. This may be because the poor and the elderly have fewer resources to mitigate the limitations imposed by urban sprawl, such as less access to individual motorized transportation. The elderly may also suffer declining physical mobility and reduced vision or hearing, and thus may be less able to navigate environments with speeding cars or wide streets. They may have more difficulty walking in sprawling cities because of the greater distances to destinations such as markets or parks. Sturm and Cohen (2004) found that the urban form may be an important contributor to elderly 'shut-ins' and sedentary lifestyles.

The Harvard University (undated) maintains that buildings, streets, and communities that encourage walking and biking; parks and playgrounds that are plentiful and appealing; and neighborhoods where people feel safe are just some of the key elements of an activity-friendly environment, which can improve health in all its dimensions by promoting physical activity and more human and social contact. It is absolutely important that planners consider the health impacts of development and transportation projects, in much the same way that they consider the environmental impacts of these projects.

It is important to realize that the social life of any neighborhood will improve with less time on the roads and more local schools, small stores, gathering spots for teens and the elderly, and other places where people can interact.

7.5.3 *Additional Remarks on the Influence of Built Environments*

The built environment has small but positive effects on the development of social capital, and the quality and type of destinations is as important as the number of walkable destinations (Croucher et al. 2012). However, urban environments may have fewer neighborhood interactions because of safety concerns and lack of familiarity with one's neighbors. Casual relationships with neighbors, merchants, or fellow employees may be less important to mental health than the social support of close relationships, such as with partners, family members, and long-standing friendships (Sturm and Cohen 2004). It is further necessary to clarify the nature of the above relationships as well as their impacts on health outcomes of different communities. For instance, it is important to determine whether these findings can be generalized to other developed countries, many of which are facing similar challenges associated with suburban sprawl, increasing car dependence, spatial and social segregation, etc. (Sturm and Cohen 2004; Croucher et al. 2012).

It has often been said that most people experience a multiplicity of places and locations where people gather and interact, including work, places to socialize, and 'third places' such as cafés, post offices, and public parks. Those places are necessary for the development strong community ties and civic engagement. If we assume that residential locations are distinguished by a stronger sense of attachment to place, we are limiting health-related human activities to a predetermined geographic boundary, which unavoidably will lead to the misclassification of context associated with health outcomes (Diez Roux 2001), or will severely underestimate the variation in contexts associated with the heath outcome(s) of interest (Rainham et al. 2010).

7.6 Health and Urban Infrastructure

In human history, cities have been important to the health of their populations for several reasons. In the 21st century, the majority of the world's population lives in cities and metropolitan areas. Cities concentrate most of the world's health problems and the conditions for their solutions, since they have the human, financial, and social capital that is needed to promote health and prevent disease, making it possible to set goals for improvement. Therefore, expanding the scope and accessibility of health promotion activities in cities is likely to increase their impact (Freudenberg 2000).

The health impact of some built environment characteristics, such as housing, traffic, environmental pollution and safety, have been widely assessed, but little is known about the impact of the primary structural characteristics of urban environments that are central to urban and local plans, such as plans for land use, building density, and the distribution of services and facilities (Melis et al. 2015).

In order to address health inequalities, urban policies should invest in the delivery of services that enhance resilience factors in a careful and equitable manner throughout the city, and above all investment should be made in a good public transportation network. Melis et al. (2015) have suggested that accessibility and transportation services could be easily modified as a compensation measure when it is impossible to provide nearby services for everyone. Accessibility to public transportation, as well as a dense urban structure, could contribute to a reduced risk of depression, especially for women and the elderly, by increasing opportunities to move around and enjoy an active social life (Melis 2016). Moreover, accessibility to transportation and a dense urban structure appear to be the two principal features of the built environment that contribute to mental health, which is considered one of the most responsive health targets of the urban structure (Melis et al. 2015).

High density is seen to increase the possibility of social interactions, because people are closer to each other. In addition, residential density has been linked to increases in physical activity, but it is insufficient on its own to influence rates of activity (Croucher et al. 2012). Nevertheless, we must recognize that residential density is important only in relation to the other elements of neighborhood design, such as mixed land use, walkable neighborhoods with street connections, and leisure, retail, or employment destinations of interest.

With respect to public transportation, research shows that job satisfaction and commitment declines with increased commuting distance on the road, but not with public transit use (Gee and Takeuchi 2004).

It is imperative that place and health researchers consider modern cities and empirically examine the diversity of places that influence health, including those places that are distant in space and time. Thus, we need to better understand how different places affect health and healthy behaviors, as well as gather information about how the structuring of social processes is associated with the structuring of the contexts in which people live (Rainham et al. 2010).

7.7 Final Comments

There is a large body of evidence that social capital is important for health, but as we have mentioned previously, specific groups may be more affected than others by the conditions in our cities, creating health inequalities.

7.7.1 Children

For children to thrive, they need schools, sports fields, friends' homes, libraries, shops, and places of worship. They also need privacy, tranquility, safety, and community (Frumkin et al. 2004). Children are more likely to develop stronger attachments to locations much closer to their place of residence; longitudinal analyses show that the quality of places early in the life course has a significant effect on health outcomes later in life (Rainham et al. 2010).

Living in car-dependent areas has very negative health effects on children, including higher rates of premature and low birth weight babies and the greater likelihood of diseases such as leukemia, and a six-fold increased risk of other cancers (OCFP 2005). In addition, children living in car-dependent areas or near highly trafficked roads are at a higher risk of suffering traffic-related injuries, and the associated restrictions on activities such as walking, cycling, and playing freely in public spaces can hinder the development of independence and increase the risk of obesity. As children develop into adolescence, social and physical bonds to places near their residence are diminished because of more relationships outside their neighborhoods, increased mobility, and independence. However, attachments to childhood places are likely to remain, and so will the health outcomes associated with these relationships in later stages of the life course (Rainham et al. 2010).

7.7.2 Women

A suburban study found that women are more likely than men to indicate problems managing stress and feelings of sadness, worthlessness, and hopelessness (Lundeen 1992). Thus, women may experience a significant amount of stress in sprawling, poorly planned communities that lack access to public transit and amenities, particularly if they have full-time jobs with long commutes, and household duties such as driving children to school and after-school activities, taking elderly dependents to the doctor, and running errands.

7.7.3 Elderly People

In general, two major issues are important for the health of elderly people: mobility and community. Both of these factors are threatened by sprawling, car-dependent communities (OCFP 2005). The elderly need access to stores, places of worship, medical offices, parks, and other recreational and cultural facilities close to home, as well as safe, well-maintained sidewalks, especially considering the fact that they will reach a point when then can no longer drive safely.

Without easy access to effective public transit, the elderly and disabled (who may be homebound) have more difficulty getting places, visiting doctors or receiving other health and social services. Overall, they are more isolated and may be lonelier than the average person. When social support is lacking, the health of the elderly is seriously compromised.

A large cohort study by Takano et al. (2002) showed that living in areas with walkable green spaces near one's residence positively influenced the longevity of urban senior citizens, independent of their age, sex, marital status, baseline functional status, and socioeconomic status.

The design of some communities can prevent people with disabilities from being physically active, and it may even prevent them from using transportation systems and being socially integrated into their community. People in wheelchairs or who use other mobility devices benefit the most from walkable, safe communities. Environmental barriers, such as lack of access to mass transit routes, bus shelters, or other public services, seriously affect the quality of life and health of the disabled.

Mobility plays an important role in the social activity patterns of older adults. Elderly who are more mobile have been found to have a larger variety of social activity locations. Stimulating their mobility by providing safe and accessible public transport and walkable neighborhoods could promote social participation and improve the health of older adults (Van den Berg et al. 2015).

A very obvious conclusion is that, in order to support healthy aging in place, residential environments should provide the necessary opportunities for social interaction among various segments of the aging population (Van den Berg et al. 2015), while considering the impact that the design of the built environment has on active community involvement.

7.7.4 Life Choices and Health

We can assume that people have varying degrees of autonomy when they decide where to live and work, with whom they socialize, and the actions they take to minimize health risks. However, the freedom to make these choices is often illusory, because we seldom account for the role that features of the context and environment play in the development of human well-being (Rainham et al. 2010).

Well-being is a concept that captures the important aspects of how people feel about and experience their daily lives; in other words, well-being encompasses more than physical health or economic indicators.

According to Platkin (2013), our quality of life can depend on many different life choices. Living near the seaside or countryside can encourage exercise, as can living in places with accessible public parks and sports facilities. Certain jobs are more physically active than others.

Many daily life activities seem insignificant, but they can have substantial impacts on health. For instance, research indicates that when people wear casual clothing, they are more active (Platkin 2013). Incorporating walking or standing activities into daily routines (using stairs, having walking meetings, standing during phone calls, walking to a coworker's desk instead of calling, etc.) can help to significantly improve health, and using pedometers has been shown to motivate people to take more steps.

Our family and social lives have tremendous influence. Getting married and having children can negatively affect physical health, because when people find that they have less time to be active and eat healthy, they are more likely to gain weight. On the other hand, having pets changes lives and can improve one's health. Cats and dogs provide affection, which can decrease the risk of disease and improve your overall health, and it has been demonstrated that dog owners walk more. We are influenced by our family and friends as well because, for instance, they can play an important role in how much we exercise and in the quality of our social interactions.

The implications of our life choices, their interrelationships and evolution in different geographical contexts, and their impacts on health need to be better understood for the proper design of living environments that contribute to health and the quality of our lives.

References

Ainsworth BE, Haskell WL, Whitt MC, Irwin ML, Swartz AM, Strath SJ, O'Brien WL, Bassett DRJ, Schmitz KH, Emplaincourt PO, Jacobs DRJ, Leon AS (2000) Compendium of physical activities: an update of activity codes and MET intensities. Med Sci Sports Exerc 32(9):S498–S504

American Planning Association (APA) (2003) How cities use parks to Improve Public Health. American Planning Association. Chicago, United States. Retrieved from: http://imaginecities.com/test/wp-content/uploads/2014/02/physicalactivitycities.pdf. Accessed 13 May 2016

Baum F (1999) Social capital and health: implications for health in rural Australia. In: Leaping the boundary fence: using evidence and collaboration to build healthier communities. Proceedings of the 5th National Rural Health Conference, Adelaide, S.A., Australia, 14–17 March

Bedimo-Rung AL, Mowen AJ, Cohen DA (2005) The significance of parks to physical activity and public health: a conceptual model. Am J Prev Med 28(2S2):159–168

Berry MS, Repke MA, Nickerson NP, Conway LG III, Odum AL, Jordan KE (2015) Making time for nature: visual exposure to natural environments lengthens subjective time perception and reduces impulsivity. PLoS ONE 10(11):e0141030

Black C (2008) Working for a healthier tomorrow. Retrieved from https://www.gov.uk/government/uploads/system/uploads/attachment_data/file/209782/hwwb-working-for-a-healthier-tomorrow.pdf. Accessed 2 June 2016

Breslow L (1999) From disease prevention to health promotion. J Am Med Assoc 281(11):1030–1033

Brownson RC, Ballew P, Dieffenderfer B, Haire-Joshu D, Heath GW, Kreuter MW, Myers BA (2007) Evidence-based interventions to promote physical activity: what contributes to dissemination by state health departments. Am J Prev Med 33(1):S66–S73

Calogiuri G, Chroni S (2014) The impact of the natural environment on the promotion of active living: an integrative systematic review. BMC Public Health 14:873

Caspersen CJ, Pereira MA, Curran KM (2000) Changes in physical activity patterns in the United States, by sex and cross-sectional age. Med Sci Sports Exerc 32(9):1601–1609

Christian TJ (2009) Opportunity costs surrounding exercise and dietary behaviors: quantifying trade-offs between commuting time and health-related activities. Available at SSRN: http://ssrn.com/abstract=1490117

City of London Corporation (2014) Best practice in promoting employee health and wellbeing in the city of London retrieved from: https://www.cityoflondon.gov.uk/business/economic-research-and-information/research-publications/Documents/Research-2014/employee-health-and-wellbeing-in-the-city-of-London-final.pdf. Accessed 5 May 2016

Cohen DA, McKenzie TL, Sehgal A, Williamson S, Golinelli D, Lurie N (2007) Contribution of public parks to physical activity. Am J Public Health 97(3):509–514

Crabtree S (2010) Wellbeing lower among workers with long commutes retrieved from: http://www.gallup.com/poll/142142/wellbeing-lower-among-workers-long-commutes.aspx. Accessed 12 Feb 2016

Croucher K, Wallace A, Duffy S (2012) The influence of land use mix, density and urban design on health: a critical literature review. The University of York, UK. Retrieved from: http://www.gcph.co.uk/assets/0000/3519/Review_of_infleunce_of_land_use_mix_density_and_urban_design_on_health_final.pdf. Accessed 5 May 2016

Diez Roux AV (2001) Investigating neighborhood and area effects on health. Am J Public Health 91(11):1783–1789

Dora C (2013) Health—a measure of performance for Urban Transport. World Health Organization. Presentation file retrieved from: http://www.uncrd.or.jp/content/documents/23228EST-P6_WHO.pdf. Accessed 13 May 2016

Dora C, Haines A, Balbus J, Fletcher E, Adair-Rohani H, Alabaster G, Hossain R, de Onis M, Branca F, Neira M (2015) Indicators linking health and sustainability in the post-2015 development agenda. Lancet 385(9965):380–391

Eakin EG, Brown WJ, Marshall AL, Mummery K, Larsen E (2004) Physical activity promotion in primary care: bridging the gap between research and practice. Am J Prev Med 27(4):297–303

Freudenberg N (2000) Health promotion: a review of current practice and future prospects in the United States. Annu Rev Public Health 21:473–503

Frumkin H (2003) Healthy places: exploring the evidence. Am J Public Health 93(9):1451–1456

Frumkin H, Frank L, Jackson R (2004) Urban sprawl and public health. Designing, planning and building for healthy communities. Island Press, Washington, DC

Gee GC, Takeuchi DT (2004) Traffic stress, vehicular burden and well-being: a multilevel analysis. Soc Sci Med 59(2):405–414

Gies E (2006) The health benefits of parks: how parks help keep Americans and their communities fit and healthy. The Trust for Public Land. (https://www.tpl.org/sites/default/files/cloudtplorg/pubs/benefits_HealthBenefitsReport.pdf. Accessed 5 May 2016

Goetzel RZ (2009) Perspective: do prevention or treatment services save money? The wrong debate. Health Aff 28(1):37–41

Grosvenor MB, Smolin LA (2012) Visualizing nutrition: everyday choices. Wiley, Hoboken, NJ

Hancock T (1993) Health, human development and the community ecosystem: three ecological models. Health Promot Int 8(1):41–47

Hancock T, Duhl L (1998) The parameters of a healthy city. Promoting Health in the Urban Context. Copenhagen, World Health Organization Regional Office for Europe. WHO Healthy Cities Papers, No. 1

Huinink J, Feldhaus M (2012) Fertility and commuting behaviour in Germany. Comparative Population Studies—Zeitschrift für Bevölkerungswissenschaft 37(3–4):491–516

Isenberg JP, Quisenberry N (2002) Play: essential for all children a position paper of the association for childhood education international (www.imaginationplayground.com//Play-essential-for-all-children.doc. Accessed 4 Feb 2016

Jimmy G, Martin BW (2005) Implementation and effectiveness of a primary care based physical activity counselling scheme. Patient Educ Couns 56(3):323–331

Jones C (2014) Four ways the built environment affects mental health Article for the web site Urbanist Link: http://urbanist.co/four-ways-the-built-environment-affects-mental-health/. Accessed 14 Dec 2015

Kahn EB, Ramsey LT, Brownson RC, Heath GW, Howze EH, Powell KE, Stone EJ, Rajab MW, Corso P (2002) The effectiveness of interventions to increase physical activity—a systematic review. Am J Prev Med 22(4):73–107

Krenichyn K (2006) The only place to go and be in the city: Women talk about exercise, being outdoors, and the meanings of a large urban park. Health Place 12:631–643

Kuo FE, Sullivan WC (2001) Environment and crime in the inner city. Environ Behav 33(3):343–367
Lee ACK, Maheswaran R (2011) The health benefits of urban green spaces: a review of the evidence. J Public Health 33(2):212–222
Lopez-Zetina J, Lee H, Friis R (2006) The link between obesity and the built environment Evidence from an ecological analysis of obesity and vehicle miles of travel in California. Health Place 12(4):656–664
Lowrey A (2011) Your commute is killing you web article for slate. http://www.primary.slate.com/articles/business/moneybox/2011/05/your_commute_is_killing_you.html. Accessed 24 Jan 2016
Lundeen S (1992) Health needs of a suburban community: a nursing assessment approach. J Community Health Nurs 9(4):235–244
Maas J, Verheij RA, Groenewegen PP, de Vries S, Spreeuwenberg P (2006) Green space, urbanity, and health: how strong is the relation? J Epidemiol Community Health 60(7):587–592
Maller C, Townsend M, Leger LS, Henderson-Wilson C, Pryor A, Prosser L, Moore M (2009) Healthy parks, healthy people : the health benefits of contact with nature in a park context. George Wright Forum 26(2):51–83. Retrieved from: http://www.georgewright.org/262maller.pdf. Accessed 5 May 2016
Matheson EM, King DE, Everett CJ (2012) Healthy lifestyle habits and mortality in overweight and obese individuals. J Am Board Family Med 25(1):9–15
Mattisson K, Håkansson C, Jakobsson K (2015) Relationships between commuting and social capital among men and women in southern Sweden. Environ Behav 47(7):734–753
Melis G, Gelormino E, Marra G, Ferracin E, Costa G (2015) The effects of the urban built environment on mental health: a cohort study in a large northern Italian city. Int J Environ Res Public Health 12(11):14898–14915
Melis G (2016) Public transport and urban density affect urban mental health link: http://www.urbandesignmentalhealth.com/blog/public-transport-and-urban-density-affect-urban-mental-health-says-italian-study. Accessed 5 Feb 2016
Novaco RW, Stokols D, Milanesi L (1990) Objective and subjective dimensions of travel impedance as determinants of commuting stress. Am J Community Psychol 18(2):231–257
Novaco RW, Kliewer W, Broquet A (1991) Home environmental consequences of commute travel impedance. Environ Ecol Psychol 19(6):881–909
OCFP (2005) The health impacts of Urban Sprawl. Ontario College of Family Physicians. Toronto, Ontario, Canada. Retrieved from: http://ocfp.on.ca/docs/committee-documents/urban-sprawl---volume-4---social-and-mental-health.pdf?sfvrsn=5. Accessed 13 May 2016
Owen N, Glanz K, Sallis JF, Kelder SH (2006) Evidence-based approaches to dissemination and diffusion of physical activity interventions. Am J Prev Med 31(4):S35–S44
Paumgarten N (2007) There and back again (retrieved from: http://www.newyorker.com/magazine/2007/04/16/there-and-back-again. Accessed 26 Jan 2016
Pearson DG, Craig T (2014) The great outdoors? Exploring the mental health benefits of natural environments. Front Psychol 5:1178
Perez Barbosa D, Zhang J, Seya H (2016) Effects of the residential environment on health in Japan linked with travel behavior. Int J Environ Res Public Health 13(2)
Pinto BM, Goldstein MG, Ashba J, Sciamanna CN, Jette A (2005) Randomized controlled trial of physical activity counseling for older primary care patients. Am J Prev Med 29(4):247–255
Platkin C (2013) Critical life choices to live healthier and have a better diet http://www.dietdetective.com/7-critical-life-choices-live-healthier-and-have-better-diet-0/. Accessed 20 Feb 2016
Putnam RD (2000) Bowling alone: the collapse and revival of american community. Simon Schuster, New York
Rabin BA, Brownson RC, Kerner JF, Glasgow RE (2006) Methodologic challenges in disseminating evidence-based interventions to promote physical activity. Am J Prev Med 31(4):S24–S34

Rainham D, McDowell I, Krewski D, Sawada M (2010) Conceptualizing the healthscape: contributions of time geography, location technologies and spatial ecology to place and health research. Soc Sci Med 70(5):668–676

Sciamanna CN, Goldstein MG, Marcus BH, Lawrence K, Pinto BM (2004) Accuracy of recall of exercise counseling among primary care patients. Prev Med 39(6):1063–1067

Smolin LA, Grosvenor MB (2005) Eating right: an introduction to human nutrition. Chelsea House Publishers, New York

Solecki WD, Welch JM (1995) Urban parks: green spaces or green walls? Landscape Urban Plann 32(2):93–106

Steptoe A, Perkins-Porras L, McKay K, Rink E, Hilton S, Cappuccio F (2003) Primary care-behavioural counselling to increase consumption of fruit and vegetables in low income adults: randomised trial. Primary Care BMJ 326(7394):1–6

Sturm R, Cohen DA (2004) Suburban sprawl and physical and mental health. Public Health 118(7):488–496

Stutzer A, Frey BS (2008) Stress that doesn't pay: the commuting paradox. Scand J Econ 110(2):339–366

Takano T, Nakamura K, Watanabe M (2002) Urban residential environments and senior citizens' longevity in megacity areas: the importance of walkable green spaces. J Epidemiol Community Health 56(12):913–918

The Harvard University (undated) environmental barriers to activity. http://www.hsph.harvard.edu/obesity-prevention-source/obesity-causes/physical-activity-environment/. Accessed 15 Feb 2016

U.S. Department of Health and Human Services (2000) Healthy people 2010: understanding and improving health, 2nd edn. U.S. Government Printing Office, Washington, DC

USDA (2005) Dietary guidelines for Americans 2005, Chapter 9: alcoholic beverages. the sixth Edition, U.S. Department of Health and Human Services and U.S. Department of Agriculture, U.S. Government Printing Office, Washington, DC. http://health.gov/dietaryguidelines/dga2005/document/pdf/dga2005.pdf. Accessed 6 May 2016

Van den Berg P, Kemperman A, de Kleijn B, Borgers A (2015) Locations that support social activity participation of the aging population. Int J Environ Res Public Health 12(9):10432–10449

Waddell G, Burton AK (2006) Is work good for your health and well-being? The Stationery Office, London

World Health Organization (1948) WHO definition of health. Preamble to the constitution of the World Health Organization as adopted by the international health conference, New York, 19–22 June, 1946; signed on 22 July 1946 by the representatives of 61 States (Official Records of the World Health Organization, no. 2, p. 100) and entered into force on 7 April 1948

World Health Organization (2000) Regional guidelines for developing a healthy cities project. WHO/WPRO, Manila

World Health Organization (2010) Global recommendations on physical activity for health. Geneva. Available from: http://apps.who.int/iris/bitstream/10665/44399/1/9789241599979_eng.pdf. Accessed 31 May 2016

World Health Organization (2011) Healthy urbanization: regional framework for scaling up and expanding healthy cities in the Western Pacific 2011–2015. http://www.wpro.who.int/health_promotion/healthy_urbanization_regional_framework_2011_2015.pdf. Accessed 5 May 2016

Zeratsky K (2014) Healthy lifestyle: nutrition and healthy eating. http://www.mayoclinic.org/healthy-lifestyle/nutrition-and-healthy-eating/expert-blog/physical-activity-habits/bgp-20085745. Accessed 5 May 2016

Zhang J (2015) The life-oriented approach and travel behavior research. A discussion paper for the Workshop "Life-Oriented Approach for Transportation Studies" at the 14th international conference on travel behaviour research, Windsor, UK, July 19–23

Chapter 8
Life-Oriented Tourism Behavior Research

Linghan Zhang, Lingling Wu and Junyi Zhang

Abstract Tourism as an extension of people's daily life is becoming prevalent in today's society. However, understanding tourists is still a demanding and changeable task, and the preference structures and decision patterns of different tourists are complex. Research on tourism behavior can help address these issues. In recent decades, research on tourism behavior has attracted considerable attention and has become a cornerstone of tourism market strategy and action. Tourism is not a transient behavior, but is repeated over time and is interrelated with daily life. To understand tourists' lifestyle and decision-making processes, long-term observations of tourism behavior are needed. A life-oriented approach cannot ignore tourism behavior because it is an important part of life. This chapter analyzes recent research on tourism behavior, summarizes the pertinent concepts, characteristics, determinants, and shortcomings in existing studies on tourism behavior, and suggests directions for future research.

Keywords Tourism behavior · Spatial and temporal choices · Social influence · Integrated behavior model · Generation theory · Medical tourism · Health · Quality of life · Qualitative research

8.1 Introduction

Tourism behavior refers to a person's decisions and actions during the tourism process. It is an activity from which people want to experience pleasure that cannot be satisfactorily experienced in their daily lives. Decisions on tourism behavior

---

L. Zhang · J. Zhang (✉)
Hiroshima University, Higashi-Hiroshima, Japan
e-mail: zjy@hiroshima-u.ac.jp; junyizh24@gmail.com

L. Wu
Institution for Transport Policy Studies, Tokyo, Japan

J. Zhang (ed.), *Life-Oriented Behavioral Research for Urban Policy*,
DOI 10.1007/978-4-431-56472-0_8

usually involve a number of separate but interdependent choices that are made over time and across space, such as destination, travel party, duration, travel route, and activity participation during travel. Some of the choices might result from long-term decisions (e.g., destination, season/duration, and travel party), which are further associated with other life choices, and others might be made during travel (e.g., travel route and shopping). The objects of research are often different types of people who take part in tourism, for example, mass tourists, business travelers, lifestyle travelers, and backpackers. The tourism industry has traditionally treated tourism behavior as consumer behavior.

Consumer behavior research deals not only with individuals, but also with groups or organizations. It is concerned with the decision-making processes consumers use to select, use, and dispose of products/services and the impacts that consumer choices have on consumers themselves and society (Swarbrooke and Horner 2007). Consumer behavior models usually consist of three stages: pre-purchase, consumption, and post-consumption (Engel et al. 1995). Consumer behavior is central to tourism decisions and to academic research. In recent decades, many tourism studies have empirically examined consumer decisions and behaviors from various perspectives (Kozak and Decrop 2009). The topic of consumer behavior in the tourism context is the key to the foundation of all marketing activities that are implemented to establish, advertise, and sell tourism products.

Tourism behavior research is interdisciplinary, often requiring knowledge from fields such as sociology, cultural studies, and psychology. Tourism behavior topics vary according to different perspectives. Research on tourism behavior has mainly focused on tourist-based, market-based, and destination-based aspects. For tourist-based research, the typology of tourists is a popular subject of debate. Swarbrooke and Horner (2007) suggested differences in the consumer behavior of tourists and travelers. Sharply (2014) noted that "tourists" often involved package tourism products and were an integral element of the tourism production process, while "travelers" were often on a limited budget. Cohen (1979) distinguished five types of tourists, i.e., recreational, diversionary, experiential, experimental, and existential tourists. Each acts differently in both tourism behavior and experience. Decrop and Snelders (2005) defined six types of vacations in the decision-making process. Developing typologies of tourists is an important means to explain tourism behavior. Research on tourists' satisfaction, motivation, and loyalty is also important for the study of tourism consumer behavior (Yoon and Uysal 2005; Del Bosque and San Martín 2008). To understand tourists better, individual influences, including consumers' demographics, personality traits, lifestyles, emotions, and values are vital concerns for the study of tourism behavior (Frew and Shaw 1999; Alexandra 2013). Market research divides tourists into groups of people who have similar needs, wants, or demands. Market segmentation is aimed at serving the needs of marketers. Johns and Gyimóthy (2002) discussed the factors that influenced tourism behavior based on an "active" and an "inactive" market. Understanding the main characteristics of different groups of tourists would help marketers to predict consumer behavior. Most consumer research in tourism is destination based (Mehmetoglu and Altinay 2006) and has evolved toward an informed empirical and theoretical basis and the widespread adoption of rigorous scientific research methods (Jafari 2005). Chen and Tsai (2007) proposed an integrated model and found that destination image had both direct and indirect effects on behavioral intentions. Questions such as why people choose a certain destination (Um and Crompton 1990; Mazzarol and Soutar 2002), how to get visitors to revisit that place (Jang and Feng 2007), and how to collect information on the destination all require the integrated analysis of tourism behavior (Gursoy and McCleary 2004). However, in the tourism industry, destination, tourists, and market are closely bound together, and any tourism behavior topic should comprehensively consider these three aspects.

8.2 Conceptual Issues

As a complex behavioral phenomenon, tourism behavior has been studied in a variety of disciplines such as geography, psychology, sociology, marketing science, regional and urban planning, transportation, archaeology, cultural anthropology, and agriculture. To draw a general picture about a tourism behavior, a comprehensive classification is helpful. Here, we roughly classify tourism behavior into the following dimensions: (1) information search and use; (2) the social aspect; (3) resources; (4) the spatial aspect; (5) activity participation; and (6) the temporal aspect.

Information search and use: Better scheduling needs reliable and comprehensive information, which includes pre-travel, during-travel, and post-travel information. Pre-travel information is used to decide on a travel, during-travel information is used to modify the planned schedule and support smooth decisions during travel. Information might also be needed after travel (i.e., post-travel information), for example, to evaluate the realized and unrealized activities and to communicate travel experiences to other people (i.e., word-of-mouth information).

Social aspect: The social aspect refers to whether and how tourists decide to travel with other people and/or make use of travel agencies/guides. In the case of traveling with other people, tourists are influenced by coupling constraint, that is, a person has to stay together with another person(s) at a specific place and time. In addition, tourists' decisions usually involve some group decisions, especially in the case of traveling with other people (e.g., family members, friends, and colleagues). Sometimes, tourists consult travel agencies as well as other experienced persons before making their decisions.

Resources: Time and money (e.g., income) are the main resources for performing travel activities. Because of the availability and scarcity values of these resources, participation in various activities is constrained and, consequently, the resources might affect where to visit (destination choice), how long to stay, with whom to travel, as well as the way in which tourists allocate their available time and money to the various activities during travel.

Spatial aspect and activity participation: Choices of destination, accommodation, travel mode, traveling route, stopping behavior, on-site activity participation (e.g., dining, shopping) are examples here. Performing on-site activities is the main purpose of travel and it is usually influenced by authority constraints such as programs of some on-site events, opening hours of attractions, shops, and stores. To realize and support the abovementioned behavioral dimensions, travel mode choice is indispensable. In this study, travel mode choice behavior is regarded as a part of spatial aspects and activity participation.

Temporal aspect: The temporal aspect refers to when and for how long spatial choices are made. The notion that tourist behavior changes over time is also relevant. This means that the temporal aspect might be correlated with all of the preceding dimensions.

It is expected that decisions related to these behavioral dimensions are interrelated from context to context, requiring the development of integrated frameworks of tourist behavior.

8.3 Information Search and Use

Information may be in a spoken, written, or in pictorial format (Goossens 2000; Van Raaij and Crotts 1994), and may come from personal/impersonal and commercial/noncommercial sources (Fondness and Murray 1997) and/or past experiences. Information needs can be classified into functional, hedonic, innovation, aesthetic, and sign (Vogt and Fesenmaier 1998). Functional needs are defined as motivated efforts that are directed at or contribute to a purpose. Hedonic needs support the view that tourists are pleasure-seekers. Innovation needs are defined by novelty seeking, variety seeking, and creativity. Information related to aesthetic needs is viewed as a stimulus to visual thinking, imagery, and envisioning of a place that is real and obtainable. Finally, the sign need describes the interpersonal, social, symbolic, or more general aspects of information acquisition and knowledge transfer.

People's primary motives for undertaking search of pre-travel information are to enhance the quality of travel (Goossens 2000) and to reduce the risk of travel decisions (Money and Crotts 2003). Pre-travel information is first used to motivate people to plan a trip. Such information can play the role of either push factors (e.g., feelings of pleasure, excitement, and relaxation) or pull factors (e.g., attractions like sunshine, friendly people, and culture). Pre-travel information is also used to make a detailed decision about primary choices such as destination (Snepenger et al. 1990) and travel party.

During-travel information is used to make on-site decisions such as choices of travel mode, attractions, locations, activities, and lodging (Snepenger et al. 1990) and choices of traveling route to, in, and/or around a destination. Especially nowadays, Internet-based information systems provide increasingly more accessible, reliable, and comprehensive travel information (Rayman-Bacchus and Molina

2001). Tourists can also easily access the necessary travel information via mobile phone during the course of travel, and car navigation systems are used widely, as in Japan, and can provide not only dynamic information for route guidance, but also information about on-site attractions, restaurants, and so on.

Roles of post-travel information have been mainly studied in the fields of tourist satisfaction and service quality. As argued by Westbrook and Oliver (1991), satisfaction is a post-consumption evaluative judgment about both destination performance and tourists' entire travel process including scheduling behavior. Satisfaction or dissatisfaction about the visited destination(s) is crucial because it may affect expectations for the next visit (Westbrook and Newman 1978; Kozak 2001). Another outcome of the post-evaluation of travel is word-of-mouth information. The influences of word-of-mouth information have been confirmed with respect to various aspects of consumer behavior (Boulding et al. 1993; Zeithaml et al. 1996). Word-of-mouth information usually plays two roles. First, tourists could enjoy post-travel pleasure by showing (talking about) their experiences to other people. Second, such information is also related to tourists' willingness to recommend the visited destinations to other people (Kozak 2001).

Thus, various studies have analyzed the role of information search and use in travel decisions. However, little has been studied with respect to the influence of travel information on tourists' scheduling behavior across space and over time.

8.4 Social Aspect

Using data on household decisions on travel involving airlines, collected in 1968, it was shown that husbands play the predominant role in initiating the idea to take a trip, suggesting a destination and selecting an airline; in contrast, the decision on where to go was a mutual decision (Davis 1976). In their vacation-sequence model, Van Raaij and Francken (1984) emphasized the importance of family members' influence on the decision-making process of tourism service purchases, and incorporated the interaction of household-related variables (e.g., lifestyle, power structure, role, and decision-making style) with individual-related factors. Cosenza and Davis (1981) showed that household members' involvement appears to vary across stages in the household life cycle. For pre-travel decisions, wives are highly involved in selection of a destination and collection of information (Zalatan 1998). Thornton et al. (1997) found that children influence the behavior of the travel party either through their physical needs or through their ability to negotiate with parents. On the other hand, Moutinho (1987) argued that travel decisions are also affected by the behavior of reference groups. Friends and relatives sometimes provide information to the individual decision-making process (Gitelson and Kerstetter 1994). The coupling constraint (Hagerstrand 1970), in which a person has to be together with other people at a certain place and time, is also related to the social aspect.

Concerning the role of travel agencies in tourists' decisions, there is no doubt that information from travel agencies has traditionally been one of major sources for the selection of tourism destinations (e.g., Baloglu and Mangaloglu 2001; Gartner and Bachri 1994; Nolan 1976). Nowadays, however, because use of the Internet to search for travel information is becoming increasingly common, many functions of travel information provision by travel agencies are being replaced by online resources (e.g., Buhalis 1998). However, travel agencies can provide not only information, but also advice. Travel agencies can perform better than travel websites in terms of the human touch and personal service (Law et al. 2004).

8.5 Spatial Aspect

Research about destination includes analysis of destination choice behavior, image making, and evaluation of destination (satisfaction, expectation, attitude, and service quality). Distance is one of the strongest influences on scheduling behavior. Distance can be regarded as a proxy variable for time in the scheduling decision. Indeed, it is quite difficult for tourists to measure accurately actual distance. Many studies have reported that cognitive distance, a mental representation of actual distance, is significantly different from actual distance (e.g., Bratfisch 1969; McNamara 1986a; Ankomah et al. 1996). It has also been noted that cognitive or subjective distance is a better indicator than actual distance when representing spatial choice behavior (e.g., Ankomah et al. 1996). Seddighi and Theocharous (2002) argue that spatial choice needs a multistep decision-making process. A tourist is usually first faced with two alternatives when deciding to take a holiday, namely whether to take a domestic or foreign vacation, and then to choose the travel mode after determining a destination. Spatial choices with different scales usually generate differing levels of time pressure on decisions.

Various models have been proposed to represent spatial choice at different spatial scales. At the international, national, or regional level, econometrics, including time series modeling, has been applied to analyze the influential factors of tourism flows (Song and Witt 2000; Gallet and Braun 2001; De Mello et al. 2002). At less aggregate spatial levels, discrete choice models under the principle of random utility maximization have been widely applied using either revealed preference data or stated preference data (e.g., Haider and Ewing 1990; Morley 1994; Crouch and Louviere 2001; Huybers 2003a, b). In line with the research stream of discrete choice models, especially focusing on how to represent observed and unobserved similarities among alternatives in the choice set, Zhang et al. (2008) developed a new choice model by integrating their proposed nested paired combinatorial logit (NPCL) model and relative utility-based model, where the former is used to describe the unobserved similarity (e.g., liking, hobby, and character) and the latter to explain the observed similarities (e.g., overlapped routes, similar attributes of destinations, and spatial closeness). The relative utility choice model argues that tourist behavior is context (or reference)-dependent (Zhang et al. 2004). Focusing on the choice interdependence between travel party and destination, Wu et al. (2009) represented the heterogeneous nested choice structure involved in the choices of these two decision aspects by combining the latent class and nested logit modeling approaches.

Stopping behavior at a particular travel facility prior to the completion of a travel segment also affects scheduling behavior. As argued by Wansink and Van Ittersum (2004), travel itself is motivated or initiated by the traveler's primary need; in contrast, stopping decisions during travel result from the secondary needs. There are likely two major types of stopping behavior; the first is to acquire information to make the next decisions or confirm the decided schedule, and the second is to meet the needs for gasoline, food, or taking a break. In such cases, tourists have to make trade-offs between the time for stopping and the time eventually allocated to their intended destinations.

In tourism research, few studies have focused on travel mode and route choice, possibly because these are usually determined together with destination. Multidestination choice is another aspect of tourism behavior that has not been well covered to date.

8.6 Temporal Aspect

Zimmermann (1982) argued that there are three temporal dimensions: period effects, life cycle, and cohort effects. Period effects refer to annual changes in tourist arrivals, which are a common concern in all countries. Life cycle relates to variations of individuals' behaviors due to family structure. Different cohorts might show a variety of behavior patterns. Clearly, all three dimensions closely relate to long-term decisions. Oppermann (1995) concluded that there were comparatively few studies on family life cycle applications in tourism and leisure, and research on generational or cohort differences in tourism patterns was rare; the situation has not changed notably since that time.

Furthermore, we believe that short-term decisions related to time allocation (use) decisions during travel should also be appropriately represented in the literature. However, there is also a dearth of work in this area. The existence of temporal constraints (e.g., available holidays and available time in a day) may force tourists to decide how to make effective use of their available and limited time during travel. The more time tourists spend traveling, the less time they spend at their destination. Even though the importance of time use research in tourism has been recognized since the late 1980s (e.g., Pearce 1988), there are few relevant studies. Fennel (1996) proposed a space-time model that describes tourists' behavior by dividing a space into core, transition, and periphery, reflecting their perceptions about the space and the pressures caused by social, environmental, and economic (SEE) impacts of the space. However, the way that the space is classified and how perceptions and SEE are defined is arbitrary. Fujiwara and Zhang (2005) applied Becker's (1965) time allocation theory to represent how a tourist allocates his/her available time to various activities during a one-day car trip within an integrated modeling framework (this is explained below). Linked with resource aspects, Zhang et al. (2009) developed a context-sensitive tourist's time use and expenditure behavior model by explicitly incorporating the influence of spatial closeness of destination and interdestination similarities, representing three types of interdestination interactions—time-to-time, expenditure-to-expenditure, and time-to-expenditure interactions—as well as the relative importance of destinations in decision making.

Another important decision aspect is timing. Timing decisions include both long-term and short-term aspects. The long-term decision concerns when to go on a trip, (e.g., which season), for what special occasions or events (e.g., wedding anniversary, birthday, or in celebration of finding a new job), or as determined by available vacation period. The short-term decision mainly refers to decisions during travel, such as when to depart from home/the hotel on the day of travel, when to visit a place, and when to go back home/to the hotel. An explicit representation of timing makes it possible to describe a meaningful value of time by focusing on momentary experience. In this context, Zhang et al. (2006) developed a multidimensional timing decision model under the principle of random utility maximization by representing the influence of timing constraints and censored timing. The derived model not only allows for the temporally varying utility of a timing decision, but also incorporates sequential correlation between the neighboring timings. The model can also endogenously specify the sequences of activities/trips as well as heterogeneous preferences about the timing.

With a focus on temporal change of tourist behavior, Jang and Feng (2007) explored the effects of tourists' novelty seeking and destination satisfaction on revisit intentions measured on short-term, mid-term, and long-term bases. However, no study has examined how to represent such temporal change.

8.7 Integrated Tourism Behavior Models

Tourism behavior involves a decision-making process with various interrelated choices. Early tourist behavior models were built in the 1950s mainly based on the so-called "grand models" of consumer behavior, which were used to explain decisions on tangible or manufactured products instead of services (Sirakaya and Woodside 2005). A tourist's decision-making process usually follows the following six steps: (1) search for information; (2) evaluation of alternatives; (3) purchase; (4) delivery; (5) consumption; and (6) post-consumption feedback (Engel et al. 1995). Traditional tourist behavior models mainly focused on a certain part of tourist behaviors rather than on a set of tourist behaviors.

Over the last four decades, discrete choice models have proven to be very powerful tools for consumer behavior analyses in various fields including tourism research. The multinomial logit (MNL) model has become the most widely used choice model, probably due to its simple mathematical structure and ease of estimation. Such discrete choice models assume that a decision maker chooses the alternative with the highest utility from the alternatives in the choice set under the principle of random utility maximization. The MNL model has been widely used to represent tourists' destination choice, travel mode choice, and route choice (Perdue 1986; Schroeder and Louviere 1999; Kemperman et al. 2009). However, because it is assumed that the error terms of the utility function are independently and identically distributed across alternatives, the MNL model is characterized by the independence of irrelevant alternatives (IIA) property, which states that the odds of choosing a particular alternative are independent of the existence and the attributes of any other choice alternative in one's choice set. To date, various non-IIA discrete choice models have been proposed to overcome the shortcomings of the MNL model. These non-IIA choice models can be classified into three categories (Zhang et al. 2004).

The first group of non-IIA models avoids the IIA property by relaxing the assumption of identically and independently distributed error terms, or allowing for different variances of error terms, or allowing for positive correlations between error terms. For example, Nicolau and Mas (2006) adopted the random coefficient logit model to analyze tourism destination choice. The model is used to deal with the unobserved heterogeneity of tourists, by assuming that the coefficients of the variables vary among tourists. Wu et al. (2013a) used a mixed logit model to represent the influence of social interactions on tourism participation behavior. The model assumed that members in the same social group share a common random parameter, which can create correlation patterns between error terms.

The second group of non-IIA models circumvents the IIA property by extending the utility specification to account explicitly for similarity between choice alternatives. To account for future dependency in tourism destination choice, Wu et al. (2012a) employed the universal logit model, which includes attributes of other alternatives in the utility function of the target alternative. Therefore, such cross effects can allow for correlations between alternatives and can avoid the IIA assumption.

The third group of non-IIA models assumes a hierarchical or sequential decision-making process. The best-known model that can be represented by a hierarchical decision structure is the nested logit (NL) model. In the tourism research field, the NL model has been used to represent sequential choices, such as tourism generation and destination-type choice (Nicolau and Mas 2008), destination and travel companion choice (Wu et al. 2011a), tourism participation, and destination and travel mode choice (Wu et al. 2012b).

In addition to discrete choice, another important aspect of tourist behavior is temporal choice, including tourist's length of stay and time use decisions on different activities. Most studies focus on the total time that tourists spend during a tour trip. These studies use a survival model to analyze a tourist's length of stay at a certain destination (Gokovali et al. 2007; Martinez-Garcia and Raya 2008; Thrane 2012).

Models have also been proposed to address some specific issues in tourist behavior. As noted above, the mixed logit model has been applied to capture the unobserved heterogeneity of tourists, by assuming that the parameters of variables vary randomly across individuals (Correia et al. 2007; Grigolon et al. 2014; Nicolau and Mas 2006). Some studies have adopted the latent class model to accommodate tourists' heterogeneous choice structures (Alegre et al. 2011; Wu et al. 2011a). To account for the mechanism of loss aversion, some models incorporate prospect theory, which argues that individuals' decisions are more sensitive to losses than to gains. Nicolau (2011, 2012) applied this theory to investigate tourists' asymmetric reactions to travel cost and its effect on destination choice.

Sirakaya and Woodside (2005) noted that one of the first foundational integrated models of travel decision making is that of Clawson and Knetsch (1966), who proposed an outdoor recreation experience model with a five-phase decision-making process starting with the anticipation phase, followed by travel to actual site, on-site experiences and activities, travel back, and concluding with recollection of experiences. Woodside and MacDonald (1994) introduced the concept of trip frame that describes a set of interdependent travel choices (i.e., destination, route/mode, accommodation, activity performance, and visiting shops), which are made at different points in time.

Dellaert et al. (1998) proposed a conceptual framework to represent and understand multifaceted tourist travel decisions that involve subsequent choices for different facets of a single trip as well as the constraints that may limit the number of feasible travel alternatives. They empirically identified some interdependencies in the following choice process after deciding to travel: (1) pre-travel choices (destination, accommodation, travel party, travel mode, departure time, and duration of travel), and (2) during-travel choices (special attractions to visit, travel route to follow, day-to-day expenditure and rest and food stop locations, and timing). Dellaert et al. argued that to account for the above interdependencies, multidimensional choice models like the NL or probit-type models can be applied. Because these choice models cannot directly incorporate timing decisions, they further suggested applying hazard-based duration models. However, duration models are statistically oriented and cannot properly reflect the behavioral mechanisms in timing decisions.

To elucidate the relationship between traveling to one destination versus to several destinations during a trip, King and Woodside (2001) undertook a qualitative comparative analysis of a travel and tourism purchase–consumption system, which is the sequence of mental and observable steps that a consumer undertakes to buy and use several products, for which some of the products purchased lead to a purchase sequence involving other products. King and Woodside also conceptualized a purchase–consumption framework for leisure travel, which begins with information search and use, followed by three sequential levels: level 1, choices of destination, activity, and attraction; level 2, choices of accommodation and mode/route to destination; and level 3, on-site shopping and dining behavior and choice of mode/route in and around the destination. Post-travel evaluation is also included in the proposed purchase–consumption system. Woodside and Dubelaar (2002) extended the King and Woodside model by defining a tourism consumption system as the set of related travel thoughts, decisions, and behaviors by a discretionary tourist prior to, during, and following a trip (Becken and Gnoth 2004).

Focusing on car tourists' one-day tours, Fujiwara and Zhang (2005) developed a new scheduling model by combining a destination/route choice model with a nested paired combinatorial logit (NPCL) structure and a time allocation (TA) model. The NPCL model represents choices of destination and route, where the lower level indicates choice of destination and the upper level refers to choice of route. In addition, utility of destination choice is influenced by the time spent at each site. Different route choices result in hourly variant level of service of the road network, which consequently gives rise to varying available time use in the TA model. These are reflected in the NPCL model. Moreover, the TA model endogenously incorporates the influence of hourly variant level of service at the site of interest, which is further affected by the allocated time. Consequently, an iteration estimation procedure is proposed to estimate consistently the parameters in the NPCL and TA models.

In terms of time allocation in tourism activities, some studies have attempted to analyze tourists' time allocation decisions using a time budget method (Cooper 1981; Fennel 1996), which is a method of measuring the duration and sequence of activities engaged in by an individual during a specific period of time. Activities that tourists participated in were recorded, including starting time and finishing time of each activity, from which tourists' space-time patterns can be derived. More recently, Wu et al. (2011b) applied a multiple discrete-continuous extreme value (MDCEV) model to analyze tourists' time-use behavior involving multiple activities. The model is used to represent simultaneously tourists' decisions on what activities to participate in and how much time to allocate to each activity.

Because tourists face many aspects of choices and have to deal with spatial and temporal constraints, tourist choice behavior is a multidimensional process and its decision-making mechanisms are complex. It is expected that interdependencies exist between different behavior aspects, and some models attempt to represent such interdependency. To represent interrelations between two discrete choices (i.e., destination and travel mode choices), Fukuda and Morichi (2002) developed a framework for modeling recreational travel behavior using a bivariate dichotomous probit model. However, their model can only be used to analyze binary choice behavior. Therefore, some studies used a NL model to incorporate more choice aspects and, at the same time, represent the relationship between them with the help of an inclusive value, which is, in fact, the maximal utility of the alternatives in the choice set of the lower level nest (Wu et al. 2012b). In addition, some models have been developed to represent interdependence between discrete and continuous choice. For example, Alegre et al. (2013) used a Heckman model to analyze households' tourism expenditure decisions, which was treated as an interrelated two-stage process: first, whether to make a trip and, second, how much to spend on it. Their model is a type of discrete-continuous choice model that uses a binary logit model to represent tourism participation behavior and ordinary least squares (OLS) regression to analyze tourism expenditure. At the same time, the model assumes the error terms in two functions follow a bivariate normal distribution. Wu et al. (2013b) employed a similar discrete-continuous choice model to represent these two choice aspects. In their study, tourism participation choice was analyzed with a Scobit model, which includes a skewness parameter to relax the assumption made in a binary logit model that the sensitivity of individuals to changes in explanatory variables is highest for those who have indifferent preferences over participation and nonparticipation.

8.8 Relationship Between Tourism Behavior and Other Life Choices

Tourism experience not only increases individuals' satisfaction with the leisure-life domain, but has also been found to influence other life domains. Trenberth et al. (1999) explored the role of tourism experience in the domain of work and showed that tourism could be useful in coping with work-related stress because of its active-challenge and passive-recuperative natures. Strauss-Blasche et al. (2002) conducted a survey of 53 company employees and found that a restful vacation may buffer occupational stress with respect to physical complaints and life satisfaction. Their survey results also suggested that leisure travel moderates stress primarily when stress levels are relatively high. Sirgy et al. (2011) described how specific tourism experiences contribute to positive and negative effects in various life domains, such as social engagement, love, culture, family, and physical well-being, which spill over to overall life satisfaction.

The relationship between tourism and other life domains also results from the fact that different life domains impose mutually exclusive demands on individuals' limited resources of time. The more time an individual expends on tourism activities, the less time they have for fulfilling their roles in other life domains. Such conflict causes a cross-domain spillover effect, which may have an impact on overall life satisfaction (Rice et al. 1992). Thompson and Bunderson (2001) indicated that conflicts between different life domains increase when individuals fail to allocate the appropriate time to work, family, community, religion, and tourism activities. High job stress, caused by work not being done during the vacation, for example, is associated with poorer well-being (Strauss-Blasche et al. 2002). On the other hand, tourism satisfaction is observed to exert a moderating effect between work/leisure conflict and quality of life (Lin et al. 2013).

8.8.1 Tourism and Generation Theory

Tourism behavior is a part of life choices and it changes over time. To compare the difference through life time, one of the most common and useful way is to classify people by their ages. However, people distinct not only in ages, but by the common events that help shape their lives (Travel Industry Association 2006, p. 8). Thus, tourism researchers try to gain insights through the lens of generation theory instead of simple classification of age. The idea of generation theory was derived from Manheim's arguments about "the problem of generations", and was expanded to apply in the social and cultural processes to classify generations for the purpose of sociological study (Pilcher 1994). Generation theory explains that the era in which a person was born affects the development of their view of the world (Codrington 2008). Lehto et al. (2008) stated that the growth of one generation is influenced by historical, political, economic and social events of the time, as well as educational opportunities and lifestyle changes. The most prevalent classification of generation is the division of American society: Silent Generation, Baby Boomers, Generation X, and Generation Y have become fairly well known and well used in recent years to describe groups of people of different ages in academic research. In generation theory, people of the same age are likely to have similar underlying value systems, which are the drivers of behavior and attitudes, and are good predictors of behavior and expectations (Codrington 2008).

In tourism research, generation theory was firstly introduced to identify homogeneous travel patterns and market segmentations, when marketers recognized the need to target different groups of tourists, rather than the whole market (Pennington-Gray et al. 2003). It is expected that better understanding of tourism behaviors of different generations could forecast the changes over time in a more accurate way. The existing studies are mainly focus on two aspects: tourism consumer behavior and tourism attitude/experience during travel. Most studies are about consumer behavior. For example, Furr et al. (2001) used data from 13,000 individuals to analyze generational consumption and behavioral patterns (including information-seeking behavior, purchase behavior and booking travel behavior) of Internet use to compare the differences in different generations and found that Generation X'ers and Baby Boomers groups were more actively online than the senior group. Beldona (2005) distinguished changes in online travel information search behavior and found that although younger people tended to be more eager for new things and quickly adapted to online behavior, elders also adopted new things earlier than traditionally assumed. Pennington-Gray et al. (2003) made an analysis of cohort and examined the changes in preferences for travel over time. Li et al. (2013a) examined the attitudes and behaviors of American international travelers using a generational analysis, and found that characteristics of generation affected travel characteristics in terms of information usage, previous destination experience and future choice. As for studies on tourism attitude/experience based on generation theory, Lehto et al. (2008) analyzed the tourism experiences sought and actual vacation activities of Silent Generation and Baby Boomer generation and found that the differences in cohort-induced lifestyles and values permeated into vacation experience and activity. Compared to the number of research on consumer behavior and generation theory, research on the perception of tourists is limited. However, the understanding of tourism attitude and experience based on generation theory appears to be a more useful basis for addressing different preferences and behaviors of tourists.

Pennington-Gray and Blair (2009) suggested that more theory-based research is needed to document different generations' travel attitudes and behavior, especially related to the four major generations in American. While we are happy to witness the increase in generational analysis in tourism literature of American tourism market, we also notice that few research in developing countries has considered the influence of generation theory on tourism. Given that different countries experienced different nationally significant events at different times, it seems impossible to develop a single generational theory that applies around the world (Codrington 2011). Codrington (2011) raised up the application of generation theory in Asian regions, unlike American society, generations in different countries have their own classifications for its social development. As more and more international tourists from developing countries have participated in tourism activities, applying the generation theory would gain more insightful understandings of their tourism attitudes and behaviors. On the other hand, existing studies about generation theory and tourism behavior are mainly focus on tourists' revealed preference, like consuming preference and information searching preference. Few of them have focused on the future choice or the decision-making process of different generations. However, research on tourists' intention or attitude of different generations may help to predict the future decision on tourism behavior, which could help destination managers gain a lead in the market in terms of strategic planning and marketing.

Above all, the current studies on tourism and generation theory are still not enough to explain the complex process of tourism behavior, more research is needed under the exploration of generation difference among different region, especially in the Eastern hemisphere.

8.8.2 Senior's Tourism Behavior

Tourists present different tourism attitudes and behaviors in different generation, among which, older generation is one of the main components. With the changing landscape of tourism industry, many academic articles have studied the market of those aged 55 or older, which includes pre-seniors (those 50–64) and seniors (65 and older), to better understand their tourism preferences and behaviors (Shoemaker 2000). The importance of seniors as a market segment in tourism has been recognized for years (Nichols and Snepenger 1988; Lehto et al. 2008). Unlike other generations, seniors have more discretionary time and disposable time, which makes them become main consumers in tourism industry.

Current studies on senior tourism behavior varies from many aspects and different regions. You and O'leary (2000) conducted a cohort analysis of older Japanese travelers and showed that older travelers demonstrated a more active participation pattern than a decade ago. Focusing on tourists in Taiwan, Huang and Tsai (2003) examined the senior travelers in Taiwan through their travel motivations, selection modes and travel satisfactions and adopted Ridit (Relative to an Identified

Distributed) analysis of destination selection attributes and factor analysis to perceive the gap between travel agents and senior travelers and predict seniors' future behavior. Chen and Shoemaker (2014) used generation theory to analyze the psychological characteristics and travel behavior of American senior leisure tourists and confirmed that changes in travel preferences, attitudes, and behaviors among seniors might be minimal, but the difference between two generations, like older senior over 65 and younger seniors under 65, is large because of physiological deterioration, which will make a more specific direction for senior tourism segmentation. Kim et al. (2015) investigated the relationship between seniors' tourism behavior and their overall quality of life and found that when they were satisfied with their trip experience, their overall quality of life would be improved.

To date, the number of senior tourism research is still increasing. Existing studies have revealed that younger and older seniors may have different attitudes and behaviors. On the other hand, such differences may change over time. It is therefore necessary to use longitudinal study to trace seniors' changes in their tourism attitudes and behaviors for better understanding the needs of senior travelers and providing better tourism services for them and improving their overall quality of life.

8.8.3 Young People's Tourism Behavior

According to the WTO, "youth travel includes all independent trips for periods of less than one year by people aged 16–29 which are motivated, in part or in full, by a desire to experience other cultures, build life experience and/or benefit from formal and informal learning opportunities outside one's usual environment" (Richards 2008).

Poon (1993) described a shift within tourism and tourism behavior, the change being from "old tourism," the mass tourism of the 1970s and 1980s, to "new tourism", a flexible, segmented, customized, and diagonally integrated market. Young people are different from older generations because they are more adventurous and seek more autonomy during their travels (Sparks and Pan 2009). Young travelers are not a homogeneous group, their travel style and motivation reflects a changing trend (Cohen 2004). Unlike the older generation, the primary motivation for young travelers is the quest for personal growth instead of leisure, which is achieved through autonomy in decision making, stimulation in daily life, learning through exposure, and detachment and transient yet intense interpersonal relationships (Vogt 1976).

Current research on young people's tourism behavior is limited. How highly developed Internet and mobile technology has changed young people's tourism decisions is one of many areas of debate (Xiang and Gretzel 2010; Bizirgianni and Dionysopoulou 2013). Bui et al. (2013) examined how young Asians construct the concept of an "imagined West" from their travel. They analyzed young independent travelers in Asia and found that novelty seeking, unique experience, cultural capital accumulation, and education were goals when traveling in Western countries. Thus, traditional tourism behavior research could not explain some choices or decisions of young people, because of the more complex demands they made of the process. Traditional areas of segmentation studies in tourism behavior (such as demographic, geographical, and socioeconomic segmentation) did not apply to all kinds of young individuals. New factors should have been studied, for example, psychological characteristics. Pizam et al. (2004) investigated 1429 students and found that high risk taking and sensation seeking had significant effects on travel behavior. Lepp and Gibson (2008) also investigated the relationship between sensation seeking and tourism behavior. Ting et al. (2015) explored young Malaysians' travel lifestyles and outbound tourism intentions based on tourists' holiday decisions.

With the development of technology and high-level exchanges of social value, young people today have distinct characteristics compared with their elders. Normative theory cannot fully explain their behavior change in tourism, and there remains significant room for the study of young people's tourism behavior from a variety of perspectives. In an effort to understand young people's behavior better, some comparisons of different generations have been traced in tourism behavior research. Beldona (2005) distinguished changes in travel information search behavior in the US market and explained strong cohort effects for the period 1995–2000. Chung et al. (2015) utilized generational cohort theory to enhance understanding of tourism motivation and experience of cross-strait (mainland China–Taiwan) tourism and found that generational differences played an important role. Research based on generation theory not only provides a new perspective on young people's tourism behavior, but also benefits knowledge about the senior tourism market (Chen and Shoemaker 2014).

In sum, the youth tourism market and young people's tourism behavior still lack relevant research. As the youth segment is an emerging market, scholars should consider the differences between mature tourism markets and youth tourism markets. The differences caused by social development, value, and lifestyle cannot simply be explained by normative criteria. Advanced models and theories should be established for young people's tourism behavior, which is a significant part of tourism behavior and will have many implications for practical market strategies. On the one hand, youth tourism is a rapidly growing segment of the tourism market. On the other hand, the preferences, personality, attitude, and lifestyle of young people toward tourism are different from traditional mass tourists. This gap between young and older tourists should be investigated through behavior study. Furthermore, because young people are often changeable and demanding, their tourism behavior is difficult to describe with a single choice model or theory. The data on young people's attitudes, emotions, cognition, and experience in tourism are difficult to collect from normative questionnaires. Thus, research on young people's behavior calls for advanced models and improved research methods.

8.8.4 Tourism and Health

In a report submitted to the OECD, Lunt et al. (2011) defined medical tourism as "when consumers elect to travel across international borders with the intention of receiving some form of medical treatment." Medical tourism has become an important part of the tourism industry. Although the treatment in medical tourism may span the full range of medical services, the most common treatments include dental care, cosmetic surgery, elective surgery, and fertility treatment (Lunt et al. 2011). According to the World Travel & Tourism Council (WTTC), in 2011 medical tourism contributed 9 % of global GDP (more than US$6 trillion) and accounted for 255 million jobs.[1] Even though individuals have travelled abroad for health benefits since ancient times (Lunt et al. 2011), no academic studies of medical tourism are found in the literature before Goodrich and Goodrich (1987). Some research regards medical tourism as a special case of patient mobility (see Glinos et al. 2010).

In an extensive study of various countries, Connell (2006) found that affordability of international flights, foreign currency exchange rates, aging of wealthy postwar baby boomers, diffusion of the Internet, existence of brokers connecting patients to hospital networks, progress of health care systems based on advanced technologies in major countries (India, Thailand, Malaysia, and Singapore) are major factors pushing the growth of medical tourism. Costly medical treatments in developed countries are further identified as an important factor for the growth of medical tourism in developing countries. Focusing on medical tourism in Pattaya, Thailand, Mechinda et al. (2010) revealed that loyalty to medical tourism is influenced by satisfaction, trust, perceived values, and familiarity with, and image of, the destination. According to Moghimehfar and Nasr-Esfahani (2011), factors affecting medical tourism destination choices include pull-and-push factors. Pull factors include tourism attractiveness of destination, advantages of cost, access to destination (distance and cost), while push factors include service quality and lack of advanced medical technologies and services at the residence location. Furthermore, it was noted that religious affinity was the most important factor when Muslim couples with infertility chose the destination for reproductive medical treatments. Hallcm and Barth (2011) showed that functional dimensions largely affect value perception of the experience of medical tourism, while Internet usage involves social values, knowledge, and functional values. As a comparative study across countries, Yu and Ko (2012) found that Korean tourists attached the highest importance to medical activities and tourism activities, Japanese tourists mainly emphasized convenience of medical treatment and care services, stay and cost, information, and insurance, while Chinese tourists were most sensitive to stay and cost. In addition, while Chinese tourists showed higher interest in minor surgery, beauty and health care, Japanese tourists were more interested

[1]http://travel.cnn.com/cheapest-facelifts-world-786941/ (accessed March 9, 2016).

While a tourism trip may contribute to tourists' psychological well-being and QOL, its impact would vary depending on different factors, such as length of stay (Neal et al. 2007) and different phases of the trip (Neal et al. 1999). For example, Neal et al. (2007) examined the moderating effect of length of stay and showed that tourism experience has a positive influence on QOL. Moreover, this positive influence is more evident for tourists with extended stays compared with tourists with shorter stays. Tourism activities potentially contribute to QOL in different stages. It is noteworthy that individuals' sense of well-being significantly increases before traveling through planning and anticipating the trip. However, the positive post-trip effects on QOL do not last very long, with some studies suggesting that tourism activities may have short-term effects on QOL. Findings indicate that the positive effects of a vacation fade within a short time (Eden 1990; Westman and Eden 1997). Strauss-Blasche et al. (2002) reported that improvement in QOL lasted no longer than five weeks.

Dolnicar et al. (2012) argued that tourism experience is not important to everyone. People assign different levels of importance to each of the life domains that determine their QOL (Scalon 1993). Some people regard family as the most important contributor to QOL, while others view their work as playing a key role. The impact of tourism experience on QOL may depend on different stages in life and other background variables that may influence the degree of importance of travel. When identifying domains that contribute to QOL constructs, Dolnicar et al. (2013) suggest that it is necessary to take into account that the hierarchy of needs varies across and within individuals over time. Models ranking domain importance should weight domain satisfaction by the importance a person attributes to that specific domain. They proposed a dynamic, individual, hierarchical model to demonstrate the role that tourism activities play in people's lives at any given point in time.

8.9.2 Indirect Effects of Tourism on QOL

Some studies have found that although tourism activity by itself may not be a strong influence on QOL, there might be some intervening variables. Neal et al. (1999) demonstrated that the influence of tourism experience on QOL occurs through the mediation effect of satisfaction with tourism services. They investigated the significance of tourism on leisure life and overall QOL, and showed that satisfaction with tourism services contributed to satisfaction in leisure life, which in turn affected overall QOL. Similarly, Chen et al. (2016) examined the relationships between tourism experiences and life satisfaction through the mediation effect of tourism satisfaction. It was found that individuals who felt relaxed and satisfied with their tourism experience were more likely to be satisfied with their life in general.

In addition to the mediation effect of tourism satisfaction, other intervening variables have also been explored. Sirgy (2010) proposed a conceptual framework that incorporates goal theory to analyze the relationship between tourism and QOL. Sirgy argued that the choice of leisure travel goals (e.g., intrinsic vs. extrinsic, abstract vs. concrete) is important, because those with more attractive and attainable travel goals and those who take actions to implement their goals are more likely to experience higher levels of subjective well-being as a consequence of their leisure travel. Nawijn (2011) found that although people were generally happier when they took a tourism trip, factors such as attitude and holiday stress can influence their levels of happiness, and overall they found no significant improvement in their life satisfaction. Woo et al. (2016) examined the link between tourism motivations and QOL among the elderly, and found that motivations were related to growth needs (knowledge seeking, rest and relaxation, social interaction, and self-fulfillment) rather than basic needs, and that these motivations positively affected their overall life satisfaction.

Although studies have generally supported the view that tourism activity contributes to overall life satisfaction, the complex relationship between tourism and QOL requires further investigation.

8.10 Determinants of Tourism Behavior

Tourism behavior is multi-faceted, including participation in tourism, choices of destination and travel party, choices of travel modes accessing destinations, time use and expenditure at destinations, etc. Generally speaking, even though various factors may affect human choice behaviors, they can be grouped into three categories: factors specific to choice alternatives, factors specific to individual decision-makers, and factors common to all decision-makers (Zhang et al. 2004). Here, determinants of tourist behavior are reviewed following this categorization.

8.10.1 Alternative-Related Determinants

People make a travel for visiting tourism resources (e.g., natural resource, historical and cultural resources, health tourism). A variety of infrastructures are expected to play diverse roles of supporting tourism visits. Accordingly, tourism resources and their supporting infrastructures are two major determinants from the perspective of tourism choice alternatives.

8.10.1.1 Tourism Resources

Natural resources

Natural resources are traditional attractions and important components of the tourism resources and of increasing significance to world tourism industry (Priskin

2001). The term nature-based tourism is generally applied to tourism activities depending on the use of natural resources which remain in a relatively undeveloped state, including scenery, topography, waterways, vegetation and wildlife (Deng et al. 2002). As people become more and more environmentally sensitive, nature-based tourism has received increasing attention from tourists. Millions of people travel to see and experience natural environment. Tourists' satisfaction with and expectation about natural resources are associated with their decisions on choosing nature-based tourism. The tourism managers often search new natural resources for satisfy tourists' diverse demand; however, natural resources are limited and cannot meet all the demand of tourists. Such dilemma calls for creating a sustainable form for balancing nature protection and tourist demand. It is also necessary to enhance tourist' awareness about negative impacts of their visiting behaviors, consequently resulting in their voluntary behavioral changes in consuming natural resources.

Historical and cultural resources
Historical and cultural resources are often linked to cultural heritages, which include both physical assets (e.g., architecture, paintings and sculptures), intangible culture (e.g., folklore), and interpretative arts (e.g., storytelling and drama). These resources can be displayed in museums, heritage sites, exhibitions, and theatres. Cultural resources can be a key sector of some local regions and helps to build unique images. Unlike natural tourism resources, the core of historical and cultural resources needs people's "feel" rather than "gaze" (Poria et al. 2003). Therefore, the links between cultural resources and tourists are more complex. Destinations with historical and cultural resources need to be better managed in a way of being understood and accepted by tourists. This is because different presentations of the resources may bring different perceptions to people, which may arouse or suppress tourists' interest in historical and cultural resources.

Health tourism
With the high cost of medical treatment in the original destination and fewer barriers to travel, the idea of availing healthcare in another city or country is gaining greater appeal to many travelers. (Carrera and Bridges 2006). The decisions to engage in health tourism is complex and are driven by patients' unmet need. Runnels and Carrera (2012) adopted a sequential decision-making process in opting for or against medical care abroad in terms of the required treatments, locations and quality and safety issues attendant to seeking care. Health tourism enhances individual's wellbeing in mind and body though medical interventions and the combination of daily healthy activities with tourism activities may also arouse people's intellectual curiosity and desire for new discoveries (Sung et al. 2012). As health tourism is becoming a new trend in tourism market, especially in senior tourism market, the traditional behavior of tourists would be changed. The aging phenomenon in many countries may contribute to the progress of health tourism, as older people have more discretionary time and are more concerned about their health than other generations.

Urban tourism
Cities, as destinations, receive the greatest volume of tourists (Ashworth and Page 2011) and are determinant attractions to some tourists. Urban tourism provides a set of tourist recourses or activities located in towns and cities, to show tourists the history, culture and modernism of the destination. The development of urban tourism can also have influence on tourists' behavior. For instance, sustainable urban tourism will encourage tourists engage in pro-environmental behaviors (recycling, green transports and green energy), changing people's behavior in city context (Miller et al. 2015). On the other hand, conflicts between urban residents and tourists should be paid enough attention in the design and management of urban tourism.

Event tourism
Events are animators of destination attractiveness and keys to marketing propositions in promotion of places to attract more tourists. Stimulated by event tourism, the destination provides a substitutable form of demand between residents and visitors. Event tourism expands the tourism potential and capacity beyond traditional leisure-based tourism (Getz and Page 2016). The types of event tourism often contain business (conventions, exhibition and marketplaces); entertainment (concerts, shows and award ceremonies); festival and culture (festivals, religious sites and art exhibitions); sports (professional leagues, participator and annual games). For some tourists the event in the destination is the only reason for travel and some destinations become famous all over the world for holding special events.

8.10.1.2 Supporting Infrastructure

Transportation network
When people decide to travel, the first thing to solve is how to get to the destination. The accessibility of tourism destination would determine whether this travel will happen or not in the first place. The essential role of transportation network in tourism development is recognized by many scholars (Prideaux 2000; Khadaroo and Seetanah 2007). It is influential to both tourism development and tourists' choices.
A good and attractive transportation system rests to a large extent on quality and availability of transportation infrastructure comprising air services and airports, land transport systems and routes and water transport infrastructures as well (Khadaroo and Seetanah 2008). It has crucial influences on the tourism attractiveness of destinations.

Because of time available to travel, most tourists prefer a destination with good transportation access. For tourists who want to visit multiple destinations during one trip, the transportation network is even crucial for their choices. Improved transport infrastructure and services (e.g., cheaper airlines, high-speed railway, road capacity improvements, reduced fuel consumption, and discounted transit fare) reduce time and cost spending on moving between places, and consequently accelerate the tourism development.

Accommodation

Accommodation is another important issue for tourists, most people prioritize accommodation when planning a trip and spend most of their planning time and effort on selecting the right option (Li et al. 2015). Many studies have been conducted to study the selection criteria that affect consumers' choice intentions. For example, Lockyer (2005) intensified factors such as location, price, facilities and cleanliness as strong factors on tourists' hotel selection. Sohrabi et al. (2012) conducted an exploratory study of Tehran hotels and found that hotel comfort factors (hotel services, room comfort, car parking and pleasure, etc.) and hotel compensatory factors (including expenditure, news information, security and protection) were often the determinant factors for accommodation choices. For the consideration of multiple criteria in hotel selection, Li et al. (2013b) introduced a new fuzzy decision support technique based on an aggregation function named the Choquet Integral to discover the preferences among travelers that affect their hotel selection. Hotel selection is a complex process as the wide range of selection criteria. Li et al. (2015) adopted Emerging Pattern Mining concept to discover changes and trends in travelers' intentions, which help the hotel managers to identify features of interest to specific groups and meet their guests' expectations.

While nowadays the most common accommodation for travelers is the standardized hotel chains, new types of accommodation have emerged when tourists seek more than just sleeping, for example, the flourish of family inn, which is also called B&B or homestay. The properties of family inn are small and personal in nature and the benefits of such new type of accommodation include quiet, private atmosphere, lower cost and closer interactions between guests and hosts (Nuntsu et al. 2004), which are the main factors affecting people's choices, especially young travelers who seek for novelty. Unlike other business modes of accommodation, there is also a free hospitality exchange network online called Couchsurfing. Travelers who choose Couchsurfing have totally different tourism behaviors compared to the mass tourists. In the study of Couchsurfing, not only traditional studies of accommodation, like selection criteria and operation mode, should be noted, more ethical and moral aspects should be considered to explain how putting trust in strangers and managing relationships by various social networking mechanisms (Molz 2013).

Restaurants, souvenirs, and other hospitality facilities/services

Eating local foods has been considered a key attraction for tourists. Many destinations attempt to provide tourists with culinary experiences (Cohen and Avieli 2004). In the decision-making process, food is becoming a key element in tourists' consumer behavior and to increase tourism satisfaction (Tsai and Wang 2016). In addition, delicate artifacts, convenient information centers and other convenient tourism facilities would also give tourists good impression about the destination and affect their choices during travel. Furthermore, with the rapid development of social media, facility managers should pay more attention to the online evaluations for creating more positive images of the destination by electronic word-of-mouth.

8.10.2 Decision Maker Related Determinants

Sociodemographic

Tourists can be categorized into different groups and types based on their sociodemographic characteristics. Segmentation studies are heavily utilized in tourism behavior research. Commonsense segmentation involves division by gender, age, origins, income, etc. (Nichols and Snepenger 1988; Frew and Shaw 1999). While segmentation studies explain some differences in tourism behavior, the criterion for categorization is sometimes viewed as unsophisticated. Expanded variables should be introduced for categorization and more discriminating criteria selected (Frochot and Morrison 2000). Park and Yoon (2009) studied Korean rural tourism empirically, segmenting the tourists by motivation. Prayag et al. (2015a, b) used bagged clustering on the push-and-pull factors of Western Europe to segment potential young Chinese travelers and offered implications for the young Chinese outbound tourism market. Segmentation criteria need to be specified to explain this new tourism market and tourist behavior.

Emotions and affective states

Tourism is mainly about recreation, feeling better both mentally and physically. Some people even treat it as a means of self-analysis. As an expenditure behavior, tourism decisions are highly emotional as well as influenced by other people (Swarbrooke and Horner 2007: 73). However, the importance of emotion seems to be ignored while tourism behavior research focuses on market segmentation and destination competition.

The main realm of emotion in tourism behavior research is satisfaction and loyalty research. The core question concerns the relevant emotional responses during the consumption or experience of different services. Studies cover tourists in general or at a particular destination (Baloglu 2001; Yoon and Uysal 2005). Emotion and destination image are another realm, and the impact of destination image influences decision making (Chi and Qu 2008). The relationship between emotion and tourism experience seems to be a rather new field. Tourists gain emotional experience through tourism activities and this may change their travel decision process and their choice of the next destination or whether to revisit the place (Prayag et al. 2015a, b).

8.10.3 Environmental Determinants

Social interaction

in Norway. They found that mobility varies from lifestyle mobility to more economic and necessity-based mobility; furthermore, they noted that without year-round jobs, it was difficult to persuade these mobile workers to reside permanently in the region.

Tourism can also contribute to resolving social exclusion issues by removing not only physical barriers, but also internal, cultural, and social barriers that hinder persons with disabilities from participating in tourism (Kastenholz et al. 2015). Engaging in tourism activities can contribute to slowing the progress of dementia in elderly people (Page et al. 2015).

References

Alegre J, Mateo S, Pou L (2011) A latent class approach to tourists' length of stay. Tour Manag 32:555–563

Alegre J, Mateo S, Pou L (2013) Tourism participation and expenditure by Spanish households: the effects of the economic crisis and unemployment. Tour Manag 39:37–49

Alexandra V (2013) Consumer behavior in tourism and the influencing factors of the decision making process. Revista Economica 65(2):186–198

Alinejad ME, Razaghi Z (2012) Culture and its role in tourism development. Life Sci J (ACTA Zhengzhou University, Overseas Edition) 9(3):1593–1597

Ankomah PK, Crompton JL, Baker D (1996) Influence of cognitive distance in vocation choice. Ann Tourism Res 23(1):138–150

Ashworth G, Page SJ (2011) Urban tourism research: recent progress and current paradoxes. Tour Manag 32(1):1–15

Baloglu S (2001) An investigation of a loyalty typology and the multidestination loyalty of international travelers. Tourism Anal 6(1):41–52

Baloglu S, Mangaloglu M (2001) Tourism destination images of Turkey Egypt Greece and Italy as perceived by US-based tour operators and travel agents. Tour Manag 22:1–9

Bansal HS, Voyer PA (2000) Word-of-mouth processes within a services purchase decision context. J Serv Res 3(2):166–177

Becken S, Gnoth J (2004) Tourist consumption systems among overseas visitors: reporting on American German and Australian visitors to New Zealand. Tour Manag 25:375–385

Becker GS (1965) A theory of the allocation of time. Econ J 75:493–517

Beldona S (2005) Cohort analysis of online travel information search behavior: 1995–2000. J Travel Res 44(2):135–142

Bizirgianni I, Dionysopoulou P (2013) The influence of tourist trends of youth tourism through social media (SM) and information and communication technologies (ICTs). Procedia-Social Behav Sci 73:652–660

Boelhouwer J, Stoop I (1999) Measuring well-being in the Netherlands. Soc Indic Res 48:51–75

Boulding W, Kalra A, Staelin R, Zeithaml VA (1993) A dynamic process model of service quality: from expectations to behavioral intentions. J Mark Res 30:7–27

Bratfisch O (1969) A further study of the relation between subjective distance and emotional involvement. Acta Psychol 29:244–255

Buhalis D (1998) Strategic use of information technologies in the tourism industry. Tour Manag 19(5):409–421

Bui HT, Wilkins HC, Lee YS (2013) The 'imagined West' of young independent travelers from Asia. Ann Leisure Res 16(2):130–148

Card J, Cole S, Humphrey A (2006) A comparison of the accessibility and attitudinal barriers model: travel providers and travelers with physical disabilities. Asia Pac J Tourism Res 11:161–175
Carrera PM, Bridges JFP (2006) Globalization and healthcare: understanding health and medical tourism. Expert Rev Pharmacoeconomics Outcomes Res 6(4):447–454
Chen SC, Shoemaker S (2014) Age and cohort effects: the American senior tourism market. Ann Tourism Res 48:58–75
Chen CF, Tsai DC (2007) How destination image and evaluative factors affect behavioral intentions? Tour Manag 28(4):1115–1122
Chen C, Huang W, Petrick J (2016) Holiday recovery experiences tourism satisfaction and life satisfaction—is there a relationship? Tour Manag 53:140–147
Chi CGQ, Qu H (2008) Examining the structural relationships of destination image tourist satisfaction and destination loyalty: an integrated approach. Tour Manag 29(4):624–636
Chung JY, Chen CC, Lin YH (2015) Cross-strait tourism and generational cohorts. J Travel Res
Clark T (1990) International marketing and national character: a review and proposal for an integrative theory. J Mark 54(4):66–79
Clawson M, Knetsch JL (1966) Economics of outdoor recreation. The John Hopkins Press, Baltimore
Codrington G (2008) Detailed introduction to generational theory. Available at: www.tomorrowtodayuk.com. Retrieved 10 May 2016
Codrington G (2011) Detailed introduction to generational theory in Asia. Tomorrow Today 1–22
Coghlan A (2015) Tourism and health: using positive psychology principles to maximise participants' wellbeing outcomes—a design concept for charity challenge tourism. J Sustain Tourism 23(3):382–400
Cohen E (1979) A phenomenology of tourist experiences. Sociology 13:179–201
Cohen E (2004) Backpacking: diversity and change. In: Richards G, Wilson J (eds) The global nomad: backpacker travel in theory and practice. Channel View Publications, Clevedon, pp 43–59
Cohen E, Avieli N (2004) Food in tourism: attraction and impediment. Ann Tourism Res 31(4):755–778
Connell J (2006) Medical tourism: sea sun sand and surgery. Tour Manag 27:1093–1100
Connell J (2013) Contemporary medical tourism: Conceptualisation culture and commodification. Tour Manag 34:1–13
Cooper C (1981) Spatial and temporal patterns of tourist behavior. Reg Stud 15:359–371
Correia A, Santos C, Barros C (2007) Tourism in Latin America: a choice analysis. Ann Tourism Res 34:610–629
Cosenza RM, Davis DL (1981) Family vacation decision making over the family life cycle: a decision and influence structure analysis. J Travel Res 17:17–23
Crouch GI, Louviere JJ (2001) A review of choice modeling research in tourism hospitality and leisure. In: Mazanec JA, Crouch GI, Brent Ritchie JR, Woodside AG (eds) Consumer psychology of tourism hospitality and leisure, vol 2. CABI Publishing, Wallingford, pp 67–86
Davis HL (1976) Decision making within the household. J Consum Res 2:241–260
De Mello M, Pack A, Sinclair T (2002) A system of equations model of UK tourism demand in neighbouring countries. Appl Econ 34(4):509–521
Decrop A, Snelders D (2005) A grounded typology of vacation decision-making. Tour Manag 26(2):121–132
Del Bosque IR, San Martín H (2008) Tourist satisfaction: a cognitive-affective model. Ann Tourism Res 35(2):551–573
Dellaert BGC, Ettema DF, Lindh C (1998) Multi-faceted tourist travel decisions: a constraint-based conceptual framework to describe tourists' sequential choices of travel components. Tour Manag 19(4):313–320
Deng J, King B, Bauer T (2002) Evaluating natural attractions for tourism. Ann Tourism Res 29(2):422–438

Dimanche F (1994) Cross-cultural tourism marketing research: an assessment and recommendations for future studies. In: Uysal M (ed) Global tourist behavior. The Haworth Press, Binghamton, pp 123–134
Dolnicar S, Yanamandram V, Cliff K (2012) The contribution of vacations to quality of life. Ann Tourism Res 39:59–83
Dolnicar S, Lazarevski K, Yanamandram V (2013) Quality of life and tourism: a conceptual framework and novel segmentation base. J Bus Res 66:724–729
Eden D (1990) Acute and chronic job stress strain and vacation relief. Organ Behav Hum Decis Process 45:175–193
Engel JF, Blackwell RD, Miniard PW (1995) Cross-cultural tourism marketing research: an assessment and recommendations for future studies. Consumer behavior, 8th edn. The Dryden Press, Florida
Fennel DA (1996) A tourist space-time budget in the Shetland Islands. Ann Tourism Res 23(4):811–829
Fondness D, Murray B (1997) Tourist information search. Ann Tourism Res 24(3):503–523
Frew EA, Shaw RN (1999) The relationship between personality gender and tourism behavior. Tour Manag 20(2):193–202
Frochot I, Morrison AM (2000) Benefit segmentation: a review of its applications to travel and tourism research. J Travel Tourism Mark 9(4):21–45
Fujiwara A, Zhang J (2005) Development of car tourists' scheduling model for 1-day tour. Transp Res Rec 1921:100–111
Fukuda D, Morichi S (2002) Recreation demand model as a mixture of interrelated travel behaviors. J Eastern Asia Soc Transp Stud 4:47–62
Furr HL, Bonn MA, Hausman A (2001) A generational and geographical analysis of Internet travel-service usage. Tourism Anal 6(2):139–147
Gallet CA, Braun BM (2001) Gradual switching regression estimates of tourism demand. Ann Tourism Res 28(2):503–507
Gartner WC, Bachri T (1994) Tour operators' role in the tourism distribution system: an Indonesian case study. J Int Consum Mark 6(3/4):161–179
Getz D, Page SJ (2016) Progress and prospects for event tourism research. Tour Manag 52:593–631
Gilbert D, Abdullah J (2004) Holidaytaking and the sense of well-being. Ann Tourism Res 31:103–121
Gitelson R, Kerstetter D (1994) The influence of friends and relatives in travel decision-making. J Travel Tourism Mark 3(3):59–68
Glinos IA, Baeten R, Helble M, Maarse H (2010) A typology of cross-border patient mobility. Health Place 16:1145–1155
Gokovali U, Bahar O, Kozak M (2007) Determinants of length of stay: a practical use of survival analysis. Tour Manag 28:736–746
Goodrich G, Goodrich J (1987) Health care tourism—an exploratory study. Tour Manag 8(3):217–222
Goossens C (2000) Tourism information and pleasure motivation. Ann Tourism Res 27(2):301–321
Grigolon A, Borgers A, Kemperman A, Timmermans HJP (2014) Vacation length choice: a dynamic mixed multinomial logit model. Tour Manag 41:158–167
Gursoy D, McCleary KW (2004) An integrative model of tourists' information search behavior. Ann Tourism Res 31(2):353–373
Gustavo NS (2010) A 21st century approach to health tourism spas: the case of Portugal. J Hospitality Tourism Manag 17:127–135
Hagerstrand T (1970) What about people in regional science? Paper Reg Sci Assoc 23:7–21
Haider W, Ewing G (1990) A model of tourist choices of hypothetical Caribbean destinations. Leisure Sci 12(1):33–47

Hall CM, Mitchell R (2000) Wine tourism in the Mediterranean: a tool for restructuring and development. Thunderbird Int Bus Rev 42(4):445–465

Hallem Y, Barth I (2011) Customer-perceived value of medical tourism: an exploratory study—the case of cosmetic surgery in Tunisia. J Hospitality Tourism Manag 18:121–129

Han H (2015) Travelers' pro-environmental behavior in a green lodging context: converging value-belief-norm theory and the theory of planned behavior. Tour Manag 47:164–177

Huang L, Tsai HT (2003) The study of senior traveler behavior in Taiwan. Tour Manag 24(5):561–574

Hudson S, Ritchie JRB (2001) Cross-cultural tourist behavior: an analysis of tourist attitudes towards the environment. J Travel Tourism Mark 10(2–3):1–22

Hunt SD (1976) The nature and scope of marketing. J Mark 40(3):17–28

Huybers T (2003a) Modelling short-break holiday destination choices. Tourism Econ 9(4):389–405

Huybers T (2003b) Domestic tourism destination choices—a choice modelling analysis. Int J Tourism Res 5:445–459

Jafari J (2005) Bridging out nesting afield: powering a new platform. J Tourism Stud 16(2):1–5

Jang SCS, Feng R (2007) Temporal destination revisit intention: the effects of novelty seeking and satisfaction. Tour Manag 28(2):580–590

Johns N, Gyimóthy S (2002) Market segmentation and the prediction of tourist behavior: the case of Bornholm Denmark. J Travel Res 40(3):316–327

Kastenholz E, Eusebio C, Figueiredo E (2015) Contributions of tourism to social inclusion of persons with disability. Disabil Soc 30(8):1259–1281

Kemperman A, Borgers A, Timmermans HJP (2009) Tourist shopping behavior in a historic downtown area. Tour Manag 30:208–218

Khadaroo J, Seetanah B (2007) Transport infrastructure and tourism development. Ann Tourism Res 34(4):1021–1032

Khadaroo J, Seetanah B (2008) The role of transport infrastructure in international tourism development: a gravity model approach. Tour Manag 29(5):831–840

Kim H, Woo E, Uysal M (2015) Tourism experience and quality of life among elderly tourists. Tour Manag 46:465–476

King RL, Woodside AG (2001) Qualitative comparative analysis of travel and tourism purchase-consumption systems. In: Mazanec JA, Crouch GI, Brent Ritchie JR, Woodside AG (eds) Consumer psychology of tourism hospitality and leisure, vol 2, CABI Publishing, Wallingford, pp 87–105

Kozak M (2001) A critical review of approaches to measure satisfaction with tourist destinations. In: Mazanec JA, Crouch GI, Ritchie JRB, Woodside AG (eds) Consumer psychology of tourism hospitality and leisure, Volume 2, CABI Publishing, Wallingford, pp 303–320

Kozak M (2002) Comparative analysis of tourist motivations by nationality and destinations. Tour Manag 23(3):221–232

Kozak M, Decrop A (2009) Handbook of tourist behavior, theory and practice. Routledge, London

Lam T, Hsu CHC (2006) Predicting behavior intention of choosing a travel destination. Tour Manag 27:589–599

Law R, Leung K, Wong J (2004) The impact of the internet on travel agencies. Int J Contemp Hospitality Manag 16(2):100–107

Lee JH (2015) The influence of well-being lifestyle on green health tourism motivation and visit attitude in Gangwon area. J Hotel Resort 14(2):279–297

Lee SH, Sparks B (2007) Cultural influences on travel lifestyle: a comparison of Korean Australians and Koreans in Korea. Tour Manag 28(2):505–518

Lee S, Tideswell C (2005) Understanding attitudes towards leisure travel and the constraints faced by senior Koreans. J Vacation Mark 11:249–263

Leggat P, Kedjarune U (2009) Dental health 'dental tourism' and travelers. Travel Med Infect Dis 7:123–124

Lehto XY, Jang SC, Achana FT, O'Leary JT (2008) Exploring tourism experience sought: a cohort comparison of baby boomers and the silent generation. J Vacation Mark 14(3):237–252
Lepp A, Gibson H (2008) Sensation seeking and tourism: tourist role perception of risk and destination choice. Tour Manag 29(4):740–750
Li X, Li XR, Hudson S (2013a) The application of generational theory to tourism consumer behavior: an American perspective. Tour Manag 37:147–164
Li G, Law R, Vu HQ, Rong J (2013b) Discovering the hotel selection preferences of Hong Kong inbound travelers using the Choquet Integral. Tour Manag 36:321–330
Li G, Law R, Vu HQ, Rong J, Zhao XR (2015) Identifying emerging hotel preferences using emerging pattern mining technique. Tour Manag 46:311–321
Lin J, Wong J, Ho C (2013) Promoting frontline employees' quality of life: leisure benefit systems and work-to-leisure conflict. Tour Manag 36:178–187
Litvin SW, Goldsmith RE, Pan B (2008) Electronic word-of-mouth in hospitality and tourism management. Tour Manag 29(3):458–468
Lockyer T (2005) Understanding the dynamics of the hotel accommodation purchase decision. Int J Contemp Hospitality Manag 17(6):481–492
López-Mosquera N, Sánchez M (2012) Theory of planned behavior and the value-belief-norm theory explaining willingness to pay for a suburban park. J Environ Manage 113:251–262
Lunt N, Smith R, Exworthy M, Green ST, Horsfall D, Mannion R (2011) Medical tourism: treatments markets and health system implications: a scoping review. Organization for Economic Co-operation and Development, Paris
Martin D, Woodside AG (2008) Grounded theory of international tourism behavior. J Travel Tourism Mark 24(4):245–258
Martinez-Garcia E, Raya J (2008) Length of stay for low-cost tourism. Tour Manag 29:1064–1075
Mazzarol T, Soutar GN (2002) "Push-pull" factors influencing international student destination choice. Int J Educ Manag 16(2):82–90
McNamara TP (1986) Mental representations in spatial relations. Cogn Psychol 18:87–121
Mechinda P, Serirat S, Anuwichanont J, Gulid N (2010) An examination of tourists' loyalty towards medical tourism in Pattaya Thailand. Int Bus Econ Res J 9(1):55–70
Mehmetoglu M, Altinay L (2006) Examination of grounded theory analysis with an application to hospitality research. Int J Hospitality Manag 25:12–33
Miller D, Merrilees B, Coghlan A (2015) Sustainable urban tourism: understanding and developing visitor pro-environmental behaviours. J Sustain Tourism 23(1):26–46
Moghimehfar F, Nasr-Esfahani MH (2011) Decisive factors in medical tourism destination choice: a case study of Isfahan Iran and fertility treatments. Tour Manag 32:1431–1434
Molz JG (2013) Social networking technologies and the moral economy of alternative tourism: the case of couchsurfing org. Ann Tourism Res 43:210–230
Money RB, Crotts JC (2003) The effect of uncertainty avoidance on information search planning and purchases of international travel vacations. Tour Manag 24:191–202
Moretti E (2011) Social learning and peer effects in consumption: evidence from movie sales. Rev Econ Stud 78:356–393
Morley C (1994) Experimental destination choice analysis. Ann Tourism Res 21(4):780–791
Moutinho L (1987) Consumer behavior in tourism European. J Mark 21(10):3–44
Nawijn J (2011) Determinants of daily happiness on vacation. J Travel Res 50:559–566
Neal J, Sirgy M, Uysal M (1999) The role of satisfaction with leisure travel/tourism services and experiences in satisfaction with leisure life and overall life. J Bus Res 44:153–164
Neal J, Uysal M, Sirgy M (2007) The effect of tourism services on travelers' quality of life. J Travel Res 46:154–163
Nichols CM, Snepenger DJ (1988) Family decision making and tourism behavior and attitudes. J Travel Res 26(4):2–6

Nicolau J (2011) Differentiated price loss aversion in destination choice: the effect of tourists' cultural interest. Tour Manag 32:1186–1195
Nicolau J (2012) Asymmetric tourist response to price: loss aversion segmentation. J Travel Res 51:568–576
Nicolau J, Mas F (2006) The influence of distance and prices on the choice of tourist destinations: the moderating role of motivations. Tour Manag 27:982–996
Nicolau J, Mas F (2008) Sequential choice behavior: going on vacation and type of destination. Tour Manag 29:1023–1034
Nolan D (1976) Tourist's use and evaluation of travel information. J Travel Res 14(2):6–8
Nuntsu N, Tassiopoulos D, Haydam N (2004) The bed and breakfast market of Buffalo City (BC) South Africa: present status constraints and success factors. Tour Manag 25(4):515–522
Oppermann M (1995) Travel life cycle. Ann Tourism Res 22(3):535552
Page SJ, Innes A, Cutler C (2015) Developing dementia-friendly tourism destinations: an exploratory analysis. J Travel Res 54(4):467–481
Pan TJ, Cheng WC (2014) Chinese medical tourists—their perceptions of Taiwan. Tour Manag 44:108–112
Park DB, Yoon YS (2009) Segmentation by motivation in rural tourism: a Korean case study. Tour Manag 30(1):99–108
Pearce DG (1988) Tourist time-budget. Ann Tourism Res 15(1):106–121
Pennington-Gray L, Blair S (2009) Nature-based tourism in North America: is generation Y the major cause of increased participation. In: Benckendorff P, Moscardo G, Pendergast D (eds) Tourism and generation Y. CABI Publishing, Wallingford, pp 73–84
Pennington-Gray L, Fridgen JD, Stynes D (2003) Cohort segmentation: an application to tourism. Leisure Sci 25(4):341–361
Perdue R (1986) Traders and nontraders in recreational destination choice. J Leisure Res 18(1):12–25
Phithakkitnukoon S, Horanont T, Witayangkurn A, Siri R, Sekimoto Y, Shibasaki R (2015) Understanding tourist behavior using large-scale mobile sensing approach: a case study of mobile phone users in Japan. Pervasive Mobile Comput 18:18–39
Pilcher J (1994) Mannheim's sociology of generations: an undervalued legacy. Br J Sociol 45(3):481–495
Pizam A, Jeong GH (1996) Cross-cultural tourist behavior: perceptions of Korean tour-guides. Tour Manag 17(4):277–286
Pizam A, Sussmann S (1995) Does nationality affect tourist behavior? Ann Tourism Res 22(4):901–917
Pizam A, Jeong GH, Reichel A, Van Boemmel H, Lusson JM, Steynberg L, State-Costache O, Volo S, Kroesbacher C, Kucerova J, Montmany N (2004) The relationship between risk-taking sensation-seeking and the tourist behavior of young adults: a cross-cultural study. J Travel Res 42(3):251–260
Pols J, Kroon H (2007) The importance of holiday trips for people with chronic mental health problems. Psychiatr Serv 58:262–265
Poon A (1993) Tourism, technology and competitive strategies. CABI Publishing, Oxon
Poria Y, Butler R, Airey D (2003) The core of heritage tourism. Ann Tourism Res 30(1):238–254
Powell LM, Tauras JA, Ross H (2005) The importance of peer effects cigarette prices and tobacco control policies for youth smoking behavior. J Health Econ 24:950–968
Prayag G, Disegna M, Cohen SA, Yan H (2015a) Segmenting markets by bagged clustering young Chinese travelers to Western Europe. J Travel Res 54(2):234–250
Prayag G, Hosany S, Muskat B, Chiappa GD (2015b) Understanding the relationships between tourists' emotional experiences perceived overall image satisfaction and intention to recommend. J Travel Res (in press)
Prideaux B (2000) The role of the transport system in destination development. Tour Manag 21(1):53–63

Priskin J (2001) Assessment of natural resources for nature-based tourism: the case of the Central Coast Region of Western Australia. Tour Manag 22(6):637–648
Rayman-Bacchus L, Molina A (2001) Internet-based tourism services: business issues and trends. Futures 33:589–605
Rice R, Frone M, McFarlin D (1992) Work-nonwork conflict and the perceived quality of life. J Organ Behav 13:155–168
Richards G (1999) Vacations and the quality of life: patterns and structures. J Bus Res 44:189–198
Richards G (2008) Youth travel matters: understanding the global phenomenon of youth travel. World Tourism Organization (WTO)
Runnels V, Carrera PM (2012) Why do patients engage in medical tourism? Maturitas 73:300–304
Sands J (1981) The relationship of stressful life events to intellectual functioning in women over 65. Int J Aging Hum Dev 74:11–22
Scalon T (1993) Value desire and quality of life (Chap. 15). In: Nussbaum M, Sen A (eds) The quality of life. Oxford University Press, New York
Schroeder H, Louviere J (1999) Stated choice models for predicting the impact of user fees at public recreation sites. J Leisure Res 31(3):300–324
Seddighi HR, Theocharous AL (2002) A model of tourism destination choice: a theoretical and empirical analysis. Tour Manag 23:475–487
Sharpley R (2014) The consumption of tourism. In: Sharpley R, Telfer DJ (eds) Tourism and development: concepts and issues (2nd edn), Channel View Publications, Clevedon, pp 358–366
Shoemaker S (2000) Segmenting the market: 10 years later. J Travel Res 39(1):11–26
Sigala M, Christou E, Gretzel U (2012) Social media in travel tourism and hospitality: theory practice and cases surrey. Ashgate Publishing, UK
Sirakaya E, Woodside AG (2005) Building and testing theories of decision making by travelers. Tour Manag 26(6):815–832
Sirgy M (2010) Toward a quality-of-life theory of leisure travel satisfaction. J Travel Res 49:246–260
Sirgy M, Joseph P, Kruger S, Lee D, Yu G (2011) How does a travel trip affect tourists' life satisfaction? J Travel Res 50:261–275
Smith M, Kelly C (2006) Wellness tourism. Tourism Recreation Res 31(1):1–4
Snepenger DJ, Meged K, Snelling M, Worrall K (1990) Information search strategies by destination-naive tourists. J Travel Res 29(2):13–16
Sohrabi B, Vanani IR, Tahmasebipur K, Fazli S (2012) An exploratory analysis of hotel selection factors: a comprehensive survey of Tehran hotels. Int J Hospitality Manag 31(1):96–106
Song HY, Witt SF (2000) Tourism demand modeling and forecasting: modern econometric approaches. Pergamon, Amsterdam
Song HJ, You GJ, Reisinger Y, Lee CK, Lee SK (2014) Behavioral intention of visitors to an oriental medicine festival: an extended model of goal directed behavior. Tour Manag 42:101–113
Sparks B, Pan GW (2009) Chinese outbound tourists: understanding their attitudes, constraints and use of information sources. Tour Manag 30(4):483–494
Strauss-Blasche G, Ekmekcioglu C, Marktl W (2002) Moderating effects of vacation on reactions to work and domestic stress. Leisure Sci 24:237–249
Sung J, Woo JM, Kim W, Lim SK, Chung EJ (2012) The effect of cognitive behavior therapy-based "forest therapy" program on blood pressure salivary cortisol level and quality of life in elderly hypertensive patients. Clin Exp Hypertens 34(1):1–7
Swarbrooke J, Horner S (2007) Consumer behaviour in tourism. Routledge, London
Thompson J, Bunderson J (2001) Work-nonwork conflict and the phenomenology of time: beyond the balance metaphor. Work Occupations 28:17–39

Thornton PR, Shaw G, Williams AM (1997) Tourist group holiday decision-making and behaviour: the influence of children. Tour Manag 18(5):287–297
Thrane C (2012) Analyzing tourists' length of stay at destinations with survival models: a constructive critique based on a case study. Tour Manag 33:126–132
Ting CS, Chiu LK, Kayat K (2015) Travel lifestyles and outbound tourism intentions of young Malaysians. Am J Tourism Manag 4(2):40–42
Travel Industry Association (2006) Travel across the generations. Travel Industry Association, Washington DC
Trenberth L, Dewe P, Walkey F (1999) Leisure and its role as a strategy for coping with work stress. Int J Stress Manag 6:89–103
Tsai CTS, Wang YC (2016) Experiential value in branding food tourism. J Destination Market Manag (in press)
Tuulentie S, Heimtun B (2014) New rural residents or working tourists? Place attachment of mobile tourism workers in finnish lapland and Northern Norway Scandinavian. J Hospitality Tourism 14(4):367–384
Um S, Crompton JL (1990) Attitude determinants in tourism destination choice. Ann Tourism Res 17(3):432–448
Uriely N, Yonay Y, Simchai D (2002) Backpacking experiences: a type and form analysis. Ann Tourism Res 29(2):520–538
Van Raaij WF, Crotts JC (1994) Introduction: the economic psychology of travel and tourism. J Travel Tourism Mark 3(3):1–19
Van Raaij WF, Francken DA (1984) Vocation destinations activities and satisfactions. Ann Tourism Res 11(1):101–112
Vogt JW (1976) Wandering: youth and travel behavior. Ann Tourism Res 4(1):25–41
Vogt CA, Fesenmaier DR (1998) Expanding the functional information search model. Ann Tourism Res 25(3):551–578
Voigt C, Laing JH (2010) Journey into parenthood: commodification of reproduction as a new tourism niche market. J Travel Tourism Mark 27(3):252–268
Wang D, Xiang Z, Fesenmaier DR (2016) Smartphone use in everyday life and travel. J Travel Res 55(1):52–63
Wansink B, Van Ittersum K (2004) Stopping decisions of travelers. Tour Manag 25:319–330
Westbrook RA (1987) Product/consumption-based affective responses and post purchase processes. J Mark Res 24(3):258–270
Westbrook RA, Newman JW (1978) An analysis of shopper dissatisfaction for major household appliances. J Mark Res 15:456–466
Westbrook RA, Oliver RL (1991) The dimensionality of consumption emotion patterns and consumer satisfaction. J Consum Res 18:84–91
Westman M, Eden D (1997) Effects of a respite from work on burnout: vacation relief and fade out. J Appl Psychol 82:516–527
Woo E, Kim H, Uysal M (2016) A measure of quality of life in elderly tourists. Appl Res Quality Life 11:65–82
Woodside A, Dubelaar C (2002) A general theory of tourism consumption systems: a conceptual framework and an empirical exploration. J Travel Res 41(2):120–132
Woodside AG, MacDonald R (1994) General system framework of customer choice processes of tourism services. In: Gasser R, Weiermair K (eds) Spoilt for choice, pp 30–59
Wu L, Zhang J, Fujiwara A (2009) A model of heterogeneously nested structure of tourists' destination and travel party choices. In: Proceedings of the 15th APTA (Asia Pacific Tourism Association) annual conference, Incheon, 9–12 July (CD-ROM)
Wu L, Zhang J, Fujiwara A (2011a) Representing tourists' heterogeneous choices of destination and travel party with an integrated latent class and nested logit model. Tour Manag 32(6):1407–1413
Wu L, Zhang J, Fujiwara A (2011b) Representing tourist's time use behavior based on a multiple discrete-continuous extreme value model. J Eastern Asia Soc Transp Stud 9:796–809

Wu L, Zhang J, Fujiwara A (2012a) A tourist's multi-destination choice model with future dependency. Asia Pacific J Tourism Res 17(2):121–132

Wu L, Zhang J, Fujiwara A (2012b) Dynamic analysis of Japanese tourists' three stage choices: tourism participation destination choice and travel mode choice. Transp Res Rec 2322:91–101

Wu L, Zhang J, Fujiwara A, Chikaraishi M (2012c) Analysis of tourism generation incorporating the influence of constraints based on a scobit model. Asian Transp Stud 2:19–33

Wu L, Zhang J, Chikaraishi M (2013a) Representing the influence of multiple social interactions on monthly tourism participation behavior. Tour Manag 36:480–489

Wu L, Zhang J, Fujiwara A (2013b) Tourism participation and expenditure behaviour: analysis using a scobit based discrete–continuous choice model. Ann Tourism Res 40:1–17

Xiang Z, Gretzel U (2010) Role of social media in online travel information search. Tour Manag 31(2):179–188

Xiang Z, Woeber K, Fesenmaier DR (2008) Representation of the online tourism domain in search engines. J Travel Res 47(2):137–150

Ye Q, Law R, Gu B, Chen W (2011) The influence of user-generated content on traveler behavior: an empirical investigation on the effects of e-word-of-mouth to hotel online bookings. Comput Hum Behav 27(2):634–639

Yoo KH, Gretzel U (2011) Influence of personality on travel-related consumer-generated media creation. Comput Hum Behav 27(2):609–621

Yoon Y, Uysal M (2005) An examination of the effects of motivation and satisfaction on destination loyalty: a structural model. Tour Manag 26(1):45–56

You X, O'leary JT (2000) Age and cohort effects: an examination of older Japanese travelers. J Travel Tourism Mark 9(1–2):21–42

Yu JY, Ko TG (2012) A cross-cultural study of perceptions of medical tourism among Chinese Japanese and Korean tourists in Korea. Tour Manag 33(1):80–88

Zalatan A (1998) Wives' involvement in tourism decision processes. Ann Tourism Res 25(4):890–903

Zeithaml VA, Berry LL, Parasuraman A (1996) The behavioral consequences of service quality. J Mark 60:31–46

Zhang J, Timmermans HJP, Borgers A, Wang D (2004) Modeling traveler choice behavior using the concepts of relative utility and relative interest. Transp Res Part B 38:215–234

Zhang J, Fujiwara A, Sawara J (2006) Multi-dimensional timing decisions: a case study in tourism behavior analysis. Tourism Anal 11:319–330

Zhang J, Hakoda Y, Fujiwara A (2008) Modeling of touring behavior along the Asian highway incorporating inter-alternative similarities: a comparative analysis between Japanese and Korean tourists. Infrastruct Planning Rev 25:783–792 (in Japanese)

Zhang J, Zhang H, Wu L, Fujiwara A (2009) Representing tourists' context-sensitive time use and expenditure behavior. In: Proceedings of the 15th APTA (Asia Pacific Tourism Association) annual conference, Incheon, 9–12 July (CD-ROM)

Zimmermann CA (1982) The life cycle concept as a tool for travel research. Transportation 11:51–69

Chapter 9
Influence of Land Use and Transport Policies on Women's Labor Participation and Life Choices

Yubing Xiong and Junyi Zhang

Abstract Across the whole world, gender inequality issues are serious, mainly because of traditional thinking about the role specification within a household. Within the context of urban policy, relevant studies are very limited. This chapter argues that women's labor participation should be further promoted for not only achieving gender equality, but also realizing sustainable economic development. Based on an extensive literature review, a case study in Japan was conducted by considering women's family responsibilities (especially, childcare), associated work–family conflict, time-related work–leisure conflict, and stress-related work–health conflict jointly. To examine women's decisions on labor participation associated with other life choices, a recursive multiequation system is used. Applying such a modeling system have several advantages: (1) to identify the barriers to women's labor participation in Japan after controlling for the effects of land use, transport, and life cycle stages; (2) to clarify the factors for women's good quality of family life, leisure life, health life, and quality of life as a whole; and (3) to provide cross-sectoral policy implications for women's labor participation and promotion of quality of life and work–life balance.

Keywords Women · Childcare · Labor participation · Life choices · Conflicts in life · Land use · Transport · Family life · Leisure · Health · Life cycle stages · Quality of life · Japan · Casual modeling

---

Y. Xiong (✉)
School of Transportation and Logistics, East China Jiao Tong University, Nanchang, China
e-mail: xiongmaozai1989@163.com

J. Zhang
Hiroshima University, Higashi-Hiroshima, Japan
e-mail: zjy@hiroshima-u.ac.jp; junyizh24@gmail.com

J. Zhang (ed.), *Life-Oriented Behavioral Research for Urban Policy*,
DOI 10.1007/978-4-431-56472-0_9

9.1 Introduction

After experiencing a demographic dividend of a rapidly growing labor force and a falling birth rate from the 1960s to 1980s, Japan is now facing the consequences of a rapidly aging society (Kumagai 2015). The consequence of this rapidly aging society is the sharpest labor force decline among advanced economies. Japan's working-age population aged 15–64 years will fall from its peak of 87 million in 1995 to about 55 million in 2050. This is approximately the size of the Japanese workforce at the end of World War II. Unless the output per worker rises at a faster rate to offset the decline in the number of workers, Japan's Gross Domestic Product (GDP) is likely to fall behind that of many of its neighbors. Japan has already ceded second place in global economic size to China, and India is not far behind. By some estimates, the economies of Japan and Indonesia will be the same size by the middle of this century (Steinberg and Nakane 2012). Additionally, young married mothers are largely absent from the workforce in Japan. Many women drop out of the workforce after marriage and childbirth. The majority of these women leave the workforce because of their family responsibilities. Women who return to work often enter part-time or temporary work with low pay and little security. To mitigate such work–family conflict, most families, especially young couples, would consider relocating to maximize their family life benefits. Women are attracted to areas that offer more job opportunities and more flexible positions in particular, and areas with more childcare or welfare facilities so that they may work without the burden of caring for their children. Compared with older couples, more and more young couples make the decision to migrate from small or local cities to the bigger cities and megacities to satisfy their demand for residences with good job availability and accessibility, and a high density of childcare or welfare facilities. This kind of out-migration behavior is currently quite popular among young Japanese adults. Much research has documented the effects of migration on the labor-force status of women (Sandell 1977; Spitze 1984; Shihadeh 1991). Furthermore, another body of research noted that many women benefit from family migration (Clark and Maas 2015). It is well known that Japan has a population that is shrinking and aging faster than that of any other developed countries. In an aging society, if increasing numbers of young adults migrate from small cities to the big cities or metropolitan areas for new jobs or residences, local areas will experience worsening depopulation issues. Recently, both academic and government agendas have increasingly focused on the national depopulation issue (Edgington 2012; Oeda et al. 2012). This depopulation is primarily driven by youth out-migration, particularly of the brightest adults (Stockdale 2006). Muilu and Rusanen (2003) claimed that young people are in a key position for the future of depopulated areas, especially in remote rural areas. An analysis of a 15–24-year-old age cohort in Finland showed that depopulated areas could not remain viable or maintain their economic functions in the long term without renewal of their population structure. Elderly experience obstacles to migrate out, especially with increasing age, which also accompanies the young adults' out-migration activity. The mobility behavior of elderly persons is affected largely by this kind of depopulation issue. As time passes and the living environment worsens in the local regions, an increasing number of women would lose jobs; therefore, an increasing number of young adults would migrate out to acquire a better life. The lives of elderly persons would become bland, which would further damage the Japanese expectancy of long life and a sustainable society in the long run. This is a vicious circle. Therefore, there is much Japan can do to promote its highly educated female population[1] to participate more actively in the workforce. This would mean not only a larger labor force, but also possibly a more skilled labor force because Japanese women on average have completed more years of education than their male counterparts. An increased female labor participation could provide an important boost to growth, but women face huge hurdles (e.g., childcare) to participating in the workforce in Japan. Japan should consider policies to provide better support for working mothers to increase the attractiveness of work. The World Economic Outlook and the International Monetary Fund estimate that raising women's labor participation rates in Japan to the level of northern Europe would increase GDP per capital permanently by approximately 8 % (Steinberg and Nakane 2012).

Therefore, to encourage more women to take up paid work in Japan, Prime Minister Shinzo Abe announced plans to extend childcare leave and expand public daycare facilities.[2] This growth strategy has clear benefits to the economy and for women who seek a career and sense of fulfillment it offers. For many women, having a career and raising a family is an either/or situation and Japanese society as a whole pays a penalty. Japanese women's labor force participation rate is 25 % below men's, which is about twice as high as in Germany and the UK and represents a significant reservoir of female power. Kathy Matsui, a Tokyo-based Goldman Sachs analyst known for her "Womenomics" reports, argues that this ongoing waste of women's human capital is shortsighted and is depressing the economy's growth potential. And, she maintains, it is unsustainable because, "… given the limited alternatives, Japan has no choice but to tap its most underutilized resource. It's hard to run a marathon with just one leg." Therefore, it is clear that if Japan seeks a better future (in terms of economic growth as well as social equity development), it needs to ensure that women are given career opportunities. For example, 74 % of college-educated women quit their jobs voluntarily, which is more than double the rate in the US (31 %) and Germany (35 %). The percentage of women who drop out of the workforce aged in their 30s is also much higher than in the US and Europe. However, it is still controversial whether the policies

[1]The younger generation of women in Japan is more highly educated than are their female peers elsewhere. In 2010, the cohort of women aged in their late 20s had on average 14.3 years of schooling, which is surpassed only by New Zealand among advanced economies.

[2]The Japanese Times. Saving Japan: promoting women's role in the workforce would help. (http://www.japantimes.co.jp/opinion/2013/04/21/commentary/saving-japan-promoting-womens-role-in-the-workforce-would-help/#.VtbxPHol2gS.nish).

Prime Minister Abe proposed can promote the women's labor participation. After women enter the workforce, work–family conflicts, time-related work–leisure conflicts, and stress-related work–health conflicts could be aggravated and reduce women's quality of life (QOL) further.

With the above considerations in mind, this chapter focuses on encouraging more women to take up paid work in Japan while simultaneously suggesting how to reduce women's work–family conflicts, work–leisure conflicts, and work–health conflicts to achieve a work–life balance, which promotes their QOL further. Specifically, the objectives of this chapter are to (1) identify the barriers to women's labor participation in Japan, after controlling for the effects of land use, transport, and life cycle stages; (2) clarify the factors on women's good quality of family life, leisure life, health life, and their QOL; (3) provide cross-sectoral policies with implications for women's job participation and promotion of QOL, which simultaneously creates work–life balance for women. This study is fully based on the idea of a life-oriented approach (Zhang 2014), as described in this book.

In the remainder of this chapter, Sect. 9.2 provides a brief review of existing studies for better positioning the present study in literature. The relevant data descriptions and method specifications are shown in Sect. 9.3. Section 9.4 shows the results based on a recursive multiequation model. Finally, the findings of this chapter are summarized in Sect. 9.5.

9.2 Literature Review

9.2.1 Women's Labor Participation, Land Use, and Transport

Although the free-market system theoretically provides all citizens with the opportunity to seek economic independence, the unstable economic situation, changes in the labor market and work structure, and the national political, legal, cultural, and institutional environment frequently decreases the possibilities for women to integrate into the labor market. First, there is much evidence on sociodemographic barriers in the literature. The presence of young children was shown to exert an increasingly negative effect on women's labor force participation in East Germany (Bonin and Euwals 2005) and Russia (Grogan and Koka 2010). Meanwhile, the negative effect on labor force participation of having elderly living in the household seemed to grow stronger over time for women in Belarus (Pastore and Veraschchagina 2008). Women's education level and wage distribution also showed an effect on the downward trend of women's labor participation in China (Hare 2016). Second, the literature notes that there are two other large obstacles associated with the transport and land-use fields. It is well known that labor markets cannot function without transport. Well-developed and efficient transport systems enable access to labor markets for both (potential) employers and (potential) employees. As transport systems are constrained by their maximum capacity, access to different modes of transport (car, bus, train, tram, metro, and bike) increases the range as well as the flexibility of the labor market. A well-developed transport system supports the reduction of unemployment, stimulates entrepreneurship and the competitiveness of companies, and consequently has a positive impact on the material well-being of society. A well-developed transport infrastructure makes a location more attractive for entrepreneurship and investment (Paradowska and Platje 2016). The majority of studies in the transport field have mentioned that job accessibility can be one hurdle for women's labor participation, and public transport represents a means to overcome employment accessibility and mobility problems. Several empirical studies have confirmed that insufficient job accessibility has a negative effect on labor market outcomes in decentralized cities, which accounts for a substantial part of the labor market penalization experienced by the most vulnerable workers (Howe and O'Connor 1982; Ihlanfeldt and Sjoquist 1998; Ihlanfeldt 2006; Zenou 2008). Matas et al. (2010) estimated the impact of residential job accessibility on female employment probability in the metropolitan areas of Barcelona and Madrid, and the results showed that low job accessibility using public transport negatively affects employment probability. The intensity of this effect tends to decrease with individual's educational attainment. A higher degree of residential segregation also reduces job probability in a significant way, which was also based on a "spatial mismatch" framework. Korsu and Wenglenski (2010) found that the low-skilled workers living in high-poverty neighborhoods and/or neighborhoods with low job accessibility were exposed to a greater risk of long-term unemployment in the Paris–Île-de-France metropolitan area, other things being equal. A significant amount of research has examined transit mobility as a limiting factor for obtaining a job, particularly in regards to private vehicle ownership. The location of economically developed neighborhoods and the siting of public transportation are conceivably codetermined and present an endogenous relationship. Tyndall (2015) further identified a significant causal effect linking public transportation access to neighborhood unemployment rates, particularly amongst subgroups dependent on public transit in US. However, even with the considerable amount of attention paid to the role of public transport in addressing inner-city mobility problems for workers over the past 30–40 years, very little evidence has been published that identifies successful mobility strategies (Sanchez et al. 2004). Previous research has yielded mixed results regarding whether job accessibility is an important factor in determining employment status. Sanchez et al. (2004) indicated that access to fixed-route transit and employment concentrations has virtually no association with the employment status of Temporary Assistance for Needy Families recipients in the six selected metropolitan areas (Atlanta, Georgia; Baltimore, Maryland; Dallas, Texas; Denver, Colorado; Milwaukee, Wisconsin; and Portland, Oregon). Bania et al. (2008) found little or no relationship between public transport access to employment locations and employment participation based on a rich longitudinal dataset in Cleveland, Ohio.

In addition, land-use patterns affect the work location (Lu et al. 2016) and job search process (Bunel et al. 2016). The place where you live can have a decisive influence on the chances of obtaining a job for several reasons (Bunel et al. 2016). First, the physical distance between the place of residence and the available jobs complicates the job search process and decreases the chances of leaving unemployment according to the so-called "spatial mismatch" effect (Gobillon et al. 2007; Hellerstein and Neumark 2011). In the context of employment decentralization in metropolitan areas in the US, Kain (1986) found that disconnections between residential and work location negatively affected employment among African Americans, who tend to be concentrated in the inner city. Second, the sociodemographic composition of the geographical area affects the chances of accessing the labor market through neighborhood, peer, or social media effects, all three of which play a major role in the search for employment (Galster 2012). Furthermore, the presence of local amenities (e.g., public facilities), notably the endowment of public sector employment and subsidized employment influence the employment and unemployment dynamics of the localities. Plenty of research in the land-use field mentioned that people who reside in low-density and isolated areas with poor public transit have fewer job opportunities and lower QOL. Matas et al. (2010) analyzed the effect of the urban structure of Barcelona and Madrid on the probability of female employment and found that job proximity is significant for women, but small and insignificant for men. This study also showed that low job accessibility using public transport negatively affects the employment probability. Gobillon and Selod (2007) concluded that the locations where the unemployment rate is highest affect the local people's job attainment. Furthermore, Dujardin et al. (2008) claimed that the employment probability in Brussels is coherent with the spatial structure of the city. Di Paolo et al. (2016) investigated the suggestion that living in segregated areas that are poorly connected to employment centers has a negative effect on labor market outcomes by analyzing the effect of job accessibility by public and private transport on labor market outcomes in metropolitan area of Barcelona. They found that job accessibility matters most to the intention to work, especially for women. Most interestingly, Bunel et al. (2016) pointed out that the resident effect in the Paris area is significant and important for the magnitude of employment discrimination. Based on statistical and econometric results, a good address can triple the chances of being invited to a job interview.

9.2.2 Women's Labor Participation and Health, Family, and Leisure Life

When women's labor participation and family demands are mutually incompatible, it will be detrimental to their mental health and leisure life. Work–family, work–health, and work–leisure conflicts occur, which adversely affects their

QOL. These conflicts affect significant proportions of the population in the US, Europe, Canada, and Australia (Duxbury and Higgins 2001; Erickson et al. 2010; Öun 2012; Skinner et al. 2012; Allen and Finkelstein 2014). Those conflicts generate strains and compromises in family life and affect when and how families interact and children's emotions (Crouter and Bumpus 2001; Parke 2004). Long and inflexible working hours, demanding and intensive work, and unpredictable work times are influential on one's mental health and leisure (Eby et al. 2005; Goodman and Crouter 2009; Carlson et al. 2011; Nohe et al. 2015). Based on a study conducted in the eastern United States, Goodman and Crouter (2009) investigated whether work pressure predicts greater perceptions of spillover for mothers employed full-time and found a need for policies to reduce levels of work stress and help mothers manage their work and family responsibilities. Carlson et al. (2011) further confirmed that work–family conflict was negatively related to both physical and mental health. The relationships between women's work–family conflict and health are unlikely to be static or one way (Westrupp et al. 2016). However, some recent studies have looked at this relationship across many time points based on longitudinal data collection (Rantanen et al. 2012; Allen and Finkelstein 2014; Westrupp et al. 2016). Using the cross-sectional data from the 2008 National Study of the Changing Workforce, Allen and Finkelstein (2014) investigated relationships between gender, age, and work–family conflict across six family life stages and found that work–family conflict was associated with family stage. In particular, Westrupp et al. (2016) investigated reciprocal effects between work–family conflict and mental health using longitudinal data across 8 years of the family life cycle. The findings revealed that work–family conflicts and psychological distress are distinctive aspects of mothers' well-being that influence each other over time. The findings suggested that employed mothers may benefit from policies and workplace practices that both promote maternal well-being and reduce conflicts between employment and childcare. Based on a longitudinal study in Australia, Cooklin et al. (2016) further contributed novel evidence that mental health is directly influenced by the work–family conflict interface, both positively and negatively, and highlighted such conflict as a key social determinant of health.

Achieving work–family balance is dependent on managing the conflict between work and family roles. In most couples, paid work and caregiving continues to be divided along gendered lines. In Australia, as in many other industrialized countries, fathers are typically employed full-time, and often for an extended long working week (Charlesworth et al. 2011; Bünning and Pollmann-Schult 2015). Despite extensive research on the effect of policies on the labor participation of mothers, little is known about how these policies affect the labor market outcomes. Bünning and Pollmann-Schult (2015) had an interesting finding that short maternal leaves are associated with shorter working hours among highly educated fathers, generous family allowances, and father-friendly parental leave schemes reduce the working hours of less-educated fathers. These family responsibilities push more mothers to cut back their work hours by seeking part-time or reduced hours in lower-status jobs or industries (Craig and Sawrikar 2009). Therefore, the majority of employed mothers work part-time as their way of managing the work–family conflicts (Charlesworth et al. 2011) and balance their work and family life well. The research on women's leisure is scarce and mainly focuses on their leisure-related physical activity engagement. Based on the data from a Japanese occupational cohort survey, Oshio et al. (2016) examined the association between job stress and leisure-time physical inactivity by focusing on the evolution of job stress and leisure-time physical inactivity within the same individual over time. The results showed that job stress, especially high job strain and effort–reward imbalance, was modestly associated with higher risks of physical inactivity, even after controlling for individual time-invariant attributes. Based on a two-wave data survey conducted in Dutch, De Vries et al. (2016) investigated the idea that reciprocal relations between leisure-related physical activity and work-related fatigue exists and found that an increase in leisure-related physical activity was associated with a decrease in work-related fatigue over time and that an increase in work-related fatigue was associated with a decrease in leisure-related physical activity over time.

In addition, Mehdizadeh (2013a) found that most policy makers are of the view that women's main problem in labor participation is the pressure they experience from performing multiple roles. As a result, the Iranian government has enacted laws that influence women's employment status with an agenda of reducing their working hours while maintaining a full salary. For example, to mitigate the above work–life, work–leisure, and work–health conflicts, some of the more relevant policies proposed in Iran are as follows (Mehdizadeh 2013b, 2016):

- Reduced hours of work with full pay and benefits for female employees.
- Job flexibility in the form of teleworking was introduced in the public sector in 2012.
- Married women who are permanent employees and whose husbands are sent on fixed missions outside the country are allowed to travel with their husbands and stay there for several years on leave without pay and can return to their previous jobs after their husbands' missions are finished.
- Both men and women can take unpaid leave for up to three years for reasons concerning family responsibility without losing their post.
- Nursing mothers are allowed one-hour paid free time per day for breastfeeding until the child is two years old. A mother with twins is allowed two hours per day. This time can be divided into two or three daily breaks.
- Maternity leave is extended from four months to six months, and to 12 months for twins and triplets.
- Job security for mothers is ensured after maternity leave and during breastfeeding.
- Paternity leave for fathers is extended to two extra days paid leave per month with increased maternity leave for mothers.
- Female students have the right to take one or two semesters' maternity leave.
- Women are offered help with childcare subsidies.
- Childcare centers and services provision.

This represents an impressive legislative attempt to ease women's reconciliation of employment and family life. As can be seen from the list above, policy measures aim to preserve and enhance mothers' family roles while at the same time allowing them to participate in the labor market. However, there are still many implementation problems because there is frequently a dichotomy between policy and practice.

9.2.3 Women's Labor Participation and QOL

In Chap. 3, we discussed a considerable amount of research that examined the relationships between ones' job, leisure, health–life aspects, and QOL (Brajša-Žganec et al. 2011; Zhao and Lu 2010; Tefft 2012; Lin et al. 2013; Curl et al. 2015; Tsai et al. 2016; Uysal et al. 2016). Working is a key part of most people's lives; therefore, knowing what makes a good working life is vital to knowing how well society is doing. Integral to worker well-being, working satisfaction affects the labor market through related decisions on whether to work, how to work, and how much effort to put into work. O'Neill et al. (1998) investigated the effect of employment on perceived QOL, social integration, and home and leisure activities for individuals with traumatic brain injuries. Their findings illustrated that employment showed a strong and consistent relationship with perceived QOL, social integration within the community, and home and leisure activities. Part-time employment may have been superior to full-time employment for individuals, and part-time workers had fewer unmet needs, were more socially integrated, and were more engaged in home activities than full-time workers were. Zahmatkesh et al. (2015) examined the relationship between work performance and QOL, and found that work performance is meaningful for QOL. Fujino et al. (2016) also supported the notion that better employment status enhances subjective QOL in patients with schizophrenia. However, examples of the way researchers analyze how unemployment affects the QOL are also meaningful. Subjective well-being measurements can tell us interesting and different things about the causes, consequences, and experience of unemployment (Myers and Diener 1996; Ettema et al. 2011; Plagnol and Scott 2011).

Moreover, the majority of research deals with the well-being of women in the workplace. As labor force participation among women continues to rise, the well-being of working women is of increasing concern. The focus on women is warranted because the issues that women face at work and at home often differ from the issues faced by men based on different work and family roles. Many occupations are considered gendered, with the lower status and lower paid positions often being associated with feminine characteristics. Women often suffered from harassment or discrimination in the workplace (Buzzanell et al. 2007; Camp et al. 2016; Combs and Milosevic 2016), which fully undermine the well-being of working women. The well-being of working women is of critical importance; it is in the best interest of communities and organizations. In one of the earliest studies examining the relationship between role experiences (work: autonomy, tedium, overload; marriage: spouse support, marital problems; parenting: positive mother experience, negative mother experience) and well-being (symptoms of psychological distress and happiness) in Malaysia, Noor (1999) showed that the work condition—job autonomy has a significant effect on both distress and happiness after controlling for demographic and personality variables. Based on a life course approach, Noor (2006) further indicated that there is a direct impact between work status and well-being for Malaysian women in the age group between 20 and 29 years.

9.3 Data and Method

9.3.1 *Survey and Data*

To understand women's decision-making mechanism related to their labor participation and life choices, particularly under the influence of land-use and transport policies, this chapter uses life choice data collected in 2010 (Zhang 2014) in Japan. The labor force mentioned here are people aged 15–64 years old.[3] Nine hundred thirty-eight valid samples of women were gathered, including the data of individual characteristics, life cycle stages, and the attributes of land use and transport sectors. The attributes of individual characteristics include age, occupation, and education level, while the attributes of life cycle stages involve no child home, one child home, two children home, child at school, child over 18 years old, no elderly home, one elderly home, two elderly home, etc. The attributes of land use are featured by the density of different infrastructure facilities, and the characteristics of travel behavior are represented by the main travel mode to engage in various activities. The description of sample data is shown in Table 9.1.

In terms of data representation in the national level, the OECD Better Life Index showed that women's well-being is higher than men's, especially for the life satisfaction indicator. Life satisfaction measures how ones evaluate their life as a whole rather than their current feelings. When asked to rate their general satisfaction with life on a scale from 0 to 10, the Japanese gave it a 5.9 grade, which was lower than the OECD average of 6.6. However, women reported being somewhat happier than men, rating their lives at 6.1, compared with 5.7 for men.[4] Our survey data matches the above evidence; women feel more satisfaction/happiness

[3]Ministry of Health, Labor and Welfare. Ministry of the young adults in Japan, which refers to the people aged from 15 to 34 years old. (In Japanese). (http://www.mhlw.go.jp/topics/2010/01/tp0127-2/12.html).

[4]OECD Better Life Index. (http://www.oecdbetterlifeindex.org/topics/life-satisfaction/).

Table 9.1 Summary of sample data characteristics

Sample characteristics (Value: %)	Women (N = 938)	Men (N = 940)	Sample characteristics (Value: %)	Women (N = 938)	Men (N = 940)
Age			Household income		
15–34 years old	25.46	24.03	<2 million yen/year	7.39	8.13
35–64 years old	74.54	75.97	2–6 million yen/year	47.63	45.29
Marital status			>6 million yen/year	44.98	46.58
Married	70.71	68.95	Car ownership		
Single	29.29	31.05	Have more than one car	27.46	26.34
Occupation			Have a private car	51.92	54.99
Employed	24.72	74.32	Have no car	20.62	18.67
Part-time job	18.80	3.14	Main travel mode		
Housewife	40.60	0.55	Cycling/walking	43.34	27.91
Student	8.12	9.33	Public transit	33.30	40.02
Unemployed	7.76	12.66	Car	19.89	27.17
Education level			Others	3.47	0.49
With a bachelor degree	59.31	67.74	Health condition		
Without a bachelor degree	40.69	32.26	Good	78.65	76.43
Household composition			Not good	21.35	23.57
No child	75.36	78.93	Life satisfaction		
One child	11.77	9.43	Satisfied (>4 point)	60.22	53.88
Two children	9.31	8.32	Not satisfied	39.78	46.12
Three children or more	3.56	3.32	Happiness		
No elderly	88.50	88.08	Happy (more than 8 score)	54.46	51.38
More than one elderly	11.50	11.92	Not Happy	45.54	48.62

compared with men, and women without a job feel more satisfaction/happiness than do men with paid work. The details obtained from our survey data are shown in Figs. 9.1 and 9.2.

In addition, the relationships between life cycle stages and women's labor participation are shown in Fig. 9.3, which indicates that the more preschool children and elderly persons (aged over 65 years old) there are at home, the higher the likelihood women would not go out to work. The description of explanatory variables for modelling are shown in Table 9.2.

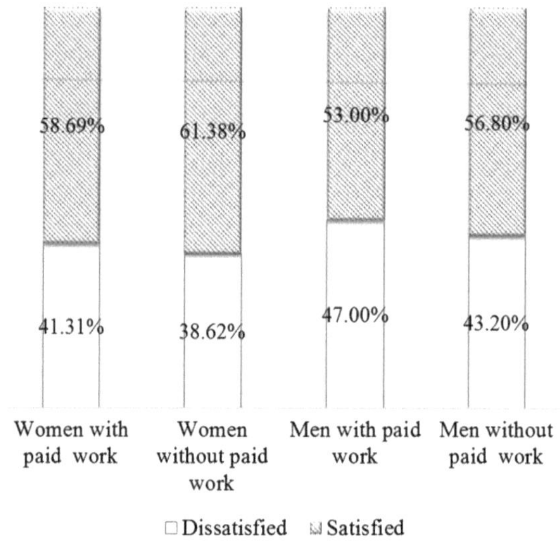

Fig. 9.1 Life satisfaction by gender

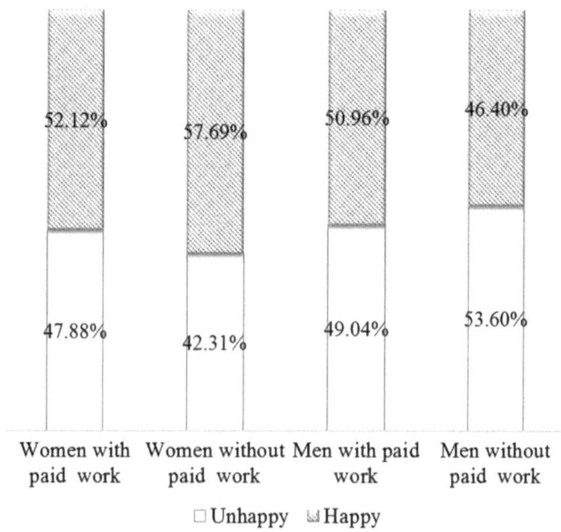

Fig. 9.2 Happiness by gender

9.3.2 Model Specification

This study employs a recursive multiequation system to illustrate the recursive impacts of land-use and transport policies on women's labor participation and their life outcomes. The structure of this multiequation system is represented in Fig. 9.4. This study focuses on five life outcomes: good family life, good leisure life, good health life, self-rated happiness, and life satisfaction. All of these outcomes are expected to be affected, directly or indirectly, by women's labor

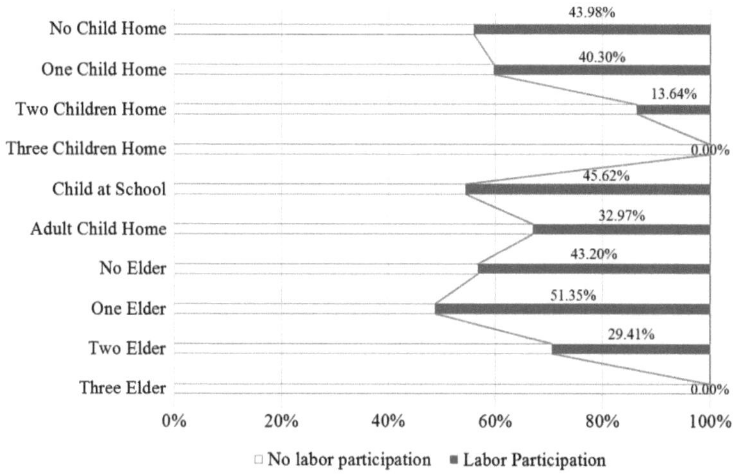

Fig. 9.3 The relationships between life cycle stages and women labor participation

participation. This life course causal model is analogous to a "pathways model" in life course epidemiology (Kuh et al. 2003). It is hypothesized that women's labor participation first directly affects their good family life attainment (high frequency of family-related activities: such as contact with family member or relatives more than once a day). Furthermore, due to time issues, women's labor participation has a straightforward relationship on their good leisure life (high frequency of leisure-related activities: such as going to the cinema, amusement park, and entertainment facilities more than twice a month). Concerning work-related time and stress, women's labor participation would also have a direct impact on their good health life (high frequency of health life-related activities: such as playing sports more than once a week). In line with the foregoing discussion, a good family life would also promote good leisure and health life. Finally, in line with our assumption to balance the women's work and life well, it is expected that women's labor participation, good family life, good leisure life, good health life, which all have a positive influence on their happiness (a score of more than 8) and life satisfaction (a score of more than 4).

To make this recursive structure of life outcomes empirically tractable, this study first dichotomizes each outcome, as discussed later in more detail. Here, we consider six binary variables: "women's labor participation," "good family life," "good leisure life," "good health life," "happiness–feeling happy," and "life satisfaction–feel satisfied." We used a recursive multivariate probit model, a full version of which is expressed in Eq. (9.1), where Y_g* is a latent variable for the binary variable Y_g, X_g is a vector of exogenous variables to explain Y_g, and ($\varepsilon_1; \ldots; \varepsilon_6$) is a vector of six-variate normally distributed error terms with var (ε_g) = 1 for $g = 1, 2, \ldots, 6$. Fifteen covariances between a pair of six error terms, which are denoted as rho$_{gk}$ (g, k = 1, 2, …, 6; g > k), are also to be estimated.

Table 9.2 Explanatory variables for modelling

Socio-demographics	*Residence choices*
Age (15–64)	Living in the megacities (1: yes, 0: no)
Role in family (1: head, 0: otherwise)	Residence duration
Marital status (1: married, 0: otherwise)	Residence property (Own = 1, 0)
Driving license (1: own, 0: otherwise)	Living area (m^2)
Number of pre-school children	Neighborhood with kindergarten (≤1 km)
Number of elderly (≥65 years old)	Neighborhood with high school (≤1 km)
Health status (1: good, 0: not good)	Neighborhood with elementary school (≤1 km)
Education level (1: bachelor, 0: otherwise)	Neighborhood with secondary school (≤1 km)
Household composition	*Travel behavior*
Household annual income	Vehicle ownership
Land use attributes (density per km^2)	Main travel model is walking/cycling (1: yes, 0: no)
Density of welfare facilities	Main travel model is public transit (1: yes, 0: no)
Density of local government facilities	Main travel model is car (1: yes, 0: no)
Density of public facilities	*Other life choices*
Density of railway stations	Job training participation (1: yes, 0: no)
Density of bus stops	Part-time job (1: yes, 0: no)
Density of employment	Professional job (1: civil servant, company employee, 0: no)
Density of medical facilities	With holiday system (1: yes, 0: no)
Life cycle stages	Vacation taken last year (days)
Child at home (1: household with pre-school child, 0: no)	Commute distance (km)
Child at school (1: household with child of school age, 0: no)	Working hours per day
Adult child at home (1: household with child of 18 years old or over, 0: no)	Work days monthly
Elderly at home (1: household with old person of 65 years old or over, 0: no)	

$$
\begin{aligned}
Y_1^* &= X_1\beta_1 + \varepsilon_1 \\
Y_2^* &= \alpha_{21}Y_1 + X_2\beta_2 + \varepsilon_2 \\
Y_3^* &= \alpha_{31}Y_1 + \alpha_{32}Y_2 + X_3\beta_3 + \varepsilon_3 \\
Y_4^* &= \alpha_{41}Y_1 + \alpha_{42}Y_2 + X_4\beta_4 + \varepsilon_4 \\
Y_5^* &= \alpha_{51}Y_1 + \alpha_{52}Y_2 + \alpha_{53}Y_3 + \alpha_{54}Y_4 + X_5\beta_5 + \varepsilon_5 \\
Y_6^* &= \alpha_{61}Y_1 + \alpha_{62}Y_2 + \alpha_{63}Y_3 + \alpha_{64}Y_4 + X_6\beta_6 + \varepsilon_6 \\
Y_g &= 1 \text{ if } Y_g > 0;\ \ Y_g = 0 \text{ otherwise, for } g = 1, 2, \ldots, 6
\end{aligned}
\tag{9.1}
$$

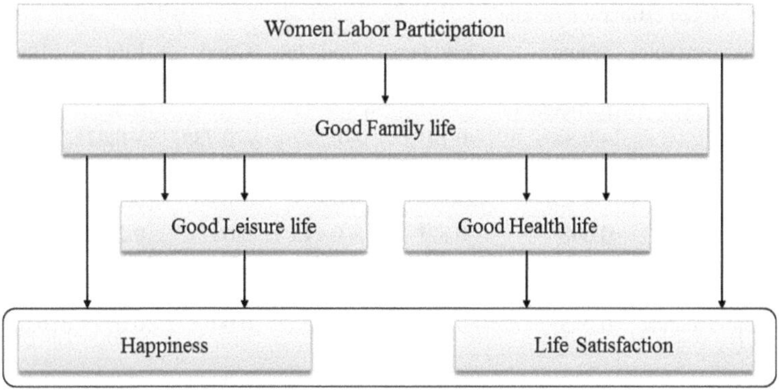

Fig. 9.4 The causal model for work and life balance

This estimation of the multivariate probit model was carried out using the software Stata Version 13.0, which applies the simulated maximum likelihood estimation method (Cappellari and Jenkins 2003). Two things should be noted regarding this six-variate probit model. First, it completely reflects the causal structure illustrated in Fig. 9.4. Second, estimation of a recursive multivariate probit model requires some considerations for the identification of the model parameters. Maddala (1983) proposed that at least one of the reduced-form exogenous variables should not be included in the structural equations as an explanatory variable. Following Maddala's approach, this study imposes exclusion restrictions: (1) to make X_1 include at least one exogenous variable that is not included in X_2, (2) to make both X_1 and X_2 include at least one exogenous variable that is not included in X_3 and X_4 (3) to make all X_1, X_2, X_3 and X_4 include at least one exogenous variable that is not included in X_5 and X_6.

9.4 Influential Factors

Table 9.3 summarizes the estimation results from the above recursive model. Based on McFadden's pseudo rho-square value, it was demonstrated that the estimation results are mainly acceptable. This study mainly focuses on the ways to promote more women to take up paid work and simultaneously balance their work and life. The estimates associated with the control variables significantly influence women's labor participation, which is in line with the results previously obtained in the literature. In terms of the attributes of life cycle stages, the results show that, as expected, a child in the family, especially one younger than 6 years old, hinder women's ability to participate in the labor workforce. However, having a child at school increases women's propensity to have paid work. The estimates associated with land-use attributes indicate that higher density of transit facilities

Table 9.3 Model estimation results

Explanatory variables	Women labor participation	Good family life	Good leisure life	Good health life	Life satisfaction	Happiness
Constant	−0.84*	−0.14*	−0.577	−0.73*	−0.22*	−0.159
Socio-demographics						
Age	−0.251*	0.30*	0.008*	−0.037	0.274*	0.173
Role in family	0.608*	−0.82*	−0.145	0.087	0.231	0.181
Marital status	−0.255*	0.569*	0.065	−0.05*	0.245*	0.286*
Driving license	0.602*	−0.03	0.096*	0.159*	−0.045	−0.115
Household annual income	0.013*	−0.03*	0.050*	0.061*	0.077*	0.070*
Health status	0.233*	0.052	0.116*	0.209*	0.749*	0.615*
Education level	0.117	−0.22*	0.037*	−0.037	0.223*	0.031
Household composition	−0.14*	0.179*	0.021	−0.20*	−0.10*	−0.10*
Number of children	−0.6*	0.320*	−0.02*	−0.11*	0.133*	0.278*
Number of elderly	−0.222*	0.366*	0.4468	−0.20*	0.282	0.281
Vehicle ownership	0.153*	0.066*	0.035*	0.035*	0.026	0.048*
Life cycle stages						
Child at home	−0.537*	0.17	−0.44*	−0.25*	−0.01*	0.046*
Child at school	0.068*	0.055*	0.22*	0.212*	0.003*	−0.077
Adult child at home	0.001	0.002	0.001	0.003	0.006	0.123*
Elderly at home	0.156	−0.64	−0.367	0.466	−0.179	−0.229
Land use attributes						
Density of railway stations	0.164*	0.055	0.398*	0.185	0.034*	0.004*
Density of bus stops	0.088*	−0.05	0.01*	0.028*	0.103*	0.085*
Density of welfare facilities	0.030	0.12*	0.078	0.115*	0.193*	−0.054
Density of local government facilities	0.109	--	--	--	0.032	−0.014
Density of medical facilities	0.010	0.021*	−0.013	0.006	0.062*	0.083*
Density of public facilities	0.021*	0.111*	0.027*	0.069*	0.007*	0.013*
Density of employment	0.344*	0.220	0.160*	0.132	0.52*	0.29*
Travel behavior						
Main travel model is walking/cycling	0.055	0.118	−0.09*	0.372*	0.225*	0.116*
Main travel model is public Transit	0.608*	−0.09	0.067*	0.371	−0.061	−0.092
Main travel model is car	0.203	0.168*	−0.049	0.142	0.002*	0.197*
Residential choices						
Megacities	0.125	−0.21*	0.025*	−0.12*	0.08*	0.145*
Residence duration	0.001	0.002	−0.008	--	0.007	0.010*
Living area	0.000	0.113*	--	0.003*	0.110*	0.004

(continued)

Table 9.3 (continued)

Explanatory variables	Women labor participation	Good family life	Good leisure life	Good health life	Life satisfaction	Happiness
Residence property	−0.079	−0.15	--	--	0.009*	−0.127
Neighborhood with kindergarten	0.023*	0.129	0.153*	0.148	0.159*	0.049*
Neighborhood with high school	0.131	0.004	−0.136	0.024	0.117	−0.014
Neighborhood with elementary school	0.194*	0.05	0.032*	0.136	0.094*	0.161*
Neighborhood with secondary school	0.421*	−0.06	0.158*	0.155	0.219*	0.129
Other life choices						
Job Training participation	0.200*	−0.01*	0.033*	0.038*	0.013	0.002*
Commute distance	–	−0.01*	−0.013*	−0.001*	−0.19*	−0.12*
Working hours per day	–	−0.04*	−0.02*	−0.01*	−0.01*	−0.03*
With holiday system	–	0.007*	0.006*	0.010*	0.002*	0.013*
Vacation taken last year	–	0.008*	0.004*	0.003*	0.020*	0.012*
Work days monthly	–	−0.154*	−0.164*	−0.01*	−0.02*	−0.01*
Professional job	–	−0.27*	0.178*	−0.76*	0.024*	−0.42*
Part-time job	–	0.146*	0.137*	0.451*	−0.19*	−0.65*
Women labor participation	–	−0.31*	−0.106*	−0.691*	0.722*	0.026*
High family life engagement	–	--	0.17*	0.133	0.227*	0.265*
High leisure life engagement	–	--	--	--	0.178*	0.287*
High health life engagement	–	--	--	--	0.272*	0.123*
Number of observation	943					
Wald Chi-square (223)	708.45					
LL0	−3251.3428					
LL1	−3130.4827					
Pseudo R-square (McFadden's)	0.1058					
P-value for Wald chi-square	0.0000					
rho21	rho31	rho41	rho32	rho43	rho53	rho65
−0.569*	−0.255*	−0.344*	0.002*	0.410*	0.131*	0.660*

Note '--' the variables weren't put into estimation for the target dependent variables; '*' statistical significance at the 5 % level

(e.g., railway station and bus stop) and public facilities have the expected effect on job acquirement for women, which suggests that these variables capture how land-use patterns favor the accessibility and availability of work. Women who consider the accessibility of the public transit in their place of residence have a higher likelihood to get paid work. Finally, women living in areas with higher employment rates have more opportunities to have paid work, which partially matches the general idea that residential segregation is often accompanied by insufficient job accessibility, especially when accompanied by poor access to public transport. Besides, in terms of the residential neighborhood, the results indicate that residence near childcare facilities, such as kindergartens, and elementary and secondary schools, have a beneficial impact on women returning to work. In other words, these primary education facilities can somewhat relieve young mothers' childcare burdens. In particular, this model considers the effect of job-training program engagement. Participating in job-training program was shown to be good for more women to obtain paid work. Therefore, the higher probability among women of being regularly employed is implicitly sensitive to women's labor participation. The labor department could offer more job-training classes to promote more women returning to work.

In addition, this study illuminates the variables beneficial to women's work–life balance, not only in women's labor participation, but also in their achievement of life outcomes and QOL promotion. The results discovered that with a child in the household, women felt happier, but were less satisfied, which negatively affects women's labor participation as well as their engagement in health- and leisure-related activities. However, having a child at school had a positive effect on women's work and life, especially enhancing their life satisfaction. Considering the land-use variables, women with a residence with higher density of transit, medical, and public facilities have a higher likelihood to feel happier and more satisfied, which is also beneficial to their leisure and healthy life pursuits. Moreover, the accessibility of welfare facilities is good for women to achieve a higher healthy lifestyle and feel more satisfied. Most importantly, the results shows that with a higher probability to obtain work, women feel more satisfied and happier about their life, while it is also detrimental to a higher quality family, health, and leisure life. The availability of childcare facilities, such as kindergartens, and elementary and secondary schools, has a beneficial impact on women's good QOL. Expectedly, based on the job characteristics, it was found that inflexible work time and long commuting distances hinder women's opportunities to work, as well as improvement of their QOL. While jobs including a sufficient holiday package, ability to take long leave, or flexible working time attracts women to participate in paid work and improve their QOL. In particular, professional women working full-time feel more satisfied with their life than do these with part-time work. The Japanese government should consider policies to increase the number of career-track female employees because it has by far the lowest rate of female managers among advanced economies worldwide.

Consistent with the above recursive assumption, the results show that women's labor participation has a negative effect on the quality of their family, leisure, and health life, which were all expected to have a positive impact on improvement of their QOL. Accordingly, the results demonstrate that women's labor participation, higher engagement in family, leisure, and health life are all beneficial to their QOL. It is also worth noting that the estimated correlations between the error terms of the five equations are always significant, which means that the interrelation between the unobservable elements that affect those five life outcomes should be taken into account to obtain a consistent estimate of the impact of women's labor participation on QOL-associated outcomes. In all, the estimation results reveal that women's labor participation has an expected persistent impact on subsequent life outcomes.

9.5 Conclusion

This study hypothesized that encouraging more women to take up paid work in Japan could cause work–family conflict, time-related work–leisure conflict, and stress-related work–health conflict, and detrimentally affect their QOL. And this study made an initial attempts to balance women's work and family life, which in accordance with the idea of a life-oriented approach (Zhang 2014). A recursive multiequation system was employed to identify the barriers to women's labor participation in Japan, after allowing for the effects of land use, transport and life cycle stages; to clarify the factors on women's good quality family, leisure, and health life, and their QOL; and to provide cross-sectoral policies' implications for women's labor participation and promotion of QOL, and simultaneously women's work–life balance.

Our empirical analysis found that women's labor participation has a persistent impact on subsequent life outcomes. In line with conventional wisdom and the results from many previous studies, women's labor participation is a hurdle for their attainment of a good family, leisure, and healthy life, while beneficial for their QOL. First, from a land-use viewpoint, job accessibility (density of employment and commute distance) and closeness of the residence to childcare facilities (such as kindergartens, elementary schools) can encourage women to obtain paid work, which is beneficial for engagement in a good leisure life, further happiness, and satisfaction. Second, considering the transport sector, despite more vehicle ownership, living in an environment with good public transit accessibility helped steer women toward the labor market. However, allowing for good healthy life attainment (engaging in more physical activities), walking or cycling rather than driving is more meaningful. The results found that the attainment of higher quality health, leisure, and family life is good for achieving a high level of QOL (happier and more satisfied). Thirdly, considering other life choices behavior, jobs with fewer working hours, fewer working days, with a sufficient holiday package, and more vacation days attract more women to go to work, and those factors improve their happiness and satisfaction. Most interestingly, participation in job-training programs also plays a prominent role in women's job, health, and leisure life, and happiness, but it is detrimental for improving family life. Japan should provide better support for working mothers. A more-flexible work environment combined with better childcare facilities and longer leave policies would help reduce the number of women who exit the workforce after childbirth. The results highlighted that land-use, transport, employment, and leave policies should cooperate to deal with the issue of women's labor participation in Japan, and simultaneously balance their work and life.

References

Allen TD, Finkelstein LM (2014) Work–family conflict among members of full-time dual-earner couples: an examination of family life stage gender and age. J Occup Health Psychol 19(3):376

Bania N, Leete L, Coulton C (2008) Job access employment and earnings: outcomes for welfare leavers in a US urban labour market. Urban Stud 45(11):2179–2202

Bonin H, Euwals R (2005) Why are labor force participation rates of East German women so high? Appl Econ Q 51(4):359

Brajša-Žganec A, Merkaš M, Šverko I (2011) Quality of life and leisure activities: How do leisure activities contribute to subjective well-being? Soc Indic Res 102(1):81–91

Bunel M, L'Horty Y, Petit P (2016) Discrimination based on place of residence and access to employment. Urban Stud 53(2):267–286

Bünning M, Pollmann-Schult M (2015) Family policies and fathers' working hours: cross-national differences in the paternal labour supply. Work Employment and Society

Buzzanell PM, Waymer D, Paz Tagle M, Liu M (2007) Different transitions into working motherhood: discourses of Asian Hispanic and African American women. J Fam Commun 7(3):195–220

Camp JK, Trzcinski E, Resko S (2016) Family and labor market policies in Germany. In: Connerley ML, Wu J (eds) Handbook on well-being of working women. Springer, Netherlands, pp 449–472

Cappellari L, Jenkins SP (2003) Multivariate probit regression using simulated maximum likelihood. The Stata J 3(3):278–294

Carlson DS, Grzywacz JG, Ferguson M, Hunter EM, Clinch CR, Arcury TA (2011) Health and turnover of working mothers after childbirth via the work–family interface: an analysis across time. J Appl Psychol 96(5):1045

Charlesworth S, Strazdins L, O'Brien L, Sims S (2011) Parents' jobs in Australia: work hours polarisation and the consequences for job quality and gender equality. Aust J Labour Econ 14(1):35

Clark WA, Maas R (2015) Interpreting migration through the prism of reasons for moves. Population Space Place 21(1):54–67

Combs GM, Milosevic I (2016) Workplace discrimination and the wellbeing of minority women: overview prospects and implications. In: Connerley ML, Wu J (eds) Handbook on well-being of working women. Springer, Netherlands, pp 17–31

Cooklin AR, Dinh H, Strazdins L, Westrupp E, Leach LS, Nicholson JM (2016) Change and stability in work–family conflict and mothers' and fathers' mental health: longitudinal evidence from an Australian cohort. Soc Sci Med 155:24–34

Craig L, Sawrikar P (2009) Work and family: how does the (gender) balance change as children grow? Gend Work Organ 16(6):684–709

Crouter AC, Bumpus MF (2001) Linking parents' work stress to children's and adolescents' psychological adjustment. Curr Dir Psychol Sci 10(5):156–159

Curl A, Thompson CW, Aspinall P (2015) The effectiveness of 'shared space'residential street interventions on self-reported activity levels and quality of life for older people. Landscape Urban Plann 139:117–125

De Vries JD, Claessens BJ, van Hooff ML, Geurts SA, van den Bossche SN, Kompier MA (2016) Disentangling longitudinal relations between physical activity work-related fatigue and task demands. Int Arch Occup Environ Health 89(1):89–101

Di Paolo A, Matas A, Raymond JL (2016) Job accessibility employment and job-education mismatch in the metropolitan area of Barcelona. In: Papers in regional science (in press)

Dujardin C, Selod H, Thomas I (2008) Residential segregation and unemployment: the case of Brussels. Urban Stud 45(1):89–113

Duxbury LE, Higgins CA (2001) Work-life balance in the new millennium: where are we?; where do we need to go? CPRN Discussion Paper No. W|12. Canadian Policy Research Network, Ottawa

Eby LT, Casper WJ, Lockwood A, Bordeaux C, Brinley A (2005) Work and family research in IO/OB: content analysis and review of the literature (1980–2002). J Vocat Behav 66(1):124–197

Edgington DW (2012) Japan's shrinking regions in the 21st Century: contemporary responses to depopulation and socioeconomic decline. Reg Stud 46(9):1275–1276

Erickson JJ, Martinengo G, Hill EJ (2010) Putting work and family experiences in context: differences by family life stage. Hum Relat 63(7):955–979

Ettema D, Gärling T, Eriksson L, Friman M, Olsson LE, Fujii S (2011) Satisfaction with travel and subjective well-being: development and test of a measurement tool. Transp Res Part F 14(3):167–175

Fujino H, Sumiyoshi C, Sumiyoshi T, Yasuda Y, Yamamori H, Ohi K, Fujimoto M, Hashimoto R, Takeda M, Imura O (2016) Predicting employment status and subjective quality of life in patients with schizophrenia. Schizophrenia Res Cogn 3:20–25

Galster GC (2012) The mechanism(s) of neighbourhood effects: theory evidence and policy implications. In: Van Ham M, Manley D, Bailey N, Simpson L, Maclennan D (eds) Neighbourhood effects research: new perspectives. Springer, Netherlands, pp 23–56

Gobillon L, Selod H (2007) The effects of segregation and spatial mismatch on unemployment: evidence from France. Research Unit Working Papers 0702, Laboratoire d'Economie Appliquee, INRA

Gobillon L, Selod H, Zenou Y (2007) The mechanisms of spatial mismatch. Urban Stud 44(12):2401–2427

Goodman WB, Crouter AC (2009) Longitudinal associations between maternal work stress negative work-family spillover and depressive symptoms. Fam Relat 58(3):245–258

Grogan L, Koka K (2010) Young children and women's labour force participation in Russia, 1992–20041. Econ Transit 18(4):715–739

Hare D (2016) What accounts for the decline in labor force participation among married women in urban China, 1991–2011? China Econ Rev 38:251–266

Hellerstein JK, Neumark D (2011) Employment in black urban labor markets: problems and solutions (No. w16986). National Bureau of Economic Research

Howe A, O'Connor K (1982) Travel to work and labor force participation of men and women in an Australian metropolitan area. Prof Geogr 34(1):50–64

Ihlanfeldt KR (2006) A primer on spatial mismatch within urban labor markets. In: Arnott RJ, McMillen DP (eds) A companion to urban economics. Blackwell Publishing, Hoboken, pp 404–417

Ihlanfeldt KR, Sjoquist DL (1998) The spatial mismatch hypothesis: a review of recent studies and their implications for welfare reform. Hous Policy Debate 9(4):849–892

Kain JF (1986) The influence of race and income on racial segregation and housing policy. Housing Desegregation and Federal Policy

Korsu E, Wenglenski S (2010) Job accessibility residential segregation and risk of long-term unemployment in the Paris region. Urban Stud 47(11):2279–2324

Kuh D, Ben-Shlomo Y, Lynch J, Hallqvist J, Power C (2003) Life course epidemiology. J Epidemiol Community Health 57(10):778–783
Kumagai F (2015) Demographic changes in Japan. In: Kumagai F (ed) Family issues on marriage divorce and older adults in Japan. Springer, Singapore, pp 11–38
Lin JH, Wong JY, Ho CH (2013) Promoting frontline employees' quality of life: leisure benefit systems and work-to-leisure conflicts. Tour Manage 36:178–187
Lu QC, Zhang J, Rahman ABM (2016) People's location change adaptation to flood and cyclone in Bangladesh. In: Compendium of papers CD-ROM, the 95th annual meeting of transportation research board, Washington, D.C., 10–14 January
Maddala GS (1983) Limited–dependent and qualitative variables in econometrics. Cambridge University Press, Cambridge, MA
Matas A, Raymond JL, Roig JL (2010) Job accessibility and female employment probability: the cases of Barcelona and Madrid. Urban Stud 47(4):769–787
Mehdizadeh N (2013a) Beyond cultural stereotypes: educated mothers' experiences of work and welfare in Iran. Crit Soc Policy 33(2):243–265
Mehdizadeh N (2013b) Measures to promote work family reconciliation in the MENA region: parental leave child care and good practices. Expert Group Meeting Doha, Qatar, 2–3 June
Mehdizadeh N (2016) Work-family balance and the well-being of educated women in Iran. In: Connerley ML, Wu J (eds) Handbook on well-being of working women. Springer, Netherlands, pp 703–716
Muilu T, Rusanen J (2003) Rural young people in regional development-the case of Finland in 1970–2000. J Rural Stud 19(3):295–307
Myers DG, Diener E (1996) The pursuit of happiness. Sci Am 274(5):70–72
Nohe C, Meier LL, Sonntag K, Michel A (2015) The chicken or the egg? A meta-analysis of panel studies of the relationship between work–family conflict and strain. J Appl Psychol 100(2):522–536
Noor NM (1999) Roles and women's well-being: some preliminary findings from Malaysia. Sex Roles 41:123–145
Noor NM (2006) Malaysian women's state of well-being: empirical validation of a conceptual model. J Soc Psychol 146(1):95–115
O'Neill J, Hibbard MR, Broivn M, Jaffe M, Sliwinski M, Vandergoot D, Weiss MJ (1998) The effect of employment on quality of life and community integration after traumatic brain injury. J Head Trauma Rehabil 13(4):68–79
Oeda Y, Asada K, Sumi T (2012) The study on daily combined activities of regular medical treatment and shopping for people who live in depopulated area. Procedia—Soc Behav Sci 43:277–283
Oshio T, Tsutsumi A, Inoue A (2016) The association between job stress and leisure-time physical inactivity adjusted for individual attributes: evidence from a Japanese occupational cohort survey. Scand J Work Environ Health 42(3):228–236
Öun I (2012) Work-family conflict in the Nordic countries: a comparative analysis. J Comp Fam Stud 43(2):165–184
Paradowska M, Platje J (2016) Key challenges facing the European Transport Labour Market. Discourse in social market economy, Discourse 2016-3. Available: http://www.ordnungspolitisches-portal.com/Diskurse/Diskurse_2016-03.pdf. Accessed 15 June 2016
Parke RD (2004) Development in the family. Annu Rev Psychol 55:365–399
Pastore F, Verashchagina A (2008) The determinants of female labour supply in Belarus. Available at SSRN 1136178
Plagnol AC, Scott J (2011) What matters for well-being: individual perceptions of quality of life before and after important life events. Appl Res Qual Life 6(2):115–137
Rantanen J, Kinnunen U, Pulkkinen L, Kokko K (2012) Developmental trajectories of work–family conflict for Finnish workers in midlife. J Occup Health Psychol 17(3):290–303
Sanchez TW, Shen Q, Peng ZR (2004) Transit mobility jobs access and low-income labour participation in US metropolitan areas. Urban Stud 41(7):1313–1331

Sandell SH (1977) Women and the economics of family migration. Rev Econ Stat 59(4):406–414

Shihadeh ES (1991) The prevalence of husband-centered migration: employment consequences for married mothers. J Marriage Fam 53(2):432–444

Skinner N, Hutchinson C, Pocock B (2012) The big squeeze: Work life and care in 2012. Australian Work and Life Index 2012. Center for Work + Life, University of South Australia. Available: http://w3.unisa.edu.au/hawkeinstitute/cwl/documents/AWALI2012-National.pdf. Accessed 15 June 2016

Spitze G (1984) The effect of family migration on wives' employment: how long does it last? Soc Sci Q 65(1):21–36

Steinberg C, Nakane M (2012) Can women save Japan? International Monetary Fund Report. Available: https://www.imforg/external/pubs/ft/wp/2012/wp12248pdf. Accessed 15 June 2016

Stockdale A (2006) Migration: pre-requisite for rural economic regeneration? J Rural Stud 22(3):354–366

Tefft N (2012) Mental health and employment: the SAD story. Econ Human Biol 10(3):242–255

Tsai SY, Lee PL, Lin JW, Lee CN (2016) Cross-sectional and longitudinal associations between sleep and health-related quality of life in pregnant women: a prospective observational study. Int J Nurs Stud 56:45–53

Tyndall J (2015) Waiting for the R train: Public transportation and employment. Urban Studies (in press)

Uysal M, Sirgy MJ, Woo E, Kim HL (2016) Quality of life and well-being research in tourism. Tour Manage 53:244–261

Westrupp EM, Strazdins L, Martin A, Cooklin A, Zubrick SR, Nicholson JM (2016) Maternal work–family conflict and psychological distress: reciprocal relationships over 8 years. J Marriage Fam 78(1):107–126

Zahmatkesh M, Rad HS, Kahaki F, Azimi S (2015) Comparison of quality of life and job performance of teachers with chronic pain and normal. The AYER 3:180–185

Zenou Y (2008) Job search and mobility in developing countries theory and policy implications. J Dev Econ 86(2):336–355

Zhang J (2014) Revisiting residential self-selection issues: a life-oriented approach. J Transp Land Use 7(3):29–45

Zhao P, Lu B (2010) Exploring job accessibility in the transformation context: an institutionalist approach and its application in Beijing. J Transp Geogr 18(3):393–401

Chapter 10
Mobility of the Elderly

Makoto Chikaraishi

Abstract This chapter briefly overviews studies on mobility of the elderly with a particular focus on its conceptualization, measurement, and evaluation. The role of mobility in the everyday life of the elderly is first explored through putting mobility discourses into a broader context. After clarifying hierarchy of travel needs, interdependencies between mobility and other life domains, and the linkage between mobility and well-being are discussed. Then, policy aspects related to mobility of the elderly are examined, aiming to draw on the potential conflicts that exist among different perspectives including social welfare, economy, and urban planning. Finally, this chapter points out the needs for conducting further cross-cutting empirical studies, establishing a clearer linkage between conceptual framework and empirical framework, developing a simple and standardized method to collectively show the importance of social aspects of transport, and exploring the potential changes in the role or position of the elderly in future.

Keywords The elderly · Mobility · Achieved mobility · Capability approach · Hierarchy of travel needs · Well-being · Measure of achievement · Measure of freedom to achieve · Social exclusion

10.1 Introduction

It is widely known that mobility decreases with aging (Fobker and Grotz 2006; Rosenbloom 2004; Whelan et al. 2006). In response to this fact, a number of transport policies to maintain or improve the mobility of the elderly have been implemented, including the introduction of low floor buses, concessionary fares on public transport, and door-to-door public transport services (Broome et al. 2012;

M. Chikaraishi (✉)
Hiroshima University, Higashi-Hiroshima, Japan
e-mail: chikaraishim@hiroshima-u.ac.jp

J. Zhang (ed.), *Life-Oriented Behavioral Research for Urban Policy*,
DOI 10.1007/978-4-431-56472-0_10

Metz 2003; Schmöcker et al. 2005). Meanwhile, it is also known that age is not just an indicator of the reduction of ability to travel (e.g., due to physical depression) but also an indicator of the reduction of travel needs (e.g., due to having less mandatory activities). This implies that the reduction of observed travel *itself* may not necessarily be linked with transportation issues. In some cases, the reduction of travel may be an issue of lacking opportunities to participate in social activities (Chikaraishi et al. 2013). This means it is important to make a clear distinction between *mobility* and *achieved mobility* in policy discussions: the former indicates the ability of the individual to travel,[1] i.e., what they can achieve, while the latter indicates the behavior they actually took, i.e., what they did. Policy focus could be substantially different depending on whether we focus on mobility or achieved mobility. For example, mobility may need to be explored when we focus on social welfare aspects of transportation, while achieved mobility may need to be focused on when we explore the economic impacts of transportation. However, such distinction has not been well made. In particular, a number of transport studies focusing on social welfare aspects have focused on achieved mobility rather than mobility, partially due to inherent difficulties in direct observation of mobility.

Another important aspect in discussing elderly mobility issues is about value judgments. We could consider that mobility *itself* has its own value, but a number of studies, especially from the viewpoint of land use and urban planning, emphasize the importance of looking at accessibility (i.e., the ability to access goods, opportunities, and services) rather than mobility. This is best reflected in the UK's social exclusion discourses (SEU 2003). On the other hand, some researchers emphasize that the value of mobility is more than the value of accessibility to some extent. For example, Rowe and Kahn (1997) emphasize that (1) low probability of disease, (2) high cognitive and physical functional capability, and (3) active engagement with life, are crucial for successful aging. From this viewpoint, a number of recent empirical studies show that mobility rather than accessibility is one of the main factors for successful aging as we will see later. In such a situation, it is becoming more and more difficult to establish a standardized policy evaluation criterion.

In this chapter, we attempt to give an overview of the current studies on mobility of the elderly with a particular focus on its conceptualization, measurement, and evaluation. We first explore the role of mobility in the everyday life of the elderly, through putting mobility discourses into a broader context: we focus on interdependencies between mobility and other life domains, followed by discussions on the linkage between mobility and well-being. We then introduce recent studies which attempt to distinguish mobility from achieved mobility. To characterize these two aspects, we adopt Sen's capability approach (Sen 1985). After

[1]The definition of "mobility" can vary across disciplines. For example, Urry (2000), a sociologist, uses mobility in a broader context: the movement of not only people, but also things, information, and ideas. In this chapter, the term mobility is used just to simply indicate the ability of the individual to travel.

that, the issues on measuring the components of mobility are explored, together with the underlying evaluative aspects. Finally, we focus on policies on mobility of the elderly. We attempt to draw on the potential conflicts that exist among different perspectives including social welfare, economy, and urban planning, calling for cross-cutting approaches to mobility issues. We conclude this chapter with some reflections on future research agenda.

10.2 Mobility in the Management of Everyday Life

Having a better understanding of the role of mobility in the management of everyday life is crucial not just in formulating transportation policies but also in formulating other relevant policies including medical, social welfare, and economic policies. This section gives an overview on the role of mobility in old people's everyday life to understand the role of mobility from a broader perspective.

10.2.1 Some Basics on Old People's Travel

A large number of studies have been conducted to characterize old people's travel, where one distinctive aspect is age-associated disability. Impaired health is reported as a significant factor that reduces mobility through giving up driving (Rimmo and Hakamies-Blomqvist 2002). Also, vehicle availability and a driving license are known as important factors determining the level of mobility (Burkhardt et al. 1998; Kim 2011a), resulting in decreasing out-of-home activities (Davey 2006). The impacts of driving cessation on trip generation is extensive: according to a case study of Hiroshima City, around 0.25 trips per day would be reduced for those who live in high accessibility areas, and around 0.5 trips per day would be reduced for those who live in low accessibility areas by driving cessation[2] (Chikaraishi et al., forthcoming). It is also pointed out that such limited mobility could contribute to an increase in depressive symptoms (Marottoli et al. 1997, 2000).

Thus, development of accessibility strategies for old people who are no longer able to drive is one of the major concerns in the elderly's mobility discourse. The main option is to provide sufficient public transport services, but the use of public transport usually involves walking from home to the bus stop or rail station, requiring a certain level of physical ability (Metz 2003). Since driving cessation usually happens due to the reduction of physical ability, conventional public transport services may not really meet old people's needs to some extent.

[2]Note that the reduction of travel needs may also be reflected in the statistics.

Existing studies show mixed results on the impacts of public transport availability on the level of mobility: some studies report the impacts are limited (Evans 2001; Schmöcker et al. 2008), while others show a significant importance (Fobker and Grotz 2006). Such gradation in the results could be partially attributed to the detailed design of public transport service. It is also shown that, even after driving cessation, transportation deficiency can be improved when they live within walking distance of places where activities are located (Kim 2011a). In this regard, providing mobility tools to support walking or replace walking by other means such as age-friendly vehicles could be an effective complementary policy option.

One important fact is that the number of active seniors in terms of the number of trips are increasing year by year on average. Figure 10.1 shows changes in the average number of trips per day by age in Japan. Clearly, the number of trips per day for those who are 65 years old or over has been increasing over the last two decades.

The reasons behind the increase in the number of trips made by old people have not yet been fully explored, but attention may need to be paid, at least, to the following two points: (1) the increase in travel needs for having basic social contacts and (2) the increase in old people who drive a car. The first point could be partially attributed to the trend toward nuclear families. It is known that maintaining a certain level of social relationships is crucial not only for keeping health conditions (Berkman 1995; Cohen 2004) but also for asking for help in case of emergency (Callahan et al. 1980; Dewit et al. 1988; Johnson and Catalano 1981). Traditionally these functions have been produced within a household, but this tends to be less possible with decreasing household size, potentially resulting in the generation of more trips. For the second point, Fig. 10.2 provides clear evidence that old people tend to rely on a car [while young male people show the opposite trend, which is consistent with Kuhnimhof et al. (2012)].

While a car is a vital source of mobility for the elderly, it is also known that the risk of traffic accidents could increase with aging (Blanchard et al. 2010; Eby et al. 2012; Hakamies-Blomqvist 1998; Keay et al. 2009; Matthews and Moran 1986). To overcome this issue, a number of actions have been taken to improve their driving skills, or to communicate with older drivers and their family members to shift from a car to other modes of travel (Ball et al. 1993; NHTSA and ASA 2007; Odenheimer et al. 1994; Owsley et al. 1991, 1998; Ross et al. 2009). However, policy interventions on driving cessation are becoming increasingly sensitive, particularly for those who heavily rely on the use of a car (Musselwhite and Haddad 2010). It would partially be induced by car-oriented land use patterns (Adams 1999).

The above mentioned current trends show that old people's travel behavior have changed both quantitatively and qualitatively. In particular, current old people are more familiar with car use and the impacts of car cessation would be much higher than for old people from the past. Such changes may affect policy decisions in various ways, calling for further understanding of their travel needs.

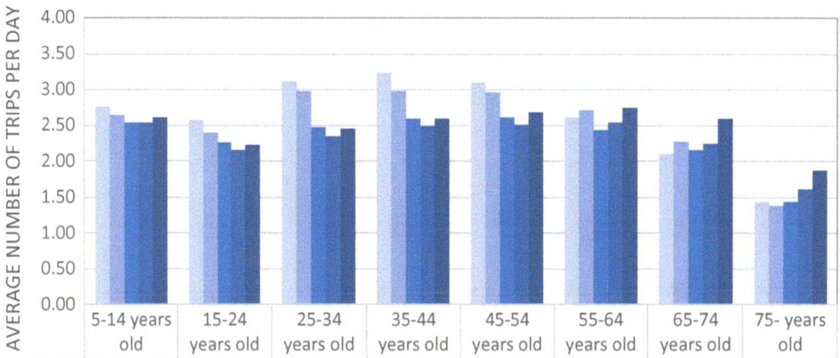

	5-14 years old	15-24 years old	25-34 years old	35-44 years old	45-54 years old	55-64 years old	65-74 years old	75- years old
1987	2.77	2.57	3.13	3.24	3.10	2.60	2.10	1.43
1992	2.65	2.40	2.97	2.98	2.96	2.71	2.28	1.38
1999	2.55	2.26	2.47	2.58	2.61	2.43	2.15	1.43
2005	2.55	2.15	2.35	2.49	2.51	2.53	2.24	1.60
2010	2.62	2.23	2.44	2.60	2.68	2.76	2.60	1.87

(a) Male

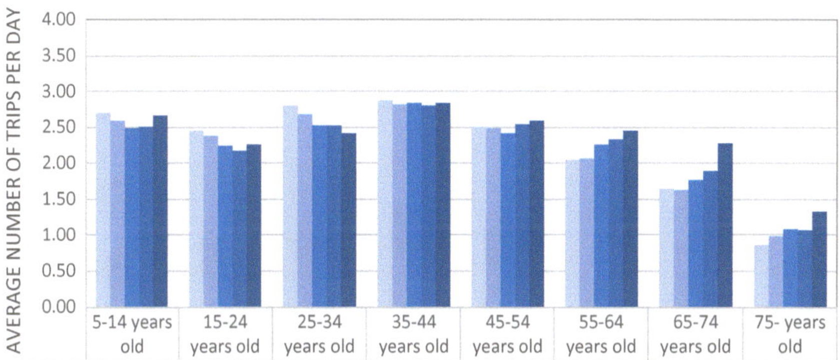

	5-14 years old	15-24 years old	25-34 years old	35-44 years old	45-54 years old	55-64 years old	65-74 years old	75- years old
1987	2.70	2.46	2.80	2.88	2.50	2.05	1.64	0.86
1992	2.60	2.38	2.68	2.83	2.49	2.06	1.64	0.99
1999	2.49	2.25	2.53	2.83	2.42	2.26	1.78	1.09
2005	2.50	2.18	2.53	2.81	2.54	2.33	1.89	1.07
2010	2.66	2.26	2.43	2.85	2.59	2.45	2.29	1.33

(b) Female

Fig. 10.1 Average number of trips per weekday by age. Data source: Nation-wide person-trip surveys (conducted by the Ministry of Land, Infrastructure, Transport and Tourism in Japan)

10.2.2 Hierarchy of Travel Needs

One fundamental question that needs to be further explored is why old people need to be mobile. The minimum answer is to satisfy the basic needs, including access to healthcare, food, water, clothing, and so forth. These are the minimum

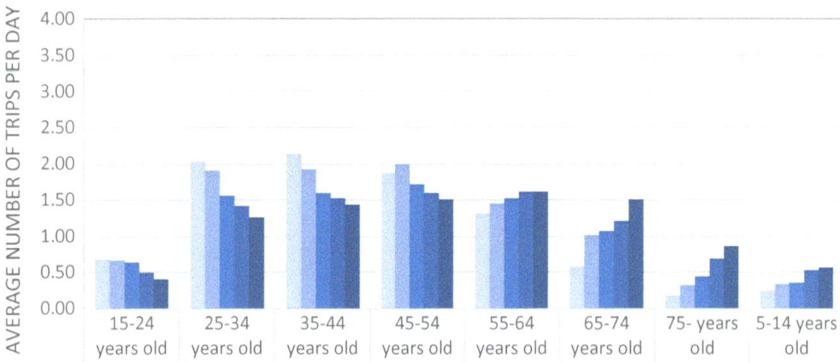

	15-24 years old	25-34 years old	35-44 years old	45-54 years old	55-64 years old	65-74 years old	75- years old	5-14 years old
1987	0.69	2.03	2.14	1.89	1.33	0.59	0.18	0.26
1992	0.68	1.92	1.92	2.00	1.45	1.01	0.32	0.33
1999	0.63	1.57	1.60	1.72	1.52	1.07	0.44	0.36
2005	0.49	1.42	1.53	1.59	1.62	1.21	0.68	0.52
2010	0.40	1.26	1.44	1.51	1.61	1.51	0.86	0.56

(a) Male

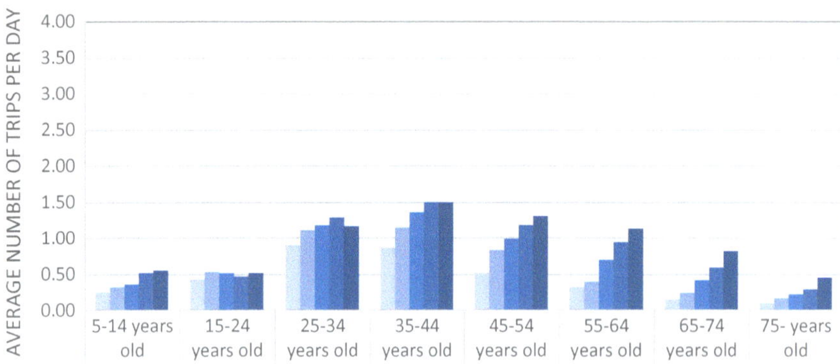

	5-14 years old	15-24 years old	25-34 years old	35-44 years old	45-54 years old	55-64 years old	65-74 years old	75- years old
1987	0.26	0.43	0.92	0.87	0.52	0.33	0.15	0.11
1992	0.33	0.54	1.12	1.16	0.84	0.41	0.24	0.17
1999	0.36	0.53	1.19	1.36	1.00	0.71	0.43	0.23
2005	0.52	0.48	1.29	1.50	1.19	0.95	0.60	0.30
2010	0.56	0.52	1.18	1.50	1.31	1.14	0.83	0.45

(b) Female

Fig. 10.2 Average number of car trips per weekday by age. Data source: Nation-wide person-trip surveys (conducted by the Ministry of Land, Infrastructure, Transport and Tourism in Japan)

resources necessary for physical well-being. On the other hand, the target of transport welfare policies is often not just for basic needs, but for a higher level of needs. To conceptually understand the needs at different levels, the hierarchy of mobility needs proposed by Musselwhite and Haddad (2010) is useful. Figure 10.3

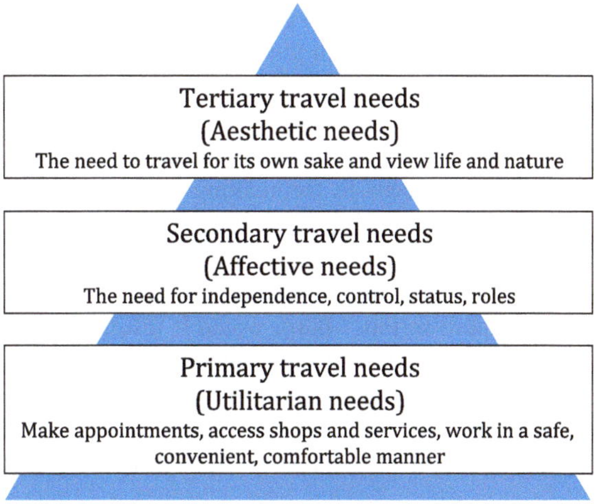

Fig. 10.3 Hierarchy of travel needs (Musselwhite and Haddad 2010)

shows Musselwhite and Haddad's hierarchy of travel needs, where so-called utilitarian needs, affective needs, and aesthetic needs are distinguished.

The primary level is utilitarian needs which consider people are traveling for an activity engagement at a destination, such as medical care at hospital or shopping at a supermarket. Though it is arguable as to what kinds of facilities should be able to be accessed to maintain a minimum living standard, this level of travel needs are directly linked with the access to basic needs. At this level, the main focus is to achieve the things they want to do at the destination, rather than traveling itself. Thus, for example, if the purpose is to get a certain food, there would be no distinction between getting it through traveling to a supermarket and getting it through a home-delivery service or even asking somebody to buy it. This type of travel needs has been intensively discussed in both practical and academic works (Kenyon et al. 2002; SEU 2003; Trinder et al. 1991).

The secondary level is affective needs, concerning whether or not one can control his or her own life. This type of need is more than accessibility in the sense that it links travel with psychological well-being associated with feeling part of society, identity, status, and roles. For example, though a shopping trip could be replaced by a home-delivery service if the purpose is to get some goods, this could lead to significant psychological issues such as feelings of depression. If we consider such aspects in policy debates, the needs for travel is going beyond the conventional accessibility needs (Marottoli et al. 1997).

The highest level is aesthetic needs, where the main concern is in access to aesthetics rather than to a practical good or service. Aesthetic needs are at the highest level in the sense that such needs are not really linked with survival and completion of ordinal tasks but rather linked with the quality of life. In the transportation field, the importance of enjoying traveling has been discussed in a number of existing literature (Mokhtarian and Salomon 2001), but it has been less focused in the analysis of old people's travel. Exploring aesthetic needs could be important, for example, to increase active seniors who could positively contribute to economic outcomes, and, in this case, the highest level of travel needs may appear in policy agenda.

Such hierarchical views on travel needs provide a useful insight to transport policy discussions: To what extent do governments have to take care of affective and aesthetic needs in formulating policies, and to what extent do they need to ensure the basic mobility that allows old people to survive and complete ordinal tasks? If the highest priority is on ensuring basic mobility and little attention is paid to the higher mobility needs, would social isolation and psychological depression be more serious? If so, would it result in increasing medical and care needs, and/or decreasing economic outcomes? Answering these questions is crucial in policy decisions, yet we do not have enough evidence. Some useful information related to such policy decisions could be obtained by looking at existing studies exploring interdependencies between mobility and other life domains.

10.2.3 Interdependencies Between Mobility and Other Life Domains

It is clear that mobility and other life domains are not independent of each other. Changes in the level of mobility would influence decisions on other life choices such as residential location, daily social contacts, and leisure activity engagement. At the same time, other life domains also affect the level of mobility. For example, health condition would determine their walking ability, residential location would determine the accessibility to public transport, and household income would be the main factor affecting the availability of personal vehicles. Thus, mobility issues may not be able to stand independently from other life domains.

Though a huge number of life domains would be linked with mobility issues, one of the critical life domains would be social engagement (including paid and unpaid work) that contributes to having an active life and reduces not only physical but also social and mental health risk. There is a two-way interaction with mobility, adding a certain difficulty when taking into account these aspects in formulating transport policies.

The importance of engagement in work has been pointed out in a number of studies. Here, work may not need to be paid but could be any kind of *productive social engagement* such as volunteering, care of family members, and informally helping friends. Existing studies show that old people who are actively engaging in productive social activities tend to remain economically active, and show better health and well-being (Curran and Blackburn 2001; Hao 2008; Siegrist et al. 2004). Whether the elderly can live such an active life or not would depend at least first on (1) whether or not they have the opportunity to be active (i.e., lack of activity opportunities), and second on (2) whether or not they have enough mobility to participate in the activity (i.e., lack of mobility). Chikaraishi et al. (2013)

conducted a small empirical study to identify which factors have larger impacts on social engagement and conclude that a lack of activity opportunities, rather than mobility, would be a main factor in hindering the elderly from active engagement.

The benefit of maintaining health is discussed not only from the viewpoint of reducing medical cost particularly from the viewpoint of active life expectancy (Katz et al. 1983; Lubitz et al. 2003) but also from the viewpoint of reducing caregivers' burden. In fact, many studies show that caregivers are most likely to experience problems with mental health and social participation (Chikaraishi et al. 2012; George and Gwyther 1986; Schulz and Beach 1999; Sisk 2000; Wiles 2003). Since the number of old people who need care are dramatically increasing [for example, the number of people who require nursing care has risen dramatically in recent years in Japan: 2.88 million people in 2001 and 4.25 million people in 2006 (Cabinet Office in Japan 2009)], the benefit of maintaining old people's health could be very high, and supporting mobility may be an important policy option toward that purpose (NHTSA and ASA 2007).

Once people cannot maintain a certain level of mobility, this could be a stimulus for changing residential location. Existing studies show that elderly households tend to move from less urbanized areas to slightly more urbanized areas (Kim 2011b) partially for better urban amenities (Speare and Meyer 1988). Also, it is pointed out that living in areas with high access to activity locations within walking distance or to well-developed transportation systems could contribute to an active life (Burkhardt 1999; Kim 2011a). In this sense, increasing residential mobility could be a powerful policy option for responding to driving cessation. On the one hand, it is found that the majority of old people live in low-density suburban areas (Chikaraishi et al. forthcoming; Kim 2011a), and residential relocation to more urbanized areas to substitute the loss of driving is not really an option for most of the elderly (Rosenbloom 2009). Urging old people to substitute the loss of driving through residential relocation needs further understanding of the residential relocation decisions taken by the elderly.

10.2.4 Mobility and Well-Being

Studies exploring the connection of mobility with well-being and quality of life has been increasing recently (Abou-Zeid and Ben-Akiva 2011; Banister and Bowling 2004; Ettema et al. 2010; Metz 2000; Mizokami et al. 2014; Musselwhite and Haddad 2010; Spinney et al. 2009). It is confirmed that active engagement of leisure activities has a positive relationship with morale, self-esteem, and self-rated perceptions of health (Misra et al. 1996; Patterson and Carpenter 1994), and thus promoting active life through enhancing mobility could be an important policy option, especially in an aging society.

Similar to Musselwhite and Haddad's (2010) assertions, Metz (2000) points out that existing analysis of travel demand and supply, focus only on benefits from improving accessibility and does not consider the so-called *destination-independent benefits*, including (1) psychological benefits, (2) exercise benefits, (3) involvement in the local community (yielding benefits from informal local support networks), and (4) potential travel (knowing that a trip could be made even if not actually undertaken). Currie and Stanley (2008) investigated such destination-independent benefits from the viewpoint of social capital. On the other hand, these studies that emphasize the importance of exploring destination-independent benefits also show difficulties in executing quantitative analysis and evaluation. Actually, we have a quite well-established evaluation tool when our objective is to minimize the generalized cost of travel (which is consistent with the microeconomic theory), but we do not really have a standardized evaluation method for destination-independent benefits. In response to this, alternative frameworks, which could take into account destination-independent benefits, have been proposed for example based on the concept of subjective well-being (Ettema et al. 2010). Meanwhile, it is known that subjective evaluation can be biased. One possible reason is that people would be reluctant to describe themselves as socially excluded (Preston and Rajé 2007). Also, it is observed that the elderly show a higher satisfaction with their current living environment and their mobility level than others (Fobker and Grotz 2006). In this sense, a subjective well-being approach has its own limitations. Nordbakke and Schwanen (2014) give an overview from a broader perspective: they explore the links between well-being and mobility under 10 different approaches to well-being (utility approach within economics, subjective well-being approach within psychology, eudaimonic approach within psychology, the basic needs approach, the resource approach, the integral needs approach, capability approaches, health-related quality of life, lay views, and an ecological approach). This study gives a clear summary on the conceptual linkage between well-being and mobility, but measuring and evaluating mobility and well-being remain unsolved issues, which are crucial for evidence-based policy decisions. In the next two sessions, we discuss the measurement aspects of mobility which involves the issues of evaluating mobility.

10.3 From a Measure of Achievement to a Measure of Freedom to Achieve

As we discussed in the Introduction, mobility and achieved mobility are different. Before reviewing existing measures of mobility, it would be better to clarify the differences between these two aspects in a conceptual way.

Mobility and achieved mobility could be distinguished by applying Amartya Sen's capability approach (Sen 1985). Figure 10.4 illustrates the concept of the capability approach. One of the core ideas of the capability approach is to make a clear distinction among the following three aspects: (1) the means

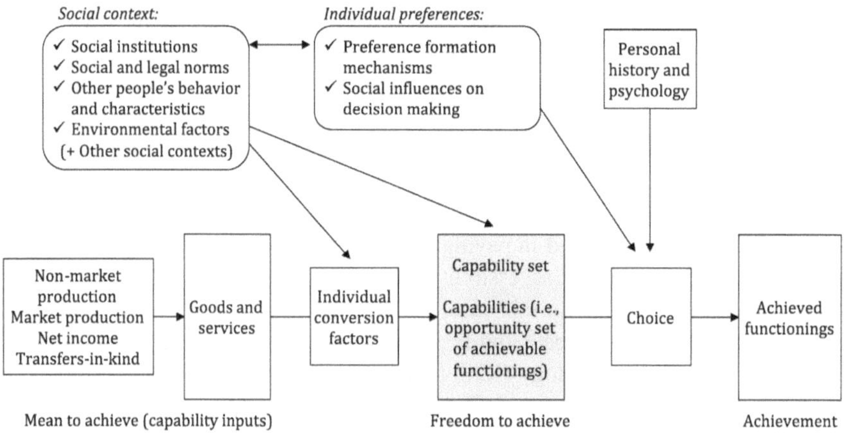

Fig. 10.4 Conceptual illustration of the capability approach (Robeyns 2005)

(i.e., commodities which would be used to achieve functionings[3]), (2) achievable functionings and capabilities (i.e., what people are effectively able to do and be), and (3) achieved functionings (i.e., outcomes such as what they did). Though all aspects could be used in policy evaluations, Sen argues that policy evaluations should focus on the second component, rather than the first and third components.

In mobility discourse, the first component would, for example, include car and bicycle ownership and the living environment such as distance to a bus stop and train station. In practice, these are widely used as proxy measures of mobility. The third component would, for example, be the number of trips made by car, bicycle, and public transport, which are also used as measures of mobility. Subjective outcomes such as subjective well-being could also be a part of the third component. Given the above first and third components, the second component may be simply defined as the ability of travel or mobility. The importance of focusing on the second component, i.e., achievable functionings, is obvious in discussions of the elderly's mobility issues. The first component may overlook the heterogeneity of physical ability among old people. For instance, the distance to a bus stop, some of the elderly may feel it is too far to walk there while others may not. One potential issue of the third component is that it reflects not only mobility but also travel needs, as we discussed in the Introduction. The number of trips made is not solely determined by the ability of travel. Thus, *if* our goal is to improve mobility, it should be understood that the first and third components are proxy measures which are potentially biased.

[3]The term "functionings" is used in Sen's (1985) work, where it means "what the person succeeds in *doing* with the commodities and characteristics at his or her command (p. 6)", or simply "what he or she manages to do or to be (p. 7)". Commodities will be used to achieve the functionings, while the achievement would be different across individuals even with the same bundle of commodities, since the ability to use the commodities are different.

Note that it is arguable whether or not the improvement of mobility is the ultimate goal of transport policies. For example, we know that too much private mobility can reduce social welfare as a whole through environmental degradation, adverse public health impacts, high accident rates, declining public transport, changes in land use and community severance (Preston and Rajé 2007). In this sense, too much emphasis on mobility needs may not be appropriate in public policy discussions. Rather than simply focus on the mobility level, the policy goal should be carefully designed in paying attention to the broader context. For example, SEU (2003) argues that accessibility rather than mobility should be the primary goal of transport policies. In this case, mobility may be understood as a means to achieve a certain level of accessibility. From this perspective, utilizing information and communication technology (ICT) tools (Kenyon et al. 2002), land use policies (Fobker and Grotz 2006), home-delivery services (Taketa et al. 2011), and residential relocation (Kim 2011a, b) could be alternative options in overcoming mobility issues. On the other hand, once we put more importance on affective and aesthetic mobility needs in policy debates, the role of mobility may be more than accessibility. Which viewpoint should be employed is a kind of normative question which may need to be answered partially through public debates (and of course through more solid theoretical/empirical analyses from a comprehensive viewpoint). We will come back to this point in Sect. 10.5. Under any normative judgments, we could say that at least the (ideal) ultimate goal of transport policies needs to be clarified before selecting evaluation measures for more informed policy decisions.

Note that a number of studies have recently utilized the capability approach in transportation policy discussions, but the ways in utilizing the capability approach can vary (Beyazit 2011; Eitoku and Mizokami 2010; Ryan et al. 2015; Smith et al. 2012). For example, travel can itself be a valuable functioning in a certain context (Nordbakke and Schwanen 2014), although it would not always be applicable. It should also be noted that achieved mobility, rather than mobility, needs to be focused on, depending on the goal of the analysis. For example, when we want to explore the economic impacts of transport policies, the number of trips actually made might be an important indicator of economic activities, rather than its potential. In summary, the capability approach would provide a useful framework for conceptualizing mobility issues, but it would not provide any normative judgments on the needs for mobility (Sen 2009). Another important note is that there would be some room needed for operationalizing the capability approach for practical use, which is common to other applications in different fields (Comim 2008; Lelli 2008; Raid el Mabsout 2011). Especially, as it is known that capability is, in general, not directly measurable. We will focus on this point in the next section.

10.4 Measuring the Components of Mobility

Even when one considers that mobility rather than achieved mobility needs to be focused on in policy debates, one would face difficulty in observing them, as we mentioned above. The data requirements for the operationalization of Sen's capability approach are heavy and the information required for its full implementation may not be available in general (Papadopoulos and Tsakloglou 2008), and thus, it would be rational to use proxy measures, such as car ownership and the number of trips the elderly made in practical contexts, in order to avoid the extreme cost of collecting the full information.

Table 10.1 summarizes some of the existing studies measuring the components of mobility. In the table, we also show the main aims for the improvement of mobility, since the selection of the measures would depend either explicitly or implicitly on the value of judgments the authors made. Although the table just shows selected studies from those that exist, there are a number of interesting observations as summarized below.

Firstly, it can be confirmed that existing indicators to measure mobility vary across case studies, indicating that there would be no standardized indicator for measuring mobility. As expected, from the viewpoint of the capability approach, it can be said that most of the indicators focus on mobility resources (e.g., car availability, public transport availability, and support networks) and/or achieved mobility (e.g., the number of trips and activity participation), rather than achievable functionings and capability. This is presumably due to the issue of observability, as mentioned above. Achievable functionings and capability are not in physical space, while mobility resources and achieved mobility are. On the other hand, some researchers make an effort to use better proxy indicators to reflect achievable functionings and capability. For example, Ryan et al. (2015) explore the achievable capability (called *mobility capability* in their paper) by observing the perception of the possibility to use public transport. Smith et al. (2012) extract the minimum requirement for mobility through a focus group. Nordbakke and Schwanen (2015) focus on the level of unmet needs for out-of-home activity. Actually, there is a growing body of literature which utilizes the capability approach to conceptualize and characterize mobility, and the above mentioned studies are doing this too.

It can also be confirmed that there is a trend to evaluate the mobility improvement in a broader context, by applying the concept of quality of life, social inclusion, and well-being. These are quite important to comprehensively capture the social impacts of transport policies. However, the evaluation results are still not comparable since the measurement unit is not standardized. One exception is the work of Stanley et al. (2011a). They attempt to monetize the value of mobility from the view of reducing the risk of social exclusion. Such monetary valuation is very powerful to put mobility discourses into much wider policy discussions where mobility and other policy options in other various sectors need to be compared.

Another interesting finding is that indicators to observe mobility do not correspond one-to-one with indicators to evaluate mobility, but there exists a certain trend. First, the use of subjective indicators in evaluating mobility has become more and more dominant, with the recent progress of theoretical works on how mobility is linked with well-being, social inclusion, and quality of life. Though this may be partially because of preferences to use subjective indicators, it is mainly because most objective indicators could not directly meet the basic requirements of the recent theoretical works. In other words, we simply do not have better objective

Table 10.1 Some empirical studies on the measurement of mobility

Authors	Study area	Travel mode covered	Main aim for improving mobility	Indicator to measure mobility	Indicator to evaluate mobility	Note
Burkhardt (1999)	US	Car	Reducing monetary, social, psychological, and mental health costs	Car availability, number of trips	Not specified (but a number of categories of indicators are shown)	Summarizing possible consequences of reducing or ceasing driving comprehensively
Marottoli et al. (2000)	New Haven, US	Car	Including but not limited to maintaining health	Car availability	Participation in out-of-home activities	The paper found the negative effects of driving cessation, i.e., decreases in out-of-home activity levels
Alsnih and Hensher (2003)	Western countries	All modes	Ensuring mobility and accessibility needs	Car availability, public transport availability, availability of support networks, residential location (amenities)	Need-based evaluation (not empirically examined)	The paper emphasizes more flexible forms of transport are needed as many seniors are seeking more flexibility in their transport services
Fobker and Grotz (2006)	Bonn, Germany	All modes	Enabling a self-determined life	Revealed travel behavior (mainly for shopping and leisure activities)	Gap between mobility and living environments (Seeking age appropriate living environments)	The paper investigates which living conditions best meet the needs of elderly people, and shows the importance of the basic facilities and public transport services within the residential environment

(continued)

Table 10.1 (continued)

Authors	Study area	Travel mode covered	Main aim for improving mobility	Indicator to measure mobility	Indicator to evaluate mobility	Note
Preston and Rajé (2007)	UK	All modes	Social inclusion (conceptualized by Sen's entitlement theory)	The level of travel in the area as a whole (area mobility), the level of travel made by particular individuals or groups (individual mobility)	Not specified (based on a matrix of area accessibility, area mobility, and individual mobility)	The paper emphasizes the importance of exploring mobility and accessibility issues at the disaggregate level
Spinney et al. (2009)	Canada	Travel is not directly dealt with	Quality of life	Mobility is not directly measured	Voluntary time outside home (as psychological benefits of mobility), sports and active leisure outside home (as exercise benefits of mobility), and community-helping and community-socializing time budget (as community benefits of mobility)	Results exhibit significant variations in transport mobility benefits by life situation and subjective well-being indices, and also indicate significant association between transport mobility benefits and quality of life. The measures used are developed from Metz's (2000) work
Musselwhite and Haddad (2010)	South West of England	Car	Quality of life	Car availability	Self-reported quality of life	The paper concludes that when older people give up driving, their self-reported quality of life is reduced which may be related to a reduction in affective and aesthetic qualities of mobility

(continued)

Table 10.1 (continued)

Authors	Study area	Travel mode covered	Main aim for improving mobility	Indicator to measure mobility	Indicator to evaluate mobility	Note
Kim (2011a)	US	All modes	Ensuring mobility and accessibility needs	Car availability, residential location, support networks	Subjective transportation deficiency	The paper points out that, in suburban areas, rather than the availability of public transport services, the placement of activity locations within walking distance would be more important in reducing transportation deficiency
Stanley et al. (2011b)	Melbourne and the Latrobe Valley, Australia	All modes	Improving well-being	Number of trips	Subjective well-being	The paper found that a lower number of trips lead to lower subjective well-being. The linkage between number of trips and well-being is assumed to be mediated by the risk of social exclusion
Smith et al. (2012)	UK	Public transport, taxi and car (in rural areas)	Capability for achieving a minimum living standard given typical accessibility conditions	The minimum requirement on mobility is set based on a focus group	Type and number of trips required to meet a minimum living standard (defined by focus group)	The main focus of this study was to identify the additional costs faced by rural households in order to achieve the same living standards as urban households. Sen's capability approach is used for conceptualization. The focus is relatively short-term in the sense that residential relocation is not considered

(continued)

Table 10.1 (continued)

Authors	Study area	Travel mode covered	Main aim for improving mobility	Indicator to measure mobility	Indicator to evaluate mobility	Note
Nordbakke (2013)	Oslo, Norway	All modes	Ensuring capability (defined as opportunities for mobility)	Not specified (based on focus group)	Not specified (based on focus group)	Based on four focus groups, they found that resources, contextual factors, and strategies are intertwined, which collectively form a "pool of capabilities for mobility"
Nordbakke and Schwanen (2015)	Norway	All modes	Well-being	Driving license, distance to public transport subjective evaluation of public transport, residential location, etc.	The level of unmet needs for out-of-home activity	Exploring factors affecting unmet needs for out-of-home activity
Ryan et al. (2015)	Stockholm, Sweden	Public transport	Not clearly mentioned but ensuring mobility (as part of capabilities)	The perception of the possibility to use public transport (mobility), the actual use of public transport (achieved mobility)	No specified (mobility capability)	Mobility and achieved mobility are distinguished by applying the capability approach

indicators (or the observation is too expensive) to fully reflect theoretical thoughts. As we discussed above, it is widely known that subjective measurements can be largely biased, particularly because elderly people eventually adjust their expectations to the reality of their situations (Fobker and Grotz 2006; Gasper 2007). If this is the case, subjective indicators would reflect personal standards, which is an undesirable property of indicators in making public policy decisions. To overcome this issue, some researchers recently use objective indicators or some other ways to extract objective mobility needs. For example, following the work of Metz (2000), Spinney et al. (2009) focus on time used to evaluate the transport mobility benefits. Smith et al. (2012) conducted a focus group to identify the minimum requirement on mobility rather than focusing on personal needs.

In summary, at this moment, we do not have a standardized method to measure and evaluate mobility from the viewpoint of social aspects of transport. It is clear that having a standardized method would be helpful to collectively emphasize the importance of the focused aspects in developing policy agendas. On the other hand, the use of the standardized method could potentially lead to misunderstanding the local context or crudely deal with context-specific issues. This is analogous to the traditional economic evaluation of mobility to some extent: while the conventional cost-benefit analysis provides a powerful rationale for taking the corresponding policy action, the local context is often not considered due to the systematic application of the established method. The locality could be more important not just because of the differences in the environment but also because of the differences in norms that the residents have. Different value judgments would lead to different criteria to select the measurement of mobility. In this sense, the selection of indicators depends on the focus to some extent which is largely affected by policy discussions. We will see this point in more detail in the next section.

10.5 Policy Goals on Mobility of the Elderly

Transport policies for the elderly often have multiple objectives. First, ensuring mobility and accessibility for social security and welfare has been considered one of the most important policy goals. In particular, declaration of a general right to transport in France was established in 1982, practical policy discussions on transport-related social exclusion issues in the UK and Australia, and the Basic Act on Transport Policy in Japan are closely linked with policies for social security and welfare (Lucas 2011; Stanley 2011). These policies may correspond to actions that ensure primary travel or utilitarian needs in the hierarchy of travel needs shown in Fig. 10.3. One key question from this perspective is how to define the minimum living standard which needs to be ensured through policy intervention, and what role transport has in ensuring the standard.

Particularly after the emergence of social exclusion discussions in the UK (SEU 2003), the role of mobility in ensuring social security and welfare has been clarified in detail. SEU (2003) notes "improving transport is not the only way to solve the 'accessibility deficits'... Over the medium- to long-term, improving local service delivery in the places where people experiencing or at risk of social exclusion live may provide a more cost-effective solution in some cases (p. 60)". From this viewpoint, in some cases mobility improvement may be able to be replaced by the use of ITC tools (Kenyon et al. 2002), and the improvement of living environment (Fobker and Grotz 2006; Kim 2011b), indicating that ensuring mobility itself would not be a primary goal of transportation policies. In other words, these focus on the right of accessibility rather than the right of mobility (Farrington 2007).

The rationale for focusing on accessibility rather than mobility is further supported by the argument of the adverse effects of mobility improvement on urban form. This is best described in the seminal work of Adams (1999): "When people acquired cars their activity patterns were transformed. They began going places previously unreachable by public transport, and travelling at times when public transport did not run. Over time, as more people acquired cars, land use patterns responded. Retailers began locating out of town for the convenience of motorists. Residential developments moved to the suburbs where there was room for garages and off-street parking. Offices moved to out-of-town business parks surrounded by car parks. And hospitals, cinemas, post offices, and warehouses all became bigger and fewer in number, and more difficult to reach by foot, bicycle or bus (p. 110)". Urry (2000) also notes that a higher requirement for mobility may result in forcing people to have a higher mobility. A number of existing studies that consider transport policies from the perspective of urban planning repeatedly emphasize that enhancing mobility could ultimately result in forcing people to have a higher mobility to satisfy basic needs. Presumably in response to such debates, some studies focus on the residential location and the living environments when exploring mobility issues (Kim 2011b).

In the meantime, as we discussed in Sect. 10.2.2, the value of mobility is sometimes considered to be more than the value of accessibility (Metz 2000; Banister and Bowling 2004; Spinney et al. 2009; Musselwhite and Haddad 2010). This is particularly true when the impacts of mobility on quality of life is the primary interest. A number of studies have confirmed that the reduction of mobility may hinder them from participating in social and leisure activities, while the minimum level of access to basic needs such as goods and health care may be maintained. One important policy question is whether policy makers should ensure not just the access to basic needs, but also the access to higher level needs such as loving, belonging, and self-actualization. Though ensuring higher level needs seem to be too much work for the government, there are some plausible reasons for it. First, it is known that satisfying higher level needs could sustain active life (Burkhardt 1999; Marottoli et al. 1997, 2000), which could contribute to increasing economic outcomes as well as reducing medical costs. One possible consequence from this viewpoint would be to help the older population keep driving as long as they can (Kim 2011a), which actually conflicts with the logical consequence from the perspective of urban form mentioned above. In this sense, a cross-cutting approach, including transport, economic, health, and urban form, is necessary to adequately formulate mobility policies. In other words, the value judgment cannot be made based solely on transportation aspects.

Such conflicting views among researchers/disciplines may be one of the major difficulties for policy decisions in a practical context, which is linked with a traditional question in sustainability discourse, i.e., how to give an appropriate weight in policy decisions to the future and the present. On the one hand, for the elderly to keep driving as long as they can, is an attractive policy option from the short-term viewpoint. On the other hand, transportation researchers and urban planners seem to generally recognize that too much private mobility can reduce social welfare as a whole through environmental degradation, adverse public health impacts, high accident rates, declining public transport, changes in land use, and community severance (Preston and Rajé 2007). Such short-term and long-term impacts need to be taken into account in the process of transport policy decisions. Unfortunately, the current policy evaluation frameworks which mainly focus on *marginal* changes in mobility. Rather than exploring the marginal changes, maximizing long-run social welfare under a certain equity constraint would need to be considered. As mentioned above, we do not have a well-established standardized method to evaluate such transport policy impacts. Though there is a certain need to set some context-dependent benefit items in policy evaluations, a standardized policy evaluation tool would be worth developing to give a solid basis for comprehensive policy evaluations on the mobility of the elderly. A standardized tool would also be helpful in comparing mobility conditions across different areas and different social groups, as well as to compare the impacts of transport policies with those in other sectors such as medical and economic. The comparison is essential, since in general resource allocation issues under a certain budget constraint (either across regions or across sectors within a region) need to be considered in policy decisions in a practical context. This is particularly true when the number of the elderly is rapidly growing, like in Japan.

10.6 Conclusions

This chapter gave a brief overview on mobility of the elderly, with a particular focus on its conceptualization, measurement, and evaluation. One clear trend is the recent expansion of the scope. Though mobility of the elderly has long been discussed with consideration of health domains, the scope further expands to put mobility into broader discourses, including social inclusion, quality of life, and well-being, contributing to a comprehensive understanding of social aspects of transport. This has also led to the development of various conceptual frameworks and measurement methods, where a number of different goals have been employed. For example, on the one hand, one can consider the ultimate goal of transport policies for the elderly is to fulfill their desires and preferences, which could minimize social exclusion and maximize the subjective well-being. On the other hand, one can consider the goal is to ensure access to basic needs rather than fulfilling their desires, which would efficiently reduce disparities across different social groups. One of the major difficulties arising from the expansion of the scope is in accommodating such different concepts and goals. As we have shown, existing studies generally show that, ensuring mobility would be a plausible policy direction from the perspective of fulfillment of desires and preferences, while ensuring accessibility would be a plausible policy direction from the perspective of fulfillment of basic needs. Clearly, such conflicting views need to be overcome to make an appropriate policy decision. To do this, further cross-cutting studies, where insights from different traditions are integrated and sublated, are necessary. The following are some research recommendations toward it.

First, further cross-cutting empirical studies which have well-established theoretical foundations are needed. As we discussed in this chapter, there is a growing body of literature which considers multiple facets of mobility of the elderly, but evidence is quite limited. For example, it is not clear how active social participation in later life contributes to the reduction of medical costs and caregivers' burdens, and to what extent transport influences this relationship, calling for cross-cutting studies which would involve researchers in the fields of transportation, economics, social science, and medical science. We also do not really know how experiences in earlier life would affect the mobility needs in later life and hence their well-being, calling for the needs of life-course studies. Second, a much clearer linkage between conceptual framework and empirical framework needs to be developed. More concretely, a clear distinction among the aim or goal of mobility improvement, an indicator to measure mobility, and an indicator to evaluate mobility is important to smoothly link theoretical and conceptual discourses with empirical works. This would provide a clear picture as to what extent theoretical thoughts are embedded into empirical analysis, and the potential of involving errors largely associated with imperfect information which is needed to fully describe theoretical thoughts. Third, from the practical point of view, we may have to consider how to put social aspects of transport into policy agenda. For this purpose, it would be better to develop a simple and standardized method to evaluate social aspects of transport. Note that such standardization also has a negative aspect, i.e., the method would be applied without careful consideration of possible fallacies and biases. This would be particularly important in discourse concerning mobility of the elderly since policy discussions are not really universal, but rather relative. Furthermore, becoming an aging society would change the role or position of the elderly. Such socio-economic changes at macro level could entirely change mobility discourse of the elderly. If this is the case, temporal and dynamic aspects also need to be seriously considered, especially when policy actions have long-term impacts.

References

Abou-Zeid M, Ben-Akiva M (2011) The effect of social comparisons on commute well–being. Transp Res Part A Policy Pract 45(4):345–361

Adams J (1999) The social implications of hypermobility. In: Proceedings of the Ottawa workshop on environmentally sustainable transport: the economic and social implications of sustainable transportation
Alsnih R, Hensher DA (2003) The mobility and accessibility expectations of seniors in an aging population. Transp Res Part A 37:903–916
Ball K, Owsley C, Sloane ME, Roenker DL, Bruni JR (1993) Visual attention problems as a predictor of vehicle crashes in older drivers. Invest Ophthalmol Vis Sci 34(11):3110–3123
Banister D, Bowling A (2004) Quality of life for the elderly: the transport dimension. Transp Policy 11(2):105–115
Berkman LF (1995) The role of social relations in health promotion. Psychosom Med 57(3):245–254
Beyazit E (2011) Evaluating social justice in transport: lessons to be learned from the capability approach. Transp Rev 31(1):117–134
Blanchard RA, Myers AM, Porter MM (2010) Correspondence between self–reported and objective measures of driving exposure and patterns in older drivers. Accid Anal Prev 42(2):523–529
Broome K, Worrall L, Fleming J, Boldy D (2012) Evaluation of flexible route bus transport for older people. Transp Policy 22:85–91
Burkhardt J (1999) Mobility changes: their nature effects and meaning for elders who reduce or cease driving. Transp Res Rec J Transp Res Board 1671:11–18
Burkhardt J, Berger A, Creedon M, McGavock A (1998) Mobility and independence: changes and challenges for loder drivers. National Academic Press, Washington DC
Cabinet Office in Japan (2009) White paper on the aging society cabinet office in Japan
Callahan JJ, Diamond LD, Giele JZ, Morris R (1980) Responsibility of families for their severely disabled elders health care. Financing Rev 1(3):29–48
Chikaraishi M, Zhang J, Fujiwara A (2012) Effects of nursing care on time use behaviour: a comparative analysis in Japan. Transportmetrica 8(3):181–208
Chikaraishi M, Fujiwara A, Kuwano M, Zhang J (2013) Functionings enhanced by social networks in elders activity participations: the capability approach. In: Compendium of papers CD-ROM, the 92nd annual meeting of the transportation research board. Washington D.C., 13–17 January
Chikaraishi M, Stanley J, Fujiwara A, Zhang J (forthcoming) Social exclusion and transport in an aging and shrinking society. In: Zhang J, Feng CM (eds) Routledge handbook of transport in Asia, Routledge
Cohen S (2004) Social relationships and health. Am Psychol 59(8):676
Comim F (2008) Measuring capabilities. In: Comin F, Qizilbash M, Alkire S (eds) The capability approach: concepts measures and applications. Cambridge University Press, Cambridge, pp 157–200
Curran J, Blackburn RA (2001) Older people and the enterprise society: age and self–employment propensities. Work Employ Soc 15(04):889–902
Currie G, Stanley J (2008) Investigating links between social capital and public transport. Transp Rev 28(4):529–547
Davey JA (2006) Older people and transport: coping without a car. Ageing Soc 27(01):49–56
Dewit DJ, Wister AV, Burch TK (1988) Physical distance and social contact between elders and their adult children. Res Aging 10(1):56–80
Eby DW, Silverstein NM, Molnar LJ, LeBlanc D, Adler G (2012) Driving behaviors in early stage dementia: a study using in–vehicle technology. Accid Anal Prev 49:330–337
Eitoku Y, Mizokami S (2010) An evaluation method of transportation policies by the quality of mobility index based on capability approach. Asian Transp Stud 1(1):77–89
Ettema D, Gärling T, Olsson LE, Friman M (2010) Out–of–home activities daily travel and subjective well–being. Transp Res Part A Policy Pract 44(9):723–732
Evans EL (2001) Influences on mobility among non–driving older Americans. Transp Res Rec Circular E–C026:151–168

Farrington JH (2007) The new narrative of accessibility: its potential contribution to discourses in (transport) geography. J Transp Geogr 15(5):319–330
Fobker S, Grotz R (2006) Everyday mobility of elderly people in different urban settings: the example of the city of Bonn, Germany. Urban Stud 43(1):99–118
Gasper D (2007) What is the capability approach?: Its core rationale partners and dangers. J Socio-Econ 36(3):335–359
George LK, Gwyther LP (1986) Caregiver Weil–Being: a multidimensional examination of family caregivers of demented adults. The Gerontologist 26(3):253–259
Hakamies-Blomqvist L (1998) Older drivers accident risk: conceptual and methodological issues. Accid Anal Prev 30(3):293–297
Hao Y (2008) Productive activities and psychological well–being among older adults. J Gerontol Ser B Psychol Sci Soc Sci 63(2):S64–S72
Johnson CL, Catalano DJ (1981) Childless elderly and their family supports. The Gerontologist 21(6):610–618
Katz S, Branch LG, Branson MH, Papsidero JA, Beck JC, Greer DS (1983) Active life expectancy. N Engl J Med 309(20):1218–1224
Keay L, Jasti S, Munoz B, Turano KA, Munro CA, Duncan DD, Baldwin K, Bandeen-Roche KJ, Gower EW, West SK (2009) Urban and rural differences in older drivers failure to stop at stop signs. Accid Anal Prev 41(5):995–1000
Kenyon S, Lyons G, Rafferty J (2002) Transport and social exclusion: investigating the possibility of promoting inclusion through virtual mobility. J Transp Geogr 10:207–219
Kim S (2011a) Assessing mobility in an aging society: personal and built environment factors associated with older peoples subjective transportation deficiency in the US. Transp Res Part F 14:422–429
Kim S (2011b) Intra–regional residential movement of the elderly: testing a suburban–to–urban migration hypothesis. Ann Reg Sci 46:1–17
Kuhnimhof T, Armoogum J, Buehler R, Dargay J, Denstadli JM, Yamamoto T (2012) Men shape a downward trend in car use among young adults—evidence from six industrialized countries. Transp Rev 32(6):761–779
Lelli S (2008) Operationalising Sen's capability approach: the influence of the selected technique. In: Comim F (ed) The capability approach: concepts, measures and application. Cambridge University Press, Cambridge, pp 310–361
Lubitz J, Cai L, Kramarow E, Lentzner H (2003) Health life expectancy and health care spending among the elderly. N Engl J Med 349(11):1048–1055
Lucas K (2011) Transport and social exclusion: where are we now? Transp Policy 20:105–113
Marottoli RA, Mendes de Leon CF, Glass TA, Williams CS, Cooney LM Jr, Berkman LF, Tinetti ME (1997) Driving cessation and increased depressive symptoms: prospective evidence from the New Haven EPESE. J Am Geriatr Soc 45(2):202–206
Marottoli RA, de Leon CFM, Glass TA, Williams CS, Cooney LM, Berkman LF (2000) Consequences of driving cessation: decreased out–of–home activity levels. J Gerontol B 55(6):334–340
Matthews ML, Moran AR (1986) Age differences in male drivers perception of accident risk: the role of perceived driving ability. Accid Anal Prev 18(4):299–313
Metz DH (2000) Mobility of older people and their quality of life. Transp Policy 7(2):149–152
Metz D (2003) Transport policy for an ageing population. Transp Rev 23(4):375–386
Misra R, Alexy B, Panigrahi B (1996) The relationships among self–esteem exercise and self–rated health in older women. J Women Aging 8(1):81–94
Mizokami S, Kawashima H, Nagata C, Yaguchi T (2014) Intervention research for quality of life improvement through the use of personal mobility mode in an aging society. Asian Transp Stud 3(1):95–107
Mokhtarian PL, Salomon I (2001) How derived is the demand for travel? Some conceptual and measurement considerations. Transp Res 35:695–719

Musselwhite C, Haddad H (2010) Mobility accessibility and quality of later life. Qual Ageing Older Adults 11(1):25–37
NHTSA and ASA (2007) Driving well: promoting older driver safety and mobility in your community. US DOT/NHTSA Pub National Highway. Traffic Safety Administration, US Department of Transportation and American Society of Aging
Nordbakke S (2013) Capabilities for mobility among urban older women: barriers strategies and options. J Transp Geogr 26:166–174
Nordbakke S, Schwanen T (2014) Well–being and mobility: a theoretical framework and literature review focusing on older people. Mobilities 9(1):104–129
Nordbakke S, Schwanen T (2015) Transport unmet activity needs and wellbeing in later life: exploring the links. Transportation 42(6):1129–1151
Odenheimer GL, Beaudet M, Jette AM, Albert MS, Grande L, Minaker KL (1994) Performance–based driving evaluation of the elderly driver: Safety reliability and validity. J Gerontol 49(4):M153–M159
Owsley C, Ball K, McGwin G Jr, Sloane ME, Roenker DL, White MF, Overley ET (1998) Visual processing impairment and risk of motor vehicle crash among older adults. JAMA 279(14):1083–1088
Owsley C, Ball K, Sloane ME, Roenker DL, Bruni JR (1991) Visual/cognitive correlates of vehicle accidents in older drivers. Psychol Aging 6(3):403–415
Papadopoulos F, Tsakloglou P (2008) Social exclusion in the EU: a capability approach. In: Comim F, Qizilbash M, Alkire S (eds) The capability approach: concepts measures and applications. Cambridge University Press, Cambridge, pp 242–267
Patterson I, Carpenter G (1994) Participation in leisure activities after the death of a spouse. Leisure Sci 16(2):105–117
Preston J, Rajé F (2007) Accessibility mobility and transport–related social exclusion. J Transp Geogr 15:151–160
Raid el Mabsout R (2011) The capability approach: from ethical foundations to empirical operationalization. Radboud University, Nijmegen Radboud University Nijmegen
Rimmo PA, Hakamies-Blomqvist L (2002) Older drivers' aberrant driving behaviour, impaired activity, and health as reasons for self-imposed driving limitations. Transp Res Part F 5(1):47–62
Robeyns I (2005) The capability approach: a theoretical survey. J Human Dev 6(1):93–117
Rosenbloom S (2004) Mobility of the elderly transportation in an aging society: a decade of experience. Technical papers and reports from a conference. Bethesda, Maryland, pp 3–21, 7–9 Nov 1999
Rosenbloom S (2009) Meeting transportation needs in an aging–friendly community generations. J Am Soc Aging 33(2):33–43
Ross LA, Clay OJ, Edwards JD, Ball KK, Wadley VG, Vance DE, Cissell GM, Roenker DL, Joyce JJ (2009) Do older drivers at–risk for crashes modify their driving over time? J Gerontol Ser B Psychol Sci Soc Sci 64B(2):163–170
Rowe JW, Kahn RL (1997) Successful aging. The Gerontologist 37(4):433–440
Ryan J, Wretstrand A, Schmidt SM (2015) Exploring public transport as an element of older persons mobility: a capability approach perspective. J Transp Geogr 48:105–114
Schmöcker JD, Quddus M, Noland R, Bell M (2005) Estimating trip generation of elderly and disabled people: analysis of London data. Transp Res Rec 1924:9–18
Schmöcker JD, Quddus MA, Noland RB, Bell MGH (2008) Mode choice of older and disabled people: a case study of shopping trips in London. J Transp Geogr 16(4):257–267
Schulz R, Beach SR (1999) Caregiving as a risk factor for mortality: the caregiver health effects study. J Am Med Assoc 282(23):2215–2219
Sen A (1985) Commodities and capabilities. Oxford University Press, Oxford
Sen A (2009) The idea of justice, Penguin
SEU (2003) Making the connections: transport and social exclusion. Final report. ODPM, London

Siegrist J, von dem Knesebeck O, Pollack CE (2004) Social productivity and well–being of older people: a sociological exploration. Soc Theor Health 2(1):1–17

Sisk RJ (2000) Caregiver burden and health promotion. Int J Nurs Stud 37(1):37–43

Smith N, Hirsch D, Davis A (2012) Accessibility and capability: the minimum transport needs and costs of rural households. J Transp Geogr 21:93–101

Speare A, Meyer JW (1988) Types of elderly residential mobility and their determinants. J Gerontol 43(3):S74–S81

Spinney JEL, Scott DM, Newbold KB (2009) Transport mobility benefits and quality of life: a time–use perspective of elderly Canadians. Transp Policy 16:1–11

Stanley JR (2011) Social exclusion. In: Currie G (ed) New perspectives and methods in transport and social exclusion research. Emerald, UK, pp 27–43

Stanley J, Hensher DA, Stanley J, Currie G, Greene WH, Vella–brodrick D (2011a) Social exclusion and the value of mobility. J Transp Econ Policy 45(2):197–222

Stanley JK, Hensher DA, Stanley JR, Vella-Brodrick D (2011b) Mobility social exclusion and well–being: exploring the links. Transp Res Part A 45(8):789–801

Taketa A, Komatsu Y, Yokomizo I (2011) The situation of and problems faced by people with the disadvantage of shopping in hilly and mountainous areas. J Rural Probl 183:255–259

Trinder E, Hay A, Dignan J, Else P, Skorupski J (1991) Concepts of equity fairness and justice in British transport legislation 1960–88. Environ Plann C 9(1):31–50

Urry J (2000) Sociologies beyond societies: mobilities for the twenty-first century. Routledge, New York

Whelan M, Langford J, Oxley J, Koppel S, Charlton J (2006) The elderly and mobility: a review of the literature report (No 255), Accident Research Centre, Monash University

Wiles J (2003) Daily geographies of caregivers: mobility routine scale. Soc Sci Med 57(7):1307–1325

Chapter 11
Risky Behaviors in Life: A Focus on Young People

Ying Jiang and Junyi Zhang

Abstract This chapter describes risky behaviors in daily life, especially focusing on young people. Driving while intoxicated, speeding, and illegal drug use are examples of risky behaviors, which often compromise health, quality of life, or life itself. People perform some risky behaviors consciously while they do others unconsciously. This chapter first depicts some typical theories of risky behaviors, including Heinrich's domino model, problem behavior theory, social development model, life history theory, and lifetime utility theory. Next, it illustrates young people's risky driving by reviewing risk homeostasis theory, applications of theory of planned behavior, influences of social networks and other persons, avoidance driving, mood during driving and driving purpose, driving and nightlife, and self-driving cars. Literature review suggests that there are some common factors (not only psychological factors, but also life choices and various habits formed in daily life) affecting different types of risky behaviors, suggesting that risky behaviors tend to covary and effects of one risky behavior may spill over to influence other risky behaviors. These imply that measures to prevent a risky behavior should jointly target multiple risky behaviors based on an integrated approach over a long period.

Keywords Young people · Problem behavior · Social development model · Life history theory · Risky driving behavior · Avoidance driving · Self-driving cars · Influences of family and peers

Y. Jiang (✉) · J. Zhang
Hiroshima University, Higashi-Hiroshima, Japan
e-mail: jiangying119@msn.com

J. Zhang
e-mail: zjy@hiroshima-u.ac.jp; junyizh24@gmail.com

J. Zhang (ed.), *Life-Oriented Behavioral Research for Urban Policy*,
DOI 10.1007/978-4-431-56472-0_11

11.1 Risky Behaviors in Daily Life

Risky behaviors are behaviors that compromise health, quality of life, or life itself (Jessor 1991). In daily life, people experience and/or perform various risky behaviors, e.g., driving while intoxicated, speeding, angry driving, illegal drug use, smoking, unsafe use of the Internet, bungee jumping, going on a jungle safari, skiing, and skating. One can even observe antisocial behavior on public transport, e.g., shouting, swearing, pushing, barging people out of the way (carelessly or aggressively), and playing loud music (Moore 2011), among the many examples that are too numerous to mention. Some risky behaviors are performed consciously, e.g., speeding, while others are done unconsciously, e.g., sitting for too long while working hard every day (which is nevertheless harmful to one's health from a long-term perspective), unhealthy diets, and unsafe use of the Internet. Some risky behaviors are not harmful to the person of interest, but may be harmful to others, e.g., throwing a glass bottle out of a car. Some risky behaviors are associated with lifestyles, e.g., smoking, working long hours, and alcohol abuse, while others are antisocial, e.g., speeding, angry driving, and illegal drug use.

Risky behaviors often result in adverse outcomes such as incarceration, loss of job, long-term illness, injury, and even death (e.g., Lane and Cherek 2000; Mason et al. 2013). The World Bank has warned that "risky behaviors—smoking, using illicit drugs, alcohol abuse, unhealthy diets, and unsafe sex—are increasing globally and pose a growing threat to the health of individuals, particularly in developing countries."[1] The Internet has dramatically improved people's lives. The Internet of Things (IoT) currently comprises 25 billion connected devices around the world and this number will grow to 50 billion worldwide by 2020, according to the World Bank.[2] These technological developments have provided people with more open, free, secure, and empowering access to goods and services; however, at the same time, issues such as privacy, safety, child protection, terrorism, and public safety have become global concerns. Importantly, use of the Internet and health are not unrelated. Indeed, Internet addiction has been recognized as an emerging behavioral problem among adolescents (American Psychiatric Association 2013; Lenihan 2007; Young 2010). Furthermore, according to the World Health Organization (WHO), the total number of road traffic deaths across the world has reached 1.25 million per year, and the highest road traffic fatality rates are observed in low-income countries[3] and tens of millions of people are injured or disabled every year.[4]

---

[1]http://www.worldbank.org/en/news/press-release/2013/11/20/risky-behaviors-growing-threats-global-health (accessed January 31, 2016).

[2]http://blogs.worldbank.org/category/tags/internet-security (accessed January 31, 2016).

[3]http://www.who.int/violence_injury_prevention/road_safety_status/2015/en/ (accessed January 31, 2016).

[4]http://www.who.int/violence_injury_prevention/road_traffic/en/ (accessed January 31, 2016).

Risky behaviors have been broadly analyzed in relation to young people. The definition of young people is culturally and historically specific, varying through time and between different societies (Cieslik and Simpson 2013: p. 45). Similar terms include younger generation, young adults, youth, adolescents, and teenagers. In general, youth refers to the period between childhood and adulthood. Several United Nations organizations treat 'youth' and 'young people' as having the same meaning, but adopt different age ranges (e.g., 15–24 years for the UN Secretariat, UNESCO and the ILO; 15–32 years for UN Habitat; under 18 years for UNICEF; and 15–35 years for the African Youth Charter).[5] UNICEF, the WHO, and UNFPA distinguish between adolescents (10–19 years), young people (10–24 years), and youth (15–24 years). In the USA, youth means the same as teenager (10–19 years). In Japan, young adults refer to those aged 15–34 years,[6] and 16–24 years in the UK.[7] According to the United Nations Population Fund (2014), there are 1.8 billion young people aged 10–24 years in the world, with currently 90 % of them living in developing countries.

This chapter is especially focused on young people's driving safety. WHO (2015) reported that road traffic accidents are a leading cause of death among young people, and the main cause of death among those aged 15–29 years. Young drivers are more likely to speed, to which alcohol is seen as an attributing factor; in particular, talking on mobile phones and texting while driving are seen as the main reasons for young people's risk of death and injury.

11.2 Theories of Risky Behaviors

Risky behaviors have been studied in various disciplines. Instead of attempting to provide a comprehensive list of theories, we select here some examples to illustrate how risky behaviors have been understood, aiming especially at clarifying the roles of domain-specific factors and social networks in explaining risky behaviors.

11.2.1 Heinrich's Domino Model

Heinrich's (1931) seminal work, known as Heinrich's Law, provided the foundation of behavior-based safety research. It claims that in a workplace, for every accident that causes a major injury, there are 29 accidents that cause minor injuries

[5]http://www.un.org/esa/socdev/documents/youth/fact-sheets/youth-definition.pdf (accessed January 31, 2016).

[6]Statistics Bureau of Japan: http://www.stat.go.jp/english/data/nenkan/1431-02.htm (accessed January 31, 2016).

[7]http://www.ukyouth.org/events/item/292-statistics-about-young-people-in-the-uk.html#.VmbxmbiLRD8 (accessed January 31, 2016).

and 300 accidents that cause no injuries, based on 5000 documented industrial accidents. Heinrich emphasized the role of human error and chance events in causing accidents. Based on observations from the 5000 accidents, Heinrich (1931) proposed the domino model, which emphasizes the worker as cause. This model argues that an accident is an end result of a chain of decision fallacies: (1) ancestry and social development; (2) fault of person; (3) unsafe act; (4) accident; and (5) injury. In other words, if one of the factors leading to an injury can be removed or corrected, then the injury will not happen. The first domino in the chain deals with a worker's undesirable personality traits (e.g., stubbornness, greed, or recklessness), which is either transferred through inheritance or has developed from a person's social environment. The second domino indicates inborn or learned character flaws (e.g., bad temper, inconsiderateness, ignorance, and recklessness) and claims that natural or environmental flaws in the *worker's family or life* cause these secondary personal defects. For example, temper means not only a tendency to become angry suddenly or easily (i.e., personal character), but also the way a person is feeling at a particular time (i.e., affective experience). Over the past decade, affective experience has been widely studied under the research framework of subjective well-being (SWB) in the field of behavioral economics (e.g., Diener 1994, 2009; Kahneman et al. 2004). Concerning personality, Diene and Lucas (1999) concluded: "One of the most consistent and robust findings in the field of subjective well-being is that the components of SWB are moderately related to personality. … The personality traits that are most consistently and strongly related to SWB are extraversion and neuroticism. Extraversion is moderately correlated with pleasant affect; neuroticism is strongly correlated with unpleasant affect. … [G]reater SWB results from the degree to which our personalities fit with our environment (p. 213)." Here, the environment in which people live is emphasized. From this perspective, as an example, bad temper may also result from an unhappy family life (a long-term affective experience), or unhappy moments experienced at home before going to work (a short-term affective experience). Thus, Heinrich was the first researcher who attached a higher importance to an individual's family or life. To reduce risky behaviors, efforts should focus on people's daily life, which is indirectly associated with the chain of the domino model.

11.2.2 Problem Behavior Theory

Risky behaviors have also been studied as a problem behavior (e.g., Miller 2008; Lam 2015). As noted by Steinberg and Morris (2001), the problem behavior theory proposed by Jessor and Jessor (1977)[8] is perhaps the most influential theory used to treat in particular adolescent problem behaviors (e.g., drug use, sexual behavior, alcohol drinking, and the problem behavior associated with excessive

[8]http://www.colorado.edu/ibs/jessor/pb_theory.html (accessed February 1, 2016).

use of alcohol). The theory explains risk taking and unconventional lifestyles in terms of three interactive systems of psychosocial influence: personality, perceived environment, and behavior (e.g., delinquency). Jessor and Jessor (1977) found that (1) there are more serious problem behaviors at the college level than at the high school level; (2) personal control has the most influence on the set of problem behaviors, followed by motivational instigations; (3) the adolescent who values academic achievement is less likely to engage in problem behavior, and the influences of *peer groups, the family, and the community* are significant. Each of these three interactive systems either serves as an instigator of, or control against, engaging in problem behavior, and the proneness to problem behavior is determined by the balance between instigators and controls across the three systems (Lam 2015). It may be assumed that these three groups of factors may be attributable to different risky behaviors in different ways.

Problem behavior theory has been applied in various fields. For example, Yu et al. (2012) noted that personality variables (e.g., positive attitudes toward tobacco use and depressive affect) and delinquent behaviors can well explain adolescent tobacco use; however, perceived environment variables (e.g., exposure to delinquent peers) cannot. Sterrett et al. (2014) observed that the trajectories of substance use, sexual behavior, and conduct problems among low-income African-American youths co-occurred with the influence of peer pressure, parental monitoring, self-worth, and belief in the inevitability of violence. Similarly, Melkman (2015) discovered that sensation seeking and deviant peer associations mainly contribute to the occurrence of problem behaviors such as delinquency, substance abuse, and risky sexual behavior, suggesting the importance of holistic group interventions addressing multiple risk factors. Lam (2015) reported that an increasing number of studies reveal the relationship between familial and parental factors and Internet addiction among adolescents, and reconfirmed existing findings empirically by showing that there was a significant relationship between parental mental health, particularly depression, and the Internet addiction status of their children.

Similarly, the US Department of Health and Human Services summarized the long-term impact of adolescent risky behaviors and family environment from a broad review of the literature (Pergamit et al. 2001). It was found that most existing studies suggest that engaging in risky behaviors as a teenager is associated with less successful adult outcomes and in most cases, earlier engagement is more likely to lead to a poor outcome as an adult. Such long-term adult outcomes are associated with parents' level of education; however, the effects of parents' help on the prevention of poor outcomes for their children differ across different domains. The influence of family on young people's risky behaviors has also been investigated by other theories/models. For example, Feinberg et al. (2013) developed a model of sibling and family influences on youth development and adjustment and showed that the sibling relationship should be reflected into practices for preventing substance use via family. The influence of family is also observed in the case of traffic safety (e.g., Taubman-Ben-Ari and Katz-Ben-Ami 2012), which will be discussed further in Sect. 9.3. Focusing on the effects of marketing on gambling, drinking, and smoking behaviors, Prentice and Cotte (2015) revealed the influence of peer group in problem driving behaviors; in addition, they clarified how casino employees' communication with casino guests affects problematic gaming behaviors. Recently, Buckley and Chapman (2016) reported that adolescents value protecting friends from harm and intervene as bystanders in friends' risky and dangerous behavior based on a model of social context for intervention.

11.2.3 Social Development Model for Representing Antisocial Behavior

The above influences of the perceived environment (e.g., peer groups, the family, and the community) on risky behaviors have been generalized under the so-called social development model (an integration of social control theory and social learning theory), which was originally conceived to prevent youth crime (Hawkins and Weis 1985). The model was developed from a life-course perspective in which four developmental periods are distinguished, namely preschool, elementary school, middle school, and high school (Elliott 1994; Catalano et al. 1996). It is argued that similar developmental processes could lead to either prosocial or antisocial outcomes, where the most important units of socialization—family, schools, peers, and community—influence behavior sequentially, both directly and indirectly (Hawkins and Weis 1985). Whether a youth's participation in each unit of socialization contributes to the development of a bond of attachment and commitment to and belief in conventional society is determined by three types of process variables: opportunities for involvement, skills, and reinforcements. Hawkins and Weis (1985) argued that opportunities for involvement are necessary, but not sufficient, for the development of a social bond, and social bonding can be achieved only if youths experience and evaluate the interventions and interactions with other members in the socialization unit positively. Their experiences and evaluations are further affected by the level of their skills and reinforcements from the environment for desired behavior. The bonding process starts in the family, where consistent rewarding is required for the development of the bond of attachment, commitment, and belief in the family. Bonding to school is conditional on how fully social bonds to the family have been developed before entering school, experiences of opportunities for involvements and skill development, as well as rewards for skillful performance at school. Similarly, bonding to peers is determined by experiences of opportunities for involvement with peers, the skills expected by peers, and rewards for interactions with peers. This bonding involves a process through which youths learn patterns of behavior, either prosocial or antisocial, from members of the socialization units, the norms and values of which are also influential (Catalano et al. 1996). It is further suggested that strong bonds to family and school reduce the likelihood of youths being attached to delinquent peers, despite exposure to high levels of risk factors. In other words, uncaring or inconsistent parents, poor school performance, and inconsistent and/or unrewarding teachers will unfortunately increase the likelihood of youths performing delinquent behaviors.

Based on the above social development model, some practical measures of risk and protective factors have been developed One of the more popular measures is the Communities That Care Youth Survey (CTC-YS) (Feinberg et al. 2007). CTC-YS broadly assesses both risk and protective factors across domains (i.e., community, family, school, and peers) that have been shown to be linked to adolescent behavior problems (violence, substance abuse, dropping out, and teen pregnancy), and support policy decisions. In total, there are 22 risk factors and nine protective factors.

A similar approach is called the participatory approach (Mason et al. 2013). It is neither top-down nor paternalistic (i.e., an approach that restricts individuals' choices in their own interests and without their consent); it is a bottom-up approach that involves youths themselves, their peers and families, and the community where they are living, with the aim of increasing healthy social bonding. This approach attempts to understand vulnerability from youths' own viewpoints, and empowers them to define the issues and develop solutions to the challenges they face. It emphasizes that risky behavior is often not an outcome of a single choice, but a series of choices in the form of lifestyle experimentation that consider various trade-offs. The usefulness of this approach is supported by the fact that community-based programs tend to be the most effective (e.g., Lantz et al. 2000). More importantly, the participatory approach involves co-creation with youths and their social networks in the design and evaluation of programming.

11.2.4 Life History Theory

According to Wang et al. (2009), risk-taking propensities are domain specific, as suggested by evolutionary psychology. Domains include social exchange, mating, parental investment, within-group competition, between-group competition, foraging, dealing with kin, and parenting. Some studies classify risk-taking domains into financial, health/safety, ethical, recreational, and social domains (e.g., Weber et al. 2002).

However, people not only make risky choices in different task domains, but also make risky choices at different stages of life. For example, existing studies reveal that adolescence is a stage of life in which children are at greatest risk of using and developing problems associated with alcohol, tobacco, and other drugs. The early onset of regular tobacco use is a good predictor of lifetime drug use (Hanna et al. 2001). Kabiru et al. (2014) reported that adverse life events increase the likelihood of delinquent behavior among adolescents living in urban slums in Kenya. Parental monitoring, religiosity, and self-esteem may moderate the effect of adversity on delinquent behavior. Such findings are also consistent with those in the context of high-income countries. Furthermore, risky lifestyles are associated with participation in a range of violent behaviors both as offenders and as victims (Baron et al. 2007). Such phenomena might be explained by life history theory, which assumes that individuals make specific trade-offs at different times in life (e.g., Stearns 2004; Kaplan and Gangestad 2005).

Aiming to provide a stronger theoretical basis for capturing such domain-specific risk-taking behaviors, Wang et al. (2009) identified five domains: between-group competition (sports watching and driving), within-group competition, environmental challenge, mating and resource allocation and fertility and reproduction. They made an initial attempt to examine the effects of life history traits on risk-taking propensity by domain, measured by subjective likelihoods of engaging in risky behaviors. As a result, it was found that risk-taking propensities in different domains are sensitive to different life history variables; furthermore, subjective life expectancy, age, and reproductive goals were identified as serving as temporal reference points that guide risk perception and risk preference. Both Heinrich's domino model and problem behavior theory emphasize the role of personality in the analysis of risky behaviors. Wang et al. (2009) suggested the need to examine whether life history traits modify personality traits. In addition, based on life history theory, Wenner et al. (2013) showed empirically that traditional assumptions in psychology about risky, deviant, and delinquent acts[9] may be incorrect and suggested that incorporating the influence of developmental contexts is crucial if we are to understand fully the ultimate causal factors driving these acts. McDonald et al. (2012) claimed that how and how much individuals engage in aggressive or antisocial behavior are a relevant outcome of one's life history strategy. Applications of life history theory have led to breakthroughs in understanding the structure of personality traits, which are, in fact, a part of life history strategy (Dunkel and Decker 2010).

11.2.5 Lifetime Utility Theory

Life history theory was developed in the sociological field. In the context of economics, a so-called lifetime utility theory (Friedman 2013) was developed to investigate the effects of distressing life events on engagement in risky behaviors as a coping response. The concept is similar, but the approach is more quantitative. Here, an individual is assumed to accumulate lifetime utility over a composite good, x_t, and behavior, b_t, where the latter contains consumption of addictive goods (e.g., cigarettes), as shown below.

$$W_t = U(b_t, x_t, S_t; H_t) + \Sigma_s \, \delta_s U(b_{t+s}, x_{t+s}, S_{t+s}; H_{t+s})$$

[9]Psychologists traditionally assume that individuals engaging in risky, deviant, and delinquent acts suffer from some form of psychopathology.

Here, W_t is the present (t) discounted value of utility over the life course with the discount rate δ. H_t indicates health capital, which is a function of one's endowment of health at birth, its depreciation and investment. When H_t falls below a critical value, it means that death ensues. S_t is one's addictive stock, which reflects past consumption of addictive substances and increases the marginal utility of addictive substances of current consumption. It is assumed that an individual chooses x_t (a composite addictive good) and x_t (other goods) to maximize his/her present discounted value of lifetime utility, incorporating the influence of health capital and life expectancy, conditional on a standard budget constraint ($Y = P_b b_t + x_t$, where P_b indicates the price of addictive goods, b, and the price of x_t normalized to 1). To represent risky behaviors, it is assumed that $\partial H_{t+s}/\partial b_t < 0$, meaning risky behaviors lead to negative investments in future health capital and it is further assumed that risky behaviors may temporarily improve immediate mental health (H_t), i.e., consuming an addictive good increases present utility. Furthermore, to represent the effects of an adverse life event (Z) on risky behaviors, the part of utility with respect to b is defined as a function of event Z and it is assumed that $\partial U_b/\partial Z > 0$, to reflect the argument that an adverse event may increase distress, which leads to an increase in risky behavior b, especially if its effects on the marginal utility of such behavior exceed those on the marginal utility of other goods, x. Friedman (2013) summarized this theory as yielding three predictions: "individuals should be more likely to try a costly behavior after a distressing event; use of positive coping mechanisms should increase after such events; and, more access to low cost coping devices should dampen the risky behavior response." To specify concretely the utility structure, Friedman (2013) applied three models of risky behavior: rational addiction, time-inconsistent preferences, and nonrational frameworks.

11.2.5.1 Rational addiction model

It is assumed that an individual chooses to consume addictive goods by maximizing his/her utility, given his/her current beliefs and information. In this model, expected risk of addiction and associated costs, and immediate benefits of addiction as well as a perceived probability of becoming addicted are reflected. Even if an individual does not think addiction desirable *ex ante*, he/she may still consume addictive substances if he/she underestimates their probability of becoming addicted. The individual considers intertemporal trade-offs with costs realized in the future in his/her utility-maximizing decision. In this context, a reduced likelihood of experiencing long-term costs can encourage risky behaviors. On the one hand, adverse events might produce this effect by lowering perceived life expectancy (e.g., in response to a violent crime); on the other hand, the impact of reduced life expectancy may depend on the expected cause of death. Expectation of a faster depletion of health capital might motivate reduced risky behavior and increased positive investments in health capital to protect or expand one's length of life. However, if the expected cause of death is a fatal event outside the individual's control (e.g., a car accident, gun violence), an earlier death may be anticipated regardless. Lowering the perceived likelihood of realizing later-life costs, would increase risky behavior.

11.2.5.2 Time-Inconsistent preference model

In this model, hyperbolic discounting is introduced into the rational addiction model by incorporating the influence of time inconsistency, where the newly introduced parameter β reflects the value placed on immediate gratification. Introducing parameter β allows the model to include the effect of stressful or distressing events on intertemporal calculations in a way that increases risky behavior.

$$W_t = U(b_t, x_t, S_t; H_t) + \beta\, \Sigma_s\, \delta_s U(b_{t+s}, x_{t+s}, S_{t+s}; H_{t+s}), \text{ where } \beta \in (0, 1)$$

11.2.5.3 Nonrational model

Here we adopt the System 1–System 2 model of cognition developed in psychology. It is argued that any decision involves two cognitive systems: one is unconscious and instinctive (System 1), and the other is conscious and deliberative (System 2). Most decisions in reality are driven by System 1 because they are habitual and involve intuitive judgment. When conscious and more deliberative processing is called for, System 2 monitors System 1 with considerable effort, even though individuals usually have a limited stock. If a certain level of effort is exceeded, individual decisions may shift to rely on System 1, leading to a variety of nonrational tendencies (e.g., reference dependence). In the case of addictive behaviors, if adverse events absorb the efforts or cause distress that increases the efforts required to engage in basic activities, they would constrain System 2, thereby increasing decisions based on System 1. As a result, overweighting of salient and near-term outcomes alongside less attention to the long run would dampen perceived disincentives to risky behaviors (Friedman 2013: p. 9).

Using data from 2002 to 2010 extracted from the National Longitudinal Survey of Youth, Friedman (2013) revealed empirically that adverse events (being a victim of a violent crime, the death of someone close to the respondent: less than 20 % in the total data) contributed clearly to an increased probability of first cigarette use and first use of an illegal drug other than marijuana for adolescents under 19 years old, based on a regression model with a first-order difference of addiction behaviors between two successive periods of time being the dependent variable. Friedman concluded that distressing events result in risky behaviors, to which a coping response is attributable.

Gardner (1993) developed a life-span rational choice theory of risk taking targeting youths' health, which is similar to the lifetime utility theory. This assumes that an individual maximizes his/her lifetime expected utility, where different attitudes toward health risks are treated as rational choices at different points in the life-span. The model also describes decisions in a life-span context that provide limited but developmentally changing information about the self and the consequences of choices.

11.3 Young People's Risky Driving

Young drivers worldwide are involved in car accidents more than any other age group (Taubman-Ben-Ari and Katz-Ben-Ami 2012). Fatalities for persons aged 16–25 are mainly caused by road accidents, which are also the second most common cause of disability for adolescents (WHO 2014). A variety of factors affect young drivers' driving safety (Scott-Parker et al. 2015a): distraction, insufficient experience, driving together with friends, sensation seeking (driving for fun, self-expression, driving for a sense of freedom, driving to feel independent), and lifestyle habits (e.g., consuming alcohol and/or illicit drugs, engagement in and awareness of religious matters). Here, lifestyle is a key concept in examining risky driving behavior.

Lifestyle has various meanings and consequently has been defined and measured in various ways (e.g., Van Acker 2016). For example, Gnardellis et al. (2008) identified five lifestyle patterns (amusement, culture, religion, sport, work) for studying vehicle accidents and confirmed that the higher the frequency of fatigue and fall-asleep incidents while driving, the greater the likelihood of causing car accidents. They further concluded that road safety measures should target drowsiness-prone drivers. According to Bina et al. (2006), male adolescents practicing risky driving tend to show a lifestyle characterized by high involvement in antisocial behaviors, tobacco smoking, and time spent in nonorganized activities with friends; girls who practice risky driving are more involved in other risk-taking behaviors, antisocial behaviors, and drug use. Thus, risky driving is not an isolated behavior but is just another risky behavior of young people. Because lifestyle is reflected in one's daily activities, these activities (some are related to driving) might be associated with risky driving behavior. In addition, because social networks and psychological factors also affect drivers' lifestyles, their influence on risky driving behavior cannot be ignored.

11.3.1 Driving Tasks

A driver needs to perform various tasks before, during, and after driving. Some tasks are completed before driving (e.g., destination and departure time), others are performed while driving (e.g., vehicle control, lane change, and car following), while the remainder are completed after driving (e.g., taking a rest before the next drive, recalling what happened during the previous drive, and review of the driving experience). Stradling (2011) summarized 10 driving tasks as follows.

(1) Strategic tasks: decisions about activity choice, travel mode, and departure time, and recognition of route alternatives and travel time.
(2) Navigation tasks: find and follow the chosen or changed route, identify and use landmarks and other cues.
(3) Road tasks: choose and maintain the correct position on the road.
(4) Traffic tasks: maintain mobility while avoiding collisions.
(5) Rule tasks: obey rules, regulations, signs, and signals.
(6) Handling tasks: use in-car controls correctly and appropriately.
(7) Secondary tasks: multitasking while driving.
(8) Speed tasks: maintain a speed appropriate to the conditions.
(9) Mood management tasks: avoid boredom and anxiety.
(10) Capability maintenance tasks: avoid compromising driver capability with alcohol or drugs, fatigue, or distraction.

Each task contributes differently to a different part of the 300–29–1 ratio (behind one serious accident lie 29 minor accidents and 300 risky actions), as suggested by Heinrich's Law (Heinrich 1931; Ward 2012). A well-prepared trip plan—part of (1) strategic task—allows a driver to concentrate more on second-by-second driving, without thinking about, for example, tasks awaiting at the destination, or choosing whether to take a toll road. Because a well-prepared trip plan may drastically reduce multitasking behavior during driving (e.g., talking on the phone, sending or reading a text message), risky actions could be reduced. Dahlen et al. (2005), O'Brien and Gormley (2013), and Le Bas et al. (2015) found that higher levels of young people's driving risks were associated with higher levels of impulsivity, implying that young drivers are less likely to prepare trip plans, and consequently supporting the importance of better trip planning before driving in promoting driving safety. Most of the above tasks (2–10) are directly related to driving; some involve habitual judgment (e.g., speed control, obeying traffic rules), while others involve second-by-second judgment (e.g., car following, lane change). Harre (2000) further classified these judgments by young drivers into five psychological risk states; that is, two desirable states: habitually cautious driving and active risk avoidance; and three undesirable states: reduced risk perception, where the actual risk is high, but the perceived risk is low; acceptance of risk as a cost, where the actual risk is high, the perceived risk is high, and risk is valued negatively; and risk seeking, where the actual risk is high, the perceived risk is high, but the risk is valued positively. Clearly, an unsafe judgment may increase the risk of an accident. For further details, refer to Sect. 11.3.2 on risk homeostasis theory.

No study has examined the role of after-driving tasks on driving safety. Even though multitasking while driving is regarded as inherently risky driving, analysis of time use while driving has been completely ignored in the literature. Dealing with a number of driving tasks at the same time involves various risks that should be avoided. Nevertheless, this experience is also useful to teach a young driver to establish a lifetime of safe driving. Huang and Winston (2011) argued that "novice teen drivers are not 'defective' or 'deficient' adult drivers. Rather, these young people are undergoing an explosive period of physical, social, emotional, and behavioral development within an expanding environmental context. … [A] dolescence is a period not only of vulnerability for teens but also of opportunity." Traffic safety measures should also benefit from such positive thinking (p. 315).

11.3.2 Risk Homeostasis Theory

Risk homeostasis theory (Wilde 1982, 1998) argues that crash rates are entirely governed by a driver's target level of risk and that the risk of an action is determined by risk perception and acceptable risk. It is assumed that the amount of risk that people prefer to take depends on expected benefits/costs of risky/safe behavior alternatives. The target level of risk is achieved when the net benefit (e.g., gaining time and increasing mobility by speeding, being punished by speeding tickets, and paying insurance surcharges caused by car repairs) is maximized. At any given moment, a driver compares the amount of risk he/she perceives with the target level of risk and adjusts his/her behavior to eliminate any discrepancies between the two. Such adjustments may lead to either more aggressive or more careful driving. Based on this theory, the annual accident rate can theoretically be calculated as the sum of injury likelihood levels resulting from all actions taken by people over a year. Note that this accident rate in turn affects the level of risk that people perceive and their subsequent decisions and actions. Because of the existence of such a target level, moderate effects of safety measures should be expected and safety measures should be taken to encourage drivers to reform their target risk levels (Hoyes et al. 1996; Hatfield et al. 2014). This theory does not claim that no safety measures will be effective; rather, it argues the ineffectiveness only of those measures for which the current risk level is desirable (Slovic and Fischhoff 1982). Because future expectations affect risky driving behavior, there is evidence to suggest that incentives may increase the perceived benefits of safe driving behavior (Wilde 1998; Bolderdijk et al. 2011). Interestingly, Bolderdijk et al. (2011) examined the effects of insurance-based incentives on speed choices of young drivers (under 30 years old; $n = 141$) over a year and found that the incentives significantly reduced speed violations of those young drivers. Thus, although the short-term effects of incentives have been observed, the long-term effects have not been elucidated.

Risk homeostasis theory also supports the argument that objective crash risk is most usefully portrayed as a function of the choices made by the driver (Wilde 1982; Harre 2000) and that this should be given appropriate attention in making decisions on traffic safety measures. From this perspective, the driving tasks listed in Sect. 11.3.1 should be reflected in decisions on various safety measures.

Just as with any other theory, risk homeostasis theory is not without limitations. For example, Chung and Wong (2012) noted that heterogeneous driver groups may exhibit structural discrepancies that reflect their various decision-making mechanisms, a point that are ignored in this theory. Trimpop (1994) argued that the theory "does not account for risk as a desirable, pleasant activity, which is actively sought out by people and offers intrinsic and extrinsic rewards, such as pleasant emotions or pleasant arousal-highs" (p. 282). The importance of paying attention to positive aspects of risky driving in promoting young people's driving safety is also supported by Huang and Winston (2011).

11.3.3 Applications of Theory of Planned Behavior

Cost-effective traffic safety measures need the support of drivers' voluntary behavioral change toward safer driving. The theory of planned behavior (TPB) (Ajzen 1988, 1991, 2011) is relevant here. It is a general theory that links beliefs and behavior. It is argued that a behavior is determined by a limited set of psychological constructs: (1) the intention (the degree to which the person intends to perform the behavior); (2) the attitude toward the behavior (one's beliefs about the likely consequences of the behavior); (3) the subjective norm (the degree to which the person thinks important others value the behavior); and (4) the perceived behavioral control (the degree to which a person thinks the behavior is under his/her personal control). Constructs (2)–(4) are interrelated and jointly affect construct (1), the intention.

Some recent studies summarize the applications of the TPB to investigate driving safety (e.g., Chorlton et al. 2012; Castanier et al. 2013; Gwyther and Holland 2015; Rowe et al. 2016). Some studies of young drivers' behavior are briefly summarized as follows.

Desrichard et al. (2007) confirmed the significant role of parents in supervising their children in France to improve their risky driving behavior and revealed that attitudes and subjective norms partially mediate the effects of age, prior behavior, and parental supervision. In a study of young drivers in Costa Rica, Leandro (2012) differed from Desrichard et al. (2007) in reporting only the significant influence of norms and perceived behavioral control on intention to reduce speed and actual speed selection. Because the original TPB did not work well, Leandro (2012) proposed to connect norms directly to speed selection and remove the direct link from perceived behavioral control to intention. In a case study in Cambodia, Brijs et al. (2014) found that helmet use was mostly determined by perceived behavioral control over a specific set of inhibiting situational factors (mostly when driving short distances, at night, or when dressed up to go out), followed by perceived behavioral control in general, perceived susceptibility, personal norms, and behavioral intentions, in decreasing order. Targeting the concealed texting of young drivers, the case study by Gauld et al. (2014) in Australia revealed that high intenders (to engage in concealed texting while driving) tended to believe more that concealed texting while driving would result in sharing information with others and using time effectively, while behavioral, normative and control beliefs showed significant differences between low and high intenders. Horvath et al. (2012) also successfully identified the significant differing impacts of these three beliefs on young drivers' speeding behaviors.

Young drivers tend to overestimate their own driving skills and underestimate the hazards involved in driving, under the influence of alcohol (Basch et al. 1989;

DeJoy 1989; Guppy 1993). Marcila et al. (2001) showed that young males' intention to drink and drive was primarily predicted by attitude, followed by perceived behavioral control, and slightly by subjective norms. In a case study of young drivers (under 35 years old) in Norway, Moan and Rise (2011) showed that the TPB variables explained just 10 % of the variance in intention not to drink and drive; they subsequently added moral and descriptive norms, which resulted in only a 2 % point increase. Based on this extended TPB, they found that perceived behavioral control was the strongest predictor of intention, followed by descriptive norm, attitude, and moral norm. Focusing on intoxicated young drivers, Moan (2013) further extended the TPB by adding past behavior, moral norm, descriptive norm, demographic variables, and frequency of alcohol use; this extension resulted in a 4 percentage point increase in the explained variance compared with the original TPB (from 19 to 23 %). Perceived behavioral control was estimated to be the strongest predictor of intention, followed by moral norm, past behavior, descriptive norm, and subjective norm. In contrast, focusing on Chinese youngsters' (19–35 years old) intention to drive after drinking, Chan et al. (2010) found that the TPB variables explained 79 % of the total variance of the intention and highlighted the youngsters' irrational beliefs of invulnerability to danger, which was added to the TPB. Focusing on young drivers in France, Cestac et al. (2011) extended the TPB by adding in the analysis drivers' past behavior, sensation seeking, comparative judgment of risk, and social image of typical deviants (self-descriptions, descriptions of typical deviants, and perceived similarity to the typical deviant). They found that attitude, normative variables, and past behavior had the most influence on the intention to speed, and the effects of perceived behavioral control on the intention increased with driving experience. Gender differences were also revealed; sensation seeking and injunctive norms showed a stronger influence on men's intention to speed than other factors, whereas self-description variables had a greater impact on women's intention. To increase the predictive power of the TPB, Cristea et al. (2013) suggested adding frequency of driving with passengers and driving while angry. Finally, given that driving is a habitual behavior, Chung (2015) observed that habit strength is a crucial mediator between intention antecedents (e.g., attitude) and the intention itself. Adding habit strength in the TPB increased the explained variance of speeding intention by about 30 %. Habit strength was measured by 12 items reflecting not only repetition of the same driving behavior but also other features such as automaticity and self-identity.

11.3.4 *Influences of Family, Peers, and Passengers on Young People's Risky Driving Behavior*

As noted by Desrichard et al. (2007), parents play a significant role in supervising their children to improve their risky driving behavior. Using Bowen's family systems theory (Bowen 1978), Miller and Taubman-Ben-Ari (2010) confirmed that driving styles of parents and their children are strongly correlated, suggesting the existence of intergenerational transmission of driving styles. Family systems theory argues that multigenerational emotional processes are transferred from generation to generation, where these processes include emotions, perceptions, attitudes, beliefs, and values. Intergenerational transferability of risky behaviors from parents to their children has also been observed elsewhere (e.g., Beck et al. 2001a, b; Ferguson et al. 2001; Bianchi and Summala 2004). In contrast, in a case study of young drivers in Israel, Guttman (2013) found that "parents tended to be optimistic about their own child's driving compared with other young drivers and were relatively unconcerned about speeding. … Most also believed many parents feel they are unable to influence young drivers' driving." Thus, the influence of parents on young drivers' risky driving behavior might differ across different cultures.

Related to the influence of parents, Taubman-Ben-Ari and Katz-Ben-Ami (2012) proposed a new concept of family climate for road safety, "which refers to the values, perceptions, priorities and practices of parents and the family in regard to safe driving, as perceived by young drivers" and is composed of seven dimensions: (1) modeling (parents' driving behavior and attitudes shown to their children); (2) feedback (parents' positive feedback and encouraging comments to their offspring in regard to safe driving); (3) communication between parents and adolescents; (4) monitoring (parental supervision and monitoring of their youngsters' driving habits); (5) parents' commitment to road safety; (6) parents' verbal safety messages; and (7) limits (the extent to which parents set systematic and clear-cut limits to their adolescents' driving behavior and discipline them for traffic violations).

Simons-Morton et al. (2008) stated that "the two most important decisions parents can make to reduce teenagers' driving risk are to delay licensure and impose limits on high-risk driving conditions (such as driving at night and with teenage passengers) during the first year of licensure." According to Bingham et al. (2006), parents in many US states are required to supervise their teenage children during 30–50 h of practice driving; moreover, graduated driver licensing programs rely on parents to supervise and monitor their teenage children's adherence to graduated driver licensing (GDL) laws.

Young people's social networks also affect their driving behavior. Pilkington et al. (2014) identified five types of young people's social driving: (1) driving as a social event in itself (i.e., without a prespecified destination); (2) driving to or from a social event; (3) driving with accompanying passengers; (4) driving late at night; (5) driving where alcohol or drugs are a feature of the journey. They further concluded that "road safety interventions need to take a more community development approach, recognizing the importance of social context and focusing on social networks of young people."

Allen and Brown (2008) stated that peers often influence young drivers' risky behaviors through direct/indirect active pressure and passive-pressure forms of intervention. Gheorghiu et al. (2015) confirmed this influence of peers. Scott-Parker et al. (2015a) concluded that both parent-specific interventions and peer-targeted interventions should be designed in a more effective way. They also emphasized that modeling safe driving behavior by parents, active monitoring of driving during novice licensure, minimization of social reinforcement, and promotion of social sanctions for risky driving should be further studied.

Fleiter et al. (2010) reported the influence on driving speed of people known to the driver (passengers and parents) and unknown other drivers. The influence of other drivers was reflected in the form of speeding to keep up with traffic flow and perceived pressure to drive faster. Chung et al. (2014) confirmed the effectiveness of an adult passenger's presence on young drivers' speed control, especially as the effect was transferred even when they drove alone afterward.

11.3.5 Avoidance Driving

Driving avoidance behavior is related to after-driving experience. Recent studies about avoidance behavior theory have mainly focused on punishment avoidance behaviors (Liourta and Empelen 2008; Scott-Parker et al. 2014) and situational avoidance behaviors (Stewart and Peter 2004; Motak et al. 2014). Punishment avoidance behavior indicates that drivers might evade detection by police by avoiding driving in police enforcement activity areas to avoid a potential traffic citation for speeding behavior due to substance-impaired driving behaviors, such as drunk driving and driving after consuming drugs (Fleiter and Watson 2005; Scott-Parker et al. 2011). Fleiter and Watson (2005) noted that traffic rule violation behavior, especially speeding behavior, is strongly correlated with the prediction of an individual's punishment avoidance behavior. This result is consistent with the findings of Scott-Parker et al. (2011), who showed that more risky driving behavior is in general practiced by punishment avoiders. Situational avoidance behavior is derived mainly from drivers' after-driving experience, especially experience of accidents while driving. Drivers tend to perform avoidance behaviors in situations in which their impairments identified or obtained from previous crash involvement might expose them to an increased risk of accident (Motak et al. 2014). Ten situations were identified by Motak et al. (2014): driving at night, at night in the rain, long distances, in the rain, in fog, during rush hour, at roundabouts, left turns, in the snow, and on highways.

In more general avoidance driving research conducted by Stewart and Peter (2004), a questionnaire for the Driving and Riding Avoidance Scale was developed. Four types of avoidance behavior—general avoidance, traffic avoidance, weather avoidance, and riding avoidance—were generated from 20 related items. Stewart and Peter (2004) also showed that stronger avoidance behaviors could be identified from drivers who experienced medical treatments from crash-related injuries than from those who were uninjured or injured and not medically treated. Naumann et al. (2011) investigated drivers' self-restriction behaviors (or avoidance behaviors) by focusing on three high-risk conditions: driving at night, driving in bad weather, and driving on highways or high-speed roads. They showed that self-restriction was not only observed in older drivers, but also in young drivers: 25 %

of drivers aged 18–24 years reported avoiding driving at night, 50 % reported avoiding driving in bad weather (the percentage was higher among young female drivers than older female drivers), and nearly 20 % reported avoiding driving on highways or high-speed roads. Le Bas et al. (2015) used the Multidimensional Personality Questionnaire 28-item harm avoidance subscale to predict young drivers' driving risk together with a series of self-report items and found that higher levels of driving risk related to higher levels of impulsivity and lower levels of harm avoidance (indicating fearlessness).

11.3.6 Mood During Driving and Driving Purpose

Because of the time and money spent on car use, transportation demand models have traditionally assumed that drivers derive negative utility from car use. However, a recent study in Denmark showed that Danish adolescents can be classified into three groups (Sigurdardottir et al. 2014): "The first group are car enthusiasts who associate cars with high instrumental, affective, symbolic and relational values, have car-oriented social networks and imagine a car-oriented lifestyle. The second group are car pragmatists, who associate cars with high instrumental and relational values, perceive car expenses as a barrier and imagine a car-oriented lifestyle only in the long term. The third group are car skeptics, who have low interest in cars and imagine a cycling-oriented future." Belgiawan et al. (2014) conducted a cross-country comparison (including both developed and developing countries) of university students' car ownership motivations and found that the emotional attachment of students to cars can be grouped into four categories: symbolic affective (whether cars allow one to distinguish oneself from others, are trendy, bring prestige, are cool, allow one to express oneself, are fun to have); independent (whether cars are convenient, give freedom to travel anytime, help one to save time when making a trip, are useful to pick up or drop off others); negative aspects (whether cars are expensive to own and maintain, disturb one's neighborhood, give an arrogant impression); and social orderliness (whether cars allow one to travel safely, are environmentally friendly). This evidence suggests that, at least for young people, car use may also involve a variety of positive feelings during driving.

In the case of risky driving, although a large body of work has accumulated on the effects of anger on driving, only a limited number of studies have focused on the effects of positive emotions on both perceptions of and experiences while driving. According to the review by Rhodes et al. (2015), (1) young male drivers tend to enjoy risky driving, (2) people in a happy mood tend to engage in less effortful information processing, leading them to engage in risky driving, and (3) individuals in a negative mood are more likely to engage in effortful and systematic processing of information, resulting in better driving. Based on a driving simulation experiment, Rhodes et al. (2015) confirmed that faster driving speed was significantly associated with driving in a happy mood and with a passenger, but that careless driving was not related to mood. As described in Sect. 11.3.1, mood management is an important driving task for drivers. Do such findings suggest that traffic safety policy makers should work out how to make drivers unhappy to avoid risky driving? Should policy makers force or encourage drivers to concentrate on driving by distracting them from enjoying a pleasant/happy driving experience? Is the implication that the role of traditional traffic safety measures in reducing risky driving is very limited, as partially indicated by the risk homeostasis theory? None of these inferences seems convincing.

Mood during driving is not only induced by driving or the driving environment. It may also come from participation in activities before and after driving (e.g., enjoying talking to a close friend before driving, or having a quarrel with a family member; anticipating talking to a close friend waiting at the destination, or going to meet a customer to apologize to them for some reason). Mood management for safe driving should go on continuously over time (i.e., before, during, and after driving). Studies of young drivers suggest that a happy mood usually results in risky driving, especially in the presence of a friend. On the other hand, experiencing risky behavior might be positive for promoting lifelong traffic safety measures because of the effects of drivers' learning behavior over time. To examine this hypothesis, it is necessary to understand better drivers' use of time and affective experience while driving.

People drive for various purposes, which may affect their mood during driving. The risky driving behavior of young people is particularly associated with psychosocial maturation during the development of their identity as a driver (Scott-Parker et al. 2015b). Scott-Parker et al. (2015b) summarized the various purposes of driving: meeting mobility needs (having a reliable, flexible, efficient, and economical means of transport; readily meeting a variety of needs; engaging in multipurpose trips); facilitating time spent with friends; driving for leisure, relaxation, fun, and excitement; the enjoyment of driving; sensation seeking; self-expression; and gaining social status, independence, and freedom. Because some of these purposes might be met by performing other activities rather than driving, it suggests that driving might be interrelated with the other activities and therefore mood management should be go on not only while driving, but also when performing the other activities.

11.3.7 Driving and Nightlife

Traffic accidents, sexually transmitted diseases, unwanted pregnancies, drunkenness, and drug use (especially of psychostimulants) are negative aspects associated with recreational nightlife (Becoña Iglesias et al. 2011). Road accidents associated with nightlife alcohol and recreational drug use are a major health problem for young people (Calafat et al. 2009a). In OECD countries in recent decades, over 8500 young drivers were killed each year in accidents that tended to occur on weekend nights and when driving under the influence of alcohol (Scagnolaria et al.

2015). Using data collected from regular nightlife users in nine European cities in 2006, Calafat et al. (2009a) found that males were more likely to be drunk and take drugs, resulting in getting a lift from someone drunk or driving drunk; drunkenness was related to risky behaviors and older young people were less likely to cause traffic accidents. Impulsivity, a preference for using a private car to get to nightlife venues, and being unemployed were associated with riding with a driver under the influence of alcohol or drugs (Calafat et al. 2009b). It seems that there are some potential associations between cultural patterns, social norms, and nightlife risk behaviors (Calafat et al. 2011). Indeed, young people admit that fines, speed cameras, and alcohol breath testing reduce risky driving; however, they also claim that a lack of public transport alternatives on weekends and at night is associated with their risky driving behavior (Ramos et al. 2008). Based on a stated preference survey, Scagnolaria et al. (2015) reported young people's greater preference for using minibuses and sharing a taxi to enjoy their nightlife; moreover, to keep young people from using their cars, they suggested the need to provide low-cost, fast, and flexible public transport to get to events and back home, which would contribute to fewer traffic accidents.

It is obviously important to change young people's attitudes toward drink-driving and to recognize more clearly the risky driving behavior involved. Smartphones may play a positive role in this respect. Pocuca et al. (2016) noted that young people's knowledge of the consequences of drink-driving and ways to avoid it may be improved with the assistance of a well-designed smartphone app. Jiang et al. (2015) reported that a GPS-enabled smartphone app (Zhang et al. 2014) that diagnoses driving safety by measuring three types of driving risks—compliance level with speed limits, abrupt acceleration and deceleration, and driving stability—was more effective in assisting drivers to comply with speed limits than in controlling acceleration and deceleration. The effects showed a large variation depending on driving propensity.

11.3.8 Self-driving Cars and Young People

Young people are always curious about new things, and self-driving cars will be no exception. A self-driving car (autonomous car, driverless car, or robotic car) is a vehicle that is able to move by itself with the assistance of various sensing and positioning technologies, without any human input while moving. It is designed for a zero-accident society. Because of the likely natural curiosity of young people, some automakers have even released a self-driving concept vehicle created for young people.[10] Other advantages of autonomous cars have been reported from the perspectives of safety, congestion, energy use, and land use (Anderson et al. 2014), even though autonomous vehicles with current technologies are still far

[10] http://www.dezeen.com/2015/10/28/mercedes-benz-autonomous-electric-concept-car-vision-tokyo-urban-hipsters/ (accessed February 13, 2016).

from the ambitious zero-accident goal. The University of Michigan's Transportation Research Institute has reported that autonomous cars were five times more likely to crash than conventional cars, with the current very low distance accumulated by autonomous cars.[11] Nevertheless, it is expected that more advanced technologies will improve further the safety level in the future.

Schoettle and Sivak (2014) conducted a public opinion survey about autonomous and self-driving vehicles in the US, the UK, and Australia. Younger respondents were more interested in having their vehicles equipped with self-driving technologies and were more willing to ride in self-driving vehicles, probably because they were more likely to expect less traffic congestion, shorter travel time, and lower insurance rates with self-driving vehicles. Somers and Weeratunga (2015) argued that younger generations, who value their time on social networks more than older generations, may be more receptive to autonomous cars. LoBello (2015) noted that 65 % of students would use a self-driving car if it was controlled by both computer and humans and over 90 % of students would use a self-driving car if auto insurance premiums were to be cut by 50 %. In contrast, Casley et al. (2013) reported that younger persons seemed to be more worried about the safety of autonomous cars and felt less comfortable in one. Young people's greater concerns about safety issues of self-driving cars were also reported by Anderson et al. (2014) and LoBello (2015).

Considering these conflicting viewpoints of young people about self-driving cars, more studies are required, especially concerning the various potential ways of using self-driving cars.

11.4 Conclusions

We recognize that there are many relevant theories and models of risky behaviors that explore a range of factors. In their systematic literature review of the relationship between risky decision making and aggression, Kuin et al. (2015) found that increased risk taking on decision-making tasks was related to higher levels of aggression, especially with respect to reactive aggression (with a premeditated aim to gain an intended advantage), as well as to proactive aggression (as a result of perceived provocation/threat or intense emotion and lack of impulse control). The two types of aggression are highly correlated. More importantly, the problems in risky decision making and reactive aggression both derive from the same underlying orbitofrontal deficit (e.g., Mehta and Beer 2010). This neurological finding suggests a potential correlation between risky decision making and aggression. Related to this argument, Kuin et al. (2015) further found that previous violent (criminal) behaviors or current aggressive feelings were significantly correlated with greater risk taking in decision-making tasks. As a concrete example, Hanna et al. (2001) showed that for young people, being a former alcohol drinker was

[11]http://fortune.com/2015/10/29/self-driving-cars-crash/ (accessed February 13, 2016).

associated with being a current smoker, which was also a strong predictor for using other drugs, implying that drinking and smoking might share some common factor inherent in an adolescent's biological or psychological makeup from childhood or birth. With a focus on low-income African-American youth, Hsieh et al. (2015) found that risks in one domain manifested as risks in the same domain across time in addition to spreading to other domains. This conclusion is consistent with the findings from studies reviewed by Hsieh et al. (2015): "high risk driving during youth is associated with other risk-taking behaviors, such as delinquency, unprotected sex, drinking, and the use of drugs". These conclusions suggest that risky behaviors tend to covary, implying that interventions should jointly target multiple risky behaviors. Indeed, this argument is supported by the concept of developmental cascades, which refer to the notion that developmental effects in one ecological domain may spill over to influence multiple domains later in development (Donovan 1993; Pharo et al. 2011).

As for risky driving, it seems that young people's various habits in daily life and at least some criteria (e.g., value of life and/or time, social norms, attitudes, and liking) for life choices are associated with driving risks and safety as well as daily security. Effective traffic safety measures for young people may also be adopted with a focus on life situations and purposes. Different life purposes are associated with different life choices, such as family formation, social networks, and residential location. Various habits formed in daily life over years may affect driving risks and/or safety. People who tend to behave in a well-planned way may arrange their daily trips following a schedule determined in advance. They may drive following a predetermined schedule and consequently may not necessarily drive very fast to reach their destination. In such cases, their driving may be safer than other types of drivers. People who purposely choose to reside in a location free of natural disasters may also drive safely, partly because their awareness of safety and security may be a prioritized criterion in their daily decisions. Individuals who are likely to be risk takers in other daily activities (e.g., always being late for work and appointments, often making decisions without careful consideration, enjoying adventurous activities) might also take risks driving. People who usually behave strictly based on rules in general may also tend to obey traffic rules. Individuals who are usually good at multitasking and/or who like to multitask to save time may be likely to do other things while driving, which is in fact dangerous behavior. Traffic safety education in primary and secondary schools is such an example, while involving young people in regular safety campaigns may be another. Other examples may include the involvement of young people in various public decisions, encouraging them to undertake more voluntary activities (both during school and work), and providing them with attractive and convenient recreational environments with good access to public transportation systems.

This literature review suggests that risky behaviors in life are not independent, which implies that understanding them demands interdisciplinary approaches. Reducing risky behaviors—which are harmful not only to people themselves but also to society—requires various sectors to collaborate with each other to enhance the efficiency and effectiveness of efforts such as laws and regulations, economic measures (both incentive-based and punishment-based measures), technological developments, and enlightenment.

References

Ajzen I (1988) Attitudes, personality, and behavior. Dorsey, Chicago, IL

Ajzen I (1991) The theory of planned behavior. Organ Behav Hum Decis Process 50:179–211

Ajzen I (2011) The theory of planned behavior: reactions and reflections. Psychol Health 26(9):1113–1127

Allen JP, Brown BB (2008) Adolescents, peers, and motor vehicles: the perfect storm? Am J Prev Med 35:S289–S293

American Psychiatric Association (2013) Diagnostic and statistical manual of mental disorders, 5th edn. American Psychiatric Association, Washington, DC

Anderson JM, Kalra N, Stanley KD, Sorensen P, Samaras C, Oluwatola OA (2014) Autonomous vehicle technology: a guide for policymakers. RAND Corporation. Available: http://www.rand.org/content/dam/rand/pubs/research_reports/RR400/RR443-2/RAND_RR443-2.pdf. Accessed 29 May 2016

Baron SW, Forde DR, Kay FM (2007) Self-control, risky lifestyles, and situation: the role of opportunity and context in the general theory. J Crim Justice 35(2):119–136

Basch CE, DeCicco IM, Malfetti JL (1989) A focus group study on decision processes of young drivers: reasons that may support a decision to drink and drive. Health Educ Q 16:389–396

Beck KH, Shattuck T, Raleigh R (2001a) Parental predictors of teen driving risk. Am J Health Behav 25(1):10–20

Beck KH, Shattuck T, Raleigh R (2001b) A comparison of teen perceptions and parental reports of influence on driving risk. Am J Health Behav 25(4):376–387

Becoña Iglesias E, López-Durán A, Fernández Del Río E, Martínez Pradeda Ú, Osorio López J, Fraga Ares J, Arrojo Romero M, López Crecente F, Domínguez González MN (2011) Drunkenness, driving and sexual relations in young cocaine and ecstasy users. Adicciones 23(3):205–218

Belgiawan PF, Schmocker J-D, Abou-Zeid M, Walker J, Lee T-C, Ettema DF, Fujii S (2014) Car ownership motivations among undergraduate students in China, Indonesia, Japan, Lebanon, Netherlands, Taiwan, and USA. Transportation 41(6):1227–1244

Bianchi A, Summala H (2004) The "genetics" of driving behavior: parents' driving style predicts their children's driving style. Accid Anal Prev 36:655–659

Bina M, Graziano F, Bonino S (2006) Risky driving and lifestyles in adolescence. Accid Anal Prev 38(3):472–481

Bingham CR, Shope JT, Raghunathan T (2006) Patterns of traffic offenses from adolescent licensure into early young adulthood. J Adolesc Health 39(1):35–42

Bolderdijk JW, Knockaert J, Steg EM, Verhoef ET (2011) Effects of Pay-As-You-Drive vehicle insurance on young drivers' speed choice: Results of a Dutch field experiment. Accid Anal Prev 43:1181–1186

Bowen M (1978) Family therapy in clinical practice. Jason Aronson, New York, London

Brijs K, Brijs T, Sann S, Trinh TA, Wets G, Ruiter RAC (2014) Psychological determinants of motorcycle helmet use among young adults in Cambodia. Transp Res Part F 26:273–290

Buckley L, Chapman RL (2016) Characteristics of adolescents who intervene to stop the risky and dangerous behavior of their friends. Accid Anal Prev 88:187–193

Calafat A, Blay N, Juan M, Adrover D, Bellis MA, Hughes K, Stocco P, Siamou I, Mendes F, Bohrn K (2009a) Traffic risk behaviors at nightlife: drinking, taking drugs, driving, and use of public transport by young people. Traffic Inj Prev 10(2):162–169

Calafat A, Adrover-Roig D, Blay N, Juan M, Bellis M, Hughes K, Mendes F, Kokkevi A (2009b) Which young people accept a lift from a drunk or drugged driver? Accid Anal Prev 41(4):703–709
Calafat A, Blay NT, Hughes K, Bellis M, Juan M, Duch M, Kokkevi A (2011) Nightlife young risk behaviours in Mediterranean versus other European cities: are stereotypes true? Eur J Pub Health 21(3):311–315
Casley SV, Jardim AS, Quartulli AM (2013) A study of public acceptance of autonomous cars. Worcester Polytechnic Institute, Bachelor Thesis
Castanier C, Deroche T, Woodman T (2013) Theory of planned behavior and road violations: the moderating influence of perceived behavioural control. Transp Res Part F 18:148–158
Catalano RF, Kosterman R, Hawkins JD, Newcomb MD, Abbott RD (1996) Modeling the etiology of adolescent substance use: a test of the social development model. J Drug Issues 26(2):429–455
Cestac J, Paran F, Delhomme P (2011) Young drivers' sensation seeking, subjective norms, and perceived behavioral control and their roles in predicting speeding intention: how risk-taking motivations evolve with gender and driving experience. Saf Sci 49(3):424–432
Chan DCN, Wu AMS, Hung EPW (2010) Invulnerability and the intention to drink and drive: an application of the theory of planned behavior. Accid Anal Prev 42:1549–1555
Chorlton K, Conner M, Jamson S (2012) Identifying the psychological determinants of risky riding: An application of an extended theory of planned behaviour. Accid Anal Prev 49:142–153
Chung YS (2015) Seemingly irrational driving behavior model: the effect of habit strength and anticipated affective reactions. Accid Anal Prev 82:79–89
Chung YS, Wong JT (2012) Beyond general behavioral theories: structural discrepancy in young motorcyclist's risky driving behavior and its policy implications. Accid Anal Prev 49:165–176
Chung EK, Choe B, Lee JE, Lee JI, Sohn YW (2014) Effects of an adult passenger on young adult drivers' driving speed: roles of an adult passenger's presence and driving tips from the passenger. Accid Anal Prev 67:14–20
Cieslik M, Simpson D (2013) Key concepts in youth studies. Sage, London
Cristea M, Paran F, Delhomme P (2013) Extending the theory of planned behavior: the role of behavioral options and additional factors in predicting speed behavior. Transp Res Part F: Traffic Psychol Behav 21:122–132
Dahlen ER, Martin RC, Ragan K, Kuhlman MM (2005) Driving anger, sensation seeking, impulsiveness, and boredom proneness in the prediction of unsafe driving. Accid Anal Prev 37(2):341–348
DeJoy DM (1989) The optimism bias and traffic accident risk perception. Accid Anal Prev 21:333–340
Desrichard O, Roché S, Bègue L (2007) The theory of planned behavior as mediator of the effect of parental supervision: a study of intentions to violate driving rules in a representative sample of adolescents. J Saf Res 38(4):447–452
Diene E, Lucas R (1999) Personality and subjective well-being. In: Kahneman D, Diener E, Schwarz N (eds) Well-being: the foundations of hedonic psychology. Russell-Sage, New York, pp 213–229
Diener E (1994) Assessing subjective well-being: progress and opportunities. Soc Indic Res 31(2):103–157
Diener E (2009) The science of well-being. Springer, New York
Donovan JE (1993) Young adult drinking-driving: behavioral and psychosocial correlates. J Stud Alcohol 54(5):600–613
Dunkel CS, Decker M (2010) Convergent validity of measures of life-history strategy. Personality Individ Differ 48:681–684
Elliott DS (1994) Serious violent offenders: onset, developmental course, and termination: the American Society of Criminology 1993 Presidential Address. Criminology 32:1–21

Feinberg ME, Ridenour TA, Greenberg MT (2007) Aggregating indices of risk and protection for adolescent behavior problems: the communities that care youth survey. J Adolesc Health 40:506–513

Feinberg ME, Sakuma K-L, Hostetler M, McHale SM (2013) Enhancing sibling relationships to prevent adolescent problem behaviors: theory, design and feasibility of siblings are pecial. Eval Program Plan 36:97–106

Ferguson SA, Williams AF, Chapline JF, Reinfurt DW, De Leonardis DM (2001) Relationship of parent driving records to the driving records of their children. Accid Anal Prev 33:229–234

Fleiter JJ, Watson B (2005) The speed paradox: the misalignment between driver attitudes and speeding behavior. In: Proceedings of the Australasian road safety research, policy and education conference. Wellington, New Zealand, 14–16 Nov 2005

Fleiter JJ, Lennon A, Watson B (2010) How do other people influence your driving speed? Exploring the 'who' and the 'how' of social influences on speeding from a qualitative perspective. Transp Res Part F 13(1):49–62

Friedman A (2013) Adverse events and risky behaviors: evidence from adolescents. Job Market Paper, Harvard University. http://scholar.harvard.edu/files/afriedman/files/jmp_abbyfriedman.pdf. Accessed 31 Jan 2016

Gardner W (1993) A life-span rational-choice theory of risk taking. In: Bell RW, Bell NJ (eds) Adolescent risk taking. Sage Publications, Newbury Park, pp 66–83

Gauld CS, Lewis I, White KM (2014) Concealed texting while driving: what are young people's beliefs about this risky behaviour? Saf Sci 65:63–69

Gheorghiu A, Delhomme P, Felonneau ML (2015) Peer pressure and risk taking in young drivers' speeding behavior. Transp Res Part F Traffic Psychol Behav 35:101–111

Gnardellis C, Tzamalouka G, Papadakaki M, Chliaoutakis JE (2008) An investigation of the effect of sleepiness, drowsy driving, and lifestyle on vehicle crashes. Transp Res Part F 11(4):270–281

Guppy A (1993) Subjective probability of accident and apprehension in relation to self-other bias, age, and reported behavior. Accid Anal Prev 25:375–382

Guttman N (2013) "My son is reliable": young drivers' parents' optimism and views on the norms of parental involvement in youth driving. J Adolesc Res 28(2):241–268

Gwyther H, Holland C (2015) An intervention encouraging planned self-regulation and goal setting in drivers across the lifespan: Testing an extended theory of planned behaviour. J Transp Health 2(2):289–301

Hanna EZ, Yi H, Dufour MC, Whitmore CC (2001) The relationship of early-onset regular smoking to alcohol use, depression, illicit drug use, and other risky behaviors during early adolescence: results from the youth supplement to the third national health and nutrition examination survey. J Subst Abuse 13:265–282

Harre N (2000) Risk evaluation, driving, and adolescents: a typology. Dev Rev 20(2):206–226

Hatfield J, Fernandes R, Soames Job RF (2014) Trill and adventure seeking as a modifier of the relationship of perceived risk with risky driving among young drivers. Accid Anal Prev 62:223–229

Hawkins JD, Weis JG (1985) The social development model: an integrated approach to delinquency prevention. J Primary Prev 6:73–97

Heinrich HW (1931) Industrial accident prevention: a scientific approach. McGraw-Hill, New York

Horvath C, Lewis I, Watson B (2012) The beliefs which motivate young male and female drivers to speed: a comparison of low and high intenders. Accid Anal Prev 45:334–351

Hoyes TW, Dorn L, Desmond PA, Taylor R (1996) Risk homeostasis theory, utility and accident loss in a simulated driving task. Saf Sci 22:49–62

Hsieh H-F, Heinze JE, Aiyer SM, Stoddard SA, Wang J-L, Zimmerman MA (2015) Cross-domain influences on youth risky driving behaviors: a developmental cascade analysis. J Appl Dev Psychol 38:11–21

Huang P, Winston FK (2011) Young drivers. In: Porter BE (ed) Handbook of traffic psychology. Academic Press, New York, pp 315–338
Jessor R (1991) Risk behavior in adolescence: a psychosocial framework for understanding and action. J Adolesc Health 12(8):597–605
Jessor R, Jessor SL (1977) Problem behavior and psychological development: a longitudinal study of youth. Academic Press, New York
Jiang Y, Zhang J, Chikaraishi M, Seya H, Fujiwara A (2015) Driving speed control behavior and safety on expressways under smart phone app based traffic safety information provision. In: Presented at the 14th international conference on travel behaviour research. Windsor, UK, 19–23 July 2015
Kabiru CW, Elung'ata P, Mojola SA, Beguy D (2014) Adverse life events and delinquent behavior among Kenyan adolescents: a cross-sectional study on the protective role of parental monitoring, religiosity, and self-esteem. Child Adolescent Psychiatry Mental Health 8:24
Kahneman D, Krueger AB, Schkade DA, Schwarz N, Stone AA (2004) A survey method for characterizing daily life experience: the day reconstruction method. Science 306(5702):1776–1780
Kaplan HS, Gangestad SG (2005) Life history theory and evolutionary psychology. In: Buss DM (ed) The handbook of evolutionarily psychology. Wiley, New York, pp 528–551
Kuin H, Masthoff E, Kramer M, Scherder E (2015) The role of risky decision-making in aggression: a systematic review. Aggression Violent Behav 25:159–172
Lam LT (2015) Parental mental health and internet addiction in adolescents. Addict Behav 42:20–23
Lane SD, Cherek DR (2000) Analysis of risk taking in adults with a history of high risk behavior. Drug Alcohol Depend 60:179–187
Lantz PM, Jacobson PD, Warner KE, Wasserman J, Larson B (2000) Investing in youth tobacco control: a review of smoking prevention and control strategies. Tobacco Control 9(1):47–63
Le Bas GA, Hughes MA, Stout JC (2015) Utility of self-report and performance-based measures of risk for predicting driving behavior in young people. Personality Individ Differ 86:184–188
Leandro M (2012) Young drivers and speed selection: a model guided by the theory of planned behavior. Transp Res Part F 15(3):219–232
Lenihan F (2007) Computer addiction—a sceptical view: invited commentary on: lost online. Adv Psychiatr Treat 13:31
Liourta E, Empelen PV (2008) The importance of self-regulatory and goal-conflicting process in the avoidance of drunk driving among Greek young drivers. Accid Anal Prev 40:1191–1199
LoBello A (2015) The implications of self-driving cars on insurance. Bryant University. Available: http://digitalcommons.bryant.edu/cgi/viewcontent.cgi?article=1020&context=honors_mathematics. Accessed 13 Feb 2016
Marcila I, Bergeron J, Audet T (2001) Motivational factors underlying the intention to drink and drive in young male drivers. J Saf Res 32:363–376
Mason MJ, Tanner JF, Piacentini M, Freeman D, Anastasia T, Batat W, Boland W, Canbulut M, Drenten J, Hamby A, Rangan P, Yang Z (2013) Advancing a participatory approach for youth risk behavior: foundations, distinctions, and research directions. J Bus Res 66:1235–1241
McDonald MM, Donnellan MB, Navarrete CD (2012) A life history approach to understanding the dark triad. Personality Individ Differ 52(5):601–605
Mehta PH, Beer J (2010) Neural mechanisms of the testosterone-aggression relation: the role of orbitofrontal cortex. J Cogn Neurosci 22(10):2357–2368
Melkman E (2015) Risk and protective factors for problem behaviors among youth in residential care. Child Youth Serv Rev 51:117–124
Miller KE (2008) Energy drinks, race, and problem behaviors among college students. J Adolesc Health 43(5):490–497

Miller G, Taubman-Ben-Ari O (2010) Driving styles among young novice drivers—the contribution of parental driving styles and personal characteristics. Accid Anal Prev 42(2):558–570
Moan IS (2013) Whether or not to ride with an intoxicated driver: predicting intentions using an extended version of the theory of planned behaviour. Transp Res Part F 20:193–205
Moan IS, Rise J (2011) Predicting intentions not to "drink and drive" using an extended version of the theory of planned behaviour. Accid Anal Prev 43(4):1378–1384
Moore S (2011) Understanding and managing anti-social behaviour on public transport through value change: the considerate travel campaign. Transp Policy 18(1):53–59
Motak L, Cabaude C, Bouge J-C, Huet N (2014) Comparison of driving avoidance and self-regulatory patterns in younger and older drivers. Transp Res Part F 26:18–27
Naumann R, Dellinger AM, Krenow M (2011) Driving self-restriction in high-risk conditions: how do older drivers compare to others? J Saf Res 42:67–71
O'Brien F, Gormley M (2013) The contribution of inhibitory deficits to dangerous driving among young people. Accid Anal Prev 51:238–242
Pergamit MR, Huang L, Lane J (2001) The long term impact of adolescent risky behaviors and family environment. Submitted to the Office of the Assistant Secretary for Planning and Evaluation, U.S. Department of Health and Human Services. Available: https://aspe.hhs.gov/report/long-term-impact-adolescent-risky-behaviors-and-family-environment. Accessed 2 Feb 2016
Pharo H, Sim C, Graham M, Gross J, Hayne H (2011) Risky business: executive function, personality, and reckless behavior during adolescence and emerging adulthood. Behav Neurosci 125(6):970–978
Pilkington P, Bird E, Gray S, Towner E, Weld S, McKibben M-A (2014) Understanding the social context of fatal road traffic collisions among young people: a qualitative analysis of narrative text in coroners' records. BMC Public Health, Vol. 14, Article Number: 78
Pocuca N, Hides L, Zelenko O, Quek L-H, Stoyanov S, Tulloch K, Johnson D, Tjondronegoro D, Kavanagh DJ (2016) Initial prototype testing of ray's night out: a new mobile app targeting risky drinking in young people. Comput Hum Behav 54:207–214
Prentice C, Cotte J (2015) Multiple Ps' effects on gambling, drinking and smoking: advancing theory and evidence. J Bus Res 68:2045–2048
Ramos P, Díez E, Pérez K, Rodriguez-Martos A, Brugal MT, Villalbí JR (2008) Young people's perceptions of traffic injury risks, prevention and enforcement measures: a qualitative study. Accid Anal Prev 40(4):1313–1319
Rhodes N, Pivik K, Sutton M (2015) Risky driving among young male drivers: the effects of mood and passengers. Transp Res Part F 28:65–76
Rowe R, Andrews E, Harris PR, Armitage CJ, McKenna FP, Norman P (2016) Identifying beliefs underlying pre-drivers' intentions to take risks: an application of the theory of planned behaviour. Accid Anal Prev 89:49–56
Scagnolaria S, Walker J, Maggia R (2015) Young drivers' night-time mobility preferences and attitude toward alcohol consumption: a hybrid choice model. Accid Anal Prev 83:74–89
Schoettle B, Sivak M (2014) A survey of public opinion about autonomous and self-driving vehicles in the U.S., the U.K., and Australia. Report No. UMTRI-2014-21, Transportation Research Institute, The University of Michigan
Scott-Parker B, Watson B, King MJ, Hyde MK (2011) Mileage, car ownership, experience of punishment avoidance and the risky driving of young drivers. Traffic Inj Prev 12(6):559–567
Scott-Parker B, Watson B, King MJ, Hyde MK (2014) "I drove after drinking alcohol" and other risk driving behaviours reported by young novice drivers. Accid Anal Prev 70:65–73
Scott-Parker B, Watson B, King MJ, Hyde MK (2015a) "I would have lost the respect of my friends and family if they knew I had bent the road rules": parents, peers, and the perilous behaviour of young drivers. Transp Res Part F 28:1–13
Scott-Parker B, King MJ, Watson B (2015b) The psychosocial purpose of driving and its relationship with the risky driving behaviour of young novice drivers. Transp Res Part F 33:16–26

Sigurdardottir SB, Kaplan S, Moller M (2014) The motivation underlying adolescents' intended time-frame for driving licensure and car ownership: a socio-ecological approach. Transp Policy 36:19–25
Simons-Morton BG, Ouimet MC, Catalano RF (2008) Parenting and the young driver problem. Am J Prev Med 35(3):S294–S303
Slovic P, Fischhoff B (1982) Targeting risks. Risk Anal 2(4):227–234
Somers A, Weeratunga K (2015) Automated vehicles: are we ready? Internal report on potential implications for main roads Western Australia. Available: https://www.mainroads.wa.gov.au/Documents/Automated%20Vehicle%20Report.RCN-D15%5E2381741.PDF. Access 29 May 2016
Stearns SC (2004) The evolution of life histories. Oxford University Press, New York
Steinberg L, Morris AS (2001) Adolescent development. Annu Rev Psychol 52:83–110
Sterrett EM, Dymnicki AB, Henry D, Byck GR, Bolland J, Mustanski B (2014) Predictors of co-occurring risk behavior trajectories among economically disadvantaged African-American youth: contextual and individual factors. J Adolesc Health 55:380–387
Stewart AE, Peter CCS (2004) Driving and risking avoidance following motor vehicle crashes in a non-clinical sample: psychometric properties of a new measure. Behav Res Therapy 42:859–879
Stradling SG (2011) Travel mode choice. In: Porter BE (ed) Handbook of traffic psychology. Elsevier, Amsterdam
Taubman-Ben-Ari O, Katz-Ben-Ami L (2012) The contribution of family climate for road safety and social environment to the reported driving behavior of young drivers. Accid Anal Prev 47:1–10
Trimpop RM (1994) The psychology of risk taking behavior. North-Holland, New York
United Nations Population Fund (2014) The power of 1.8 billion: Adolescents, youth and the transformation of the future. Available: https://www.unfpa.org/sites/default/files/pub-pdf/EN-SWOP14-Report_FINAL-web.pdf. Accessed 31 Jan 2016
Van Acker V (2016) Lifestyles and life choices. In: Zhang J (ed) Life-oriented behavioral research for urban policy. Springer, Chapter 3
Wang XT, Kruger DJ, Wilke A (2009) Life history variables and risk-taking propensity. Evol Hum Behav 30:77–84
Ward RB (2012) Revisiting Heinrich's law [online]. In: Chemeca 2012: quality of life through chemical engineering, Wellington, New Zealand, vol 2012. A.C.T.: Engineers Australia, Barton, 23–26 Sept 2012, pp 1179–1187
Weber EU, Blais AR, Betz NE (2002) A domain-specific risk attitude scale: measuring risk perceptions and risk behaviors. J Behav Decis Making 15:263–290
Wenner CJ, Bianchi J, Figueredo AJ, Philippe Rushton J, Jacobs WJ (2013) Life history theory and social deviance: the mediating role of executive function. Intelligence 41:102–113
WHO (World Health Organization) (2014) Health for the World's Adolescents. A second chance in the second decade, www.who.int/adolescent/second-decade
WHO (World Health Organization) (2015) Global status report on road safety 2015
Wilde GJS (1982) The theory of risk homeostasis: Implications for safety and health. Risk Anal 2(4):209–925
Wilde GJS (1998) Risk homeostasis theory: an overview. Inj Prev 4:89–91
Young K (2010) Internet addiction over the decade: a personal look back. World Psychiatry 9:91
Yu M, Nebbitt VE, Lombe M, Pitner RO, Salas-Wright CP (2012) Understanding tobacco use among urban African American adolescents living in public housing communities: a test of problem behavior theory. Addict Behav 37:978–981
Zhang J, Jiang Y, Sasaki K, Tsubouchi M, Matsushita T, Kawai T, Fujiwara A (2014) A GPS-enabled smart phone app with simplified diagnosis functions of driving safety and warning information provision. In: Proceedings of the 21st world congress of intelligent transport systems. Detroit, USA, 7–11 Sept 2014

Chapter 12
Adaptation of Behavior to Overcome Natural Disasters

Qing Chang Lu, Junyi Zhang, Lingling Wu and A.B.M. Sertajur Rahman

Abstract This chapter deals with how people adapt their lives to natural disasters, such as flood, cyclone, extreme weather events, earthquake, and sea level rise. With the changing global climate, the disasters would appear more frequently and seriously. However, it is still uncertain where the disasters will occur nearby personal daily activity areas, and how great the impacts on human life will be. Surprisingly, literature review suggests that relevant studies are very limited, especially in the context of developing countries. Targeting Bangladesh, one of the most vulnerable countries in the world to climate and the sixth most vulnerable to floods, this chapter describes three case studies on people's adaptation behaviors under the impacts of different flooding and cyclone scenarios in future by focusing on intercity travel behavior, job and residential location choice behavior, and tourism behavior respectively. Various findings are derived, which are useful to help identify the barriers to the adoption of adaptation measures, the roles of different stakeholders in implementing adaptation measures, and the directions of adaptation measures in the future.

Keywords Climate-related disasters · Flood · Cyclone · Bangladesh · Adaptation behavior · Residential behavior · Intercity travel · Tourism behavior · Stated preference survey · Discrete choice models

---

Q.C. Lu (✉)
Shanghai Jiao Tong University, Shanghai, China
e-mail: qclu@sjtu.edu.cn

J. Zhang
Hiroshima University, Higashi-Hiroshima, Japan

L. Wu
Institution for Transport Policy Studies, Tokyo, Japan

A.B.M. Sertajur Rahman
Roads and Highways Department, Dhaka, Bangladesh

J. Zhang (ed.), *Life-Oriented Behavioral Research for Urban Policy*,
DOI 10.1007/978-4-431-56472-0_12

12.1 Natural Disasters and Adaptation Behavior

There has been an increasing trend in the number of natural disasters over recent years. Climate-related disasters are the most common disaster events, and they have long affected human lives in various ways (Begum et al. 2014). The National Research Council (2008) has identified five types of climate-related disasters: very hot days and heat waves, increases in arctic temperature, rising sea levels, intense precipitation, and extreme hurricanes. These disasters are predicted to appear more frequently and to become more severe this century. According to Peterson et al. (2008), there is a greater than 90 % probability that more intense, longer, and more frequent periods of extreme heat and heat waves will occur in the United States. The IPCC (2007) has predicted that arctic warming and rising sea levels at the global level are virtually certain with a probability of greater than 99 %; more intense and frequent precipitation events will occur in the United States with over 90 % probability, and more intense tropical storms are likely (with over 66 % probability) around the globe in the next century. These climate-related disasters may increase the vulnerability of many societies and communities worldwide, especially those that are already vulnerable (UNDP 2011). To address such vulnerability issues, both disaster risk management (disaster risk reduction and disaster management) and climate change adaptation are required to make individuals, communities, and societies more resilient and less vulnerable to disasters (GAR 2011; Field et al. 2012; Johansson et al. 2013). There is connection between disaster risk management and climate change adaptation; however, this chapter only focuses on climate change adaptation.

The IPCC (2007) defines climate change adaptation as "adjustment in natural or human systems in response to actual or expected climatic stimuli or their effects, which moderates harm or exploits beneficial opportunities" (p. 750). At the individual/household level, agriculturalists may adapt various practices through techniques such as agronomic management, crop intensification, increasing food production based on suitable environmental conservation techniques, and water resource exploitation (Oluoko-Odingo 2011; Habiba et al. 2012). After a natural disaster, fish farmers may temporarily suspend fishing activities to help recover fishery resources and ecosystems, and/or transfer their aquaculture cages from high-risk areas to waters unaffected by the disaster (Chang et al. 2013). Households may migrate to other places (Klaiber 2014), elevate their ground floors to avoid exposure to water and change their travel modes (Ling et al. 2015), secure food and income (Nguyen and James 2013), enhance their adaptation ability through education and employment and with the support of social capital (Ding et al. 2014), and so on. Through such adaptations, people attempt to alleviate or avoid the negative impacts of climate-related disasters.

From a policy-making perspective, adaptations to climate-related disasters include responses in operations, design, planning, investment, and land use control (Transportation Research Board 2008). It is of great importance to understand people's behavior in adapting to disasters associated with climate change.

Government policies, investments, construction, shelters, and other measures should assist people to adapt to the impacts of climate-related disasters. However, the mismatch between people's needs/behavior and adaptation measures in practice could result in ineffective and failed responses to disasters. For example, people may have different preferences and make dissimilar decisions concerning residential relocation in response to disasters of varying types and intensity. Governments should be aware of these behavioral differences, propose population migration policies, and plan shelters accordingly. Another example is the adaptation of daily travel to disasters. Transportation infrastructure and travel activities are especially exposed to climate-related disasters and people's travel behavior may differ according to types of natural disasters and their impacts on transportation infrastructure. As a result, the planning, design, and construction of transportation infrastructure, as well as traffic management, should include behavioral responses so that such adaptation is more effective. Another important form of behavior that is easily affected by climate-related disasters is tourism. Tourists may simply cancel trips to an affected destination and go somewhere else; however, in this case, the affected destination will suffer from a serious reduction in tourism revenue, which may worsen the adaptation of the region to disasters. Tourists may delay visits, but this affects the planning and management of tourist destinations.

The purpose of this chapter is to understand how people will respond to future climate-related disasters. We focus on three types of adaptation behavior in the context of Bangladesh: (1) intercity travel, (2) residential relocation and job changes, and (3) tourism.

12.2 Case Study Area: Bangladesh

Bangladesh is one of the most vulnerable countries in the world to climate, and the sixth most vulnerable to floods based on the number of deaths per 100,000 people exposed to cyclones or floods (UNDP 2004). Floods, tropical cyclones, storm surges, and droughts are likely to become more frequent and severe in the coming years. Bangladesh's high vulnerability to climate change is due to a number of hydrogeological and socioeconomic factors, which include: (a) geographical location in South Asia; (b) flat deltaic topography with very low elevation; (c) extreme climate variability, governed by monsoons, which results in acute differences in water distribution over space and time; (d) high population density and poverty incidence; and (e) the dependence of the majority of its population on crop agriculture, which is strongly influenced by climate variability and change (Ahsan 2006). Most parts of Bangladesh are located on the delta of three of the largest rivers in the world. The flood plains of its three large rivers cover about 80 % of the country's land, while 25 % is flooded every year (Alam et al. 2002). Only 10 % of Bangladesh is one meter or more above the global mean sea level and one-third is under tidal influence (Karim and Mimura 2008). It is susceptible to river and rainwater flooding, and in lower lying coastal areas, to tidal flooding during storms. The most common water-related and climate-induced natural disasters on a deltaic floodplain such as those in Bangladesh are caused by floods. On average 6000 people die from flooding and storms each year (Schiermeier 2014). Flooding in Bangladesh is a result of a complex series of factors. These include a huge inflow of water from upstream catchment areas coinciding with heavy monsoon rainfall in the country, a low floodplain gradient, congested drainage channels, the convergence of major rivers inside Bangladesh, tide and storm surges in coastal areas, and polders that increase the intensity of floods outside protected areas. Different combinations of these factors give rise to different types of flooding. The most recent exceptional flood in 2007 inundated 62,300 km^2 of land (42 % of the total area) and caused severe damage to lives and property, and the most serious mega flood occurred in 1998, causing nearly 70 % of land to be inundated (Dasgupta et al. 2010). The impacts of sea level rise (SLR) are also serious. There are approximately 31 million people living along the coastal area, and it is estimated that about half of the population lives within the risk area.[1]

As shown in Fig. 12.1, it is predicted that the average SLR in Bangladesh in the future will be 1.8 meters in 2050 and 2.0 m in 2080 (Lee[2] 2013). Note that both global warming and storm surges were incorporated into the prediction. Based on the predicted sea levels, it is further predicted that 60.61 and 62.86 % of roads along the coastal area will be affected in 2050 and 2080, respectively, and the corresponding percentages for the whole country will be 23.48 and 24.35 %, respectively. Thus, the impacts of disasters resulting from climate change in Bangladesh are huge, and will become even worse in the future.

Mahmud and Prowse (2012) investigated the impacts of cyclone Aila in 2009 in Kulna, Bangladesh, and estimated that 99 % of households suffered losses. Nelson (2003) assessed the environmental health impact of floods, SLR, storm surges, and cyclones in Bangladesh caused by global climate change using the disability-adjusted life-year method, and found that children and young people are particularly vulnerable to its health impacts. To understand future SLR impacts in western Bangladesh, Karim and Mimura (2008) created eight flooding scenarios, identified the high-risk areas, and estimated the number of additional shelters needed to accommodate the affected people. In Bangladesh, the government has constructed a large number of refugee shelters and embankments in coastal areas, while the early warning system needs further improvement and more shelters are required for people at risk (Karim and Mimura 2008). Mahmud and Prowse (2012) investigated the adaptation measures taken in Bangladesh before and after cyclone Aila and concluded that predisaster interventions such as early

[1]See http://www.cegisbd.com/.

[2]Dr. Lee was a collaborating researcher on an interdisciplinary research project led by the second author, supported by the Global Environmental Leaders (GELs) Education Program for Designing a Low-Carbon World, MEXT Special Coordination Funds for Promotion of Science and Technology, from October 2008 to September 2012. He made this prediction during that project.

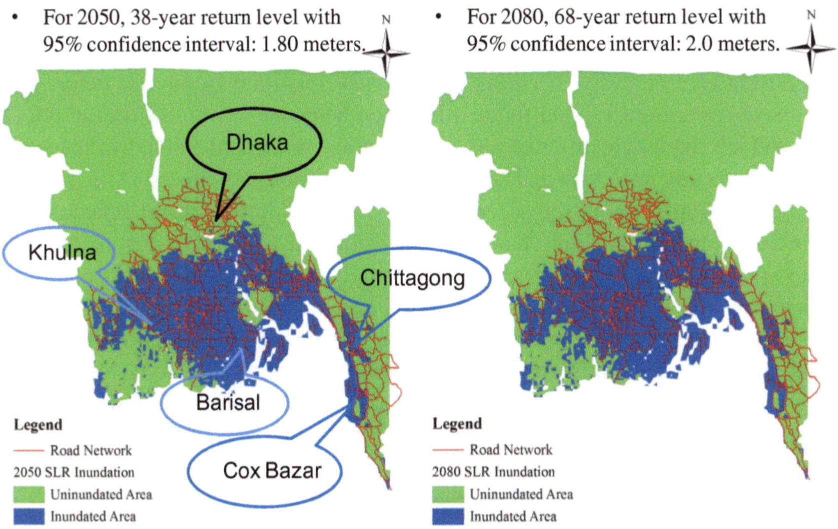

SLR impacts on road infrastructure of the costal areas

Scenarios	Affected Road Segments	Total Length (Km)	Total Study Area Road Length (Km)	Percentage (%)
1.8 m (2050)	1935	4745.02	7828.47	60.61
2.0 m (2080)	2007	4920.97	7828.47	62.86

SLR impacts on road infrastructure of the whole country

Scenarios	Affected Road Segments	Total Length (Km)	Total National Road Length (Km)	Percentage (%)
1.8 m (2050)	1935	4745.02	20205.96	23.48
2.0 m (2080)	2007	4920.97	20205.96	24.35

Fig. 12.1 Predicted sea level rise (=global warming + storm surge) in future Bangladesh

warning systems and disaster preparedness training gave better results than post-disaster relief. Because of climate-related disasters in Bangladesh, transportation networks are frequently interdicted, creating barriers to economic activities and having huge impacts on people's daily lives. Ecosystems (e.g., wetlands, forests, and coastal areas) could also be seriously influenced by climate disasters. From a long-term perspective, mitigation measures in both Bangladesh and other countries around the world are definitely required, but these appear to be difficult to achieve. Accordingly, adaptation measures should be given a higher priority in the medium and short term.

In this study from the end of January to the beginning of March 2013, we conducted two questionnaire surveys with respect to adaptation to future climate-related disasters in inland and coastal areas of Bangladesh. The first survey concerns travel behavior, residential relocation, and job changes, while the second survey investigates tourist behavior. Both surveys concern floods and cyclones as climate-related disasters.

In the first survey, question items include people's experiences and understanding of climate disasters, predisaster adaptive behavior, responses during disasters, and postdisaster recovery. It covers barriers and important factors for behavior in the above circumstances, and future adaptation behavior (travel, residential relocation, and job change) in different disaster scenarios, household and individual attributes, and other factors. Approximately 1000 respondents participated in the survey.

The question items in the second survey include tourists' travel schedules for their current trip to Bangladesh and their subjective evaluation of destinations visited (when they were interviewed), adaptation to previous climate disasters, travel experiences during the previous year, stated preferences regarding their responses as visitors to Bangladesh to various flood and cyclone scenarios, as well as information such as their individual and household characteristics. As a result, 1000 valid questionnaires were obtained. It was observed that 64.3 % of the respondents were male, of whom three-quarters were under 40 years old, almost half were international tourists, and about two-thirds were traveling with family or friends.

Detailed explanations of the above surveys are provided in Sects. 3 and 4.

12.3 Literature Review

Because of differences in individual characteristics such as knowledge, education, income, and government policies, people's choices in adapting to disasters resulting from global climate change also differ. Patt and Schoter (2008) found that people rarely choose evacuation and resettlement to adapt to floods because of their perceptions of climate change. Artur and Hilhorst (2012) analyzed the adaptation measures adopted by people in the flood-prone areas of Mozambique, and pointed out that people's adaptive strategies, ranging from flood-proofing houses to everyday behavior such as investment strategies, are much more diverse than those mentioned by Osbahr et al. (2008). Sahin and Mohamed (2013) consulted three types of stakeholders. Residents preferred improved building design and protective structures, politicians favored improved building design and resettlement, and the experts believed that improved building design and public awareness were the best choices.

Various factors affect individual choices concerning adaptation to climate change disasters. Adger et al. (2003) stated that adaptation to climate change was a function of individuals' access to resources, and that access to information played an important role in choosing resources (Phillips 2003). A stronger perception of climate change risks prompts stronger responses to adapt to climate change (Barnett and Adger 2003; Hess et al. 2008). Adaptation is also affected by psychological factors such as ambiguity aversion (fear) and ambiguity seeking (hope) (Viscusi and Chesson 1999). Grothman and Patt (2005) focused on the psychological factors of people's risk perceptions and perceived adaptive capacity as the main factors influencing individuals' adaptation choices, and showed the importance of sociocognitive factors in adaptation behavior. Other factors, such as personal experience, values, morals, and culture also play important roles in adaptation choices, including those of experts and decision makers (Sundblad et al. 2007). Adaptation responses entail people adjusting their behavior to cope more effectively with the impacts of climate change disasters (Mozumder et al. 2011). Jin and Francisco (2013) found that people as well as local governments in the Zhejiang coastal area of China have little knowledge about SLR and adaptation strategies, and that their knowledge increases and attitudes change significantly when they are provided with information brochures.

12.3.1 Analysis of Intercity Travel Behavior Associated with Climate-Related Disasters

Travelers are completely exposed to the weather and disasters during extreme weather events. During adverse or serious weather events, people adjust their travel plans to avoid or alleviate the impacts. Travel plans may be canceled or changed, and travel may be delayed. It is important to understand changes in travel behavior caused by climate change because transportation network performance depends largely on responses to traffic conditions (Khattak and Palma 1997; Lu and Peng 2011; Lu et al. 2012). Travel behavior analysis under adverse weather conditions attracts the most attention from the literature reviewed for this study. Khattak and Palma (1997) reported that half of the automobile travelers among their respondents changed their travel patterns under adverse weather conditions in Brussels, Belgium, and observed that bad weather had a stronger influence on departure time than did route and mode changes. Heavy rain was found to reduce traffic volume in Melbourne, Australia by 2–3 % (Keay and Simmonds 2005), and the impacts of weather on travel demand have also been noted in other studies (e.g., Van et al. 2006). Moreover, weather information was found to change the behavior of travelers in Flanders, Belgium significantly (Cools and Creemers 2013), and these changes depended greatly on trip purpose (Cools et al. 2010). A study in Toronto, Canada confirmed the significant impact of weather on mode of travel, especially walking and cycling among younger travelers (Saneinejad et al. 2012). Ahmed et al. (2013) found that weather conditions are a paramount factor in decisions made about cycling in Victoria, Australia. Evidence was also found for a correlation between climate change and choice of transport and distance traveled in the metropolitan Randstad region of the Netherlands. Switching from open-air modes of travel such as cycling and walking to alternatives such as private cars and mass transit rail is an especially common effect of climate change (Böcker et al. 2013b). There is little doubt that people's travel behavior is affected by climate change, and daily travel behavior is changed accordingly.

However, it is agreed that because of the diversity of climate change regimes and culture/habituation in different countries, travel behavior in response to climate change differs between regions (Khattak and de Palma 1997; Böcker et al. 2013b; Cools and Creemers 2013). As shown above, adaptation of travel behavior to climate change is mainly researched in developed countries. As a global threat, climate change poses the same or even greater risks on developing countries, and the capacity of those countries to adapt may be much lower than that of developed countries because of poor transportation planning and infrastructure as well as their developing economies (Lu et al. 2014). Thus, understanding travel responses to climate change in developing countries may be as important as it is in developed countries or even more so. Furthermore, even in the same country, people in coastal areas may respond to climate change events such as intense storm surges, hurricanes, and SLR in a different way to those in inland regions. In addition, almost all the literature reviewed addresses the behavioral adaptation of intracity travel, emphasizing the use of private cars, buses, bicycles, and walking (Aultman-Hall et al. 2009; Elieas et al. 2013); changes in intercity travel receive less attention. Moreover, intercity travel differs from intracity travel in terms of distance, purpose, and alternative routes (that is, there are fewer redundant travel routes in intercity than in intracity travel), and intercity transportation infrastructure may have greater exposure to climate change because there are fewer buildings and shelters (Böcker et al. 2013a). These all make travel behavior under conditions of climate change different from intracity travel.

12.3.2 Analysis of Life Adaptation to Climate-Related Disasters

In recent years, changes of residence and job location have attracted scholars' attention, especially in connection with changes in the environment. Mortreux and Barnett (2009) divided the factors influencing residence or job location choice into three groups: factors at the point of origin including the environment, the economy, or government policies; factors at the destination involving social networks, the economy, or government policies; and intervening obstacles such as distance or institutional constraints. From an agent-based simulation model, Kniveton et al. (2011) found that the migration or change in residential location is obviously affected by the environment, that is, whether it is dry or wet. They also suggested that the impact of rainfall on choice of location is expressed via its influence on other drivers such as employment opportunities, access to natural resources, national policies and incentives, ecological vulnerability, political instability, and infrastructure. Joarder and Miller (2013) discussed four groups of factors that affect temporary and permanent migration as a result of environmental change, and found that more factors have significant effects on temporary migration than on decisions concerning permanent migration. After a review of empirical research on migration and climate change, Klaiber (2014) confirmed that household relocation arises because of changes in economic opportunities and climate amenities resulting from climate change. Saldana-Zorrilla and Sandberg (2009) found that declining income, better education, and an increasing number of natural disasters led to higher levels of out-migration in response to climate-related disasters in Mexico. On the basis of evidence from two communities in Canada, Wolf et al.

(2013) argued that values such as tradition, freedom, harmony, safety, and unity shape different interpretations of climate change impacts, and as a result lead to distinct adaptation decisions, including migration or relocation. Transportation between residence and job location is an important factor in residence or job location choice. In transportation studies, residence or job location choice are usually addressed in terms of factors such as their relationship with public transport accessibility, travel costs, travel modes, traffic congestion, and departure times (Arentze and Timmermans 2007; Nurlaela and Curtis 2012). However, in reality, decisions to change residence or job location depend on many other socioeconomic factors, such as personal or family attributes and government policies. For example, the balance of residence and job location choices is found to be associated with the population patterns of cities and traditional residence and job location policies (Wang and Chai 2009; Loo and Chow 2011). The influences of physiological factors and gender on residence location choice have also been investigated in the literature (Sermons and Koppelman 2001; Choocharukul et al. 2008). Other studies have investigated many other factors or reasons, and have identified factors such as lack of education, strong attachments to land, age, family size, and the availability of transport infrastructure (Mortreux and Barnett 2009; Doevenspeck 2011; Gray 2011). It could be concluded that although factors that influence decisions to change residence or job location may vary between studies or countries, there is little doubt that people's relocation behavior is associated with climate change.

Most of the above literature focuses on household or residence location choice in response to climate change. However, people may consider changing job location first and residence location thereafter because it is more difficult to move families. There is a consensus that because of the diversity of climate change regimes and culture/habituation in different countries, people's location choice behavior under conditions of climate change may differ (Cools et al. 2010; Böcker 2013a, b). Thus, understanding such choices in different countries is necessary, especially those of developing and vulnerable countries. Given the uncertainties of climate change, people's residence and job location change choice decisions may vary according to different climate change scenarios or in response to events such as rain, river or coastal flooding, and cyclones. All these issues should be addressed with detailed investigations of people's preferences for location choices in various climate change and impact scenarios.

To address the above research gaps, we aim to identify factors that explain the connected choices of residence and job location, including personal and family socioeconomic factors and previous experiences in Bangladesh.

12.3.3 Adaptive Behavior of Tourists Associated with Climate-Related Disasters

The World Tourism Organization (2003) has identified extreme weather events resulting from climate change as a critical threat to tourism, especially in coastal regions and developing countries. Damage to destination infrastructure and ecosystems has a devastating impact on tourism demand and may ultimately influence the long-term sustainability of tourism destinations (Gómez Martín 2005; Nicholls 2006).

With regard to the influence of extreme weather events on tourist behavior, most of the existing studies have focused on risks perceived by tourists. Some researchers have found that the perceived influence of travel risks resulting from climate change varies among tourists according to their sociodemographic variables (Lepp and Gibson 2003; Park and Reisinger 2010; Gössling et al. 2012). For instance, some studies show that older people are more sensitive to the risk of weather extremes than younger people (Moreno 2010). Perceptions of weather risks during travel were found to differ according to family status, with single tourists far more resilient to weather than families with children (Limb and Spellman 2001). A study conducted by Denstadli et al. (2011) revealed that foreign tourists perceived the risks from weather conditions to be higher than domestic tourists did. In addition, some external factors have been found to influence tourists' risk perceptions. For example, media coverage of extreme weather events can create a negative image of a destination (Gómez Martín 2005; Perry 2006).

However, tourists' actual and potential response to the impacts of extreme weather events is still an under-researched area (Gössling and Hall 2006; Eugenio-Martin and Campos-Soria 2010; Moore 2010). With increases in the frequency and intensity of extreme weather events (floods, cyclones, droughts, etc.) in recent years, the importance of understanding the impacts of extreme weather events on tourist behavior in policy decisions on future risk management in the development of the tourism industry has been recognized (Law 2006; Gössling et al. 2012). Therefore, this study aims to fill the gap by investigating the adaptation of tourist behavior to climate disasters in the context of Bangladesh.

12.4 Residents' Adaptation Behavior in Bangladesh: Survey

Focusing on climate-related disasters in Bangladesh, we attempt to clarify how people adapted in the past and will adapt in the future to the effects of such disasters. For this purpose, we designed a questionnaire survey that covers people's experiences and understanding of climate disasters, predisaster adaptive behavior, response behavior during disasters, postdisaster recovery behavior, barriers to and important factors in the above behavior, and future adaptive behavior in different disaster scenarios, as well as variables such as household and individual attributes. We administered the survey to residents in the coastal and inland areas in January and February 2013.

12.4.1 Survey Design and Implementation

Here, the term "climate-related disasters" refers to floods, cyclones, storm surges, SLR, tornados, droughts, and other events. The following items are included in the questionnaire survey.

(1) Experience of climate-related disasters: impacts of flood, cyclone, and tornado experienced in the past; number of injured family members, average monetary loss in terms of livestock, housing, farmland, crops, and other property; depth, duration and date of the most serious river flood, rainfall flood, and SLR; frequency that house and land were affected by floods or cyclones, and the average cost of damage on each occasion.
(2) Understanding of climate-related disasters: perception of negative impacts of disasters on quality of life, and perception of frequency and seriousness of disasters in recent years.
(3) Adaptation of behavior to damage.

- Predisaster adaptation behavior.
  - Concern about future risks of disasters to family, house, property, etc.
  - Response measures to the potential risks of disasters: (1) do not prepare, (2) elevate the house, (3) strengthen the house, (4) protect the house using walls, dikes, or similar structure, (5) move to a cyclone/flood shelter, (6) move family, livestock, and property to a safe place, and return after the flood/cyclone, (7) consider a permanent move to a safe place, (8) consult experienced people, and (9) take other measures.
  - Confidence in preparation.
  - Cost of preparation.

- Adaptation during disasters (with respect to the most serious disasters).
  - Measures adopted in addition to those above.
  - Places to move in the case of measures (6) or (7) above: homes of relatives or friends/colleagues, the roadside, a place provided by the government, or another place.
  - A source of disaster information: newspapers, cellphone, radio, TV, Internet, or other sources.
  - Information providers: government, community, neighborhood, own experience, etc.
  - The timing of information: when disaster information is received.
  - Means of evacuation: walking, carts, ox carts, bicycles, rickshaws, and/or motorized vehicles.
  - Help from the government, community, and neighborhood: rescue, food, tents, quilts, clean water, money, and shelter, or no help was received.

  - Help offered to the neighborhood: rescue, food, tents and quilts, clean water, money, or shelter, or no help was offered.
  - Cost of responses during a disaster.

– Predisaster adaptation behavior.

  - Concern about future risks of disasters to family, house, property, etc.
  - Response measures to the potential risks of disasters: (1) do not prepare, (2) elevate the house, (3) strengthen the house, (4) protect the house using walls, dikes, or similar structure, (5) move to a cyclone/flood shelter, (6) move family, livestock, and property to a safe place, and return after the flood/cyclone, (7) consider a permanent move to a safe place, (8) consult experienced people, and (9) take other measures.
  - Confidence in preparation.
  - Cost of preparation.

(4) Satisfaction with the measures before, during, and after a flood inundation, cyclone, SLR, sea water intrusion, drought, tornado, or other events (if they had had no such experience, respondents did not need to answer).
(5) The relative importance of predisaster preparation, responses during a disaster, and postdisaster recovery.
(6) The greatest difficulties in adapting to the impacts of disasters: lack of money, lack of knowledge, lack of government policy, lack of help from the government, lack of help from the community, lack of help from the neighborhood, etc.
(7) The relative importance of the roles of government, community, neighborhood, and self-help throughout the process of resisting disasters.
(8) Priority levels of the following measures for different stakeholders (government, community, and neighborhood): predisaster measures (building dikes/seawalls, elevated roads, or shelters, elevating houses, or establishing an early warning system), responses during a disaster (reinforcing houses, evacuation assistance, moving to safe places, sourcing quilts and groceries, medical care, or money), and postdisaster actions (repairing houses, finding vacant land for relocation, finding jobs in the city, or finding jobs abroad).
(9) Future plans to adapt to natural disasters.

  – Possible adaptation choices: (1) do not prepare, (2) elevate the house, (3) strengthen the house, (4) protect the house using walls, dikes, or similar, (5) move to a cyclone/flood shelter, (6) move family, livestock, and property to a safe place, and return after the flood/cyclone, (7) consider a permanent move to a safe place, (8) consult experienced people, etc.
  – Estimation of the impact of disasters when constructing or retrofitting houses.
  – Estimation of the potential impact of disasters when choosing a new job.
  – Important factors affecting the choice of adaptation measures: cost, effectiveness, ease of implementation, level of risk, previous experience, etc.

– Willingness to accept compensation from the government if it could not properly protect the respondents' house, land, and/or work from disasters.

(10) Stated adaptation behaviors in various flood or cyclone scenarios with respect to intercity travel and life choices: 16 scenarios were designed for floods or cyclones, based on a stated preference (SP) survey. Each respondent was asked to report their adaptation choices with respect to both floods and cyclones, each with four scenarios. In other words, the above 16 scenarios were divided into four groups to reduce the burden on respondents. For detailed descriptions, refer to Sect. 5.

We administered the survey to residents living in the coastal and inland areas of Bangladesh from the end of January to the beginning of March 2013. In the SP survey, future scenarios of disasters are assumed with respect to floods and cyclones separately, based on an orthogonal experiment, where SP attributes include frequency and intensity of floods and cyclones, and four attributes describing flood/cyclone impacts (inundation, damage to residential areas, damages to roads, and salinity intrusion). Note that salinity intrusion is only introduced into the coastal scenarios. In total, 16 SP profiles are derived. To reduce the answering burden, each respondent was randomly assigned four SP profiles. These attributes and their levels were assumed based on historical data in Bangladesh. Under each scenario, every respondent was requested to choose one out of six choices: Choice 1 (do not change job, do not change residential location, and do not reinforce the house), Choice 2 (do not change job, do not change residential location, but reinforce the house), Choice 3 (change job, do not change residential location, and do not reinforce the house), Choice 4 (change job, do not change residential location, but reinforce the house), Choice 5 (do not change job, but change residential location), Choice 6 (change job and change residential location). A total of 998 respondents participated in the survey.

There were three survey teams. Each team consisted of one supervisor and several interviewers who conducted the survey in various parts of Bangladesh. Each survey team had one local interpreter to avoid communication difficulties in the local language. We conducted the survey in the following 14 districts, which are frequently affected by cyclone and flood disasters: Chittagong, Cox's Bazar, Khulna, Bagerhat, Satkhira, Barisal, Noakhali, Faridpur, Patuakhali, Bhola, Jessore, Bogra, Gaibandha, and Sirajgonj (see Fig. 12.2).

Most cities are located in the central southern area, along the east coast and its largest river, which are the country's low-lying areas. The nine coastal cities lie on the central eastern coast; they include Chittagong, the nation's second biggest city, and Cox's Bazar, a tourism city. The western coastal region is a mangrove area, and no city in that area was included. The five inland cities include three in the eastern part of the country, one in the north, and one in the west.

Because many of the respondents could not read and/or write, we decided to ask interviewers to interview respondents and fill in the questionnaire forms themselves instead of asking respondents to do so. The respondents were given gifts in the form of food/clothing in return for their time on the survey. For difficult

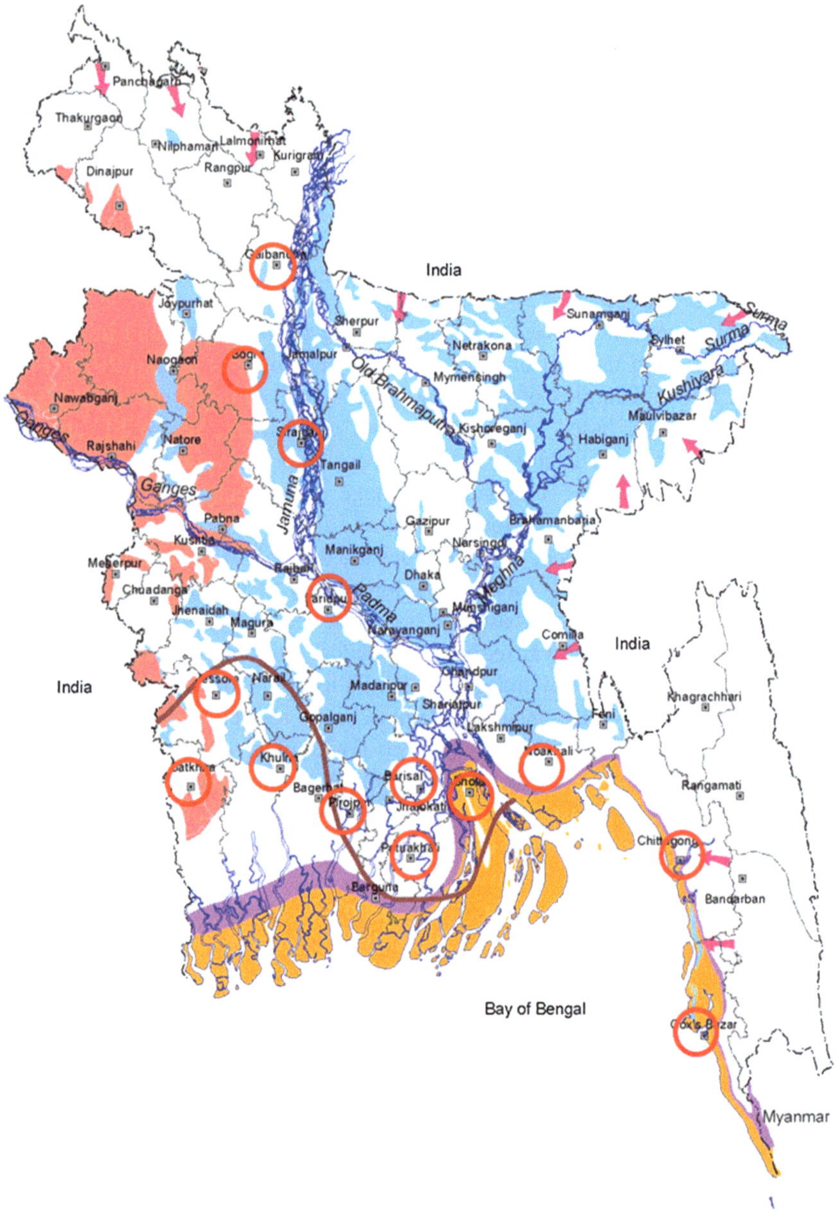

Fig. 12.2 Distribution of survey areas in disaster-prone regions in Bangladesh

questions (e.g., the SP parts, or those on perceptions and capability), the questions were first explained with examples before the respondents answered.

Profiles of respondents and their households are shown in Fig. 12.3. As for the respondents' ages, 27 % were in their 20s, 32 % were in their 30s, and 22 % were

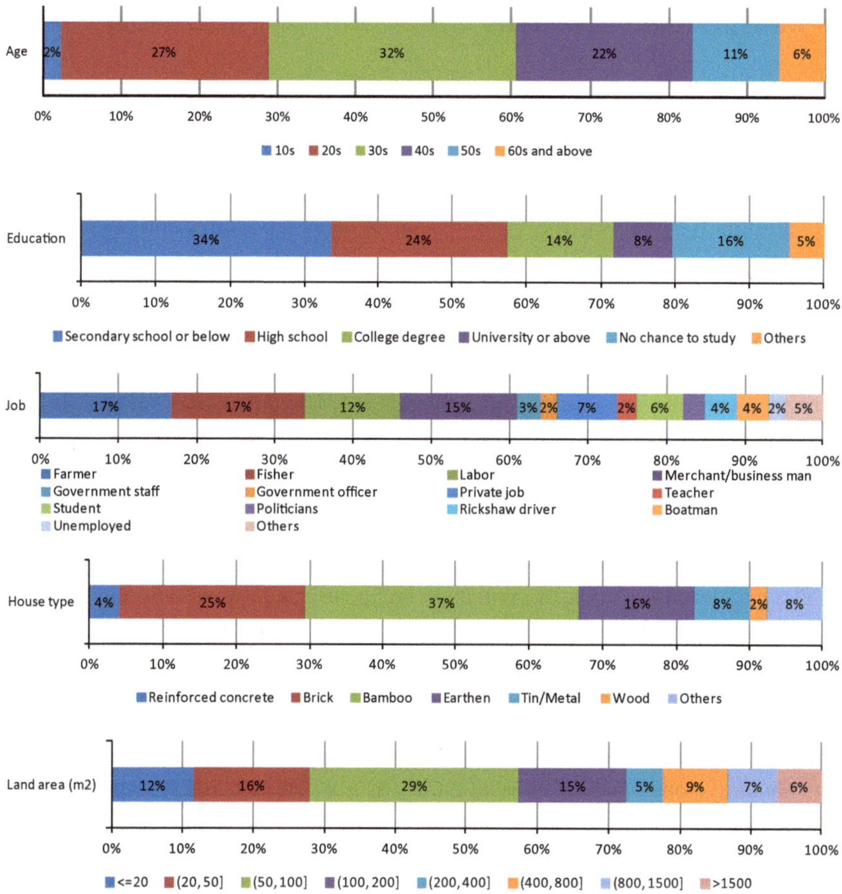

Fig. 12.3 Profiles of respondents and their households

in their 40s. The largest group of respondents were those with secondary school education or less (34 %), and 16 % had had no opportunity to study. High school graduates were the second largest group of respondents (24 %). Those who had graduate or postgraduate education accounted for just 22 %. Concerning occupation, farmers and fishers each accounted for 17 %; 12 % were laborers, 15 % were merchants and businessmen, 4 % were rickshaw drivers, and only 5 % of respondents worked in government offices. Among the respondents, 37 % lived in bamboo houses (the largest group), 25 % in brick houses, and 16 % in earthen houses. Only 4 % of respondents lived in reinforced concrete houses. Among the respondents, 28 % had a piece of land of no more than 50 m^2 in area. Respondents with between 50 and 100 m^2 of land were the largest group, and 22 % of respondents owned more than 400 m^2 of land.

12.4.2 Aggregation Analysis

We start with an analysis of people's understanding and experience of natural disasters, and then explore how people prepared for and adapted to natural disasters in the past. After that, we examine how people intend to adapt to future natural disasters in different scenarios. Here we aim to identify the barriers to adaptation measures in Bangladesh, the roles of stakeholders in implementing adaptation measures, and future directions for adaptation measures.

Experiences and Understanding of Climate Change Disasters

The numbers of people injured by floods, cyclones, and tornados in the past are shown in Fig. 12.4. Floods and tornados injured similar numbers of people: 8 % of respondents had one injured family member, 4 % had two, and 1 % had three or more family members who had suffered injury.

Regarding damages to property caused by floods, cyclones, and tornados, respectively, (1) 47, 62, and 15 % of households suffered loss of livestock; (2) 53, 73, and 22 % of households suffered damage to their houses, and (3) 44, 57, and 13 % of households suffered from farmland and crop damage.

The incidences of houses and land being affected by floods and cyclones are shown in Fig. 12.5. We found that only 2–3 % of respondents had not been affected frequently by floods and cyclones, and 47 % were affected by floods and 41 % by cyclones at least once a year. Even though cyclones do not occur every year, a large number of respondents still report damage. This surely indicates the seriousness of water disasters, but at the same time, it suggests misunderstandings about cyclones. As for impacts on life as a whole, we asked respondents "to what extent do you think disasters negatively affect your quality of life, including daily travel?" (see Fig. 12.6). Almost all the coastal people endure the impacts of disasters, and more than 80 % of them are at least seriously affected. This is different from the answers of the inland people, of whom only half report more serious effects, and more than 20 % report that their quality of life is not affected at all. More than three times the number of respondents in the coastal area report negative effects than in the inland area. As a result, there are obvious differences between coastal and inland areas in the answers to the first question. As for future

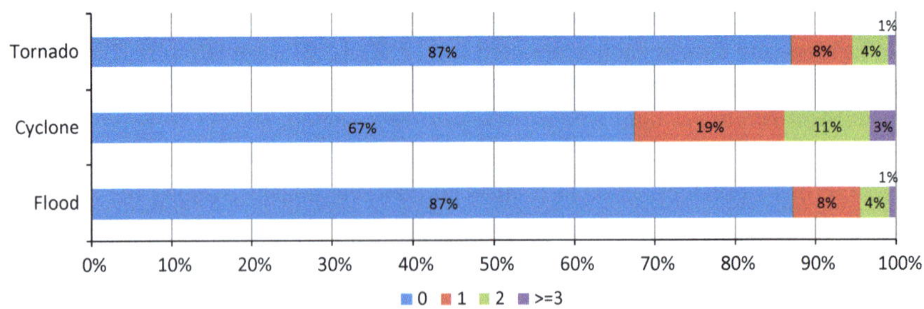

Fig. 12.4 Numbers of injured people caused by flood, cyclone, and tornado in the past

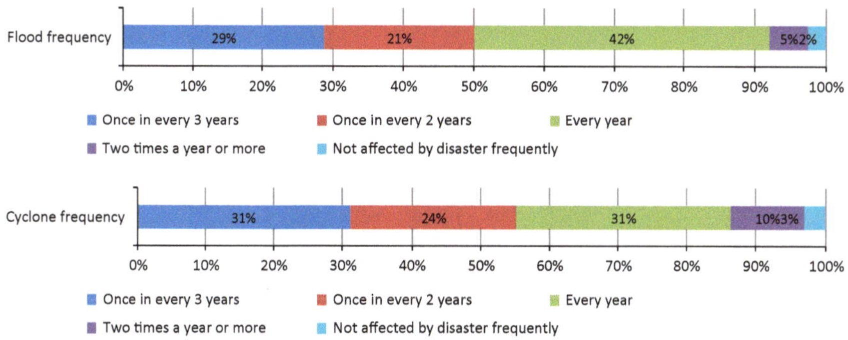

Fig. 12.5 Frequencies that houses and land are affected by flood and cyclone

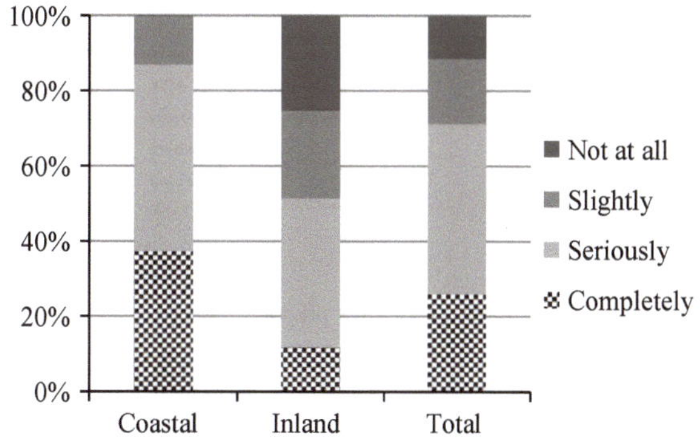

Fig. 12.6 Flood impacts on people's quality of life

impacts, we asked one further question: "Do you think that climate-related disasters have become more frequent and severe in recent years?" (Fig. 12.7). More than 60 % of people believed that disasters were becoming more frequent and severe in both areas, and this percentage was slightly higher in the inland areas than in the coastal area. However, fewer people on the coast are sure about their responses, whereas a higher percentage of people gave a negative answer in the inland area. This indicates that the climate varies much more on the coast than in the inland area, and the inland people are more sensitive to climate change and accept the reality of more frequent and serious disasters in recent years. Comparing the answers of coastal and inland people, we find more differences in Fig. 12.6 than in Fig. 12.7. A general conclusion drawn from the above results is that most people are affected by disasters related to climate change and believe the impacts are more serious in the coastal areas than in the inland areas of Bangladesh.

Adaptation Measures

Adaptation measures taken before disasters are shown in Fig. 12.8. It is found that more than 30 % of respondents did not prepare for climate disasters. Of those who

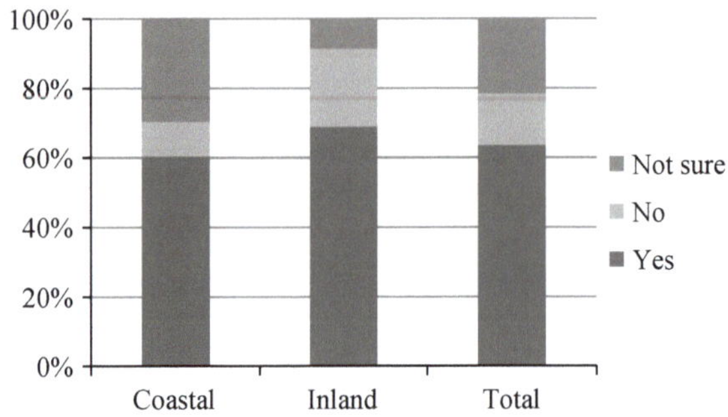

Fig. 12.7 People's attitude towards climate change

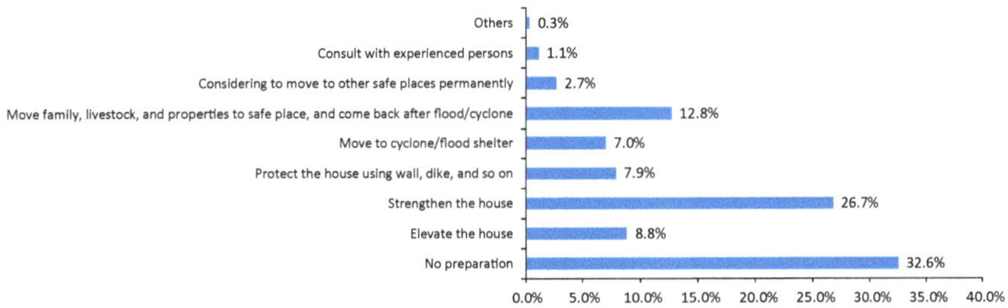

Fig. 12.8 Adaptation measures prepared before disasters

did, 26.7 % strengthened their houses; 12.8 % moved their families, livestock, and property to safe places and returned after a disaster; 8.8 % elevated their houses; and 7.9 % protected their houses using walls, dikes, and similar measures.

Unlike the measures taken before disasters, 32.6 % of respondents, which is the largest proportion, moved their families, livestock, and property to safe places and returned after a disaster; 15.1 % moved to cyclone/flood shelters; and 27.9 % strengthened their houses and remained there (14.2 %), protecting their houses using walls, dikes, and similar measures (8.8 %), or elevating their houses (4.9 %). These percentage values are shown in Fig. 12.9. As for the means of evacuation during disasters (see Fig. 12.10), 64.5 % of respondents evacuated on foot; only 7.6 % used motorized vehicles, and others used very slow travel modes including carts (4.2 %), cattle (4.2 %), bicycles (5.3 %), and rickshaws (14.3 %). Figure 12.11 shows help received and offered during disasters. It is observed that 21.0, 35.1, and 70.9 % of respondents did not receive any help from the government, the community, and the neighborhood. It is also revealed that 79.0 % provided no help to their neighbors. Nearly 40 % of respondents received food, but only 22.4 % received it from the community. As for clean water, 23.4 and 22.5 % of respondents received clean water from the government and communities, respectively. Mutual help within neighborhoods was not popular in the sense that only a very low percentage of respondents received help from and provided help

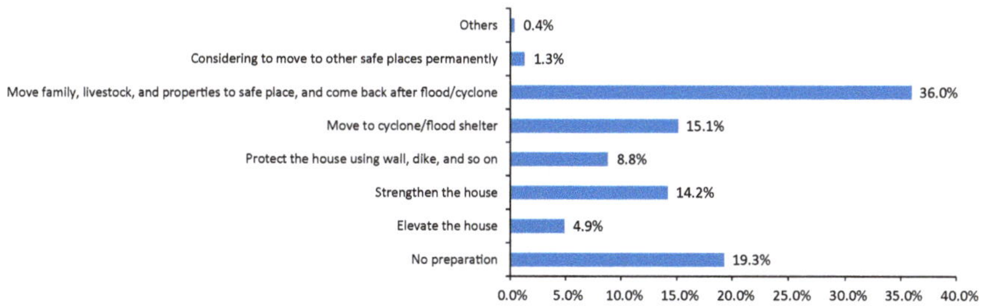

Fig. 12.9 Adaptation measures taken during disasters

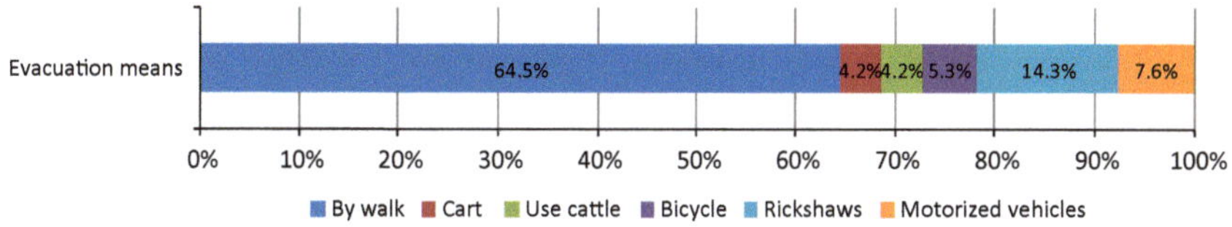

Fig. 12.10 Evacuation means during disasters

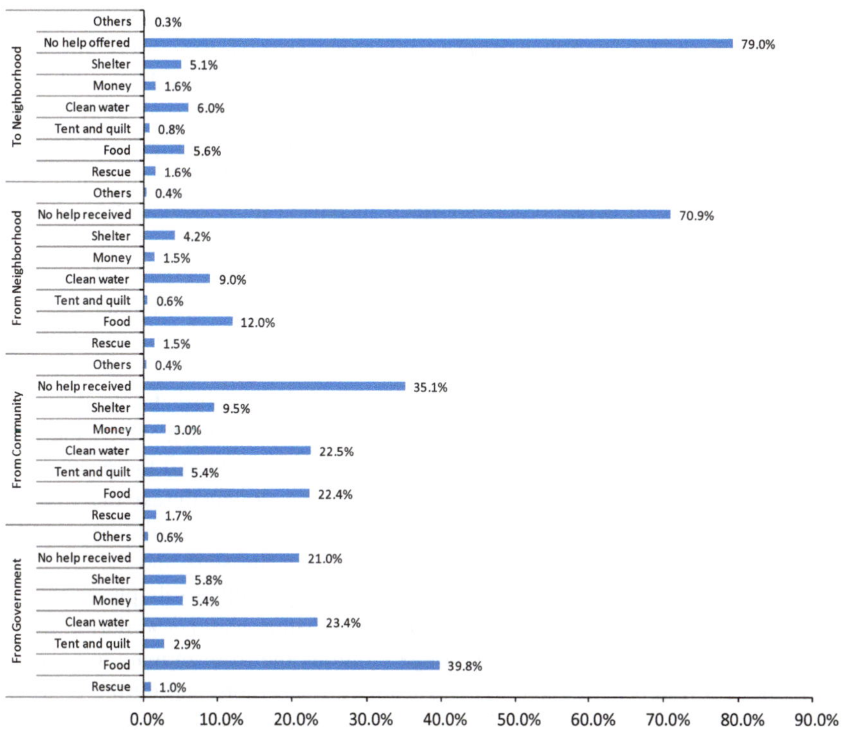

Fig. 12.11 Help received/offered during disasters

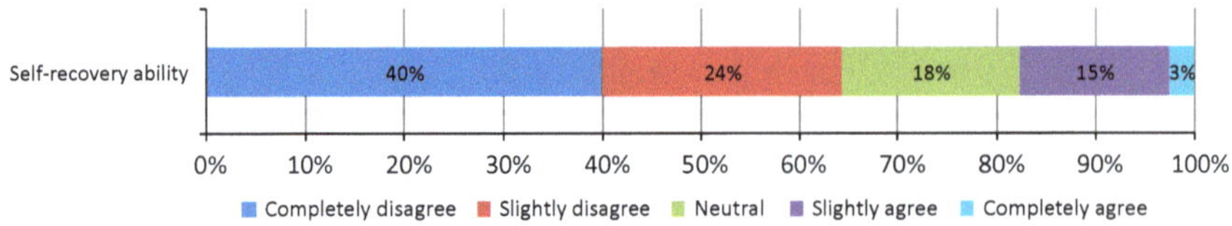

Fig. 12.12 Evaluation of self-recovery ability

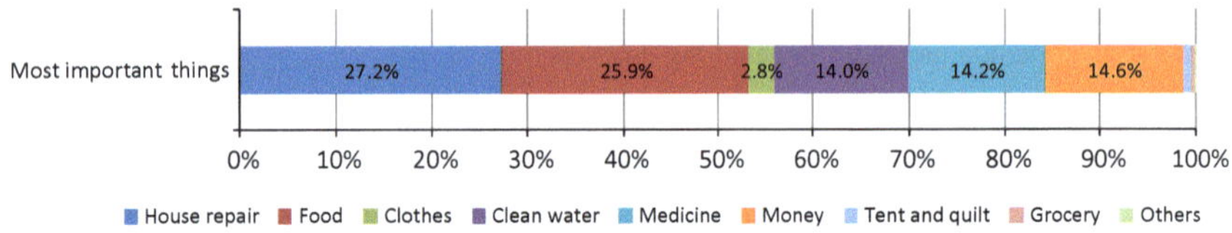

Fig. 12.13 The most important things during the recovery evaluated by respondents

to their neighbors. Communities provided shelter to 9.5 % of respondents, but the government provided it to only 5.8 %.

Figure 12.12 shows the respondents' evaluations of their ability to recover after disasters. We found that only 18 % of respondents are capable of recovering. Respondents reported that the most important aspects of recovery are house repairs (27.2 %), food (25.9 %), money (14.6 %), medicine (14.2 %), and clean water (14.0 %) (see Fig. 12.13). As time passes after a disaster, more people receive help from the government and communities (those who received no help decreased to 13.9 and 24.9 %, respectively, compared with the periods during disasters), but not from neighborhoods (which increased to 77.8 %, compared with the periods during disasters) (see Fig. 12.14).

As for future adaptation plans (Fig. 12.15), it is found that 26.0 % of respondents want to strengthen their houses; 16.8 % want to move their families, livestock, and property to safe places and return after disasters; but 24.6 % were unprepared.

Comparisons among predisaster adaptation measures, those during disasters, and those planned for the future are shown in Fig. 12.16, from which the item "consult with experienced people" before disasters is deleted and the percentages of other items recalculated. We found that past experiences encourage more people to protect their houses using measures such as walls and dikes (the corresponding share of respondents increases from 8.0 % before disasters and 8.8 % during disasters to 13.6 in the future) and to consider moving to other safe places permanently (the share increases from 2.7 % before disasters and 1.3 % during disasters to 4.8 % in the future), but discourage more people from moving to cyclone/flood shelters (the percentage decreases from current before and during disasters of 7.1 and 15.1 % to future 5.6 %). A moderate proportion of respondents make adaptation plans for the periods before and during disasters with respect to other measures.

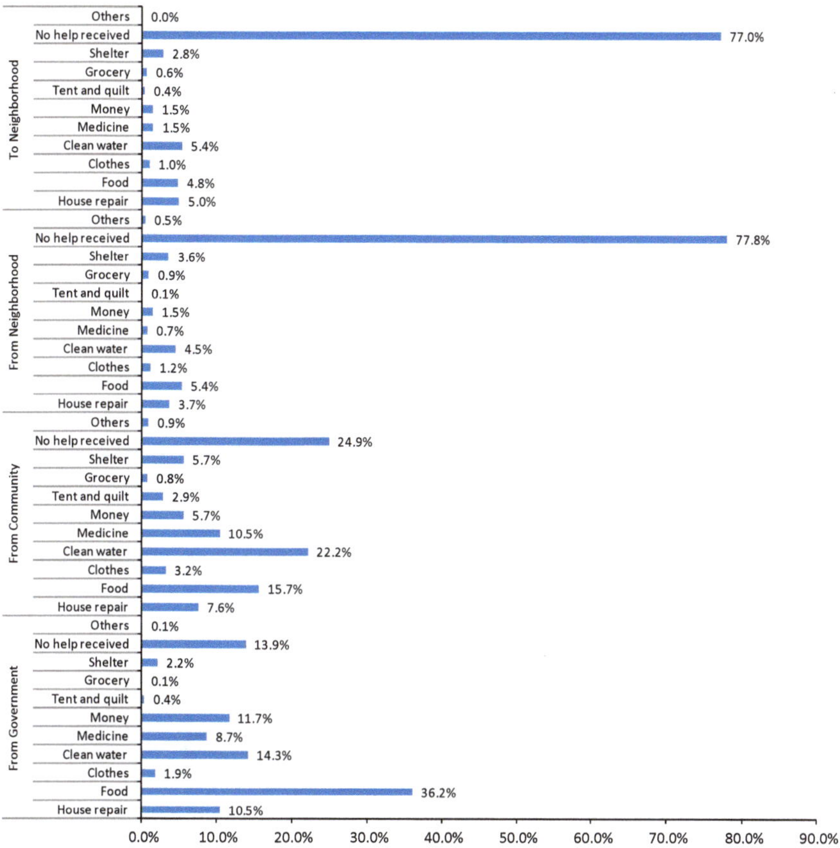

Fig. 12.14 Help received/offered after-disasters recovery

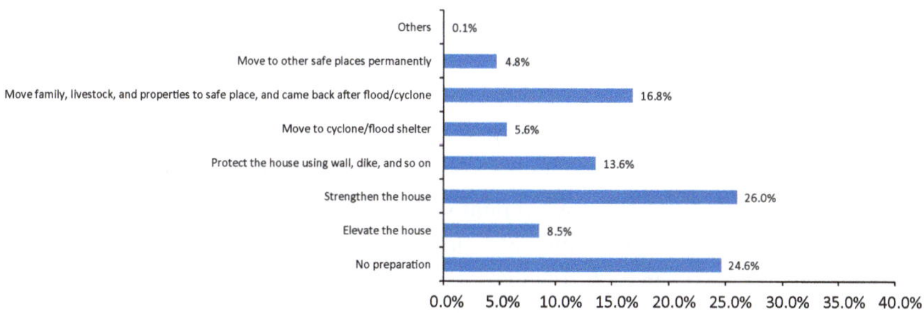

Fig. 12.15 Future adaptation plans

Barriers and Capability of Adaptation Measures

It is observed (see Fig. 12.17) that the current major difficulties in adapting to the impacts of climate disasters include lack of money (reported by 32.9 % of

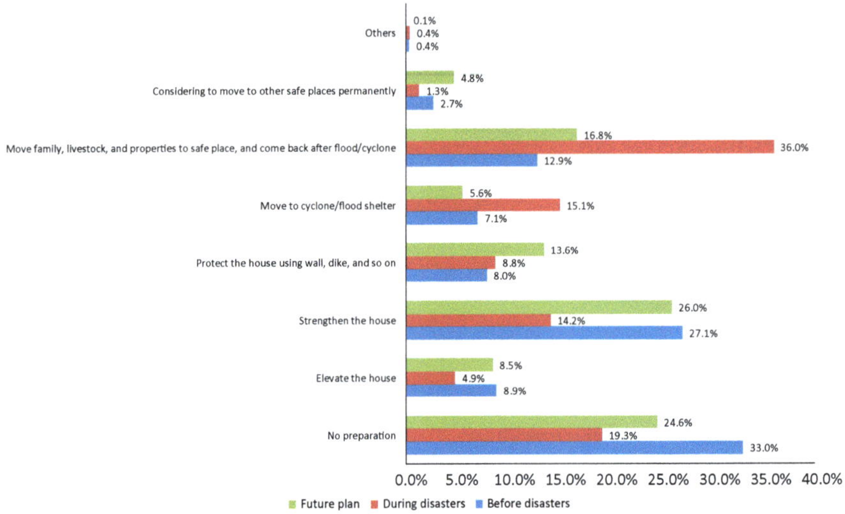

Fig. 12.16 Comparisons between before-disasters, during-disasters, and future adaptation measures

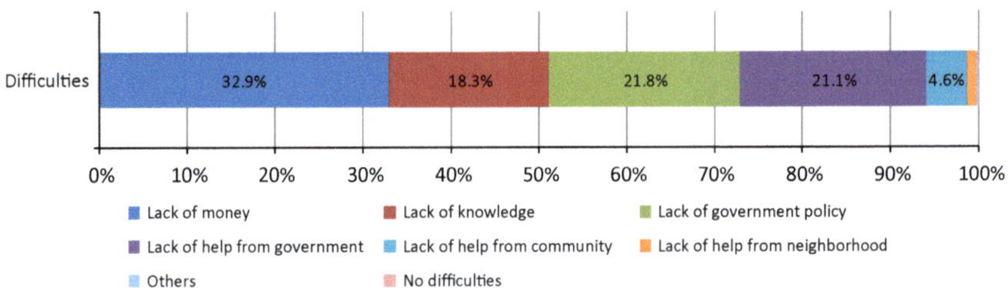

Fig. 12.17 Current major difficulties in adapting to the impacts of climate disasters

respondents), lack of government policy (21.8 %), lack of help from the government (21.1 %), and lack of knowledge (18.3 %). It is obvious that more than 40 % of difficulties come from the government side.

Figure 12.18 shows that some respondents are capable of dealing with adaptation measures in terms of finances, physical strength, family structure, help from neighbors, knowledge of countermeasures, and time. It is confirmed that 53.1 % of respondents are entirely unable to manage financially, and for 47.6 % of respondents no such help is available from neighbors. Figure 12.17 shows that very few people report difficulties arising from lack of help from neighbors, probably because no such help is available. In other words, this may indicate that many people have only limited resources for themselves, so they cannot provide any help for their neighbors. Other capability indicators show that about 10–20 %

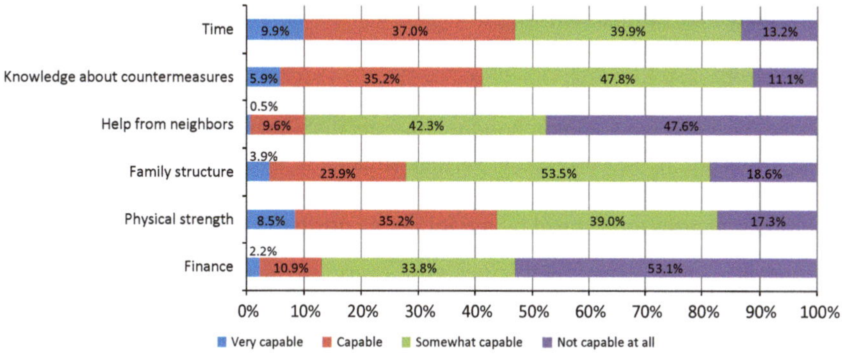

Fig. 12.18 Capabilities in dealing with adaptation measures

of respondents surely have insufficient capability, and few people are confident in their capabilities in terms of family structure compared with other indicators.

12.5 Stated Household Adaptation to Disasters in Bangladesh

In the above questionnaire survey, household adaptation is divided into two types: intercity travel and more general life adaptation (including job, residential location, and housing). Here, only the SP data are used to understand how households will adapt to future floods and cyclones. Because the impacts of these climate-related disasters may differ considerably between the coastal area and the inland area, we conducted the survey in both areas.

12.5.1 Stated Intercity Travel Behavior Analysis

To quantify the influence of future disasters on intercity travel behavior, we designed an SP survey. Because cyclones often occur in the coastal areas of Bangladesh, we prepared future scenarios for both floods and cyclones for respondents residing in the coastal area, but only flooding scenarios for the inland respondents.

First, as for the choice set in the SP survey, respondents were asked to choose one of the following five alternatives for various disaster scenarios:

(1) continue to travel as usual;
(2) cancel the trip;
(3) change the travel mode/route;

(4) change the destination;
(5) change the departure time.

Second, the disaster scenarios are designed as follows. The SP attributes were selected based on the common flooding impacts that people in Bangladesh are currently enduring, those observed in various streams of literature, and future predictions by Lee (2013).

Flood scenarios are defined by the following attributes at different levels:

- frequency (three levels): once every year, every two years or every three years;
- intensity represented in terms of water depth (three levels): on an adult of average size; water reaches knees, waist, or chest or above;
- whether permanent/frequent inundation occurs (two levels): yes or no;
- whether the residential area is isolated by water (two levels): yes or no;
- whether roads to other cities are destroyed permanently (two levels): yes or no.

Cyclone scenarios are defined by the following attributes at different levels:

- frequency (three levels): twice a year, every year, once every two years;
- intensity (three levels): some structural damage to houses, complete collapse of some houses, or complete failure of many houses;
- whether permanent/frequent inundation occurs (two levels): yes or no;
- whether the residential area is isolated by water (two levels): yes or no;
- whether roads to other cities are destroyed permanently (two levels): yes or no.

Based on an orthogonal experiment, we obtained a total of 16 disaster scenarios. To reduce the burden on respondents, these 16 scenarios were divided into four groups. Each respondent received only one group of four scenarios. The four groups were distributed equally among the survey respondents, so that each scenario would be presented to a quarter of the total sample during the implementation stage. Unfortunately, at the data collection stage, equal sample sizes for groups could not be guaranteed. For each scenario, the respondent was asked to choose one of the aforementioned five alternatives: i.e., (a) continue to travel as usual, (b) cancel the trip, (c) change the travel mode/route, (d) change the destination, or (e) change the departure time.

Before the questions on intercity travel behavior were answered, current behavior was also reported with respect to three main destinations (destination name, trip purpose, frequency of visits, main travel mode, travel cost, and travel time).

12.5.1.1 Aggregation Analysis

Figure 12.19 shows the results of people's intercity travel behavior responses as a whole, in all given disaster scenarios derived from the orthogonal experiment design. Among all the travel choices under flooding, more people in both coastal and inland areas chose "(a) continue to travel as usual" than other alternatives. A higher percentage of people in the coastal area indicated they would not change

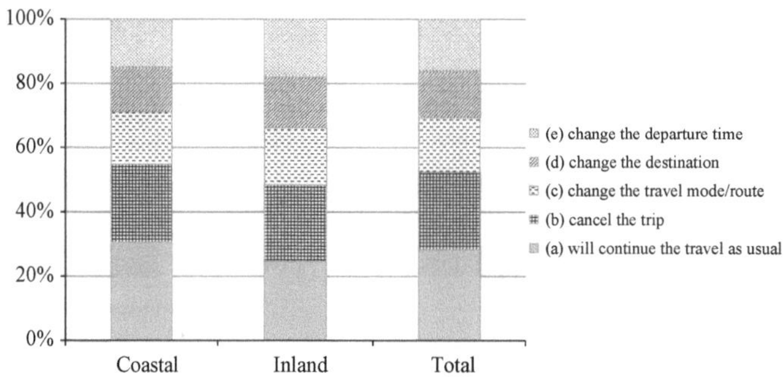

Fig. 12.19 Discriptive of people's intercity travel choice under flooding as a result of climate change

their behavior, indicating that coastal people are more passive and accustomed to the impacts of flooding. The proportions that chose other travel choices such as "(c) change travel mode/route" and "(e) change departure time" were slightly higher in the inland area, but the proportion of respondents who chose "(b) cancel the trip" was similar in both areas. This suggests that people in the inland area are slightly more inclined to change their travel plans if flood conditions change, and coastal people may be more sophisticated in adapting their travel behavior. However, the area makes no difference in the choice to cancel trips. Generally, more people would either travel with no change or cancel trips than make other changes, as the "(a) continue to travel as usual" and "(b) cancel the trip" choices account for more than 50 % of the responses.

Figures 12.20, 12.21 and 12.22 show the reported adaptations to intercity travel behavior associated with different impacts of disasters.

Comparing these three figures, one can easily observe that in many cases, "(a) continue to travel as usual" shows the largest proportion of respondents. In other words, even in severe disasters, a large proportion of people would still continue their intercity trips as usual. This suggests that participating in these intercity trips as usual is important to their lives. Similarly, the proportion that chose "(b) cancel the trip" is also high. For disaster frequency, there is a larger gap between the proportions selecting alternatives (a) and (b), associated with "once every three years", "once every two years", and "every year."

The alternatives "(c) change the travel route", "(d) change the destination", and "(e) change the departure time" indicate that people continue to make intercity trips, but change the way they do so. These three alternatives account for the largest share of responses, and in many cases their total share exceeds 50 %. Among the three alternatives, "(e) change the departure time" is influenced less by disasters than are the other two alternatives.

As for trip cancelation, when the flood reaches the waist of an average-sized adult in the inland area, the largest proportion of trip cancelations is reported (40 %). This may be because in the inland area, if the water level just reaches the

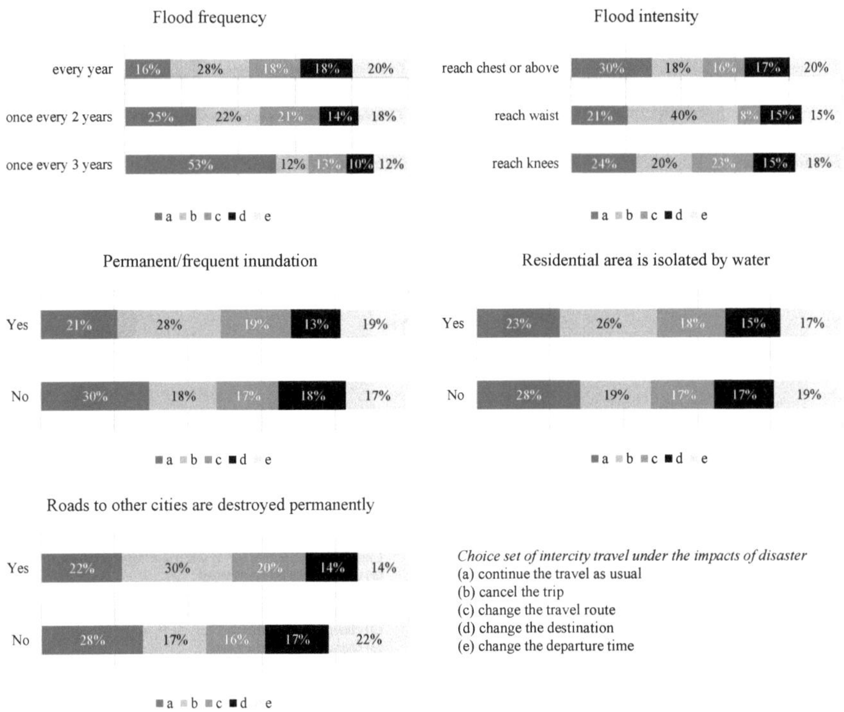

Fig. 12.22 Intercity travel adaptation behavior in the inland area and flood **a** Flooding and cyclone frequency. **b** Flooding and cyclone intensity. Note: IFLF means inland flood frequency which decreases from IFLF1 to IFLF3; CFLF denotes coastal flood frequency which decreases from CFLF1 to CFLF3; CLF means coastal cyclone frequency which decreases from CLF1 to CLF3; IFLI denotes inland flood intensity which increases from IFLI1 to IFLI3; CFLI means coastal flood intensity which increases from CFLI1 to CFLI3; CLI denotes coastal cyclone intensity which increases from CLI1 to CLI3

(1. very capable, 2. capable, 3. somewhat capable, 4. not capable at all), help available from neighbors (1. very available, 2. available, 3. somewhat available, 4. not available at all), knowledge of countermeasures against disaster (1. much knowledge, 2. moderate knowledge, 3. a little knowledge, 4. no knowledge), time available (1. much time, 2. some time, 3. little time, 4. no time);

- Mutual help and public help variables (i.e., social capital variables): help from government during the recovery period, help from community during the recovery period, and help from neighborhood during the recovery period in terms of: 1. house repair, 2. food, 3. clothes, 4. clean water, 5. medicine, 6. money, 7. tent and quilts, 8. grocery, 9. shelter, 10. no help received, 11. other help;
- Recovery variables: recovery time, recovery cost (recover to normal life from the impacts of disaster).

As a measure of model accuracy (see Tables 12.1, 12.2 and 12.3), McFadden's rho-squared values range between 0.1047 and 0.1071. This is not sufficiently high,

Table 12.1 Estimation results of household intercity travel adaptation behavior model: flood at the coastal area

Reference alternative in estimation: (e) change the departure time	(a) will continue the travel as usual				(b) cancel the trip			
Explanatory variable	Param	t-score		VR (%)	Param	t-score		VR (%)
Constant term	1.945	2.813	**		−1.301	−1.784	+	
Disaster frequency	−0.684	−3.004	**	7.2	0.566	2.409	*	9.8
Disaster intensity	−0.109	−1.325		1.8	−0.107	−1.276		2.7
Inundation	−0.011	−0.078		0.01	0.232	1.667	+	4.8
Isolated by water	−0.682	−4.764	**	22.6	−0.258	−1.781	+	5.9
Road destroyed	−0.572	−4.145	**	15.8	0.427	3.049	**	12.6
Financial ability	0.189	1.670	+	3.1	0.251	2.156	*	10.7
Physical strength	0.098	0.931		1.0	0.139	1.279		4.3
Capability of family structure	−0.176	−1.574		2.9	−0.095	−0.822		1.6
Available help from neighborhood	−0.159	−1.452		1.7	−0.149	−1.318		3.5
Knowledge about disaster	0.372	3.461	**	12.1	0.203	1.865	+	7.8
Available time to tackle disaster	0.061	0.645		0.4	0.240	2.442	*	10.8
Help from government during recovery	−0.454	−2.200	*	7.8	−0.208	−0.960		2.6
Help from community during recovery	−0.493	−2.832	**	10.7	−0.432	−2.423	*	14.7
Help from neighborhood during recovery	−0.671	−3.542	**	9.6	−0.333	−1.739	+	5.1
Recovery time	0.003	1.187		2.0	0.003	0.993		2.9
Recovery cost	−0.066	−1.073		1.2	0.025	0.379		0.3
Reference alternative in estimation: (e) change the departure time	(c) change the travel route				(d) change the destination			
Explanatory variable	Param	t score		VR (%)	Param	t-score		VR (%)
Constant term	−0.924	−1.167			−1.189	−1.435		
Disaster frequency	−0.041	−0.159		0.03	0.977	3.516	**	13.9
Disaster intensity	−0.123	−1.297		1.5	0.014	0.140		0.02
Inundation	0.085	0.558		0.3.	0.782	4.809	**	24.9
Isolated by water	0.067	0.428		0.2	−0.011	−0.067		0.01
Road destroyed	1.288	8.099	**	74.3	0.594	3.685	**	14.3
Financial ability	0.219	1.765	+	4.3	0.017	0.132		0.02
Physical strength	−0.192	−1.646	+	4.8	−0.282	−2.330	*	8.7
Capability of family structure	0.000	0.002		0.00	−0.009	−0.073		0.01

Table 12.1 (continued)

Reference alternative in estimation: (e) change the departure time	(c) change the travel route				(d) change the destination			
Available help from neighborhood	0.079	0.658		0.4	0.327	2.588	**	6.1
Knowledge about disaster	0.133	1.117		1.5	0.309	2.486	*	7.3
Available time to tackle disaster	0.085	0.801		0.8	−0.079	−0.719		0.6
Help from government during recovery	−0.021	−0.092		0.01	−0.055	−0.233		0.1
Help from community during recovery	−0.207	−1.063		1.6	−0.457	−2.318	*	8.0
Help from neighborhood during recovery	0.126	0.637		0.5	−0.295	−1.347		2.1
Recovery time	0.005	1.720	+	4.0	−0.001	−0.149		0.02
Recovery cost	−0.120	−1.837	+	5.7	−0.187	−2.838	**	14.0

Initial log-likelihood: −3836.900; Final log-likelihood: −3435.248; McFadden's Rho-squared: 0.1047; Adjusted McFadden's Rho-squared: 0.0983; Sample size: 2384 SP responses
Note + Signicant at the 10 % level; *Signicant at the 5 % level; **Signicant at the 1 % level; *VR* variance ratio in the total variance

Table 12.2 Estimation results of household intercity travel adaptation behavior model: Cyclone at the coastal area

Reference alternative in estimation: (e) change the departure time	(a) will continue the travel as usual				(b) cancel the trip			
Explanatory variable	Param	t-score		VR (%)	Param	t-score		VR (%)
Constant term	3.142	4.442	**		−0.211	−0.331		
Disaster frequency	−0.682	−6.269	**	23.6	0.039	0.398		0.2
Disaster intensity	−0.501	−5.798	**	19.0	−0.296	−4.040	**	22.9
Inundation	−0.139	−1.011		0.6	0.615	4.975	**	33.0
Isolated by water	−0.866	−5.831	**	20.2	−0.114	−0.879		1.2
Road destroyed	−0.618	−4.361	**	10.0	0.375	3.005	**	2.5
Financial ability	0.217	1.840	+	2.5	0.136	1.324		3.4
Physical strength	0.015	0.143		0.01	0.017	0.173		0.1
Capability of family structure	−0.041	−0.355		0.1	0.038	0.376		0.2
Available help from neighborhood	−0.232	−2.031	*	2.2	−0.210	−2.115	*	7.0
Knowledge about disaster	0.184	1.695	+	1.9	0.060	0.634		0.7
Available time to tackle disaster	−0.014	−0.145		0.0	0.162	1.885	+	5.1

Table 12.2 (continued)

Reference alternative in estimation: (e) change the departure time	(a) will continue the travel as usual				(b) cancel the trip			
Help from government during recovery	−0.695	−3.470	**	12.2	−0.194	−1.040		2.2
Help from community during recovery	−0.295	−1.738	+	2.4	−0.010	−0.068		0.01
Help from neighborhood during recovery	−0.586	−2.939	**	4.3	−0.083	−0.494		0.4
Recovery time	0.003	1.049		0.8	0.005	1.978	*	9.5
Recovery cost	−0.029	−0.484		0.2	0.057	1.054		1.8
Reference alternative in estimation: (e) change the departure time	(c) change the travel route				(d) change the destination			
Explanatory variable	Param	t-score		VR (%)	Param	t-score		VR (%)
Constant term	−0.807	−1.051			−0.352	−0.437		
Disaster frequency	−0.050	−0.430		0.2	0.129	0.996		2.0
Disaster intensity	−0.432	−4.790	**	26.6	−0.163	−1.664	+	4.0
Inundation	0.170	1.162		1.6	0.860	5.347	**	45.7
Isolated by water	0.205	1.359		2.3	0.301	1.788	+	5.7
Road destroyed	1.005	6.712	**	49.1	0.662	4.145	**	28.3
Financial ability	0.085	0.702		0.8	−0.001	−0.012		0.00
Physical strength	0.008	0.075		0.01	−0.141	−1.171		3.5
Capability of family structure	0.213	1.785	+	5.1	−0.089	−0.696		1.0
Available help from neighborhood	0.028	0.240		0.1	−0.086	−0.701		0.8
Knowledge about disaster	−0.136	−1.204		2.1	0.082	0.664		0.8
Available time to tackle disaster	0.021	0.208		0.1	0.011	0.097		0.02
Help from government during recovery	−0.007	−0.031		0.00	−0.206	−0.894		2.1
Help from community during recovery	0.140	0.771		0.9	0.186	0.962		2.0
Help from neighborhood during recovery	−0.131	−0.656		0.5	−0.194	−0.900		1.6
Recovery time	0.006	2.365	*	9.7	0.002	0.676		0.8
Recovery cost	−0.049	−0.794		1.0	−0.058	−0.911		1.8

Initial log-likelihood: −3836.900; Final log-likelihood: −3425.993; McFadden's Rho-squared: 0.1071; Adjusted McFadden's Rho-squared: 0.1007; Sample size: 2384 SP responses

Note + Signicant at the 10 % level; *Signicant at the 5 % level; **Signicant at the 1 % level; *VR* variance ratio in the total variance

Table 12.3 Estimation results of household intercity travel adaptation behavior model: flood at the inland area

Reference alternative in estimation: (e) change the departure time	(a) will continue the travel as usual				(b) cancel the trip			
Explanatory variable	Param	t-score		VR (%)	Param	t-score		VR (%)
Constant term	1.738	2.387	*		−3.041	−3.916	**	
Disaster frequency	−2.344	−6.802	**	39.0	0.325	0.940		1.4
Disaster intensity	−0.038	−0.370		0.1	−0.004	−0.039		0.00
Inundation	−0.213	−1.128		0.9	0.246	1.314		2.9
Isolated by water	−0.434	−2.314	*	3.7	0.575	3.057	**	14.5
Road destroyed	0.367	2.008	*	2.7	0.977	5.408	**	45.2
Financial ability	0.054	0.411		0.2	0.345	2.576	**	14.3
Physical strength	−0.027	−0.216		0.04	0.194	1.551		6.6
Capability of family structure	−0.327	−2.555	*	6.0	0.059	0.453		0.5
Available help from neighborhood	−0.079	−0.635		0.3	−0.031	−0.248		0.1
Knowledge about disaster	0.398	2.856	**	7.1	−0.008	−0.062		0.01
Available time to tackle disaster	0.470	4.105	**	16.1	0.148	1.308		3.9
Help from government during recovery	−0.656	−2.672	**	7.8	−0.212	−0.857		2.0
Help from community during recovery	0.233	1.112		1.1	−0.118	−0.569		0.7
Help from neighborhood during recovery	−0.148	−0.568		0.2	−0.182	−0.696		0.7
Recovery time	0.016	2.726	**	13.0	0.008	1.344		6.5
Recovery cost	−0.097	−1.653	+	1.9	0.047	0.767		0.8

Reference alternative in estimation: (e) change the departure time	(c) change the travel route				(d) change the destination		
Explanatory variable	Param	t-score		VR (%)	Param	t-score	VR (%)
Constant term	0.171	0.216			−1.536	−1.863 +	
Disaster frequency	−0.972	−2.706	**	10.8	0.194	0.517	1.1
Disaster intensity	−0.358	−3.345	**	14.7	−0.014	−0.127	0.1
Inundation	0.358	1.854	+	4.7	−0.379	−1.890 +	15.2

(continued)

Table 12.3 (continued)

Reference alternative in estimation: (e) change the departure time	(c) change the travel route				(d) change the destination		
Explanatory variable	Param	t-score		VR (%)	Param	t-score	VR (%)
Isolated by water	0.003	0.015		0.00	0.084	0.431	0.7
Road destroyed	0.833	4.413	**	25.4	0.298	1.526	9.4
Financial ability	−0.076	−0.539		0.5	0.091	0.616	1.8
Physical strength	0.003	0.024		0.00	−0.139	−0.992	6.8
Capability of family structure	−0.234	−1.713	+	4.2	−0.075	−0.539	1.4
Available help from neighborhood	0.107	0.793		0.9	0.232	1.643	11.3
Knowledge about disaster	0.181	1.234		2.7	0.080	0.529	1.4
Available time to tackle disaster	0.243	1.968	*	6.3	0.283	2.253 *	27.4
Help from government during recovery	0.002	0.008		0.00	−0.086	−0.307	0.6
Help from community during recovery	0.912	3.986	**	25.6	0.330	1.424	10.5
Help from neighborhood during recovery	−0.182	−0.667		0.6	0.280	1.090	5.7
Recovery time	−0.002	−0.274		0.1	−0.014	−1.612	6.0
Recovery cost	−0.089	−1.448		3.4	−0.022	−0.360	0.7

Initial log-likelihood: −2303.106; Final log-likelihood: −2058.804; McFadden's Rho-squared: 0.1061; Adjusted McFadden's Rho-squared: 0.0953; Sample size: 1431 SP responses
Note + Signicant at the 10 % level; *Signicant at the 5 % level; **Signicant at the 1 % level; *VR* variance ratio in the total variance

but acceptable as a model, to identify influential factors. There are many statistically significant parameters, and most parameters have the expected sign (positive or negative). All these results suggest that the MNL model is still applicable to such adaptation behavior, although it suffers from the Independence of Irrelevant Alternatives (IIA) property.

(1) ***Intercity travel adaptation behavior in the coastal area: Flood scenarios***

Table 12.1 shows that flood affects most of a household's choice alternatives for intercity travel. The permanent destruction of roads to other cities is among the three most influential factors in terms of statistical significance and variance ratio on intercity choice alternatives. The permanent destruction of roads is estimated to result in trip cancelations, changes of travel route and destination, and to hinder people from making their usual intercity trips. Destruction of roads is especially decisive in relation to the "(c) change the travel route" alternative because it explains 74.3 % of the total variance. These findings reconfirm that roads are a crucial form of infrastructure that support daily life. Isolation of residential areas by water markedly reduces the likelihood that a household will continue intercity travel as usual, because it shows the largest variance ratio (22.6 %) of the total variance of the alternative "(a) continue to travel as usual". Inundation mostly affects "(d) change the destination" (variance ratio: 24.9 %): people are more likely to change the destination of their intercity trips if inundation occurs, while the effect of disaster frequency is ranked in the second place (13.9 %), together with that of recovery cost (14.0 %). Disaster intensity does not influence any alternative of the intercity trip. Disaster frequency does not affect "(c) change the travel route", while inundation is not related to "(a) continue to travel as usual" and "(c) change the travel route" because their parameters are all insignificant.

Trip cancelation should be regarded as having the most serious impact on household life. In line with this, the alternative "(b) cancel the trip" is mostly influenced by help from the community during the recovery period (house repairs, food, clothes, clean water, medicine, money, tents and quilts, groceries, shelter, or other assistance), for which the variance ratio (VR) is 14.7 % and which has a negative influence. This suggests that receiving help from the community during the recovery period may mitigate the impacts of floods markedly, because households are less likely to cancel intercity trips. In other words, if households cannot obtain help from the neighborhood during the recovery period, they mostly cancel their intercity trips. Household capability (mainly time available to respond to the impacts of disasters and financial ability) is also strongly associated with trip cancelation. Households with lower financial capacity and less available time are more likely to cancel intercity trips, suggesting that policies to improve household capability in the face of disasters should be promoted to mitigate the impacts of disasters on people's lives.

Regarding social capital, help from the government, communities, and neighborhoods have the greatest influence on decisions to "(a) continue to travel as usual" and "(b) cancel the trip" than on other choices. Recovery time and cost are irrelevant to "(a) continue to travel as usual" and "(b) cancel the trip".

(2) ***Intercity travel adaptation behavior in the coastal area: Cyclone scenarios***

As shown in Table 12.2, in contrast to the case of flooding, the most influential factors are all cyclone-related attributes. This result is intuitive. The top three factors in decisions to "(a) continue to travel as usual" are disaster frequency (VR = 23.6 %), isolation by water (VR = 20.2 %), and disaster intensity (VR = 19.0 %), while those on "(b) cancel the trip" are inundation (VR = 33.3 %), disaster intensity (VR = 22.9 %), and the destruction of roads (VR = 12.5 %). The option "(c) change the travel route" is affected most strongly by the destruction of roads (VR = 49.1 %) and disaster frequency (26.6 %), while "(d) change the destination" is affected most by inundation (VR = 45.7 %) and the destruction of roads (28.3 %). Again, we reconfirm the critical influence of roads on people's lives because of the larger variance ratios. The influence of household capacity is very limited, because only six of 24 relevant parameters are statistically significant. Help from the government, community and neighborhood only affect "(a) continue to travel as usual". Households experiencing longer recovery time are more likely to cancel their trips and/or change their travel route in response to cyclones.

(3) ***Intercity travel adaptation behavior in the inland area: Flood scenarios***

As Table 12.3 shows, influential factors in intercity travel are similar to those of floods in the coastal area. There are four groups of factors: disaster related, household capability related, external help, and recovery time and cost. It is observed that some factors from all four groups affect intercity travel behavior. Unlike the flood case in the coastal area, the impacts of flooding are not extensive. We only found significant influences of disaster frequency (VR = 39.0 %) on "(a) continue to travel as usual", road destruction (VR = 45.2 %) and isolation by water (VR = 14.5 %) on "(b) cancel the trip", road destruction (25.4 %) and disaster frequency (VR = 10.8 %) on "(c) change the travel route", and inundation on "(d) change the destination". Larger influences are observed for household capability with respect to time available to respond to the impacts of disasters on "(a) continue to travel as usual" (VR = 16.1 %) and on "(d) change the destination" (VR = 27.4 %), financial ability (VR = 14.3 %) on "(b) cancel the trip", and available help from neighborhood (VR = 11.3 %) on "(d) change the destination".

(4) ***Summary***

A comparison of the three cases above shows that people living in the coastal area of Bangladesh are more vulnerable than those in the inland area. This is partly because the land nearby the coastal area is very low, and consequently more easily inundated by water. Improving household capability to adapt to the impacts of floods and cyclones is more effective in the coastal area than in the inland area. Help from the government, community, and neighborhood has a stronger influence on adaptation to the impacts of floods in the coastal and inland areas; in contrast, the influence of help on adaptation to cyclones is very limited. Limited influences are also observed with respect to recovery time and cost.

12.5.2 Stated Adaptation to Floods and Cyclones in Bangladesh

We investigated household life adaptation behavior in the SP survey by asking respondents to choose one of the following six alternatives in different disaster scenarios:

(a) change neither job nor residential location, and do not reinforce the house (Choice 1: Job0_Res0_Hou0);
(b) change neither job nor residential location, and reinforce the house (Choice 2: Job0_Res0_Hou1);

(c) change jobs, do not change residential location, and do not reinforce the house (Choice 3: Job1_Res0_Hou0);
(d) change jobs but not residential location, and reinforce the house (Choice 4: Job1_Res0_Hou1);
(e) do not change jobs, but change residential location (Choice 5: Job0_Res1);
(f) change both job and residential location (Choice 6: Job1_Res1).

The SP attributes are the same as those in the previously mentioned SP survey of intercity travel behavior, that is, 16 SP scenarios divided into four groups. Each respondent answered questions for only one group, which includes four scenarios. As a result, a total of 788 valid respondents (3152 responses) were surveyed for this part of the analysis: 487 respondents (1948 SP responses) from the coastal area and 301 respondents (1204 SP responses) from the inland area.

12.5.2.1 Reported Features of Life Adaptation Behavior

The descriptive analysis results show that more people would choose to relocate their residence rather than change their job location in response to flooding and cyclone impacts, which underlines the seriousness of impacts on people's houses. In the proposed flooding scenarios, more people (almost 50 % of the respondents) from the inland region chose no response or would just reinforce their houses. However, more coastal people would choose to change residence location in response to flooding impacts. This indicates that coastal people suffer more from flooding impacts, and changing residence location may be their best choice when adapting to coastal flooding. People's choices in response to hypothetical flood and cyclone frequency and intensity are shown in Fig. 12.23. Figure 12.23(a) shows people's responses to different flood and cyclone frequencies. With a decrease in frequency, the percentage of people choosing no response (Choice 1) increases, and this increase under conditions of flood is greater than that of cyclones. The number of people who would change residence location (Choices 5 and 6) decreases when there is a decrease in flood or cyclone frequency. The number of people who choose job location change and house reinforcement (Choices 2, 3, and 4) increases with a decrease in frequency; however, this change is not as obvious as that for Choices 1, 5, and 6. Similar results can be observed for people's choices for different levels of flood and cyclone intensity, as shown in Fig. 12.23(b). The number of people who choose to change residence location (Choices 5 and 6) increases with flood or cyclone intensity, and the percentages of people who indicate no response or house reinforcement alone decrease with an increase in intensity. As illustrated in Fig. 12.23, more people would choose residence relocation when flood or cyclone frequency and intensity increase, and almost 50 % of the respondents would select Choices 5 and 6 under the highest level of frequency and intensity. More than half of the respondents would choose no response or just house reinforcement (Choices 1 and 2) given the lowest flood and cyclone frequency, but this percentage is a little lower (around

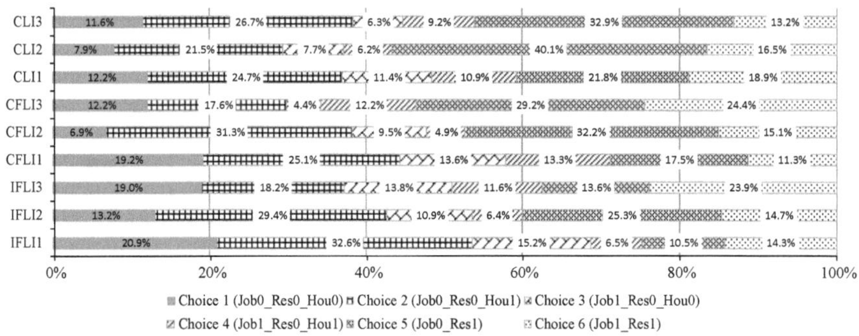

(a) Flooding and cyclone frequency.

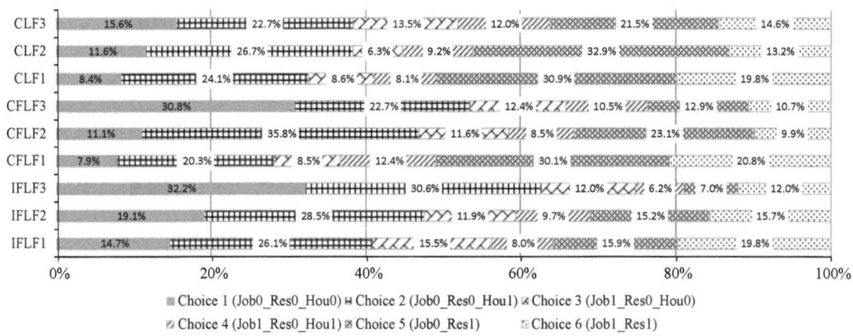

(b) Flooding and cyclone intensity.

Fig. 12.23 People's location change choices under different **a** flooding and cyclone frequency, and **b** flooding and cyclone intensity

40 %) for Choices 1 and 2 with the lowest flood and cyclone intensity; the percentages of people who select job relocation choices (Choices 3 and 4) are the lowest among all the six choices; more people would choose residence relocation change given cyclone frequency changes than those who would do so for changes in flood frequency.

12.5.2.2 Reported Life Adaptation Associated with Disaster Attributes

Analyses in this section are based on the results shown in Figs. 12.24, 12.25 and 12.26.

Disaster Frequency

In the three cases (floods and cyclones in the coastal area, and floods in the inland area), the alternative "(a) change neither job nor residential location, and do not reinforce the house" (i.e., the status quo) is sensitive to flood frequency in a similar way: the proportions of respondents making this choice range from a frequency of about 10 % (a flood every year) to about 30 % (once every three years). These

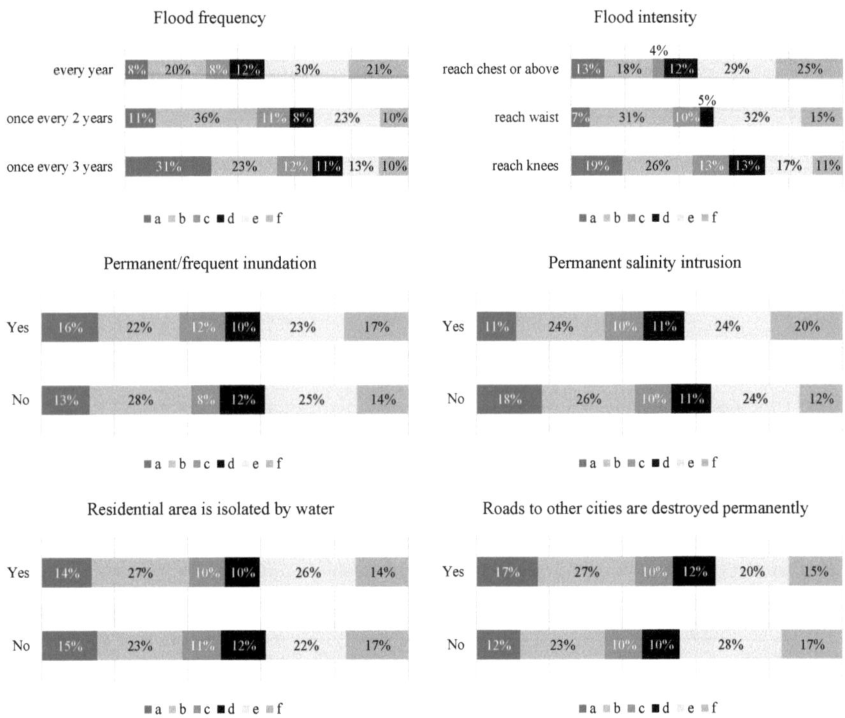

Fig. 12.24 Life adaptation behavior in the coastal area under the influence of flood

proportions are higher in the inland area than in the coastal area. The alternative "(f) change both job and residential location" (the most drastic change) shows the opposite response pattern, which is also similar across the three cases: the proportion of respondents ranges from about 10 % (once every three years) to about 20 % (every year). As for residential relocation (i.e., "(e) do not change job, but change residential location" and "(f) change both job and residential location"), consistent with our expectation, cyclones would result in more people changing their residential location than would flooding, while in the two flood cases, a coastal flood would lead to more relocation of households than would an inland flood. Concerning job change (i.e., the alternatives "c", "d" and "f"), variations in respondent proportions are smaller across the three disaster cases, ranging from about 30 % (once every two years) to 40 % (twice a year).

Disaster Intensity

Floods and cyclones are measured differently: by water level for floods and by damage to housing for cyclones. A comparison of floods in the two areas shows that floods in the coastal area have less influence on people's lives than on those in the inland area, because the choice shares for alternative (a) range from 7 to 19 % in the coastal area, and those in the inland area from 14 to 20 %. As for the most

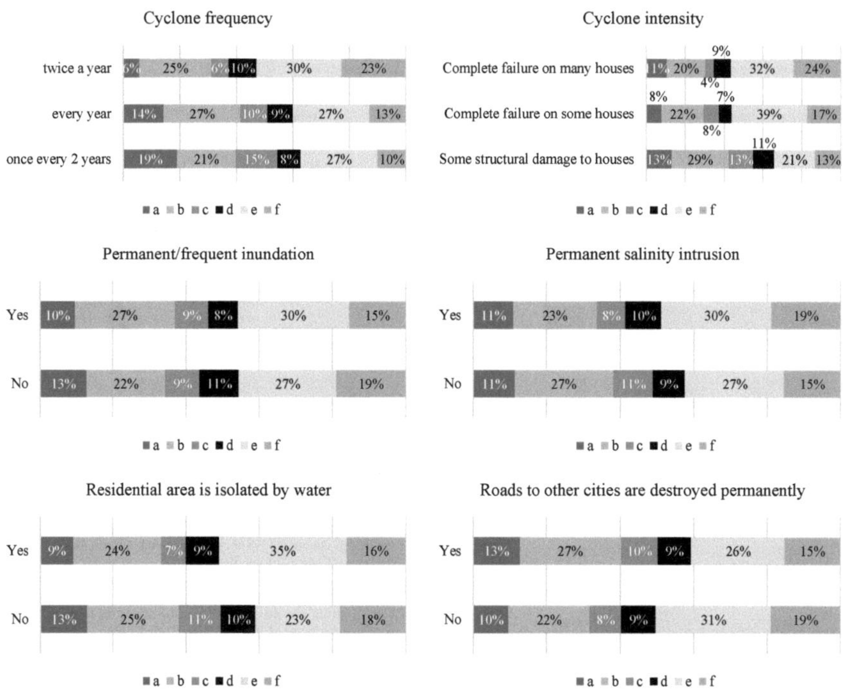

Fig. 12.25 Life adaptation behavior in the coastal area under the influence of cyclone

serious impact (i.e., alternative (f): change both job and household location), the variations of response proportions across the three cases are small, approximately between 10 and 25 %. Cyclones would force more people to change their residential locations than would floods, while the impacts of inland floods are smallest among the three scenarios in terms of residential relocation choices [i.e., alternatives (e) and (f)]. What are the impacts on job change? From a comparison of total choice proportions of alternatives (c), (d), and (f), it is found that half of the respondents in the inland area would have to change jobs when the water level reached chest level or above. In the case of coastal disasters (floods and cyclones), about 40 % of respondents would have to change their jobs if a cyclone caused the complete collapse of many houses in the area and floodwater levels reached chest level or above.

Permanent/Frequent Inundation of Houses

Impacts of permanent/frequent inundation of houses would result in the largest number of households (30 %) changing residential locations, but not changing jobs [i.e., alternative (e)] in the case of a coastal cyclone. A similar proportion of responses would be observed in the case of an inland flood with respect to alternative (b): "change neither job nor residential location, and reinforce the house" (28 % of responses). Note that similar proportions of responses have different

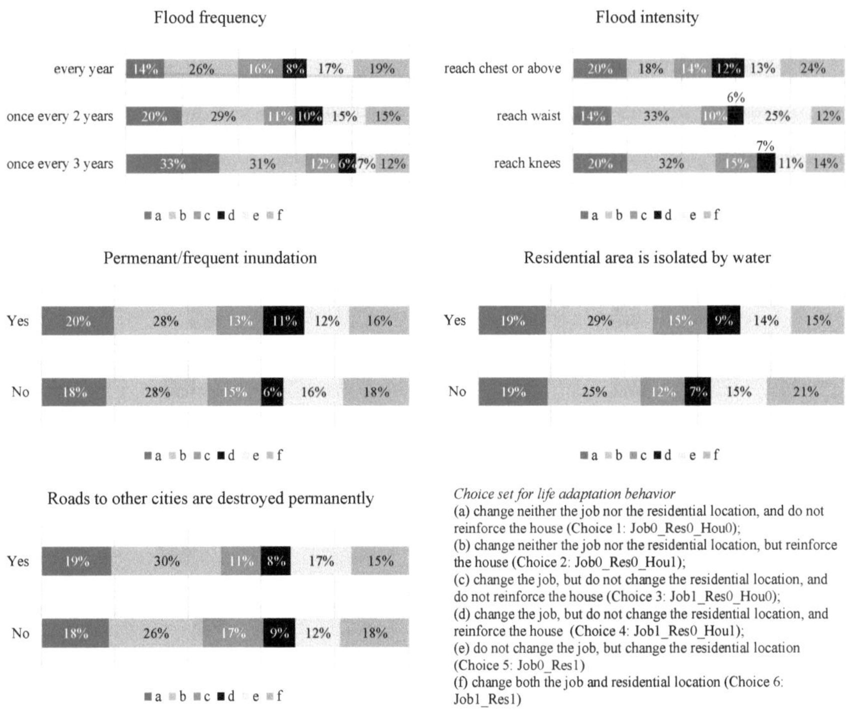

Fig. 12.26 Life adaptation behavior in the inland area under the influence of flood

meanings for disaster impacts. It would be fair to state that the impact of a cyclone is greater than that of an inland flood, because more people have to change residential location, which is costlier than reinforcing their houses. The most serious impact would be the job change. From this viewpoint, it is found that floods in both coastal and inland areas would result in about 40 % of respondents changing their jobs, while this proportion would be just 10 points lower in the case of a cyclone. This may be because of the fact that inundation caused by a flood lasts longer than that of a cyclone.

Permanent Salinity Intrusion

The impacts of salinity intrusion seem similar for floods and cyclones (only in the coastal area), where the only differences are the choices of "(c) change job, do not change residential location, and do not reinforce the house" and "(e) do not change job, but change residential location". Cyclones would lead to 30 % of respondents changing jobs, but they would see no need to change their residential location or reinforce their houses. In comparison, this proportion would drop to 24 % in a flood.

Isolation of Residential Area by Water

Isolation of residential areas by water from cyclones seems to have the largest impact on people's lives, because more people have to adapt to some extent, and because the proportion of respondents choosing "(a) change neither job nor residential location, and do not reinforce the house" is the lowest (just 9 %) among the two cases: 14 % in a coastal flood and 19 % in an inland flood. As for job change, an inland flood would result in 39 % of respondents changing jobs, while 32 % would do so in a cyclone, and 34 % in a coastal flood. Concerning residential relocation, a cyclone would force more than 50 % of households to relocate; in contrast, about 30 % would do so in the two flood cases.

Permanent Destruction of Roads to Other Cities
It is expected that road damage would markedly reduce the accessibility of households to various places, consequently forcing more people to change jobs. From the survey results, the total proportion of those who would change jobs with respect to alternatives (c), (d), and (f) is 37 % for a coastal flood, 34 % for a cyclone, and 34 % for an inland flood. In fact, the impacts on residential relocation measured by the proportion of respondents who chose alternatives (e) and (f) are similar to those for job change.

12.5.2.3 Choice Model Analysis

In the modeling analysis, the following variables are used:

- flood and cyclone attributes: all SP attributes including disaster frequency (once a year, once every two years, once every three years), disaster intensity (flood reaches knees, reaches waist, reaches chest or above on an adult of average size; cyclone: some structural damage to houses, complete collapse of some houses, complete collapse of many houses), permanent salinity intrusion (yes or no: only for life adaptation behavior in the coastal area), permanent or frequent inundation (yes or no), whether residential area is isolated by water (yes or no), whether roads to other cities are destroyed permanently (yes or no).
- self-help variables: financial ability (1. very capable, 2. capable, 3. somewhat capable, 4. not capable at all), physical strength (1. very capable, 2. capable, 3. somewhat capable, 4. not capable at all), capability of family structure (1. very capable, 2. capable, 3. somewhat capable, 4. not capable at all), help available from neighbors (1. very available, 2. available, 3. somewhat available, 4. not at all available), knowledge about countermeasures against disaster (1. much knowledge, 2. moderate knowledge, 3. a little knowledge, 4. no knowledge), available time (1. much time, 2. some time, 3. little time, 4. no time).
- mutual help and public help variables: help from the government during the recovery period, help from the community during the recovery period, help from the neighborhood during the recovery period—1. house repair, 2. food, 3. clothes, 4. clean water, 5. medicine, 6. money, 7. tents and quilts, 8. groceries, 9. shelter, 10. no help received, 11. other help.
- recovery variables: recovery time, recovery cost (to return to normal life following the impacts of a disaster).

The model estimation results (Tables 12.4, 12.5 and 12.6) with respect to the three cases revealed larger influences of disaster-related factors on people's lives in the coastal areas than those of the inland areas, while larger influences are also observed in terms of household capabilities, social capital, and recovery time and cost, in the inland area. To be specific, the most influential factors on life adaptation behavior in cases of coastal floods are flood frequency, flood intensity, and salinity intrusion, while in cyclones, inundation is the most influential factor.

(1) ***Life adaptation behaviors under the impacts of coastal flooding***

The strongest influence on "(a) change neither job nor residential location, and do not reinforce the house", is flood frequency, because the variance ratio is largest with a value of 46.1 %, followed by flood intensity (VR = 27.7 %) and salinity intrusion (VR = 14.9 %). These are also the major factors in "(b) change neither job nor residential location, and reinforce the house". Concerning "(c) change job, do not change residential location, and do not reinforce the house" and "(d) change job but not residential location, and reinforce the house", flood frequency and intensity share the top two factors. Unexpectedly, isolation of residential areas by water does not affect any life adaptation behavior. Even though the influences are smaller in magnitude, permanent road destruction results in more people choosing the status quo, i.e., the alternative "(a) change neither job nor residential location, and do not reinforce the house", and it further reduces the probability that people will not change their jobs, but will change their residential location.

Capability-related factors have much smaller influences on adaptation to cyclones. Higher capability related to family structure leads to a lower probability that people will choose the status quo (no change) and change their jobs, but will not change their residential locations and jobs. In contrast, help available from the neighborhood is associated with the probability that people will choose the status quo. As for social capital, i.e., external help, help from the community during the recovery period, has no influence at all on any choices. Help from the government during the recovery period affects alternatives (a), (b), and (e), and help from the neighborhood during the recovery period only influences (a). The parameter of help from the neighborhood in alternative (a) is negative, which indicates that with the help of their neighborhood, households attempt to change their behavior to mitigate the impacts of a cyclone. Similarly, help from the government also reduces the probability of people choosing the status quo. In contrast, with the help of the government, respondents tend to reinforce their houses [alternative (b)] and change their residential locations, but not to change their jobs.

The time-consuming nature of recovery results in fewer people reinforcing their houses (but not changing jobs or residential locations) or changing their jobs (but not their residential locations or reinforcing their houses) in the sense that the relevant parameters are negative and statistically significant. On the other hand, the financial demands of recovery lead to more people changing jobs, but not changing their residential location and reinforcing their houses, because the parameter of recovery cost is positive for alternative (d).

Table 12.4 Estimation results of household life adaptation behavior model: flood at the coastal area

Reference alternative in estimation: (f) will change both the job and residential location	(a) will change neither the job nor the residential location, and will not reinforce the house				(b) will change neither the job nor the residential location, but will reinforce the house				(c) will change the job, but will not change the residential location, and will not reinforce the house			
Explanatory variable	Param	t-score		VR (%)	Param	t-score		VR	Param-	t-score		VR (%)
Constant term	6.494	7.145	**		4.545	5.963	**		4.289	4.498	**	
Disaster frequency	−3.317	−10.761	**	46.1	−1.865	−7.440	**	35.3	−1.901	−5.999	**	29.7
Disaster intensity	−0.896	−7.795	**	27.7	−0.614	−7.043	**	27.4	−1.010	−8.339	**	43.8
Inundation	−0.282	−1.585		1.0	−0.449	−3.084	**	6.2	0.313	1.718	+	2.2
Salinity intrusion	−1.124	−6.306	**	14.9	−0.699	−4.801	**	15.1	−0.464	−2.551	*	5.0
Isolated by water	0.037	0.200		0.0	−0.045	−0.300		0.1	−0.203	−1.075		1.0
Road destroyed	0.472	2.828	**	2.7	0.213	1.483		1.4	0.056	0.318		0.1
Financial ability	−0.022	−0.156		0.01	−0.129	−1.050		1.0	−0.108	−0.725		0.5
Physical strength	0.080	0.639		0.2	0.008	0.071		0.00	0.075	0.557		0.4
Capability of family structure	−0.232	−1.713	+	1.4	−0.113	−0.964		0.7	−0.481	−3.278	**	9.6
Available help from neighborhood	−0.219	−1.655	+	1.1	0.075	0.653		0.3	−0.052	−0.373		0.1
Knowledge about disaster	−0.158	−1.222		0.6	−0.119	−1.082		0.9	−0.145	−1.044		1.1
Available time to tackle disaster	0.072	0.635		0.1	0.184	1.868	+	2.8	0.122	0.994		0.8
Help from government during recovery	−0.430	−1.760	+	1.7	−0.419	−1.993	*	4.3	0.050	0.185		0.03
Help from community during recovery	0.181	0.891		0.4	0.139	0.798		0.5	−0.070	−0.323		0.1
Help from neighborhood during recovery	−0.419	−1.750	+	1.0	−0.016	−0.080		0.00	0.211	0.881		0.7
Recovery time	−0.004	−1.260		0.6	−0.006	−2.173	*	2.8	−0.007	−2.001	*	3.3
Recovery cost	−0.085	−1.207		0.5	−0.070	−1.162		1.2	0.099	1.212		1.6

(continued)

Table 12.4 (continued)

Reference alternative in estimation: (f) will change both the job and residential location	(d) will change the job, but will not change the residential location, and will reinforce the house				(e) will not change the job, but will change the residential location			
Explanatory variable	Param	t-score		VR (%)	Param	t-score		VR (%)
Constant term	−0.129	−0.133			3.010	4.025	**	
Disaster frequency	−0.683	−2.285	*	10.4	−0.072	−0.278		0.1
Disaster intensity	−0.453	−4.469	**	40.3	−0.114	−1.355		2.3
Inundation	−0.266	−1.536		4.4	−0.264	−1.808	*	4.6
Salinity intrusion	−0.360	−2.081	*	8.1	−0.547	−3.753	**	19.9
Isolated by water	−0.248	−1.385		3.8	0.156	1.017		1.6
Road destroyed	0.267	1.549		4.4	−0.383	−2.670	**	9.5
Financial ability	−0.033	−0.211		0.1	−0.413	−3.435	**	27.2
Physical strength	0.220	1.645		5.9	0.082	0.768		1.2
Capability of family structure	0.063	0.437		0.4	−0.159	−1.376		3.8
Available help from neighborhood	−0.005	−0.036		0.0	0.091	0.804		0.8
Knowledge about disaster	−0.150	−1.109		2.5	−0.165	−1.537		3.7
Available time to tackle disaster	−0.084	−0.697		0.9	0.177	1.827	+	4.9
Help from government during recovery	0.369	1.296		3.3	−0.481	−2.312	*	12.2
Help from community during recovery	−0.100	−0.484		0.5	0.240	1.413		3.5
Help from neighborhood during recovery	0.357	1.561		4.9	−0.291	−1.463		3.0
Recovery time	0.000	−0.050		0.01	−0.003	−1.163		1.6
Recovery cost	0.201	2.275	*	10.0	−0.015	−0.242		0.1

Initial log-likelihood: −4271.555; Final log-likelihood: −3798.506; McFadden's Rho-squared: 0.1107; Adjusted McFadden's Rho-squared: 0.1040; Sample size: 2384 SP responses

Note + Significant at the 10 % level; *Significant at the 5 % level; **Significant at the 1 % level; *VR* variance ratio in the total variance

Table 12.5 Estimation results of household life adaptation behavior model: cyclone at the coastal area

Reference alternative in estimation: (f) will change both the job and residential location	(a) will change neither the job nor the residential location, and will not reinforce the house				(b) will change neither the job nor the residential location, but will reinforce the house				(c) will change the job, but will not change the residential location, and will not reinforce the house			
Explanatory variable	Param	t-score		VR (%)	Param	t-score		VR (%)	Param	t-score		VR (%)
Constant term	3.762	4.276	**		2.453	3.465	**		3.543	3.633	**	
Disaster frequency	−1.414	−10.187	**	67.3	−0.464	−4.151	**	14.1	−1.085	−7.457	**	42.3
Disaster intensity	−0.333	−3.074	**	7.6	−0.539	−6.534	**	31.6	−0.779	−6.383	**	26.3
Inundation	−0.033	−0.183		0.02	0.548	3.889	**	12.0	0.210	1.122		0.9
Salinity intrusion	−0.460	−2.554	*	4.9	−0.511	−3.638	**	10.7	−0.691	−3.686	**	10.0
Isolated by water	−0.594	−3.138	**	7.8	−0.223	−1.551		2.0	−0.520	−2.664	**	5.3
Road destroyed	0.391	2.306	*	3.5	0.301	2.167	*	3.7	0.274	1.521		1.6
Financial ability	0.001	0.004		0.00	−0.134	−1.129		1.5	−0.079	−0.515		0.2
Physical strength	−0.218	−1.649	+	2.6	−0.348	−3.252	**	12.8	−0.209	−1.492		2.5
Capability of family structure	−0.033	−0.235		0.0	0.167	1.472		2.3	0.181	1.217		1.4
Available help from neighborhood	0.129	0.942		0.6	0.186	1.686	+	2.0	0.032	0.220		0.0
Knowledge about disaster	0.013	0.099		0.01	0.116	1.112		1.2	−0.272	−1.926	+	3.0
Available time to tackle disaster	−0.178	−1.531		1.6	0.088	0.926		0.8	−0.174	−1.386		1.5
Help from government during recovery	−0.313	−1.250		1.7	−0.115	−0.557		0.4	−0.339	−1.238		1.5
Help from community during recovery	−0.152	−0.725		0.5	−0.179	−1.059		1.2	0.221	0.955		0.8
Help from neighborhood during recovery	−0.367	−1.553		1.6	−0.304	−1.640		2.1	0.063	0.263		0.1
Recovery time	−0.001	−0.392		0.1	0.000	0.008		0.00	−0.003	−1.080		1.0

(continued)

Table 12.5 (continued)

Reference alternative in estimation: (f) will change both the job and residential location	(a) will change neither the job nor the residential location, and will not reinforce the house				(b) will change neither the job nor the residential location, but will reinforce the house				(c) will change the job, but will not change the residential location, and will not reinforce the house			
Explanatory variable	Param	t-score		VR (%)	Param	t-score		VR (%)	Param	t-score		VR (%)
Recovery cost	−0.034	−0.462		0.2	−0.074	−1.250		1.6	0.122	1.376		1.5

Reference alternative in estimation: (f) will change both the job and residential location	(d) will change the job, but will not change the residential location, and will reinforce the house				(e) will not change the job, but will change the residential location			
Explanatory variable	Param	t-score		VR (%)	Param	t-score		VR (%)
Constant term	1.068	1.149			3.312	**		
Disaster frequency	−0.413	−2.945	**	20.1	−4.100	**		22.8
Disaster intensity	−0.417	−3.986	**	36.6	−0.737			0.6
Inundation	0.050	0.278		0.2	3.082	**		11.6
Salinity intrusion	−0.145	−0.815		1.5	−1.786	+		3.9
Isolated by water	−0.129	−0.703		1.2	1.972	*		5.1
Road destroyed	0.122	0.692		1.1	−1.025			1.3
Financial ability	0.043	0.275		0.2	−2.242	*		10.3
Physical strength	−0.103	−0.748		2.0	−3.016	**		17.1
Capability of family structure	0.193	1.312		5.2	1.592			4.0
Available help from neighborhood	0.010	0.067		0.01	1.305			2.0
Knowledge about disaster	−0.080	−0.581		0.8	1.323			2.3
Available time to tackle disaster	−0.338	−2.775	**	18.5	−0.319			0.1
Help from government during recovery	−0.091	−0.339		0.3	−2.004			8.3
Help from community during recovery	−0.273	−1.276		4.7	0.775			0.9
Help from neighborhood during recovery	0.148	0.648		1.0	−2.739	**		8.5
Recovery time	0.002	0.574		1.0	−0.083			0.01
Recovery cost	0.116	1.371		5.6	−0.857			1.3

Initial log-likelihood: −4271.555; Final log-likelihood: −3798.506; McFadden's Rho-squared: 0.1107; Adjusted McFadden's Rho-squared: 0.1040; Sample size: 2384 SP responses

Note + Signicant at the 10 % level; *Signicant at the 5 % level; **Signicant at the 1 % level; *VR* variance ratio in the total variance

Table 12.6 Estimation results of household life adaptation behavior model: flood at the inland area

Reference alternative in estimation: (f) will change both the job and residential location	(a) will change neither the job nor the residential location, and will not reinforce the house				(b) will change neither the job nor the residential location, but will reinforce the house				(c) will change the job, but will not change the residential location, and will not reinforce the house			
Explanatory variable	Param	t-score		VR (%)	Param	t-score		VR (%)	Param	t-score		VR (%)
Constant term	4.065	4.663	**		2.949	3.615	**		1.356	1.465		
Disaster frequency	−2.139	−5.659	**	23.5	−1.106	−3.232	**	13.3	−0.099	−0.252		0.2
Disaster intensity	−0.354	−3.140	**	5.9	−0.570	−5.596	**	26.5	−0.317	−2.733	**	20.8
Inundation	0.214	1.023		0.7	0.140	0.755		0.6	−0.042	−0.197		0.1
Isolated by water	0.113	0.550		0.2	0.310	1.706	+	2.7	0.498	2.370	*	13.8
Road destroyed	0.203	1.019		0.6	0.295	1.651	+	2.8	−0.306	−1.465		5.7
Financial ability	0.170	1.163		1.6	0.215	1.602		4.1	0.256	1.655	+	8.5
Physical strength	0.046	0.314		0.1	0.067	0.499		0.3	0.112	0.722		2.5
Capability of family structure	−0.224	−1.580		2.1	−0.233	−1.778	+	4.2	−0.186	−1.239		6.0
Available help from neighborhood	−0.414	−2.795	**	5.8	−0.190	−1.376		2.6	−0.174	−1.097		3.5
Knowledge about disaster	0.116	0.773		0.5	−0.282	−2.098	*	6.1	−0.250	−1.628		9.7
Available time to tackle disaster	0.162	1.322		1.2	0.238	2.102	*	6.7	0.185	1.431		8.2
Help from government during recovery	−1.436	−4.952	**	29.0	−0.511	−1.847	+	5.9	−0.124	−0.383		0.6
Help from community during recovery	−0.078	−0.332		0.1	−0.315	−1.491		3.2	−0.333	−1.355		7.0

(continued)

Table 12.6 (continued)

Reference alternative in estimation: (f) will change both the job and residential location	(a) will change neither the job nor the residential location, and will not reinforce the house				(b) will change neither the job nor the residential location, but will reinforce the house				(c) will change the job, but will not change the residential location, and will not reinforce the house			
Explanatory variable	Param	t-score		VR (%)	Param	t-score		VR (%)	Param	t-score		VR (%)
Help from neighborhood during recovery	−0.456	−1.536		1.2	−0.043	−0.170		0.0	−0.369	−1.225		4.0
Recovery time	0.025	3.609	**	25.8	0.019	2.739	**	20.9	0.004	0.421		0.4
Recovery cost	−0.112	−1.768	+	1.8	−0.008	−0.133		0.02	−0.104	−1.599		9.1

Reference alternative in estimation: (f) will change both the job and residential location	(d) will change the job, but will not change the residential location, and will reinforce the house				(e) will not change the job, but will change the residential location				
Explanatory variable	Param	t-score		VR (%)	Param	t-score			VR (%)
Constant term	0.205	0.186			1.445	1.548			
Disaster frequency	−0.959	−2.088	*	8.0	0.245	0.618			1.6
Disaster intensity	−0.003	−0.024		0.00	−0.088	−0.771			2.0
Inundation	0.995	3.876	**	25.9	−0.178	−0.833			2.9
Isolated by water	0.457	1.817	+	5.0	0.198	0.975			3.6
Road destroyed	0.252	1.033		1.8	0.337	1.652	+		10.6
Financial ability	0.056	0.307		0.2	0.229	1.493			10.8
Physical strength	0.093	0.514		0.7	−0.116	−0.754			3.4
Capability of family structure	−0.563	−3.169	**	21.2	−0.199	−1.362			8.8
Available help from neighborhood	0.144	0.733		0.9	−0.455	−3.006	**		42.2
Knowledge about disaster	−0.250	−1.335		4.1	0.045	0.296			0.4
Available time to tackle disaster	0.312	1.990	*	10.8	0.028	0.214			0.2
Help from government during recovery	0.035	0.090		0.02	−0.259	−0.802			3.8
Help from community during recovery	0.169	0.583		0.7	−0.017	−0.069			0.03

Table 12.6 (continued)

Reference alternative in estimation: (f) will change both the job and residential location	(d) will change the job, but will not change the residential location, and will reinforce the house				(e) will not change the job, but will change the residential location				
Explanatory variable	Param	t-score		VR (%)	Param	t-score			VR (%)
Help from neighborhood during recovery	−0.635	−1.654	+	4.8	−0.154	−0.529			1.2
Recovery time	0.011	1.124		2.2	0.009	1.074			6.4
Recovery cost	−0.178	−2.345	*	13.6	−0.046	−0.692			2.1

Initial log-likelihood: −2486.962; Final log-likelihood: −2224.902; McFadden's Rho-squared: 0.1054; Adjusted McFadden's Rho-squared: 0.0943; Sample size: 1388 SP responses
Note + Significant at the 10 % level; *Significant at the 5 % level; **Significant at the 1 % level; *VR* variance ratio in the total variance

(2) ***Life adaptation to the impacts of cyclones in the coastal area***

The impacts of a cyclone are observed with respect to the choices of "(b) change neither job nor residential location, and reinforce the house" and "(c) change job, do not change residential location, and do not reinforce the house", where cyclone frequency, intensity, inundation, and salinity intrusion are identified as the most influential factors in terms of statistical significance and the explained variance ratios. Specifically, cyclone frequency is decisive in the choice of alternative (a), because its variance ratio is 67.3 %, which is much larger than that of any other factor. Cyclone intensity mostly affects alternatives (b), (c), and (d), with variance ratios being 31.6, 26.3, and 36.6 %, respectively. The influences of salinity intrusion on (b) and (c) are also relatively large, with variance ratios being about 10 %. Isolation of residential areas by water is influential on (a), (c), and (e), but the variance ratios are just 7.8, 5.3, and 5.1 %, respectively, which is much smaller than those for other cyclone attributes, except for road damage. Road damage influences (a) and (b), although its influence is even smaller.

The third largest influence on (b) is physical strength, and that on (d) is time available to respond to disasters. Other capability-related factors are estimated to affect life adaptation behavior to a statistically significant extent, such as time available to respond to disasters influencing (b), and knowledge about disasters affecting (c); however, these influences are quite small. As for help-related factors, receiving help from the neighborhood during the recovery period reduces the probability that households will choose "(e) will not change jobs, but will change residential location". Finally, recovery time and cost do not affect any adaptation behavior.

(3) ***Life adaptation behaviors under the impacts of inland flooding***

All flood attributes affect some life adaptation behaviors in the inland area, but their influences are limited in terms of variance ratios. As for "(a) change neither job nor residential location, and do not reinforce the house", the most influential factor is help from the government during the recovery period (VR = 29.0 %), followed by recovery time (VR = 25.8 %) and flood frequency (VR = 23.5 %). In contrast, "(b) change neither job nor residential location, and reinforce the house", "(c) change job, do not change residential location, and do not reinforce the house", and "(d) change job but not residential location, and reinforce the house" are mostly affected by flood attributes: (b) and (c) by flood intensity (26.5 and 20.8 %, respectively), and (d) by inundation (VR = 25.9 %). In the case of "(e) do not change jobs, but change residential location", available help from the neighborhood is most influential (VR = 42.2 %), followed by financial ability (VR = 10.8 %) and road damage (VR = 10.6 %).

Other major influential factors are isolation of residential area by water (VR = 13.8 %) on alternative (c), capability of family structure on (d) (VR = 21.2 %), recovery time on (b) (VR = 20.9 %), and recovery cost (VR = 13.6 %) and available time to tackle disasters (10.8 %) on (d). Knowledge about disasters is also found to influence alternative (b), even though its influence is limited (VR = 6.1 %).

12.6 Tourists' Stated Adaptation in Response to Floods and Cyclones

12.6.1 Data

12.6.1.1 Questionnaire Design

For the purpose of this study, a questionnaire consisting of four main parts was designed. The first part includes questions regarding tourists' travel schedule for their current trips in Bangladesh (such as destination choice, travel date, travel mode, size of travel party, duration of stay, and expenditure) and their subjective evaluation of destinations visited.

The second part investigates tourists' SP responses regarding visitor behavior in Bangladesh in different flood and cyclone scenarios (i.e., their reported behavior in the hypothetical scenarios). The factors and levels describing these scenarios were developed in consultation with local experts involved either professionally or academically with disaster management.

The flood scenarios are defined by:

- frequency (three levels: every year, once every two years, or once every three years).
- intensity (three levels: reaches knees, reaches waist, or reaches chest or above).
- permanent/frequent inundation (two levels: yes or no).
- permanent salinity intrusion (two levels: yes or no).

- visited area is isolated by water (two levels: yes or no).
- roads to other cities are destroyed permanently (two levels: yes or no).

The cyclone scenarios are defined by:

- frequency (three levels: twice a year, once a year, or once every two years).
- intensity (three levels: some structural damage to houses, complete structural collapse in a small number of houses, or complete collapse in many houses).
- frequent inundation (two levels: yes or no).
- permanent salinity intrusion (two levels: yes or no).
- area visited is isolated by water (two levels: yes or no).
- roads to other cities are destroyed permanently (two levels: yes or no).

The choice set included five alternatives: (1) still travel as planned, (2) cancel the trip, (3) change to other destinations, (4) change travel modes/routes, (5) change the stay duration and/or timing. A fractional factorial experimental design was used in the generation of the choice situations. As a result, 16 SP profiles were generated for flood and cyclone scenarios. To reduce the burden on each respondent, each questionnaire included only four SP profiles for either flood or cyclone.

The third part investigates respondents' adaptation behavior to previous climate disasters. Respondents were asked to provide information about two recent trips that were influenced by climate disasters, including the disaster type, their information source, the timing of the disaster (i.e., before or during their trip), their travel schedule (destination country, travel date, travel purpose, companion, travel mode, duration of stay, expenditure, etc.), and their response to the disaster.

The fourth part collects information on individual and household characteristics, including gender, age, education level, occupation, household annual income, and travel experiences during the previous year (i.e., the number of tourism trips taken in the previous year, including both domestic and international travels).

12.6.1.2 Survey Implementation

The survey was conducted between the middle of January and the first week of February, 2013, which was the peak season for both domestic and international tourism. The survey focused on two main tourism regions of Bangladesh: one in the southeastern part, which has the world's longest natural sea beach, and the other in the southern part, which has the largest mangrove forest in the world.

The survey was carried out in nine zones of the above two regions by two survey teams. Each survey team consisted of one supervisor and several interviewers. The questionnaire was designed in English. For international tourists, the questionnaire was filled out by the tourists themselves. For domestic tourists, the survey was conducted through face-to-face interviews, and the questionnaire was filled out by the interviewers.

12.6.1.3 Data Description

As a result, 1000 valid questionnaires were obtained (537 domestic tourists and 463 international tourists). The data characteristics are summarized in Table 12.7. It is observed that 64.3 % of the respondents are male, three-quarters of whom were under 40 years of age, and about two-thirds of whom traveled with family or friends. In comparison with domestic tourists, international tourists have a more equal gender distribution, and are wealthier, older, and have more travel experience.

12.6.2 Aggregation Analysis

Figure 12.27 shows the cross aggregation analysis of several individual characteristics and tourists' adaptation behavior in response to floods and cyclones. The findings are summarized below:

(a) Gender: Male tourists are less likely to cancel their travel plans in response to climate disasters.
(b) Age: The probability of canceling or changing travel plans increases with age.
(c) Type of tourist: International tourists are more likely than domestic tourists to cancel or change their travel plans.
(d) Travel experience: Tourists with more travel experience are less likely to cancel their plans or change their travel timing.
(e) Traveling companions: Tourists who travel alone are more likely to cancel their plans.
(f) Travel mode: Tourists who travel by private car are more likely to cancel their plans in response to climate disasters.

12.6.3 Modeling Analysis

In this section, tourists' reported adaptation behavior in response to climate disasters is analyzed using an MNL model, which includes five alternatives: (1) still travel as planned, (2) cancel the trip, (3) change to other destinations, (4) change travel modes/routes, and (5) change the stay duration and/or timing of travel.

Because the cross aggregation revealed that gender, age, travel experience, type of tourist, companions, and travel mode have significant influences on responses to climate disasters, these variables are included as explanatory variables to represent reported behavior. Additionally, it is expected that tourist satisfaction with their travel may influence their future behavior as well. In the survey, respondents were asked to report their travel schedule for their current trip to Bangladesh

Table 12.7 Summary of survey data characteristics

Selected items	Domestic (537) (%)	International (463) (%)	Total (1000) (%)
Gender			
Male	71.1	56.4 %	64.3 %
Female	28.9	43.6	35.7
Age			
<30 years old	50.8	25.1	38.9
30 ~ 39 years old	33.7	38.9	36.1
40 ~ 49 years old	9.9	27.0	17.8
> = 50 years old	5.6	9.0	7.2
Annual household income			
<10,000 USD	67.4	17.3	44.2
10,000–50,000 USD	28.3	44.9	36.0
50,000–100,000 USD	3.5	18.8	10.6
>100,000 USD	0.8	19.0	9.2
Education level			
University or above	62.4	56.6	59.7
Others	37.6	43.4	40.3
Travel experience (Including both domestic and international travel)			
None	77.5	18.1	50.0
Once	16.4	33.1	24.1
More than once	6.1	48.8	25.9
Travel companion			
Alone	5.9	11.2	8.4
With family	37.6	34.1	36.0
With friends	37.8	28.9	33.7
With colleagues	7.6	9.3	8.4
Group travel	9.7	11.2	10.4
Others	1.4	5.3	2.9

and their subjective evaluation of destinations visited. The respondents were also asked to evaluate the tourism destination on a five-point scale, anchored by "1" indicating least satisfied and "5" indicating most satisfied. Twelve individual components and overall satisfaction were included in the questionnaire to obtain the tourists' subjective evaluations. Given that the satisfaction levels of different components would be correlated, only overall satisfaction level is used as the explanatory variable in the analysis. Furthermore, tourists' previous behavior is included as an explanatory variable to examine whether there is habit persistence in tourists' adaptation behavior in response to disasters.

As mentioned above, the survey covers two types of disasters (i.e., floods and cyclones). Tourists' responses to these two disasters are analyzed separately. Six attributes that describe the disaster scenarios are included in the model to examine the impact of disaster severity on tourist behavior. Table 12.8 lists the explanatory variables in the analysis of tourists' stated adaptation behavior.

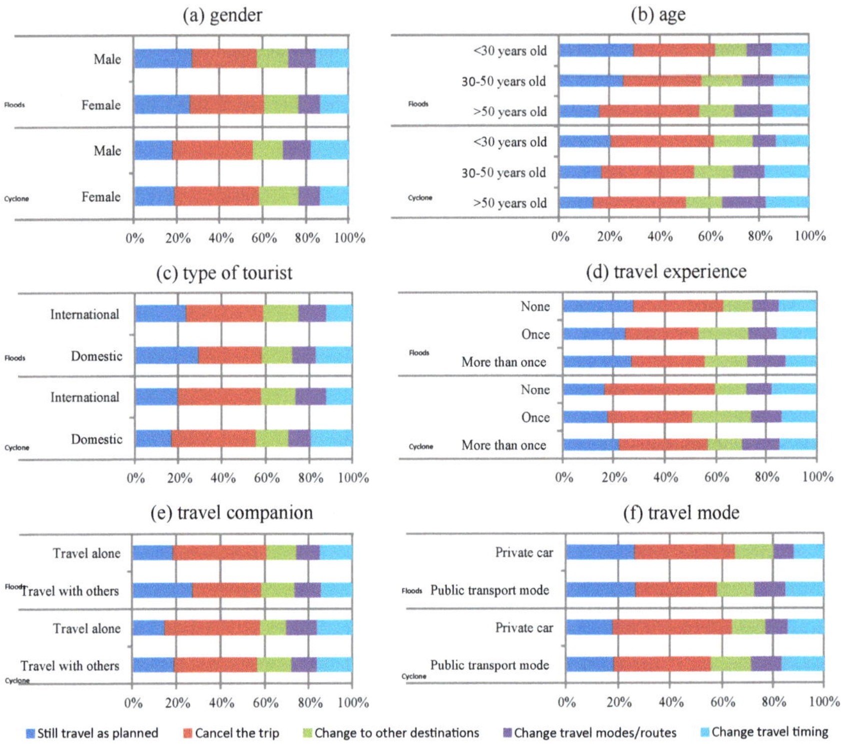

Fig. 12.27 Cross aggregation between individual characteristics and tourist's adaptation behavior

Tables 12.9 and 12.10 display model estimation results for tourist behavior in response to flood and cyclone disasters, respectively. For both flood and cyclone, most of the explanatory variables are statistically significant at the 95 or 90 % levels. The estimated parameters for individual characteristics and trip-related variables, including gender, age, travel experience, type of tourist, companion, and travel mode, show similar results to the cross aggregation. It is worth noting that satisfaction level has a significant influence on tourist behavior under climate disasters. This suggests that tourists with higher satisfaction levels are less likely to cancel their trips or change to other destinations when they experience climate disasters. Tourists' previous adaptation behavior has a significant influence on the alternative of "cancel the trip". The positive parameter indicates that tourists who canceled their trips in response to climate disasters previously are more likely to behave similarly when confronted by climate disasters in the future.

In terms of attributes related to the severity of floods, almost all the parameters show positive influences. It can be concluded that tourists are more likely to cancel or change their travel plans if floods become more severe. It is interesting that while the frequency of floods significantly increases tourists' probability

Table 12.8 List of explanatory variables

Explanatory variables	Description
Individual and trip related variables	
Gender	1: Male; 0: Female
Age	Actual age
Travel experience	Numbers of tourism trips last year
Type of tourist	1: International trip; 0: Domestic trip
Travel companion	1: Alone; 0: Otherwise
Travel mode	1: Private car; 0: Public transport mode
Satisfaction	Overall satisfaction level on a scale from 1 to 5
Previous adaptive behavior	1: Chose this adaptation alternative in the past; 0: Otherwise
Disaster scenarios	
Frequency	Frequency every year
Intensity (flood)	1: Reach waist or above; 0: Otherwise
Intensity (cyclone)	1: Complete house structure collapse; 0: Otherwise
Frequent inundation	1: Yes; 0: No
Permanent salinity intrusion	1: Yes; 0: No
Isolated by water	1: Yes; 0: No
Transportation is destroyed	1: Yes; 0: No

Table 12.9 Model estimation result for tourist behavior under flood disaster

Explanatory variable	Cancel		Change to other destinations		Change travel modes/routes		Change travel timing	
	Parameter		Parameter		Parameter		Parameter	
Individual and trip related variables								
Gender	−0.15	*	−0.09		0.19		0.01	
Age	0.31	**	0.27	**	0.37	**	0.22	**
Travel experience	−0.05	**	−0.01		−0.03		−0.08	**
Type of tourist	0.16	*	0.23	*	0.31	**	−0.10	
Travel companion	0.50	**	0.12		0.07		0.41	**
Travel mode	0.29	**	0.01		−0.38		−0.06	
Satisfaction	−0.62	**	−0.27	**	−0.01		−0.01	
Previous adaptation behavior	0.17	*	−0.02		0.14		0.08	
Disaster scenarios								
Frequency	1.73	**	1.32	**	1.52	**	1.62	**
Intensity	0.05		-0.29		−0.13		0.25	*
Frequent inundation	0.43	**	0.35	**	0.28	**	0.38	**

Table 12.9 (continued)

Explanatory variable	Cancel		Change to other destinations		Change travel modes/routes		Change travel timing	
	Parameter		Parameter		Parameter		Parameter	
Permanent salinity intrusion	0.35	**	0.19	*	0.26	**	0.06	
Isolated by water	0.56	**	0.26	*	0.01		0.07	
Transportation is destroyed	0.56	**	0.41	**	0.23	**	0.31	**
Initial log-likelihood	−6418.43							
Converged log-likelihood	−4783.42							
McFadden's Rho-squared	0.25							

*significant at the 90 % level, **significant at the 95 % level

of canceling or changing their travel plans, the intensity of floods only influences the alternative of "change travel timing". This indicates that when flood intensity increases, tourists are more likely to change their travel timing rather than to cancel their trip.

The results for cyclones are similar to those for floods, except that intensity significantly affects tourists' decisions to cancel their trip in response to cyclone disasters. This suggests that while the increased intensity of floods would increase the probability of tourists changing their travel timing, they would be more likely to cancel their trip if the intensity of cyclones increased.

12.6.4 Summary

This study investigated tourist adaptation behavior in response to climate disasters in Bangladesh. The findings can be summarized as: (1) there are more factors influencing the cancelation of trips than other types of adaptation behavior. This indicates that trip cancelation behavior would easily be influenced by various individual and trip attributes. Therefore, the question of how to reduce trip cancelations should receive close attention in tourism policy decisions in Bangladesh. (2) Most variables related to disaster severity (e.g., frequency, inundation, and damage to transportation networks) have statistically significant influences on adaptation behavior. (3) If climate disasters were to become more serious, one could expect more cancelations and changes of destination, especially for international

Table 12.10 Model estimation result for tourist behavior under cyclone disaster

Explanatory variable	Cancel		Change to other destinations		Change travel modes/routes		Change travel timing	
	Parameter		Parameter		Parameter		Parameter	
Individual and trip related variables								
Gender	−0.03		−0.23	**	0.24	*	0.18	
Age	0.28	**	0.21	**	0.34	**	0.39	**
Travel experience	−0.04	*	−0.05	*	−0.07	**	−0.05	
Type of tourist	0.42	**	0.15		0.13		0.72	**
Travel companion	0.26		−0.10		0.25		0.25	
Travel mode	0.41	**	−0.02		−0.19		0.09	
Satisfaction	−0.47	**	−0.21	**	−0.07		−0.01	
Previous adaptation behavior	0.21	*	0.10		−0.15		0.11	
Disaster scenarios								
Frequency	0.78	**	0.66	**	0.91	**	0.77	**
Intensity	0.15	*	0.02		0.12		0.03	
Frequent inundation	0.60	**	0.57	**	0.58	**	0.59	
Permanent salinity intrusion	0.07		0.05		0.01		0.17	
Isolated by water	0.27	**	0.11		0.32	**	0.22	*
Transportation is destroyed	0.41	**	0.08		0.21	**	0.14	
Initial log-likelihood	6436.14							
Converged log-likelihood	4757.64							
McFadden's Rho-squared	0.26							

*significant at the 90 % level, **significant at the 95 % level

tourists. This indicates that the national government should pay more attention to preparation for future disasters in tourism policy decisions. To improve resilience in overseas markets, it is recommended that regional planning be coordinated to promote alternate destinations within the country as a means of attracting international tourists who, as this research suggests, are more likely to switch destinations in the face of climate disasters. Satisfaction with travel is influential in decisions on both trip cancelation and change of destination. This suggests the importance of enhancing tourism service quality in Bangladesh.

12.7 Conclusions

Climate-related disasters have caused various kinds of damage to human lifelines, such as houses, roads, schools, agricultural land, factories, electric power stations, water supply facilities, and other public facilities. Without these lifelines, people could not survive, and damage to these lifelines would seriously affect people's lives. For example, as Kotzee and Reyers (2016) noted in a review, "studies on the impacts of severe flood events in the last decade report on unpredictable, usually rapid onset events that lead to substantial financial losses, destruction of infrastructure, displacement, and death." (p. 45). Such impacts are especially serious in low-income countries where various types of infrastructure are underdeveloped, even for current needs (Conway and Schipper 2011; Thakur et al. 2011; Arndt et al. 2012; Schweikert et al. 2014). Various studies have examined the impacts of climate change on human life, economic activity, physical assets, and the environment, and demonstrate the need to address these impacts proactively to minimize the damage to current and future development (Schweikert et al. 2014). Some researchers have pointed out that the literature on climate change impacts and adaptation in the infrastructure sector is primarily qualitative (e.g., Arndt et al. 2012). Various studies have shown quite a high probability that climate-related disasters will occur in the future (IPCC 2007). However, it is still uncertain where the disasters will occur nearby personal daily activity areas, and how great the impacts on human life will be. Under such uncertain situations, households must make difficult decisions on whether to continue their current lives as usual or to adapt themselves to uncertain future disasters at the expense of various monetary and mental costs. In particular, because jobs and residences currently meet people's most fundamental needs in life, changing these in response to climate-related disasters implies that people must simultaneously change other life behaviors, such as children's education, members' social networks, and/or various daily activities, accordingly. On the other hand, participating in international tourism activities has become an essential part of many people's lives in developed countries. This phenomenon will continue, and provide many developing countries with special economic development opportunities via the promotion of international tourism. Considering the negative impacts of climate-related disasters observed in various literature studies, it is obvious that providing disaster-resilient tourism is crucial for developing countries vulnerable to disasters, such as Bangladesh.

Climate change is a reality to which societies need to respond with appropriate and sustainable adaptive actions. However, little is known about how households, especially those in developing countries vulnerable to climate-related disasters, adapt themselves to survive with the future impacts of the disasters. In this study in the context of Bangladesh, we made an initial attempt to examine quantitatively adaptation behaviors and measures in a country at an ever-increasing risk of climate disasters at the household and individual levels by focusing on intercity travel adaptation, life adaptation, and tourism adaptation behaviors. A utility-based discrete-choice model was adopted to estimate how households and tourists would change their behavior in response to future impacts of floods and cyclones using a stated preference survey. The findings are useful to help identify the barriers to the adoption of adaptation measures, the roles of different stakeholders in implementing adaptation measures, and the directions of adaptation measures in the future, even though further studies are required to derive more robust conclusions based on advanced modeling techniques with more realistic decision-making mechanisms.

In the face of disasters, people have to make various decisions and take various actions to return to normal life. However, the question is whether their lives return to normal with these efforts. These efforts may or may not be made depending on their capabilities, the availability of social support, future concerns, or other considerations. People in countries such as Bangladesh have often experienced climate-related disasters. Whether people are capable of adapting to them depends not only on personal efforts, but also on external support. Even if people are capable of adapting to the disasters, they may still face difficult decisions, depending on how they perceive the uncertainty of future disasters at the level of their daily action space. Disaster-adaptive behavior is closely related to social exclusion issues, i.e., unequal treatment and situations of different population groups in society (e.g., Jones and Boyd 2011; Ruiz Meza 2014; Ensor et al. 2015). In this regard, adaptive capacity becomes a key concern. This is defined as the ability of social actors to make deliberate changes that influence the resilience of their complex social–ecological systems (Walker et al. 2004; Ruiz Meza 2014). Feasible adaptation measures should be proposed, considering people's acceptance of various interventions and examined by integrating insights from both interdisciplinary and cross-sectoral studies. On the other hand, climate-related disasters sometimes bring benefits. For example, land may become more fertile after a flood. Such positive impacts should also be identified and fully exploited in adaptation measures. Because climate-related disasters damage various sectors simultaneously, joint efforts from these sectors are required. It is necessary to clarify the kinds of cross-sectoral approaches that are more effective at various time scales: long term, medium term, and short term.

Acknowledgments The above researches are funded by Ministry of Education, Culture, Sports, Science & Technology (MEXT) in Japan under the Special Coordination Funds for Promotion of Science and Technology at Hiroshima University.

References

Adger WN, Huq S, Brown K, Hulme M (2003) Adaptation to climate change in the developing world. Prog Dev Stud 3(3):179–195

Ahsan UA (2006) Bangladesh: climate change impacts and vulnerability—a synthesis. Department of Environment, Government of Bangladesh, Climate Change Cell

Ahmed F, Rose G, Jakob C (2013) Examining the impact of changes in weather on commuter cyclist's travel behavior. Compendium of Papers CD-ROM, the 92nd annual meeting of the Transportation Research Board, Washington D.C., 13–17 Jan 2013

Alam MJB, Hoque Alamgir M, Hoque MdM (2002) Assessment of economic loss caused by flood damaged transportation network in engineering concerns of floods a 1998 perspective. Directorate of Advisory, Extension and Research Services, BUET, Dhaka, Bangladesh
Arentze T, Timmermans HJP (2007) Congestion pricing scenarios and change of job or residential location: results of a stated adaptation experiment. J Transp Geogr 15:56–61
Arndt C, Chinowsky P, Strzepek K, Thurlow J (2012) Climate change, growth and infrastructure investment: the case of Mozambique. Rev Dev Econ 16(3):463–475
Artur L, Hilhorst D (2012) Everyday realities of climate change adaptation in Moazambique. Glob Environ Change 22:529–536
Aultman-Hall L, Lane D, Lambert RR (2009) Assessing the impact of weather and season on pedestrian traffic volumes. Transp Res Rec 2140:35–43
Barnett J, Adger WN (2003) Climate dangers and atoll countries. Clim Change 61:321–337
Begum RA, Sarkar MSK, Jaafar AH, Pereira JJ (2014) Toward conceptual frameworks for linking disaster risk reduction and climate change adaptation. Int J Disaster Risk Reduct 10(A):362–373
Böcker L, Dijst M, Prillwitz J (2013a) Impact of everyday weather on individual daily travel behaviours in perspective: a literature review. Transp Rev 33(1):71–91
Böcker L, Prillwitz J, Dijst M (2013b) Climate change impacts on mode choice and traveled distances: a comparison of present with 2050 weather conditions for the Randstad Holland. J Transp Geogr 28:176–185
Chang Y, Lee M-A, Lee K-T, Shao K-T (2013) Adaptation of fisheries and mariculture management to extreme oceanic environmental changes and climate variability in Taiwan. Marine Policy 38:476–482
Choocharukul K, Van HT, Fujii S (2008) Psychological effects of travel behavioural preference of residential location choice. Transp Res Part A 42:116–124
Conway D, Schipper ELF (2011) Adaptation to climate change in Africa: challenges and opportunities identified from Ethiopia. Glob Environ Change 21(1):227–237
Cools M, Creemers L (2013) The dual role of weather forecasts on changes in activity-travel behavior. J Transp Geogr 28:167–175
Cools M, Moons E, Creemers L, Wets G (2010) Changes in travel behavior response to weather conditions. Transp Res Rec 2157:22–28
Dasgupta S, Pandey K, Huq M, Khan ZH, Masud MS, Ahmed MMZ, Mukherjee N (2010) Climate proofing infrastructure in Bangladesh: the incremental cost of limiting inland monsoon flood damage. The WORLD BANK. http://siteresources.worldbank.org/INTEAER/Resources/Inland.pdf. Accessed 29 May 2016
Denstadli J, Jacobsen J, Lohmann M (2011) Tourist perceptions of summer weather in Scandinavia. Annals Tourism Res 38:920–940
Ding W, Ren W, Li P, Hou X, Sun X, Li X, Xie J, Ding Y (2014) Evaluation of the livelihood vulnerability of pastoral households in Northern China to natural disasters and climate change. Rangeland J 36(6):535–543
Doevenspeck M (2011) The thin line between choice and flight: environment and migration in rural Benin. Int Migr 49:50–68
Elias W, Albert G, Shiftan Y (2013) Travel behavior in the face of surface transportation terror attacks. Transp Policy 28:114–122
Ensor JE, Park SE, Hoddy ET, Ratner BD (2015) A rights-based perspective on adaptive capacity. Glob Environ Change 31:38–49
Eugenio-Martin JL, Campos-Soria J (2010) Climate in the region of origin and destination choice in outbound tourism demand. Tour Manag 31(6):744–753
Field CB, Barros V, Stocker TF, Qin D, Dokken DJ, Ebi KL, Mastrandrea MD, Mach KJ, Plattner G-K, Allen SK, Tignor M, Midgley PM (2012) IPCC, 2012: Managing the risks of extreme events and disasters to advance climate change adaptation. A Special report of working groups I and II of the intergovernmental panel on climate change. Cambridge University Press, Cambridge, UK, 582 pp

GAR (2011) 2011 Global assessment report on disaster risk reduction: revealing risk, redefining development. United Nations International Strategy for Disaster Reduction (UNISDR)
Gómez Martín MB (2005) Weather, climate and tourism a geographical perspective. Annals Tourism Res 32(3):571–591
Gössling S, Hall CM (2006) Uncertainties in predicting tourist flows under scenarios of climate change. Clim Change 79(3–4):163–173
Gössling S, Scott D, Hall CM, Ceron JP, Dubois G (2012) Consumer behaviour and demand response of tourists to climate change. Annals Tourism Res 39(1):36–58
Gray C (2011) Soil quality and human migration in Kenya and Uganda. Glob Environ Change 21:421–430
Grothmann T, Patt A (2005) Adaptive capacity and human cognition: the process of individual adaptation to climate change. Glob Environ Change 15:199–213
Habiba U, Shaw R, Takeuchi Y (2012) Farmer's perception and adaptation practices to cope with drought: perspectives from Northwestern Bangladesh. Int J Disaster Risk Reduct 1:72–84
Hess JJ, Malilay JN, Parkinson AJ (2008) Climate change: the importance of place. Am J Prev Med 35:468–478
IPCC (2007) Summary for policymakers. In: Parry ML, Canziani OF, Palutikof JP, van der Linden PJ, Hanson CE (eds.) Climate change 2007: impacts, adaptation and vulnerability. contribution of working group II to the fourth assessment report of the intergovernmental panel on climate change. Cambridge University Press, Cambridge, UK, pp 7–22
Jin J, Francisco H (2013) Sea-level rise adaptation measures in local communities of Zhejiang Province, China. Ocean Coast Manage 71:187–194
Joarder MAM, Miller PW (2013) Factors affecting whether environmental migration is temporary or permanent: evidence from Bangladesh. Glob Environ Change 23:1511–1524
Johansson M, Nyberg L, Evers M, Hansson M (2013) Using education and social learning in capacity building—the IntECR concept. Disaster Prev Manage 22(1):17–28
Jones L, Boyd E (2011) Exploring social barriers to adaptation: insights from western Nepal. Glob Environ Change 21(4):1262–1274
Karim MF, Mimura N (2008) Impacts of climate change and sea-level rise on cyclonic storm surge floods in Bangladesh. Glob Environ Change 18:490–500
Keay K, Simmonds I (2005) The association of rainfall and other weather variables with road traffic volume in Melbourne, Australia. Accid Anal Prev 37:109–124
Khattak AJ, Palma A (1997) The impact of adverse weather conditions on the propensity to change travel decisions: a survey of Brussels commuters. Transp Res Part A 31(3):181–203
Klaiber HA (2014) Migration and household adaptation to climate: a review of empirical research. Energ Econ 46:539–547
Kniveton D, Smith C, Wood S (2011) Agent-based model simulations of future changes in migration flows for Burkina Faso. Glob Environ Change 215:34–40
Kotzee I, Reyers B (2016) Piloting a social-ecological index for measuring flood resilience: a composite index approach. Ecol Ind 60:45–53
Law R (2006) The perceived impact of risks on travel decisions. Int J Tourism Res 8:289–300
Lee HS (2013) Estimation of extreme sea levels along the Bangladesh coast due to storm surge and sea level rise using EEMD and EVA. J Geophys Res Oceans 118:4273–4285
Lepp A, Gibson H (2003) Tourist roles, perceived risk and international tourism. Annals Tourism Res 30(3):606–624
Limb M, Spellman G (2001) Evaluating domestic tourists' attitudes to British weather. A qualitative approach. In: Proceedings of the first international workshop on climate, tourism and recreation. Halkidiki, Greece, 5–10 Oct 2001
Ling FH, Tamura M, Yasuhara K, Ajima K, Trinh CV (2015) Reducing flood risks in rural households: survey of perception and adaptation in the Mekong delta. Clim Change 132(2):209–222
Loo BPY, Chow ASY (2011) Jobs-housing balance in an era of population decentralization: an analytical framework and a case study. J Transp Geogr 19:552–562

Lu QC, Peng ZR (2011) Vulnerability analysis of transportation network under the scenarios of sea level rise. Transp Res Rec 2263:174–181
Lu QC, Peng ZR, Du R (2012) Economic analysis of sea-level rise impacts and adaptation strategies in transportation. Transp Res Rec 2273:54–61
Lu QC, Zhang J, Peng ZR, Rahman ABMS (2014) Inter-city travel behaviour adaptation to flooding and climate change. J Transp Geogr 41(12):148–153
Mahmud T, Prowse M (2012) Corruption in cyclone preparedness and relief efforts in coastal Bangladesh: lessons for climate adaptation? Glob Environ Change 22:933–943
Moore WR (2010) The impact of climate change on Caribbean tourism demand. Curr Issues Tourism 13(5):495–505
Moreno A (2010) Mediterranean tourism and climate change: a survey-based study. Tour Plan Dev 7:253–265
Mortreux C, Barnett J (2009) Climate change, migration and adaptation in Funafuti, Tuvalu. Glob Environ Change 19:105–112
Mozumder P, Flugman E, Randhir T (2011) Adaptation behavior in the face of global climate change: survey responses from experts and decision makers serving the Florida Keys. Ocean Coast Manag 54(1):37–44
National Research Council (2008) Potential impacts of climate change on U.S. transportation. Transportation Research Board Special Report 290. http://onlinepubs.trb.org/onlinepubs/sr/sr290.pdf. Accessed 1 March 2016
Nelson DI (2003) Health impact assessment of climate change in Bangladesh. Environ Impact Assess Rev 23:323–341
Nicholls S (2006) Climate change, tourism and outdoor recreation in Europe. Manag Leisure 11:151–163
Nguyen KV, James H (2013) Measuring household resilience to floods: a case study in the Vietnamese Mekong River Delta. Ecol Soc 18(3): Article Number: 13
Nurlaela S, Curtis C (2012) Modeling household residential location choice and travel behaviour and its relationship with public transport accessibility. Procedia Social Behav Sci 54:56–64
Oluoko-Odingo AA (2011) Vulnerability and adaptation to food insecurity and poverty in Kenya. Ann Assoc Am Geogr 101(1):1–20
Osbahr H, Twyman C, Adger WN, Thomas DSG (2008) Effective livelihoods adaptation to climate change disturbance: scale dimensions of practice in Mozambique. Geoforum 39:1951–1964
Park K, Reisinger Y (2010) Differences in the perceived influence of natural disasters and travel risk on international travel. Tourism Geographies 12(1):1–24
Patt A, Schroter D (2008) Perceptions of climate risk in Mozambique: implications for the success of adaptation strategies. Glob Environ Change 18:458–467
Perry A (2006) Will predicted climate change compromise the sustainability of Mediterranean tourism? J Sustain Tourism 14(4):367–375
Peterson TC, McGuirk M, Houston TG, Horvitz AH, Wehner MF (2008) Climate variability and change with implications for transportation. Transportation Research Board Special Report 290. http://onlinepubs.trb.org/onlinepubs/sr/sr290Many.pdf. Accessed 1 March 2016
Phillips J (2003) Determinants of forecast use among communal farmers in Zimbabwe. In: O'Brien K, Vogel C (eds) Coping with climate variability: the use of seasonal climate forecasts in Southern Africa. Ashgate, Aldershot, UK, pp 110–128
Ruiz Meza LE (2014) Adaptive capacity of small-scale coffee farmers to climate change impacts in the Soconusco region of Chiapas, Mexico. Clim Dev 7(2):100–109
Sahin O, Mohamed S (2013) A spatial temporal decision framework for adaptation to sea level rise. Environ Model Softw 46:129–141
Saldana-Zorrilla SO, Sandberg K (2009) Impacts of climate-related disasters on human migration in Mexico: a spatial model. Clim Change 96:97–118
Saneinejad S, Roorda MJ, Kennedy C (2012) Modeling the impact of weather conditions on active transportation travel behavior. Transp Res Part D 17:129–137

Schiermeier Q (2014) Holding back the tide. Nature 508:164–166
Schweikert A, Chinowsky P, Espinet A, Tarbert M (2014) Climate change and infrastructure impacts: comparing the impact on roads in ten countries through 2100. Procedia Eng 78:306–316
Sermons MW, Koppelman FS (2001) Representing the differences between female and male commuting behaviour in residential location choice models. J Transp Geogr 9:101–110
Sundblad EL, Biel A, Garling T (2007) Cognitive and affective risk judgments related to climate change. J Environ Psychol 27:97–106
Thakur PK, Maiti S, Kingma NC, Hari Prasad V, Aggarwal SP, Bhardwaj A (2011) Estimation of structural vulnerability for flooding using geospatial tools in the rural area of Orissa, India. Nat Hazards 61(2):501–520
Transportation Research Board (2008) Potential impacts of climate change on U.S. transportation. Transportation Research Board Special Report 290. Available: http://onlinepubs.trb.org/onlinepubs/sr/sr290.pdf. Accessed 29 May 2016
UNDP (2004) A Global report "reducing disaster risk: a challenge for development". John S. Swift Co., New York, USA
UNDP (2011) Human development report 2011: sustainability and equity—a better future for all. United Nations Development Programme (UNDP), New York
Van Berkum E, Weijermars W, Hagens A (2006) The impact of weather on urban travel demand in the Netherlands. Paper Presented at the EURO working group for transportation conference, Bari, Italy, 245–252
Viscusi WK, Chesson H (1999) Hopes and fears: the conflicting effects of risk ambiguity. Theor Decis 47(2):153–178
Wang D, Chai Y (2009) The jobs-housing relationship and commuting in Beijing, China: the legacy of Danwei. J Transp Geogr 17:30–38
Walker B, Holling CS, Carpenter SR, Kinzig A (2004) Resilience, adaptability and transformability in social–ecological systems. Ecol Soc 9(2):5
Wolf J, Allice I, Bell T (2013) Values, climate change, and implications for adaptation: evidence from two communities in Labrador, Canada. Glob Environ Change 43:548–562
World Tourism Organisation (2003) Climate change and tourism. In: Proceedings of the first international conference on climate change and tourism. Djerba, Tunisia, April 9–11

Chapter 13
Mobility Biographies and Mobility Socialisation—New Approaches to an Old Research Field

Joachim Scheiner

Abstract This chapter investigates mobility biographies and mobility socialization, which are especially useful to capture long-term life choices. In the past decade, a research approach has been developed to better understand daily mobility by framing it in the context of individual life courses, their path dependencies and their social, economic and space-time links. This chapter briefly reviewed this approach and its origins. The concept of mobility biographies is introduced first, including a discussion of the role of routines (habits), life domains linked to mobility, and key events and transitions in the life course. A further step puts individual mobility biographies in a wider social context by referring to the concepts of socialization and linked lives. The importance of historical context for studying mobility biographies is briefly sketched. The chapter concludes with an outlook on future research.

Keywords Mobility socialisation · Mobility biography · Life events · Habits · Learning process · Linked lives · Travel behaviour · Path dependence · Transition · Context · Qualitative-hermeneutic approach

13.1 Introduction

In the last decade, a new, dynamic perspective on mobility[1] has developed, which has been labelled the 'mobility biography' (Lanzendorf 2003; Scheiner 2007) or 'life course oriented' (Chatterjee et al. 2013; Sharmeen et al. 2014) or 'life

[1]The term mobility is used here to capture the multitude of dimensions of travel behaviour (trip frequencies, travel distances, mode choice etc.) as well as the availability of mobility tools, such as cars, bicycles, or public transport season tickets.

J. Scheiner (✉)
Technische Universität Dortmund, Dortmund, Germany
e-mail: joachim.scheiner@tu-dortmund.de

J. Zhang (ed.), *Life-Oriented Behavioral Research for Urban Policy*,
DOI 10.1007/978-4-431-56472-0_13

trajectory' (Oakil 2013) approach to travel. Multiple methods are used in this framework to study trends in mobility on the individual level. The new perspective was facilitated by the household panel travel surveys that were established from the 1980s in the US, the Netherlands, the UK, and Germany. Two reasons may justify this approach.

Firstly, there is strong uncertainty about the direction of cause and impact between mobility and its correlates. Cross-sectional associations cannot establish cause and impact, or they can only do so to a limited extent on the basis of strong theories. The debate on the endogeneity of residential choice to mobility (residential self-selection) may serve as an example. While it was typically assumed for a long time that the urban environment—characterised by land-use structures and transport systems—at a household's residence impacts upon household mobility, the idea of residential self-selection suggests that households choose their urban environment according to their mobility and access preferences (Holz-Rau and Kutter 1995; Handy et al. 2005; Scheiner 2009; Cao and Cao 2014; Ettema and Nieuwenhuis 2015). By contributing to the clarification of the sequential structures of changing conditions and behavioural changes, life course oriented approaches provide better evidence on cause and impact structures, although in some cases 'lead effects' in mobility (see below) may make cause-impact structures even less obvious.

Secondly, the breaking of routines and changing of behaviour as an outcome of key events or transitions in the life course opens up chances for policy interventions targeted at such transitions, e.g. by offering public transport trial tickets or travel information to people when they change workplace, change residence, or retire. In this way, life course studies on mobility can contribute to research on the effectiveness of such interventions and the sensitivity of different population groups towards them. On the other hand, if mobility turns out to be relatively unaffected even by substantial changes in relevant conditions, policy efforts to change these conditions are likely to have little effect. Policy perspectives aimed at life course changes have been increasingly developed in recent years, e.g. by motivating the elderly to use public transport (Kasper et al. 2009), evaluating cycling concepts (Chatterjee et al. 2013), or informing households who intend to relocate about the negative accessibility and transport consequences of choosing a non-integrated residential location in order to affect their preferences (Holz-Rau et al. 2010; Rodriguez et al. 2011).

Since the term mobility biographies was introduced by Lanzendorf (2003) a large number of related empirical studies have emerged worldwide, in Germany (Prillwitz et al. 2006; Tully and Baier 2011; Harms and Lanzendorf 2007; Ottmann 2009; Scheiner 2009; Lanzendorf 2010; Scheiner and Holz-Rau 2013a, b), Switzerland (Axhausen et al. 2006; Beige and Axhausen 2012), the Netherlands (Van der Waerden et al. 2003; Oakil 2013; Sharmeen et al. 2014), the UK (Chatterjee et al. 2013), Sweden (Frändberg 2006), Japan (Zhang et al. 2014), Australia (Bonham and Wilson 2012) and the US (Rasouli et al. 2015; Mjahed et al. 2015; Klein and Smart 2015).

This chapter presents a brief review. The concept of mobility biographies is introduced in the following. The relevance of (1) routines (habits), (2) life domains that are linked to mobility, and (3) transitions and key events in the life course is highlighted. A further step is made to link individual mobility biographies to a wider social context by referring to the concepts of socialisation and linked lives. The importance of historical context for mobility biographies is touched upon briefly. The chapter concludes with an outlook to further research.

13.2 The Concept of Mobility Biographies

Biographical approaches to mobility benefit from a number of research strands. Life course and lifetime approaches have a long tradition in biology, where they were developed using the term 'reproductive success' (Clutton-Brock 1988; Rockwell and Barrowclough 1995), and in economics, where the focus is on the utility maximisation of households or individuals over the life course (Merton 1969; Samuelson 1969; Mussa 1976) or their labour market success (Fortin 2005; Raz-Yurovich 2013). In psychology and sociology a broad spectrum of topics are studied using the concepts of life course, life cycle, life span, life history, or biography [for a discussion of terms see Elder et al. (2006); for a distinction between life course and biography see Sackmann (2007); on the relevance of critical life events from a psychological perspective see Filipp (1995)]. These topics include socialisation, learning theory, personality development, the development of attitudes, personal ties and partnerships (Arránz Becker 2013).

The mobility biography approach has a closer relationship with sociological and geographical migration studies because of the shared interest in spatial mobility. In these studies life course oriented and biographical approaches can be traced back at least to the 1980s [Mulder 1993; Halfacree and Boyle 1993; Willekens 1999; Coulter 2013; for Germany see Wagner (1989), ARL (1992), Birg et al. (1998), Gerber (2011)]. At the same time, this field explicitly takes into account other life course domains that are important for mobility biographies, such as the family (Michielin and Mulder 2008; Mulder and Cooke 2009) and employment (Mulder and Ham 2005, Pailhé and Solaz 2008), as well as path dependencies, previous experiences and the impact of socialisation on mobility (Myers 1999; Feijten et al. 2008; Blaauboer 2011).

Another worthwhile link is time geography, where life course approaches were developed no later than the 1970s. These perspectives are based on Hägerstrands (1970) idea of space-time paths. Such paths were almost exclusively studied on the daily level in geography and transport studies [with the rare exceptions of studies looking at paths spanning several weeks: Hanson and Hanson (1980)]. However, the concept may well be applied to the life span, as has been proposed by Hägerstrand (1970) and explicitly applied by Martensson (1979).

In the 1980s and 1990s, early studies used the upcoming panel data to look at longer-term variability in mobility (Goodwin 1989; Zumkeller et al. 1998), and ideas were developed for biographical concepts relevant to travel. For example, household car ownership biographies were collected in Stuttgart in 1992 by Holz-Rau and Kutter (1995), while Scheiner (2000) studied the role of biographical factors in destination choice in reunited Berlin. However, these early attempts were not fully worked out into biographical or life course oriented approaches. Only after the turn of the millennium did the idea of a process-oriented, biographical approach to travel emerge more or less simultaneously in several universities (Axhausen 2002; Lanzendorf 2003; Scheiner 2003; Van der Waerden et al. 2003). The theoretical ideas of this approach are based on three main elements:

(1) Habits, which are reflected in the routine character of daily (travel) action, resulting in strong behavioural stability over a long time,
(2) Close relationships between individual mobility biographies and other domains of the life course,
(3) Significant changes in mobility that are motivated by transitions, events and learning processes over an individual's biography, and breaks in routines.

There has been less emphasis in this approach on 'linked lives' (Elder et al. 2006)—the links between an individual's mobility biography and other persons in the social environment. Such links suggest socialisation being at work in mobility. Accordingly, one could add a fourth element:

(4) The impact of socialisation agents in mobility that suggest interpersonal links in biographical processes in mobility.

The majority of empirical work focuses on the third point. The emphasis of these studies is on the impact of key events (or life events, life-cycle events, life course events) and transitions on mobility, i.e. mostly on mode choice. The reliance on statistical significance of cause-impact relationships has raised criticism of the mobility biographies approach. Miles et al. (2013) claim that to date the potential of the approach has not been fully developed because most studies are limited to statistical measures. Instead, 'deeper' qualitative-hermeneutic approaches could improve understanding of people's behaviour in time and space, and of related changes in mobility. Such approaches emerge in the most recent literature (Rau and Manton 2016; Sattlegger and Rau 2016).

Indeed most mobility biography studies fit better with life course research than with biography research. The life course is typically conceived as a sequence of events and role transitions that a person lives through from birth to death (Elder et al. 2006). In contrast, a biography is understood as a subject's self-reflective, meaningful action within the temporal structure of his or her own life (Sackmann 2007). Accordingly, biography studies reconstruct subjective meaning while life course studies attempt to objectively measure sequences and structures in people's lives, e.g. by asking for pre-defined stations, events or sequences. Nevertheless this paper stays with the term mobility biography as it has been used widely for related research in the past decade.

13.2.1 Habits

One of the key assumptions of transport research is the strong habitualisation of travel behaviour (Gärling/Axhausen 2003). Recurring destinations, and travel modes and transport systems being available in the long term are typical of daily trip making. Accordingly, daily travel is not characterised by permanent scrutinising and self-reflection, but by routine action. These habits are empirically reflected in path dependency in mobility, i.e. strong associations between mobility at a given point in time and earlier mobility. To put it plainly: the strongest impact factor affecting mode choice to work is mode choice to work the day before.

The idea of habitualised daily action has been deeply rooted in sociological theories of action ever since the work of Max Weber (1921) and Alfred Schütz (1932). It can also be integrated into more recent rational choice models of action (Esser 1991). Action theoretical approaches have been explicitly developed for and applied to travel (Scheiner 2000; Guell et al. 2012; Congleton 2014; Cass and Faulconbridge 2015). Habits make acting easier and less risky. Individuals use them when they assume that searching for alternatives will involve overly high search costs, or if the expected utility of searching is too limited or too uncertain (Gärling and Axhausen 2003). Routines manifest themselves in the repeated realisation of action sequences, even though repetition is not a sufficient criterion to define an action as routine. A constitutive attribute of routines is the unscrutinised, schematic performance of a pre-stored action pattern that works as a 'recipe' (Esser 1991: 61ff).

In the past ten years the day-to-day variability of mobility has become a notable field of research, challenging the idea of strong routines. Detailed analysis suggests a high degree of variability (Schlich et al. 2004; Chikaraishi et al. 2009). On the other hand, Susilo and Kitamura (2005) find relatively robust individual activity spaces over a period of six weeks, particularly on weekdays. Bhat et al. (2005) find recurring weekly rhythms in activity patterns. By and large, mobility can be considered stable in the short to mid term (Thøgersen 2006). The residence location as well as many destinations (the workplace, residences of friends and kin, leisure places, doctors' surgeries, etc.) and associated trip lengths do not change on a short term basis. Mode choice is relatively robust as well, as long as transport conditions do not change on an origin-destination relation, even though mode choice may have become more variable over recent decades, as suggested by increasing levels of car ownership and heavy investment in public transport in many (European) cities. This is reflected in more multimodal behaviour among young adults (Buehler and Hamre 2015; Heinen and Chatterjee 2015). One may ask whether multimodality may be considered an action routine on a more complex level: take the bicycle when the weather is fine, but the bus when it rains. Yet multimodal behaviour has been shown to be associated with a higher likelihood for behavioural change (Kroesen 2014; Heinen and Ogilvie 2016).

13.2.2 Domains of the Life Course: Housing, Employment, Household and the Family

Two basic approaches have been developed to identify life domains relevant for mobility biographies. Lanzendorf (2003) adapts a model by Salomon (1983) to distinguish three domains: lifestyle, accessibility, and mobility. The lifestyle domain includes a demographic career (or path), an employment career, and a leisure career. The accessibility domain depends on the lifestyle domain, and it includes decisions on basic nodes in daily activity space: the residence, workplace, and leisure places. The mobility domain in turn depends on the accessibility domain. It includes mobility tool ownership (car, season ticket) and travel behaviour.

A second, somewhat similar suggestion has been made by Scheiner (2007). Based on his own studies that suggested only limited relevance of lifestyles for travel (Scheiner 2009), he dismisses the lifestyle aspect, focusing instead on the family and household biography, employment biography, and residential biography.[2] Each of these three life domains (or 'partial biographies') is related to the mobility biography, which again includes mobility tool ownership and travel behaviour.

Events and transitions in family and household biography, employment biography, and residential biography must not be considered in isolation. Rather they may be linked to each other in myriad ways, as demographic and sociological studies on residential biographies shows (Birg et al. 1998; Sackmann and Wingens 2001; Mulder and Ham 2005; Mortimer and Shanahan 2006; Michielin and Mulder 2008; Mulder and Cooke 2009; Cooke et al. 2009). This has practical implications for mobility biography studies. For instance, the close relationship between residential relocations and household composition changes implies that the study of relocation effects on travel behaviour needs to take such household changes into account to avoid misspecifications in models and false interpretations.

Mobility biographies may also affect other life domains, such as the residential biography. For instance, the residential location options of zero-car households are clearly limited (Van Wee et al. 2002; Hesse and Scheiner 2009). Partnership and family biographies can be impaired by mobility: long commute trips are known to be burdensome not only for commuters, but also for their families, and they can even reduce fertility (Schneider et al. 2002; Stutzer and Frey 2008, van der Klis 2009; Sandow 2014).

[2]These 'partial biographies' have also been named cycles in research (family cycle, employment cycle). This term suggests a more or less predefined, closed course that may be subdivided into a limited number of typical stages. Research on individualisation and lifestyles suggests, however, that this idea no longer matches societal reality.

13.2.3 Transitions and Key Events in the Life Course

The moments in a life course when behaviour potentially changes significantly, are considered key events, life events or (in cases of unexpected events and with a flavour of crisis), 'critical incidents' (Van der Waerden et al. 2003). Key events mark the moment of 'transition' (Chatterjee et al. 2013), when a state changes into another state [see Müggenburg et al. (2015) and Chatterjee and Scheiner (2015) for discussions of related terms]. While key events refer to a more or less precisely defined point in time, transitions may last longer, and they may be linked to longer-term experiences and learning processes. As transitions may also occur suddenly, key events may be considered to mark a special case of transition. For instance, individuals classing themselves as 'old-aged' may result from a health-related key event, an accident, or the death of a partner. The individual transition to old age may however just as well be a slow process of adaption to age.

Transitions may have asymmetrical implications for mobility. For instance, Krämer-Badoni and Kuhm (2000) argue that the activity options permitted by the car cannot be reversed easily. The probability of car purchase after an event (e.g. income increase, residential suburbanisation) should therefore be higher than the probability of car disposal after the reverse event [for empirical evidence see Dargay (2001), Beige (2008), Rasouli et al. (2015), Clark et al. (2016a) on commute mode changes; Chi (2016) on fuel price changes], but the evidence is not consistent (Clark et al. (2016b) find the reverse to be true). Accordingly, the effects of transitions on mobility should be studied separately for two/various directions of events.

Studies of the effects of key events on mobility account for a large proportion of research on mobility biographies. A number of key events in three life domains have been found to exhibit significant effects (empirical studies in brackets).

- Family and household biography: Leaving the parental home; forming a household; birth of a child; separation from one's partner; a child moving out of the parental home (Dargay 2001; Dargay and Hanly 2007; Clark et al. (2016a, b) on changes in household composition and size; Zwerts et al. (2007) and Lanzendorf (2010) on childbirth; Oakil (2013) and Scheiner and Holz-Rau (2013a) on various household and family events).
- Employment biography: Start of apprenticeship or studying; entering the labour market (Harms and Lanzendorf 2007); change of workplace (Kalter 1994; Oakil 2013; Clark et al. 2016a); income change (Dargay 2001; Clark et al. 2016b); transition between employment and unemployment (Kroesen 2014; Clark et al. 2016b; Rasouli et al. 2015); retirement (Ottmann 2009; Oakil 2013).
- Residential biography: Residential relocation and associated changes in accessibility (Krizek 2003; Dargay and Hanly 2007; Scheiner 2005; Handy et al. 2005; Prillwitz et al. 2006; Oakil 2013; Clark et al. 2016a; Aditjandra et al. 2016).

It has to be noted that the acquisition of a driving license as well as the purchase or disposal of a car may be considered parts of a mobility biography, rather than its determinants.

Other studies have focussed on ‘external’ events, or incidents, caused by transport system disturbances, new infrastructure or changes in the urban layout that may promote (short-term or long-term) behavioural changes, e.g. temporary closures of a major road (Fujii and Gärling 2003; Yun et al. 2011), changes in parking at the workplace (Scheiner and Holz-Rau 2013a) or new cycling (Chatterjee et al. 2013) or public transport infrastructure (Heinen et al. 2015; Pnevmatikou et al. 2015; Termida et al. 2016). Little is known, however, about whether behavioural changes are lasting [see Termida et al. (2016) for mid-term effects seven months after the extension of a tram line].

Sequential structures between life course events and mobility have received little attention to date. Rare evidence suggests delayed effects result from income changes (Dargay 2001), while behavioural changes caused by anticipated key events (‘lead effects’) were recently studied by Oakil (2013). Lagged and lead effects may be expected particularly in those dimensions of mobility that do not require instant behavioural adaption, those that require large investment, and those that appear reasonable from the perspective of a household as a whole. For instance, entering the labour market is linked to an immediate change in time use. In contrast, a car may be purchased in anticipation of the birth of a child, but also long after the birth and associated learning processes related to changed daily needs.

Events in a mobility biography may themselves be understood as key events for other life domains. For instance, the loss of a driving license has been found to be linked to substantial decreases in quality of life (Kieschke et al. 2010). Gerontological studies have highlighted driving cessation as a critical incident that may negatively affect life satisfaction, health, mobility and activity levels, but with inconsistent results (see Scheiner 2006; Curl et al. 2013; Chihuri et al. 2015).

13.3 Mobility Socialisation and Linked Lives

People’s life courses are not isolated from other people’s life courses. They are embedded in social structures on the personal level, in family, kin, friendship and neighbourhood networks, as well as in economic, political or administrative organisations on a ‘system’ level. The ‘life world’ dimension of these embeddings is studied in sociology and psychology using the term ‘linked lives’ (Elder et al. 2006).

The integration of individuals in society over the course of their lives by means of the impact of significant others (individuals, groups or organisations) is studied in social psychology using the term socialisation. Socialisation is “the adoption of a group’s (typical) behaviours, opinions and values by an individual” (Herkner 1991: p. 41, author’s translation) so that thus “an individual capable of social acting emerges” (Tully and Baier 2011: p. 195, author’s translation). Sociological socialisation research highlights the learning and practising of social roles (Bahrdt 1994: p. 78f). Hence, socialisation may be understood as mutual interaction that enables group integration. This may refer to a small group, such as a family or a clique, or a society as a whole. Socialisation agents—peers groups or others—may be individuals or organisations. Typical socialisation agents are parents and the family, media, or schools.

It is likely that there are socialisation impacts on mobility (Flade and Limbourg 1997; Baslington 2008; Tully and Baier 2011; Mjahed et al. 2015) that are transmitted by parental mobility, school mobility education, adolescents' cliques, or partners (Kroesen 2015). There is evidence for such transmission of behaviour from parents to children in residential choice (Myers 1999; Blaauboer 2011) as well as in demographic life paths (Liefbroer and Elzinga 2012). This suggests 'linked lives' in terms of interpersonal links in mobility biographies. However, the idea of mobility socialisation presupposes that mobility is a relevant phenomenon for group integration; otherwise there would be no pressure to adjust mobility. The high relevance of mobility may well be assumed for adolescents—the first moped/scooter, gaining a driving license, and owning a car are associated with considerable subjective and objective liberty (Mienert 2003; Tully and Baier 2011). However, for societal integration as a whole this cannot be assumed likewise. Even if mobility is a basic dimension that structures modern societies, the size of activity space, or the use of the car, the train or the bicycle are not necessarily linked to social inclusion or exclusion and the need to adjust behaviour. On the other hand one may assume that forced constraints in activity spaces because of a lack of mobility options may cause exclusion tendencies. Research also needs to take into account that the transmission of behaviours from one generation to the next is not only caused by socio-psychological norms and learning, but also has an economic background (e.g. inheritance of residential property).

The link between mobility socialisation and mobility biographies lies in the fact that socialisation needs to be understood as a process over time. Mobility socialisation in childhood and adolescence can therefore be considered a 'pre-structuring' of the later mobility biography. The relevant 'temporal window' is, however, not limited to childhood and adolescence. Rather, socialisation processes span the whole life course, although the most formative stages are in childhood and adolescence, while preferences and behaviours may change slower in later life due to inertia and stronger path dependencies. The formation of behaviours is not limited to mode choice and distance sensitivity; flexibility, adaptability and the variety of routines may also be shaped by socialisation.

Asking about the relevance of socialisation for mobility opens up a range of interesting research questions in any case. These include, for instance, the structure of interactions within households and families, between generations, and in personal networks. Generation specific mobility biographies could be a worthwhile field of investigation not only from an intra-family perspective, but also in terms of cohorts. Examples are the collective experience of early tourism to the Mediterranean in the central European post-war generation, or the significance of the social norm of stays abroad among young adults now. What is more, the idea of (municipal or national) mobility cultures (Klinger et al. 2013) is an approach that enables the study of the possible effects of the wider socio-spatial environment on mobility (e.g., the idea of 'slow cities').

13.4 The Importance of Context

The examples just mentioned above make it clear that life courses are embedded in historical trends. Therefore external conditions need to be taken into account to adequately interpret life courses.[3] Such conditions may be reflected statistically in cohort or period effects (Weis and Axhausen 2009; Scheiner and Holz-Rau 2013a). Their interpretation requires consideration of economic, social, technological and political conditions in a study period. Otherwise investigation of individual experiences and changes in mobility over time would probably fall short of recognising the role of context for the individual. For instance, emigration and long-distance commuting were not just individual but collective experiences among East Germans after German reunification in 1990. Also, the young German families who travelled to Italy with their first cars for the first time in the 1960s shared a collective experience.

Reconstructing historical states and trends is a considerable challenge for mobility biography studies. For instance, the increase in mass motorisation over the past century may be reconstructed easily, but this is true only on the national level, not on a spatially or socially disaggregated level (see Scheiner (2012) for an attempt). At what point in time, and to what degree, a social norm of car ownership emerged from this trend is far more difficult to reconstruct. Another example is the recent trend of delayed licensing among young adults (Delbosc 2016) and associated increased public transport use, which can only be understood adequately (for Germany) against the background of the introduction of the semester ticket since the 1990s in many universities. These examples may serve to illustrate that considerable knowledge of historical context and great care are required when long-term trends in mobility are interpreted.

13.5 Consequences for Research

Mobility biographies—or mobility life courses—have emerged as a promising research area with multiple dimensions over the past few years. A number of important questions have rarely been studied to date in this field [see also the reviews of Müggenburg et al. (2015), Chatterjee and Scheiner (2015)], and a number of conclusions can be drawn for future research.

- Existing studies are mostly limited to typical, widely used measures of travel behaviour, especially mode choice. Trip purposes, distances covered, activity patterns and trip chaining have hardly been touched upon [but see Scheiner (2014) for the latter two points, Rasouli et al. (2015) for shopping duration, Kroesen 2014 for multimodality].

[3]External conditions here do not refer to conditions on the individual or household level that may change over the life course, but to macro-economic, social, technological and political conditions that are relevant for a population as a whole.

- Some important key events have gained much attention, such as residential relocation, while others have been investigated less often. Interactions between various key events as well as interactions between different persons and the key events they experience (e.g. the partner entering the labour force) have largely been neglected [though some studies include gender interactions or differences in the effects of key events, e.g., Scheiner (2014), Oakil (2016)]. Within-household interactions have emerged as a vibrant research field in transport studies (Srinivasan and Athuru 2005; Auld and Zhang 2013), but without looking at the life course.
- Between-group differences in the effects of key events on mobility have been largely ignored. Existing group-specific studies lack systematic comparison between groups.
- The impact of socialisation on mobility has not gained much attention to date [but see Baslington (2008), Haustein et al. (2009), Kroesen (2015)].
- Sequential structures between life course events and mobility have not been studied in depth. Rare findings suggest lagged effects of income changes (Dargay 2001). Lead effects have been found by Oakil (2013), e.g. car acquisition in anticipation of a child being born.
- Most studies in the field focus on discrete events or on short segments of people's life courses. Observing longer-term trajectories offers more potential to fully develop a biographical perspective and understand the development of travel behaviour and the factors that motivate individuals to take different paths (Jones et al. 2014).
- There is a striking lack of hermeneutic approaches to the meaning of mobility and its embedding in key events, socialisation, experience, learning, and wider social and geographical contexts. The subjective perspectives of individuals and their own reconstructions of their mobility biographies have received little attention (Miles et al. 2013; Rau and Manton 2016; Sattlegger and Rau 2016). Looking at mobility biographies from the perspective of respondents and reflecting on their statements and narratives against other historical material could contribute to broadening theoretical perspectives on mobility biographies, and further enhance understanding of the development of travel behaviour over the life course.

Acknowledgments This research was funded by the German Research Foundation (DFG) as part of the project 'Veränderungen der Mobilität im Lebenslauf: Die Bedeutung biografischer und erreichbarkeitsbezogener Schlüsselereignisse' (Travel behaviour changes over the life course: the role of biographical and accessibility-related key events, 2015–2018).

References

Aditjandra PT, Cao X, Mulley C (2016) Exploring changes in public transport use and walking following residential relocation: a British case study. J Transp Land Use 9(3):1–19

ARL (Akademie für Raumforschung und Landesplanung) (1992) Regionale und biographische Mobilität im Lebensverlauf. Forschungs- und Sitzungsberichte der Akademie für Raumforschung und Landesplanung 189, ARL, Hannover
Arránz Becker O (2013) Effects of similarity of life goals, values, and personality on relationship satisfaction and stability: findings from a two-wave panel study. Pers Relat 20:443–461
Auld J, Zhang L (2013) Inter-personal interactions and constraints in travel behavior within households and social networks. Transportation 40:751–754
Axhausen KW (2002) A dynamic understanding of travel demand: a sketch. Arbeitsbericht Verkehrs- und Raumplanung des Instituts für Verkehrsplanung, Transporttechnik, Straßen- und Eisenbahnbau 119: ETH, Zürich
Axhausen KW, Frei A, Ohnmacht T (2006) Networks, biographies and travel: first empirical and methodological results. Paper presented at the 11th international conference on travel behaviour research, Kyoto, 16–20 Aug 2006
Bahrdt HP (1994) Schlüsselbegriffe der Soziologie, 6th edn. C.H Beck, München
Baslington H (2008) Travel socialization: a social theory of travel mode behavior. Int J Sustain Transp 2:91–114
Beige S (2008) Long-term and mid-term mobility decisions during the life course. Doctoral Dissertation, ETH Zürich, Institut für Verkehrsplanung und Transportsysteme (e-collection.library.ethz.ch/eserv/eth:30645/eth-30645-02.pdf. Accessed 18 Nov 2015
Beige S, Axhausen KW (2012) Interdependencies between turning points in life and long-term mobility decisions. Transportation 39:857–872
Bhat CR, Srinivasan S, Axhausen KW (2005) An analysis of multiple interepisode durations using a unifying multivariate hazard model. Transp Res Part B 39:797–823
Birg H, Flöthmann E-J, Heins F, Reiter I (1998) Migrationsanalyse. Empirische Längsschnitt- und Querschnittanalysen auf der Grundlage von Mikro- und Makromodellen für die Bundesrepublik Deutschland. Materialien des Instituts für Bevölkerungsforschung und Sozialpolitik 43, Universität, Bielefeld
Blaauboer M (2011) The impact of childhood experiences and family members outside the household on residential environment choices. Urban Stud 48:1635–1650
Bonham J, Wilson A (2012) Bicycling and the life course: the start-stop-start experiences of women cycling. Int J Sustain Transp 6:195–213
Buehler R, Hamre A (2015) The multimodal majority? driving, walking, cycling, and public transportation use among American adults. Transportation 42:1081–1101
Cao J, Cao X (2014) The impacts of LRT, neighbourhood characteristics, and self-selection on auto ownership: evidence from Minneapolis-St. Paul Urban Stud 51:2068–2087
Cass N, Faulconbridge J (2015) Commuting practices: new insights into modal shift from theories of social practice. Transp Policy 45:1–14
Chatterjee K, Scheiner J (2015) Understanding changing travel behaviour over the life course: contributions from biographical research. A resource paper for the workshop "life-oriented approach for transportation studies". Presented at IATBR (14th international conference on travel behaviour research), Windsor, UK, 19–23 Jul 2015
Chatterjee K, Sherwin H, Jain J, Christensen J, Marsh S (2013) A conceptual model to explain turning points in travel behaviour: application to bicycle use. Transp Res Rec 2322:82–90
Chi J (2016) Long- and short-run asymmetric responses of motor-vehicle travel to fuel price variations: new evidence from a nonlinear ARDL approach. Transp Policy (in press)
Chihuri S, Mielenz TJ, DiMaggio CJ, Betz ME, DiGuiseppi C, Jones VC, Li G (2015) Driving cessation and health outcomes in older adults: a longroad study. AAA Foundation for Traffic Safety, Washington
Chikaraishi M, Fujiwara A, Zhang J, Axhausen KW (2009) Exploring variation properties of departure time choice behavior using multilevel analysis approach. Transp Res Rec 2134:10–20
Clark B, Chatterjee K, Melia S (2016a) Changes in level of household car ownership: the role of life events and spatial context. Transportation 43(4):565–599

Clark B, Chatterjee K, Melia S (2016b) Changes to commute mode: the role of life events, spatial context and environmental attitude. Transp Res Part A 89:89–105
Clutton-Brock TH (1988) Reproductive success. Studies of individual variation in contrasting breeding systems. University of Chicago, Chicago
Congleton C (2014) Strategic social interaction in travel mode choice: a case study of UC Davis campus travel. Compendium of papers CD-ROM, the 93rd annual meeting of transportation research board. Washington 12–16 Jan 2014
Cooke TJ, Boyle P, Couch K, Feijten P (2009) A longitudinal analysis of family migration and the gender gap in earnings in the United States and Great Britain. Demography 46:147–167
Coulter R (2013) Wishful thinking and the abandonment of moving desires over the life course. Environ Plann A 45:1944–1962
Curl AL, Stowe JD, Cooney TM, Proulx CM (2013) Giving up the keys: how driving cessation affects engagement in later life. Gerontol. doi:10.1093/geront/gnt037
Dargay J (2001) The effect of income on car ownership: evidence of asymmetry. Transp Res Part A 35:807–821
Dargay J, Hanly M (2007) Volatility of car ownership, commuting mode and time in the UK. Transp Res Part A 41:934–948
Delbosc A (2016) Delay or forgo? A closer look at youth driver licensing trends in the United States and Australia. Transportation (in press)
Elder GH Jr, Johnson MK, Crosnoe R (2006) The emergence and development of life course theory. In: Mortimer J, Shanahan MJ (eds) Handbook of the life course. Springer, Berlin, pp 3–19
Esser H (1991) Alltagshandeln und Verstehen. Zum Verhältnis von erklärender und verstehender Soziologie am Beispiel von Alfred Schütz und "Rational Choice", Mohr Siebeck, Tübingen
Ettema D, Nieuwenhuis R (2015) Residential self-selection effects and TOD development: how does relocation motivation influence the effect of built environment? Compendium of papers CD-ROM, the 94th annual meeting of the transportation research board, Washington, 11–15 Jan 2015
Feijten P, Hooimeijer P, Mulder CH (2008) Residential experience and residential environment choice over the life-course. Urban Stud 45:141–162
Filipp S-H (ed) (1995) Kritische Lebensereignisse. Beltz, Weinheim
Flade A, Limbourg M (1997) Das Hineinwachsen in die motorisierte Gesellschaft. Institut für Wohnen und Umwelt, Darmstadt
Fortin NM (2005) Gender role attitudes and the labour-market outcomes of women across OECD countries. Oxford Rev Econ Policy 21:416–438
Frändberg L (2006) International mobility biographies: a means to capture the institutionalisation of long-distance travel? Current Issues Tourism 9:320–334
Fujii S, Gärling T (2003) Development of script-based travel mode choice after forced change. Transp Res Part F 6:117–124
Gärling T, Axhausen KW (2003) Introduction: habitual travel choice. Transportation 30:1–11
Gerber K (2011) Räumliche Mobilität im Wandel: wanderungen im Lebenslauf und ihre Auswirkungen auf die Stadtentwicklung in Nordrhein-Westfalen. VS Verlag, Wiesbaden
Goodwin PB (1989) Family changes and public transport use 1984–1987. Transportation 16:121–154
Guell C, Panter J, Jones NR, Ogilvie D (2012) Towards a differentiated understanding of active travel behaviour: using social theory to explore everyday commuting. Soc Sci Med 75:233–239
Hägerstrand T (1970) What about people in regional science? Papers Reg Sci 24:7–21
Halfacree KH, Boyle PJ (1993) The challenge facing migration research: the case for a biographical approach. Prog Hum Geogr 17:333–348
Handy S, Cao X, Mokhtarian P (2005) Correlation or causality between the built environment and travel behavior? evidence from Northern California. Transp Res Part D 10:427–444

Rodriguez DA, Levine J, Weinstein A, Song J (2011) Can information promote transportation-friendly location decisions? a simulation experiment. J Transp Geogr 19:304–312
Sackmann R (2007) Lebenslaufanalyse und Biografieforschung. VS Verlag, Wiesbaden
Sackmann R, Wingens M (2001) Strukturen des Lebenslaufs: Übergang - Sequenz - Verlauf. Juventa, Weinheim, München
Salomon I (1983) Life styles—a broader perspective on travel behaviour. In: Carpenter S, Jones P (eds) Recent advances in travel demand analysis. Gower, Aldershot, pp 290–310
Samuelson PA (1969) Lifetime portfolio selection by dynamic stochastic programming. Rev Econ Stat 51:239–246
Sandow E (2014) Til work do us part: the social fallacy of long-distance commuting. Urban Stud 51:526–543
Sattlegger L, Rau H (2016) Carlessness in a car-centric world: a reconstructive approach to qualitative mobility biographies research. J Transp Geogr 53:22–31
Scheiner J (2000) Eine stadt—zwei Alltagswelten? Ein Beitrag zur Aktionsraumforschung und Wahrnehmungsgeographie im vereinten Berlin. Abhandlungen Anthropogeographie 62, Reimer, Berlin
Scheiner J (2003) Housing mobility and travel behaviour: a process-oriented approach to spatial mobility. evidence from a new research field in Germany. Paper presented at the RGS-IBG International Annual Conference "Geography, serving society and the environment", London, 3–5 Sept 2003
Scheiner J (2005) Auswirkungen der Stadt- und Umlandwanderung auf Motorisierung und Verkehrsmittelnutzung: ein dynamisches Modell des Verkehrsverhaltens. Verkehrsforschung Online 1:1–17
Scheiner J (2006) Does the car make elderly people happy and mobile? settlement structures, car availability and leisure mobility of the elderly. Eur J Transp Infrastruct Res 6:151–172
Scheiner J (2007) Mobility biographies: elements of a biographical theory of travel demand. Erdkunde 61:161–173
Scheiner J (2009) Sozialer Wandel, Raum und Mobilität. VS Verlag, Wiesbaden
Scheiner J (2012) A century of motorisation in urban and rural contexts: paths of motorisation in German cities. Erdkunde 66:313–328
Scheiner J (2014) The gendered complexity of daily life: effects of life-course events on changes in activity entropy and tour complexity over time. Travel Behav Soc 1:91–105
Scheiner J, Holz-Rau C (2013a) A comprehensive study of life course, cohort, and period effects on changes in travel mode use. Transp Res Part A 47:167–181
Scheiner J, Holz-Rau C (2013b) Changes in travel mode choice after residential relocation: a contribution to mobility biographies. Transportation 40:431–458
Schlich R, Schönfelder S, Hanson S, Axhausen KW (2004) Structures of leisure travel: temporal and spatial variability. Transp Rev 24:219–237
Schneider NF, Limmer R, Ruckdeschel K (2002) Berufsmobilität und Lebensform. Sind berufliche Mobilitätserfordernisse in Zeiten der Globalisierung noch mit Familie vereinbar? Kohlhammer, Stuttgart
Schütz A (1932/1981) Der sinnhafte Aufbau der sozialen Welt, 2 ed, Suhrkamp, Frankfurt am Main
Sharmeen F, Arentze T, Timmermans H (2014) An analysis of the dynamics of activity and travel needs in response to social network evolution and life-cycle events: a structural equation model. Transp Res Part A 59:159–171
Srinivasan K, Athuru S (2005) Analysis of within-household effects and between-household differences in maintenance activity allocation. Transportation 32:495–521
Stutzer A, Frey BS (2008) Stress that doesn't pay: the commuting paradox. Scand J Econ 110:339–366
Susilo YO, Kitamura R (2005) Analysis of day-to-day variability in an individual's action space: exploration of 6-week Mobidrive travel diary data. Transp Res Rec 1902:124–133

Termida NA, Susilo YO, Franklin JP (2016) Observing dynamic behavioural responses due to the extension of a tram line by using panel survey. Transp Res A 86:78–95

Thøgersen J (2006) Understanding repetitive travel mode choices in a stable context: a panel study approach. Transp Res Part A 40:621–638

Tully CJ, Baier D (2011) Mobilitätssozialisation. In: Schwedes O (ed) Verkehrspolitik. VS Verlag, Wiesbaden, pp 195–211

Van der Klis M (2009) Commuter partnerships. balancing home, family, and distant work. Doctoral dissertation, Faculty of Social and Behavioural Sciences, University of Amsterdam (http://dare.uva.nl/document/2/64928). Accessed 18 Nov 2015

Van der Waerden P, Timmermans H, Borgers A (2003) The influence of key events and critical incidents on transport mode choice switching behaviour: a descriptive analysis. Paper presented at the 10th international conference on travel behaviour research (IATBR), Lucerne, 10–15 Aug 2003

Van Wee B, Holwerda H, van Baren R (2002) Preferences for modes, residential location and travel behaviour: the relevance for land-use impacts on mobility. Eur J Transp Infrastruct Res 2:305–316

Wagner M (1989) Räumliche Mobilität im Lebensverlauf. Ferdinand Enke, Stuttgart

Weber M (1921/1972) Wirtschaft und Gesellschaft. Grundriß der verstehenden Soziologie, 5 ed, J.C.B. Mohr, Tübingen

Weis C, Axhausen KW (2009) Induced travel demand: evidence from a pseudo panel data based structural equations model. Res Transp Econ 25:8–18

Willekens FJ (1999) The life course: models and analysis. In: Van Wissen LJG, Dykstra PA (eds) Population issues. Kluwer, New York, pp 23–51

Yun M, van Herick D, Mokhtarian PL (2011) Nonwork travel behavior changes during temporary freeway closure: the Fix 1-5 project in Sacramento, California. Transp Res Rec 2231:1–9

Zhang J, Yu B, Chikaraishi M (2014) Interdependences between household residential and car ownership behavior: a life history analysis. J Transp Geogr 34:165–174

Zumkeller D, Chlond B, Lipps O (1998) Konstanz / Variabilität des Verkehrsverhaltens bei gleichen Personen. Endbericht (BMV FE 70.595/1998), Institut für Verkehrswesen, Karlsruhe

Zwerts E, Janssens D, Wets G (2007) How the presence of children affects parents' travel behaviour. Compendium of papers CD-ROM, the 86th annual meeting of the transportation research board, Washington, 21–25 Jan 2007

Chapter 14
Biographical Interactions Over the Life Course: Car Ownership, Residential Choice, Household Structure, and Employment/Education

Biying Yu and Junyi Zhang

Abstract This chapter focuses on interdependent decisions on car ownership mobility, residential choice mobility, household structure mobility, and employment/education mobility over the life course. This study represents the above interdependencies based on a multilinear utility model and make an empirical study based on data from a web-based life history survey. Each of the four mobility domains is simply described as a set of episodes. Dependent variables in the model are the duration of each episode between two consecutive changes in each mobility domain. By using the multilinear utility functions, interepisode interactions within each mobility domain and interdomain interactions are simultaneously incorporated. The survey was conducted in 2010 and 1000 households provided valid data, and may well be the first life history survey with such a large sample size and comprehensive coverage in the transportation literature. Estimation results show a competitive relationship between the duration of episodes in the same domain, while a synergistic relationship between the duration of episodes in different domains exists. Furthermore, the biographical interactions in the life course are found to be substantial, contributing almost 95 % to total household utility, implying that mobility decisions are likely to be intertwined over the life course.

Keywords Biographical interactions · Car ownership mobility · Residential choice mobility · Household structure mobility · Employment/education mobility · Cross-/within-domain interactions

---

B. Yu (✉)
Beijing Institute of Technology, Beijing, China
e-mail: yubiying_bj@bit.edu.cn

J. Zhang
Hiroshima University, Higashi-Hiroshima, Japan

J. Zhang (ed.), *Life-Oriented Behavioral Research for Urban Policy*,
DOI 10.1007/978-4-431-56472-0_14

14.1 Introduction

In the behavioral sciences, the importance of relationships between long-term choices and short-term choices is emphasized. For example, Ben-Akiva and Lerman (1991), define long-term decisions as employment location, residential location, and housing type; medium-term decisions as automobile ownership and mode of travel to work; and short-term decisions as nonwork travel (frequency, destination, and mode). Many researchers have recognized that employment, residential, and travel choices are not independent of each other and individuals or households alter their lifestyle by collectively adjusting their varied dimension behaviors to land-use and transportation policies (Eliasson and Mattsson 2000; Waddell 2001). Once a transportation system is built or a land-use policy is carried out, it influences people's travel behavior and life in other domains (e.g., residential, household structure, housing, employment, and education) for a long time period. Consequently, understanding people's decisions on various interrelated life choices from the long-term perspective is one of the most fundamental requirements for urban policy makers. In other words, there is a need for life course dynamic analysis, which links different domains of life together and sheds light on the mobility biography.

The life course approach has been applied by demographic and housing researchers in a number of fields (Mayer and Tuma 1990; Wissen and Dykstra 1999). From their diverse viewpoints, behavior can be explained by its continuity over a person's lifetime and by specific events that involve major changes in other domains of life. Moreover, the life course is further subdivided into a series of trajectories that are comprised of a sequence of events and episodes (defined as the period between two consecutive events) in certain domains of life. The term 'mobility biography' refers to the total of an individual's longitudinal trajectories over their life course in the mobility domain. To date, the key interest of life course researchers has been to analyze the biographical interactions of different life course trajectories (Ommeren et al. 1999; Wissen and Dykstra 1999; Dieleman 2001), which are essentially twofold: on the one hand, there is an intraevent or interepisode interaction in the same domain caused by historical experience or future expectations. Mobility history and the different durations that a person maintained a situation in former episodes are of some importance because prior mobility is strongly correlated with current mobility. In each episode, because there is a gap between ideal and reality, people usually have some expectations about the future, which might also influence decisions about the current period. On the other hand, there are sometimes interactions between different domains. Events in one domain are frequently connected to changes in other domains. For example, moving to a suburban area will increase the probability of car ownership and therefore travel behavior. Our analysis will include differences in timing, duration, rates of change, and probabilities of the occurrence of certain events within a period of time as well as explanatory variables (Beige and Axhausen 2008).

In this chapter, to study travel behavior from a long-term perspective, the mobilities for our four main domains—residential, household structure, employment/education, and car ownership—are extracted from the life course to understand better individuals' travel behavior reactions to changes occurring in their personal and household life, professional career, spatial structures, as well as travel modes. Note that the research entry point is the duration of the episode between two consecutive events in each domain. By explicitly accommodating the above two types of interactions, a multilinear utility function is adopted to represent each individual's utility in his/her life that consists of the subutilities of each episode in all four domains. To our knowledge, the analysis in this chapter is the first attempt to formulate and apply such a comprehensive methodological framework for jointly modeling mobility in the four main domains in the life course from a behavioral perspective. Because dealing with life course dynamics requires longitudinal data, a web-based retrospective life story survey covering each respondent's life from 18 years old to the survey date was carried out at the end of 2010 in Japan and 1000 valid responses were obtained. In the survey, for all domains, mobility timing and frequency were obtained and then for each episode, detailed information was collected. The proposed model is estimated using these data.

The remainder of this chapter is organized as follows. Section 14.2 elucidates the interaction mechanisms between the four mobilities. Section 14.3 presents the structure of the multilinear utility model that explicitly incorporates the interepisode interaction in one domain as well as the interepisode interaction between different domains. Section 14.4 introduces the survey and the data it collected. The model is estimated and explained in Sect. 14.5. Section 14.6 concludes with a discussion of further research issues.

14.2 Biographical Interactions Between Mobilities

It is argued in the life course approach that various domains of people's lives are mutually interrelated. It suggests that mobility is not arbitrary but is related to important key events in the life course that trigger such changes. To date, many studies have confirmed that a person's mobility biography has to be seen in the collective context of his/her residential, household structure, employment/education, and car ownership biographies. Mobilities in these biographies are further found intertwined across the life course.

Residential mobility is a special biographical moment, in which familiar routines are always broken (Scheiner 2006). Its consequences are likely to include changes in the accessibility of opportunities, such as workplace, transport systems, retail and leisure facilities, and relatives' places of residence (Van der Waerden et al. 2003). The motivation of residential mobility might be a change of household structure, employment, or travel mode. Alternatively, these changes could also be the result of residential migration. For instance, residential change was found to correspond closely with events in employment and household biographies, such as household formation, a child's birth, or workplace change (Dieleman and Mulder 2002). In relation to car ownership mobility, some efforts have been made to explain residential mobility over the life course by underlying travel demand (Van Ommeren et al. 2000; Lanzendorf 2003, 2010; Scheiner 2006). These studies concluded that travel behavior and long-term residential mobility are intertwined decision flows within the life course. As an example, Scheiner (2006) argued that residential location is not only a predetermined condition of an individual's travel behavior but also an outcome of a household decision and that this decision manifests itself as either staying or moving. Moreover, travel behavior, travel changes, and accessibility of opportunities may also be criteria or even constraints on the residential mobility decision. Beige and Axhausen (2008) analyzed residential mobility and the ownership of mobility tools by using retrospective survey data covering information from 1984–2005 for each respondent. They found a strong interrelation between these two aspects of mobility.

Household structure mobility is strongly related to age and generation. This mobility is usually reflected in change of household size, the number of children, or the number of older people. These changes have been found to play a major role in the mobility of households. For example, household mobility often occurs with increase or decrease of the number of adult household members (Dargay 2001; Mohammadian and Miller 2003; Dargay and Hanly 2007; Scheiner 2007). Household structure mobility is also found concomitant with changes of residential location and job. Lanzendorf (2003) noted that the presence of children in households and their ages affect in a fundamental way the assignment of household responsibilities, employment, car availability, ownership, and ultimately travel. In particular, Lanzendorf (2003) argued that activity patterns of the parents change greatly after the birth of a child. Indeed, it has also been observed that long commuting trips, a result of car ownership mobility, in turn lead to serious burdens for commuters themselves and their families, which significantly lower subjective well-being, health, and fertility (Novaco et al. 1990; Scheiner 2007; Stutzer and Frey 2008).

Employment/education mobility comprises a job/education pause and the beginning of a new job or education course. Some studies have shown that the effects of a job pause due to the birth of a child on travel by women are obvious and these not only result in activity pattern change for women but also for other household members (Lanzendorf 2003). Another pause is retirement, which allows for a new arrangement of lifestyle choices. More free time makes new time arrangements available that might also affect travel (Kaiser 2003). The start of a new job/education is probably concomitant with an increase of income, which allows a broader range of travel options, or with a location change that might require the household/individual to move to a more convenient residential location or buy a car to save on commuting time without changing residence (Lanzendorf 2010). It is evident that the employment/education change is interdependent with travel behavior and household structure as well as residential location. However, it should be noted that this relationship is not one way. In other words, the availability of a car together with the household structure and residential location can adversely affect job search. If no car is available, the residential location is far away, or there are young children who need care, the probability of finding an adequate job is limited to jobs in the vicinity or those that are easy to access by public transport.

Based on the above interpretation, a complex relationship structure is sketched out. However, little has been done with respect to biographical interactions among the above four mobility domains.

14.3 Methodology

Our literature review suggests complex biographical interactions between car ownership, residential choice, household structure, and employment/education mobilities in the life course. To represent these biographical interactions, it is necessary to adopt modeling approaches that can simultaneously deal with all these mobility biographies by properly reflecting the inherent behavioral mechanisms. Recognizing that some methods are likely able to capture such complex mechanisms, this study attempts to explore the possibility of utility-maximizing approaches in describing the biographical mobilities over the life course. Under the utility-maximizing principle, it is assumed that an individual/household wants to maximize his/her lifetime utility derived from residential choice, car ownership, household structure, and employment/education mobilities to achieve the most satisfied life to date. We recognize that, in reality, it is difficult for a person to maximize his/her utility obtained from different life choices over a life course; our model is simply an approximation of people's actual decisions. That said, the concept of lifetime utility has already been proposed and applied in a number of fields, e.g., career development, labor economics, and risky behavior.

For this purpose, a multilinear utility function (Zhang et al. 2002; Zhang and Fujiwara 2006) is adopted here and household k's lifetime utility (i.e., U_k) is derived from the subutility of residential episode u_{ki}^R, car ownership episode u_{kj}^C, household structure episode u_{km}^F, and employment/education episode u_{kn}^E. Episode here is defined as the period between two consecutive changes in a life trajectory. The duration of the episode is the decision variable (i.e., dependent variable) in the following optimization problem:

$$Max \quad U_k = g(u_{ki}^R, u_{kj}^C, u_{km}^F, u_{kn}^E) \tag{14.1}$$

subject to

$$T_k = \sum_i t_{ki}^R, \quad T_k = \sum_j t_{kj}^C, \quad T_k = \sum_m t_{km}^F, \quad T_k = \sum_n t_{kn}^E$$
$$t_{ki}^R > 0, \quad t_{kj}^C > 0, \quad t_{km}^F > 0, \quad t_{kn}^E > 0 \tag{14.2}$$

where $g(u^R_{ki}, u^C_{kj}, u^F_{km}, u^E_{kn})$ is the household utility function with respect to $u^R_{ki}, u^C_{kj}, u^F_{km}, u^E_{kn}$, and $t^R_{ki}, t^C_{kj}, t^F_{km}, t^E_{kn}$ are respectively the *i*th residential episode duration, the *j*th car ownership episode duration, the *m*th household structure episode duration, and the *n*th employment/education episode duration. Note that the number of episodes *i, j, m, n* is not fixed and differs across households. If there is no change in the life course, then only one episode is observed (equal to the whole life to date, T_k); that is, *i, j, m, n* are equal to or larger than 1. The utility function $g(u^R_{ki}, u^C_{kj}, u^F_{km}, u^E_{kn})$ is specified as

$$\begin{aligned} g(u^R_{ki}, u^C_{kj}, u^F_{km}, u^E_{kn}) = & \sum_i u^R_{ki} + \sum_j u^C_{kj} + \sum_m u^F_{km} + \sum_n u^E_{kn} + \lambda^R \sum_i \sum_{i'} u^R_{ki} u^R_{ki'} \\ & + \lambda^C \sum_j \sum_{j'} u^C_{kj} u^C_{kj'} + \lambda^F \sum_m \sum_{m'} u^F_{km} u^F_{km'} + \sum_n \sum_{n'} u^E_{kn} u^E_{kn'} \\ & + \lambda^{RC} \sum_i \sum_j u^R_{ki} u^C_{kj} + \lambda^{RF} \sum_i \sum_m u^R_{ki} u^F_{km} + \lambda^{RE} \sum_i \sum_n u^R_{ki} u^E_{kn} \\ & + \lambda^{CF} \sum_j \sum_m u^C_{kj} u^F_{km} + \lambda^{CE} \sum_j \sum_n u^C_{kj} u^E_{kn} + \lambda^{FE} \sum_m \sum_n u^F_{km} u^E_{kn} \end{aligned} \tag{14.3}$$

where, $\lambda^R, \lambda^C, \lambda^F, \lambda^E$ are the interepisode interaction parameters for each domain, and $\lambda^{RC}, \lambda^{RF}, \lambda^{RE}, \lambda^{CF}, \lambda^{CE}, \lambda^{FE}$ are the interepisode interaction parameters for a pair of domains. Here, the domain refers to residential choice, car ownership, household structure, or employment/education.

It is further assumed that the marginal utility with respect to the duration of each episode is positive and has a diminishing property, i.e., the marginal utility of an increase of duration decreases. To meet such conditions, the utility function for each episode is defined as follows:

$$u^R_{ki} = \rho^R_{ki}\, ln(t^R_{ki}) \tag{14.4}$$

$$u^C_{kj} = \rho^C_{kj}\, ln(t^C_{kj}) \tag{14.5}$$

$$u^F_{km} = \rho^F_{km}\, ln(t^F_{km}) \tag{14.6}$$

$$u^E_{kn} = \rho^E_{kn}\, ln(t^E_{kn}). \tag{14.7}$$

Here, $\rho^R_{ki}, \rho^C_{kj}, \rho^F_{km}, \rho^E_{kn}$ are introduced to represent the heterogeneous baseline utilities of residential episode *i*, car ownership episode *j*, household structure episode *m*, and employment/education episode *n* across households. To guarantee the positivity of the utility function, an exponential form is then applied to the above four equations:

$$\rho^R_{ki} = exp(\beta^R x^R_{ki} + \varepsilon^R_{ki}) \tag{14.8}$$

$$\rho^C_{kj} = exp(\beta^C x^C_{kj} + \varepsilon^C_{kj}) \tag{14.9}$$

$$\rho_{km}^{F} = exp(\beta^{F} x_{km}^{F} + \varepsilon_{km}^{F}) \tag{14.10}$$

$$\rho_{kn}^{E} = exp(\beta^{E} x_{kn}^{E} + \varepsilon_{kn}^{E}) \tag{14.11}$$

where x_{ki}^{R} is a vector of observed household attributes and residential-specific factors in duration i; x_{kj}^{C} is a vector of observed household attributes and car ownership-specific factors in duration j; x_{km}^{F} is a vector of observed household attributes and residential-specific factors in duration m; and x_{kn}^{E} is a vector of observed household attributes and employment/education-specific factors in duration n. $\beta^{R}, \beta^{C}, \beta^{F}, \beta^{E}$ are unknown parameters for corresponding $\{x\}$. The error terms $\varepsilon_{ki}^{R}, \varepsilon_{kj}^{C}, \varepsilon_{km}^{F}, \varepsilon_{kn}^{E}$ are used to describe the influence of unobserved factors (e.g., attitude, lifestyle preference, social interaction, etc.) on the residential, car ownership, household structure, and employment durations, respectively.

The optimization problem in Eq. (14.1) can be solved by forming the Lagrangian and applying the Kuhn–Tucker (KT) conditions. The Lagrangian function is:

$$L = U_k + \gamma^{R}(T_k - \sum_{i} t_{ki}^{R}) + \gamma^{C}(T_k - \sum_{j} t_{kj}^{C}) + \gamma^{F}(T_k - \sum_{m} t_{km}^{F}) + \gamma^{E}(T_k - \sum_{n} t_{kn}^{E}) \tag{14.12}$$

where $\gamma^{A}(A = R, C, F, E)$ is the Lagrangian multiplier associated with the time constraint for household k. Subsequently, by taking the first episode of each domain as the reference, the KT first-order conditions can be given by

$$\widehat{\varepsilon}_{ki}^{R} = ln(\widehat{\Omega}_{k1}^{R}) - ln(\widehat{\Omega}_{ki}^{R}) + ln(t_{ki}^{R}) - ln(t_{k1}^{R} + 1) \tag{14.13}$$

$$\widehat{\varepsilon}_{kj}^{C} = ln(\widehat{\Omega}_{k1}^{C}) - ln(\widehat{\Omega}_{kj}^{C}) + ln(t_{kj}^{C}) - ln(t_{k1}^{C} + 1) \tag{14.14}$$

$$\widehat{\varepsilon}_{km}^{F} = ln(\widehat{\Omega}_{k1}^{F}) - ln(\widehat{\Omega}_{km}^{F}) + ln(t_{km}^{F}) - ln(t_{k1}^{F} + 1) \tag{14.15}$$

$$\widehat{\varepsilon}_{kn}^{E} = ln(\widehat{\Omega}_{k1}^{E}) - ln(\widehat{\Omega}_{kn}^{E}) + ln(t_{kn}^{E}) - ln(t_{k1}^{E} + 1) \tag{14.16}$$

where

$$\hat{\Omega}_{ki}^{R} = (1 + \lambda^{R} \sum_{i'} u_{ki'}^{R} + \lambda^{RC} \sum_{j} u_{kj}^{C} + \lambda^{RF} \sum_{m} u_{km}^{F} + \lambda^{RE} \sum_{n} u_{kn}^{E}) \cdot exp(\beta^{R} x_{ki}^{R}) \tag{14.17}$$

$$\hat{\Omega}_{kj}^{C} = (1 + \lambda^{C} \sum_{j'} u_{kj'}^{C} + \lambda^{RC} \sum_{i} u_{ki}^{R} + \lambda^{CF} \sum_{m} u_{km}^{F} + \lambda^{CE} \sum_{n} u_{kn}^{E}) \cdot exp\,(\beta^{C} x_{kj}^{C}) \tag{14.18}$$

$$\hat{\Omega}^F_{km} = (1 + \lambda^F \sum_{m'} u^F_{km'} + \lambda^{RF} \sum_i u^R_{ki} + \lambda^{CF} \sum_j u^C_{kj} + \lambda^{FE} \sum_n u^E_{kn}) \cdot exp(\beta^F x^F_{km}) \tag{14.19}$$

$$\hat{\Omega}^E_{kn} = (1 + \lambda^E \sum_{n'} u^E_{kn'} + \lambda^{RE} \sum_i u^R_{ki} + \lambda^{CE} \sum_j u^C_{kj} + \lambda^{FE} \sum_m u^F_{km}) \cdot exp(\beta^E x^F_{kn}). \tag{14.20}$$

The utility terms in Eqs. (14.17)–(14.20) correspond to those whose error terms have been thrown out. The error terms in Eqs. (14.13)–(14.16) $\widehat{\varepsilon}^R_{ki}, \widehat{\varepsilon}^C_{kj}, \widehat{\varepsilon}^F_{km}, \widehat{\varepsilon}^E_{kn}$ are the composite products that have merged with the error terms in the utility components in Eqs. (14.17)–(14.20). Although in this way these error terms become very complicated and are difficult to explain, they are always operable from a mathematical viewpoint. Besides, the interaction that comes from the unobserved factors is not of interest in this analysis; clarification of the error terms is left as a future research issue. By assuming $\widehat{\varepsilon}^R_{ki}, \widehat{\varepsilon}^C_{kj}, \widehat{\varepsilon}^F_{km}, \widehat{\varepsilon}^E_{kn}$ are independent of each other and follow the normal distribution with mean zero and variances $(\sigma^R_{ki})^2, (\sigma^C_{kj})^2, (\sigma^F_{km})^2, (\sigma^E_{kn})^2$, respectively, the likelihood can be derived as:

$$P_k = \left\{\prod_i \left[\frac{1}{\sigma^R_{ki}} \cdot \phi\left(\frac{\widehat{\varepsilon}^R_{ki}}{\sigma^R_{ki}}\right)\right]\right\} \cdot \left\{\prod_j \left[\frac{1}{\sigma^C_{kj}} \cdot \phi\left(\frac{\widehat{\varepsilon}^C_{kj}}{\sigma^C_{kj}}\right)\right]\right\} \cdot \left\{\prod_m \left[\frac{1}{\sigma^F_{km}} \cdot \phi\left(\frac{\widehat{\varepsilon}^F_{km}}{\sigma^F_{km}}\right)\right]\right\} \cdot \left\{\prod_n \left[\frac{1}{\sigma^E_{kn}} \cdot \phi\left(\frac{\widehat{\varepsilon}^E_{kn}}{\sigma^E_{kn}}\right)\right]\right\} \tag{14.21}$$

where ϕ denotes the probability density function of the standard normal distribution, and Φ denotes the cumulative density function of the standard normal distribution.

14.4 Data

To study the interactions between mobility decisions (including residential location mobility, car ownership mobility, household structure mobility, and employment/education mobility) over the life course, longitudinal data are required. The standard method is to conduct a panel survey; in this way, relatively reliable data can be collected. However, panel surveys are time-consuming if one is to obtain enough information about long-term behavioral changes. As an alternative to a panel survey, a retrospective approach is used, which asks respondents to recall past information. Based on retrospective reports, life history surveys have been developed and applied for many years in the social sciences to capture human behavior over the life course (Freedman et al. 1988; Belli 1998; Belli et al. 2007).

Because the reliability of retrospective data is one key problem, some studies have argued that people tend to remember major events, such as residential moves or personal and familial events, better than other events (Hollingworth and Miller 1996). In light of these considerations, in November 2010, a web-based life story survey covering the life of each respondent from 18 years old to the survey date was carried out in Japan. The web survey was implemented with the help of a major web survey company with more than 1.4 million registered panels. As a result, 1000 questionnaires were collected from the registered panels living in major Japanese cities, in which age, gender, and residential distributions across the whole population in Japan are guaranteed. The survey contents cover the four domains in which we are interested, namely residential, household, employment/education, and car ownership trajectories. First, for each domain, the frequency of changes and the exact mobility timing during the observed period were elicited, and then detailed information about each episode was reported as follows:

- residential trajectory: location, income, house property, accessibility (in terms of distance) of various facilities (including railway station, bus stop, primary, junior, and high schools, hospital, park, supermarket, city hall) in each episode;
- household trajectory: size, information on each household member in each episode (age, gender, relation to householder);
- employment/education trajectory: job category, commuting time to job/school, accessibility to job/school, travel mode in each episode;
- car ownership trajectory: number of cars, main user, car efficiency, purpose and frequency of use in each episode.

Note that we only asked respondents to include mobility in the four domains if the duration of an episode was at least one year. Moreover, only information about the previous four changes was collected. Mobility timing information allowed us to calculate the duration of each episode. For each individual, the number of episodes was one to no more than five. Individuals without any change in their past life then had only one episode and the duration was from 18 years old to the survey date. For respondents with four or more changes in their past life, five episodes were allotted including the episode before the first mobility to that from the fourth mobility to the survey date. Corresponding to each episode for the four examined domains, the specific attributes were added to the model as explanatory variables for that episode.

In Table 14.1, we show the distribution of mobility frequency for each cohort during the life course. Almost 90 % of the population experienced mobility in residential location, household structure, and employment/education. In contrast, car ownership mobility was less frequent compared with the other three domains. Households without car ownership change in the life course accounted for 36 % (166 individuals), which is far larger than the other domains. Further aggregation showed that of the 166 individuals, fewer than half had never owned a car. In other words, more than 80 % of individuals owned or used to own a car or cars.

Next, we examined the frequency of change of car ownership. Figure 14.1 shows the duration distribution of residential, car ownership, household structure,

Table 14.1 Distribution of the mobility frequency for each cohort during the life course

Change times	1940 cohort (%)	1950 cohort (%)	1960 cohort (%)	1970 cohort (%)	1980 cohort (%)	Total (%)
	10	33	31	15	11	100
Residential location change						
Zero	10	17	9	14	28	14
Once	15	16	12	24	21	18
Twice	18	20	24	23	27	23
Three	14	12	16	15	13	15
≥Four	43	35	38	24	12	30
Car ownership change						
Zero	36	34	27	37	55	36
Once	20	12	19	24	32	21
Twice	10	7	13	13	9	11
Three	5	7	11	11	2	9
≥Four	30	39	30	15	3	23
Household structure change						
Zero	5	10	12	21	29	16
Once	10	11	17	28	37	22
Twice	8	22	23	20	15	19
Three	20	21	20	15	11	17
≥Four	57	37	28	16	8	26
Employment/Education change						
Zero	20	13	11	15	23	15
Once	18	18	11	19	23	17
Twice	11	14	12	10	21	13
Three	11	15	13	14	18	14
≥Four	39	40	54	42	15	42

and employment/education episodes. A left-skewed distribution is clearly present for all four domains. Overall, 3097 residential, 2482 car ownership, 2954 household structure, and 3314 employment/education episodes were observed in the sample. On average, these episodes lasted 7.7, 9.7, 8.2, and 7.3 years with a standard deviation of 7.8, 9.6, 7.8, and 8.6 years, respectively. Roughly 70 % of all episodes lasted up to 10 years. For all four domains, the most frequent episode lasted 2–3 years. We then analyzed the changes occurring during the life course. Figure 14.2 displays the mobility timing of residential location, car ownership, household structure, and employment/education in the life course, grouped by five years. For all four domains, the peak period of mobility clearly lies between the ages of 20 and 35 years. The co-occurrence of mobility for residential location, car ownership, household structure, and employment/education can be captured by similar curves. For car ownership, the curve is relatively even compared with the other domains.

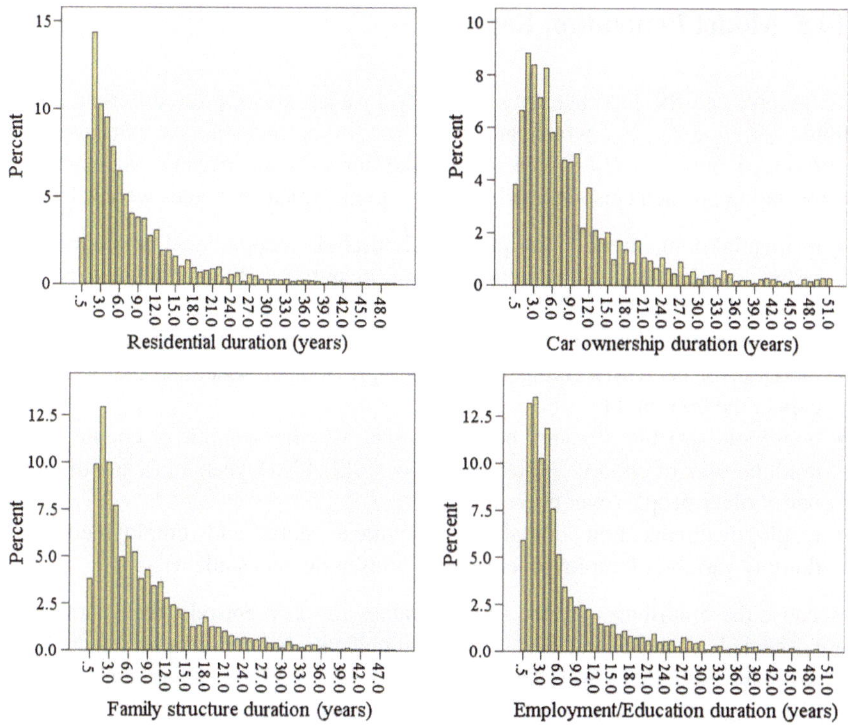

Fig. 14.1 Duration distribution of the residential, household structure, employment/education, car ownership episodes

Fig. 14.2 Mobility timing in residential, household structure, employment/ education, car ownership during the life course

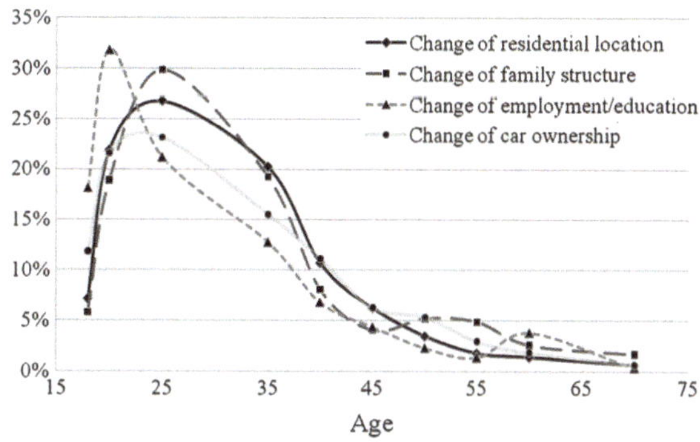

14.5 Model Estimation Results

To incorporate the heterogeneity of utility in each episode for different households, $\rho_{ki}^{R}, \rho_{kj}^{C}, \rho_{km}^{F}, \rho_{kn}^{E}$, which are composed of episode-specific attributes, are introduced into Eqs. (14.8)–(14.11). In the survey data, because we have rich information on each episode in all domains, some typical attributes were selected:

- residential domain: the house property, household income level, accessibility to railway station, bus stop, primary school, hospital, park, supermarket, and the CBD;
- car ownership domain: ownership of a car license, whether car ownership increases or decreases compared with the previous episode, and the number of cars in the household;
- household structure domain: household size, whether a single or couple household, number of children (younger than 6, 6–12, 13–18 years old), and the number of older people (over 60 years);
- employment/education domain: employment state, and employment type dummy variables (employee, employer, housewife, and student).

Because these attributes are the specific values for each episode, their parameters are assumed to be the same across different episodes but different across domains. The model estimations were carried out using the standard maximum likelihood method generated by GAUSS 9.0 software. The results are presented in Table 14.2.

14.5.1 Interepisode Biographical Interactions

All the biographical interaction terms are statistically significant at the 95 % confidence level. This supports the assumption that different domains in the life course are not independent. Specifically, the interepisode interaction term for each domain is negative, indicating that the longer the previous episode continued (or the future episode is going to continue), the shorter is the current episode. This competitive relationship might be caused by the limit on total lifetime. Such competitive relationships have often been observed in the context of short-term time allocation behavior (e.g., time allocation within a day or a week). To our knowledge, this is the first time this research literature has been able to clarify such competitive relationships over the life course based on utility-maximizing approaches. With respect to the interepisode interaction terms for pairs of domains, a synergistic relationship is present in the sense that all the relevant interaction parameters are positive. This signifies that the longer the duration of an episode in one domain is, the longer it is likely to be for other domains, suggesting the co-occurrence of the four domains over the life course. In other words, the occurrence of any life event might induce the occurrence of all four mobilities.

Table 14.2 Model estimation results

Explanatory variable	Coefficient	t-score	
Interaction terms between the mobility durations			
Intra-residential episodes	−1.200	−17.872	**
Intra-car ownership episodes	−0.723	−3.089	**
Intra-household structure episodes	−1.161	−8.728	**
Intra-employment episodes	−1.022	−9.179	**
Residential & car ownership	0.920	18.632	**
Household structure & car ownership	0.638	5.592	**
Car ownership & employment	0.522	5.854	**
Residential & household structure	1.178	9.508	**
Residential & employment	0.773	20.289	**
Household structure & employment	1.261	8.087	**
Attributes reflecting the heterogeneous utility of residential location duration			
House property (1: own, 0: otherwise)	0.410	16.156	**
Belong to middle income group (3 ~ 8 Million yen) (1: yes, 0: no)	−0.024	−0.712	
Belong to high income group (>8 Million yen) (1: yes, 0: no)	0.005	2.359	**
Accessibility to railway station	−0.163	−6.473	**
Accessibility to bus stop	−0.046	−2.717	**
Accessibility to primary school	0.013	0.326	
Accessibility to hospital	−0.031	−0.809	
Accessibility to park	−0.038	−2.021	**
Accessibility to supermarket	−0.048	−2.293	**
Accessibility to central area (i.e., city hall)	0.044	1.563	
Attributes reflecting the heterogeneous utility of car ownership duration			
Whether have car license (1: yes, 0: no)	0.109	6.095	**
Number of cars in the household	0.134	3.712	**
Compared with previous episode, whether the car ownership increase (1: yes, 0: no)	0.068	1.126	
Compared with previous episode, whether the car ownership decrease (1: yes, 0: no)	0.129	4.329	**
Attributes reflecting the heterogeneous utility of household structure duration			
Household size	0.095	4.734	**
Whether single household (1: yes, 0: no)	0.000	0.015	
Whether couple household (1: yes, 0: no)	−0.145	−11.869	**
Number of children younger than 6 years old	−0.262	−5.858	**
Number of children belong to 6 ~ 12 years old	0.060	4.351	**
Number of children belong to 13 ~ 18 years old	0.038	0.522	
Number of elder people older than 60 years old	0.027	1.923	
Attributes reflecting the heterogeneous utility of employment/education duration			
Whether is employed in the duration (1: yes, 0: no)	−0.139	−3.388	**
Whether is private-company employer (1: yes, 0: no)	0.486	11.219	**
Whether is private-company employee (1: yes, 0: no)	0.310	3.844	**

(continued)

Table 14.2 (continued)

Explanatory variable	Coefficient	t-score	
Whether is housewife (1: yes, 0: no)	0.634	7.908	**
Whether is student (1: yes, 0: no)	−0.298	−2.963	**
Variance			
Variance of duration before the newest residential change	0.967	2.834	**
Variance of duration before the second newest residential change	0.955	1.363	
Variance of duration before the third newest residential change	0.941	6.083	**
Variance of duration before the forth newest residential change	1.195	2.659	**
Variance of duration before the newest household structure change	1.189	9.154	**
Variance of duration before the second newest household structure change	1.238	9.351	**
Variance of duration before the third newest household structure change	1.398	1.852	
Variance of duration before the forth newest household structure change	1.623	2.170	**
Variance of duration before the newest employment change	1.188	9.757	**
Variance of duration before the second newest employment change	1.202	7.468	**
Variance of duration before the third newest employment change	1.267	3.771	**
Variance of duration before the forth newest employment change	1.416	12.057	**
Variance of duration before the newest car ownership change	1.210	2.981	**
Variance of duration before the second newest car ownership change	1.346	8.095	**
Variance of duration before the third newest car ownership change	1.581	1.582	
Variance of duration before the forth newest car ownership change	1.971	9.151	**
Initial log-likelihood	−20359.4		
Converged log-likelihood	−12219.7		
Rho-square	0.3998		
Adjusted Rho-square	0.3972		

**Significant at the 5 % level

14.5.2 Utility Components

The utility components were calculated and the results are shown in Fig. 14.3. It is evident that the total additive utility [sum of the first four terms in the right-hand side of Eq. (14.3)] is very small, only accounting for about 5 % of total household utility (absolute value) over the life course. In other words, the pure utility of each

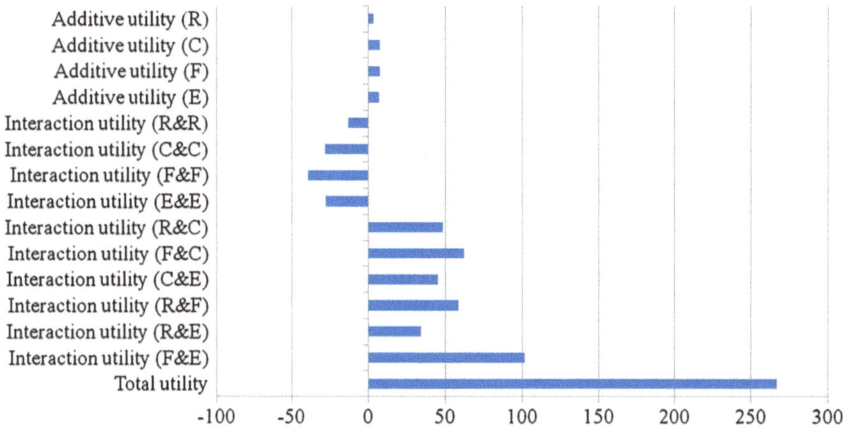

Fig. 14.3 Utility composition in the proposed model

domain contributed little to the household's life satisfaction. In contrast, the overall interaction utility accounts for almost 95 % of the total utility (absolute value) (23 % of the total is intraepisode interaction in the same domain and 72 % of the total is interdomain interactions), implying that households tend to make decisions on a set of mobilities; consequently, decisions on different mobilities are not independent but jointly made. The car ownership domain has a very strong interaction with residential, household structure, and employment/education domains, accounting for almost 40 % of the total utility (absolute value). Thus, considering travel behavior from the life course perspective can contribute to a better understanding of the dynamic mechanism.

14.5.3 Explanatory Variables

Most of the explanatory variables involved in the baseline preferences are estimated to be statistically significant. A positive sign means that the corresponding variable is associated with a longer duration of the episode and a negative sign implies the opposite.

In the residential mobility domain, the house property has a positive influence on the duration of episode, meaning that households are more likely to move if they do not own a house in that episode. Households with a high annual income (more than 8 million yen) are inclined to reside in a place longer than those from low- and middle-income groups. This might result from high-income households choosing their "dream home" location earlier, thus obviating the need for frequent house moves. Accessibility to a railway station, bus stop, park, and supermarket is found to be negatively related to the duration of a residential episode, indicating that the farther people live away from the above facilities, the more they will move residence, which may be associated with the inconvenience of daily life.

With respect to the car ownership mobility domain, the number of cars owned in a household and whether car ownership increases or decreases compared with the previous episode show a positive influence on episode duration for a specific car ownership state. If a household owned more cars in this episode, their satisfaction with cars might be higher than other households; the need to change this state would therefore be less. In addition, compared with the previous episode, if the household disposed of one or more cars, they would be inclined to keep this state for a longer time, which might be associated with a reduced demand for car usage in daily life. To some extent, this variable represents the effect of sequential choices of car ownership over the life course.

In the household structure mobility domain, large households prefer to maintain the current episode of household structure. Couple households are more willing to change their structure, probably because of the desire for a child. Households with children younger than 6 years old never maintain this state for very long, while households with children 6–12 years old are less likely to change. This might be explained by couples usually thinking to have their second or third child when they are still young. However, after the children enter primary school, due to the burden of expenditure and limited vigor, they do not expect any mobility of the household structure.

In the employment/education mobility domain, if household members are currently employed, then households will not continue this episode for very long, probably because they are looking for a better job or they move to the next education degree. But for household members who are a private-company employer or a private-company employee, they will maintain their current work longer compared to other jobs. While for household members who are a housewife or househusband, they are more likely to maintain their current status (unemployed) longer than others. Students show a more changeable life in the employment/education domain; this may be due to the confliction between studying and having a part-time job, or the predetermined graduation time.

Based on these results, it can be seen that through changing accessibility to fundamental facilities such as a railway station, bus stop, park, and supermarket, the duration of a residential episode will change. Because of the evident interaction among different mobility domains, the decision on mobility in car ownership, household structure, and employment/education could also be influenced indirectly. The policies that encourage people to dispose voluntarily of their old cars can directly reduce car ownership change which may further influence the mobility decisions in other life domains. By packaging these two types of policies, the mobility behavior of households in the life course might be explicitly regulated.

14.6 Conclusion

When formulating long-term transport policies, changes of people's behaviors over the life course cannot be ignored. To predict whether policies could result in the desired changes in the future, policy makers need to understand how people behave in response to the policies under study as well as to other factors over a longer time period. Unfortunately, very few studies have been conducted using longer time observations, due to the difficulties of collecting relevant data and representing relevant behaviors.

This study aims to represent biographical interactions between car ownership mobility, residential mobility, household structure mobility, and employment/education mobility over the life course. Recognizing that there are various types of biographical interactions, this study focuses only on the interactions between major mobility domains from the perspective of mobility duration between two consecutive changes of a domain. Four mobility domains are examined, namely car ownership, residential choice, household structure, and employment/education, which are closely related to travel behavior and are important factors when evaluating transport policies. The biographical interactions are modeled by using a multilinear utility function, which can flexibly incorporate various interactions as well as independent utility components simultaneously within a unified utility-maximizing modeling framework. As an empirical analysis, a web-based retrospective life story survey covering the life of each respondent from 18 years old to the survey date was carried out at the end of 2010 in Japan, with 1000 households providing valid data. Findings obtained from the empirical analysis are summarized as follows.

- The effectiveness of the proposed model to represent biographical interactions was confirmed, implying that the adopted utility-maximizing approach was acceptable to capture behaviors over the life course in this case study.
- It was found that among the duration of episodes in the same domain, a significant competitive relationship exists for residential mobility, car ownership mobility, household structure mobility, and employment/education mobility.
- The interdomain interactions in the life course were substantial. The overall interaction utility derived from residential mobility, car ownership mobility, household structure mobility and employment/education mobility accounted for almost 72 % of the total, implying that households prefer to make a decision on a set of mobilities when considering changing residence, car ownership, household structure, or employment/education. In other words, the mobility decision is likely to be intertwined with mobility in other domains.
- Policies for changing accessibility to fundamental facilities (e.g., railway station, bus stop, park, and supermarket) and encouraging people to dispose voluntarily of their old cars were found to be effective in altering household decisions on the mobility of these main domains in the life course.

Some limitations should be noted here. As one of the first attempts to deal with the life course dynamics in transportation from the behavioral perspective, the methodology adopted in this chapter can capture to some extent the interactions between different mobility domains. However, the assumptions made in our model might be not very consistent with realities, including the utility-maximizing principle and the diminishing marginal utility of duration of each episode. The most important issue is how to build a model with more realistic features. Another problem is that mobility over the life course is a sequential decision process. To accommodate such behavioral mechanisms, it is necessary to introduce the occurrence timing of each episode. Finally, the most important policy-related issue might be how to make effective use of such life course data to support transport policy decisions.

References

Beige S, Axhausen KW (2008) Long-term and mid-term mobility decisions during the life course: experiences with a retrospective survey. IATSS Res 32(2):16–33

Belli RF (1998) The structure of autobiographical memory and the event history calendar: potential improvements in the quality of retrospective reports in surveys. Memory 6(4):383–406

Belli RF, Smith LM, Andreski PM, Agrawal S (2007) Methodological comparisons between CATI event history calendar and standardized conventional questionnaire instruments. Public Opin Q 71(4):603–622

Ben-Akiva M, Lerman SR (1991) Discrete choice analysis: theory and application to travel demand. The MIT Press, Cambridge

Dargay J (2001) The effect of income on car ownership: evidence of asymmetry. Transp Res Part A 35:807–821

Dargay J, Hanly M (2007) Volatility of car ownership, commuting mode and time in the UK. Transp Res Part A 41(10):934–948

Dieleman F (2001) Modelling residential mobility: a review of recent trends in research. J Hous Built Environ 16:249–265

Dieleman FM, Mulder CH (2002) The geography of residential choice. In: Aragonés JI, Francescato G, Gärling T (eds) Residential environments: choice, satisfaction, and behavior. Bergin & Garvey, Westport, Connecticut, pp 35–54

Eliasson J, Mattsson L (2000) A model for integrated analysis of household location and travel choices. Transp Res Part A 34(5):375–394

Freedman D, Thornton A, Camburn D, Alwin D, Young-DeMarco L (1988) The life history calendar: a technique for collecting retrospective data. Sociol Methodol 18:37–68

Hollingworth BJ, Miller EJ (1996) Retrospective interviewing and its application in study of residential mobility. Transp Res Rec 1551:74–81

Kaiser B (2003) FRAME-Freizeitmobilität älterer Menschen. Paper presented at the annual meeting of the working group transportation of the German association of geographers, Wuppertal, 5–7 June

Lanzendorf M (2003) Mobility biographies: a new perspective for understanding travel behaviour. Paper presented at the 10th international conference on travel behaviour research, Lucerne, 10–15 Aug

Lanzendorf M (2010) Key events and their effect on mobility biographies: the case of child birth. Int J Sustain Transp 4(5):272–292

Mayer KU, Tuma NB (1990) Event history analysis in life course research. University of Wisconsin Press, Madison

Mohammadian A, Miller EJ (2003) Dynamic modeling of household automobile transactions. Transp Res Rec 1831:98–105

Novaco RW, Stokols D, Milanesi LC (1990) Subjective and objective dimensions of travel impedance as determinants of commuting stress. Am J Community Psychol 18:231–257

Ommeren JNV, Rietveld P, Nijkamp P (1999) Job mobility, residential mobility and commuting: a search perspective. J Urban Econ 46:230–253

Scheiner J (2006) Housing mobility and travel behaviour: a process-oriented approach to spatial mobility. evidence from a new research field in Germany. J Transp Geogr 14(4):287–298

Scheiner J (2007) Mobility biographies: elements of a biographical theory of travel demand. Erdkunde 61(2):161–173

Stutzer A, Frey B (2008) Stress that doesn't pay: the commuting paradox. Scand J Econ 110(2):339–366

Van der Waerden P, Timmermans H, Borgers A (2003) The influence of key events and critical incidents on transport mode choice switching behaviour: a descriptive analysis. Paper presented at the 10th international conference on travel behaviour research (IATBR), Lucerne, 10–15 Aug

Van Ommeren J, Rietveld P, Nijkamp P (2000) Job mobility, residential mobility and commuting: A theoretical analysis using search theory. Ann Reg Sci 34:213–232

Waddell P (2001) Towards a behavioral integration of land use and transportation modeling. In: Hensher D (ed) Travel behavior research: the leading edge. Pergamon, New York, pp 65–95

Wissen LJG, Dykstra PA (1999) Population issues. An interdisciplinary focus. Kluwer Academic/Plenum Publishers, New York

Zhang J, Fujiwara A (2006) Representing household time allocation behavior by endogenously incorporating diverse intra-household interactions: a case study in the context of elderly couples. Transp Res Part B 40:54–74

Zhang J, Timmermans H, Borgers A (2002) A utility-maximizing model of household time use for independent, shared and allocated activities incorporating group decision mechanisms. Transp Res Rec 1807:1–8

Chapter 15
Household Time Use Behavior Analysis: A Case Study of Multidimensional Timing Decisions

Junyi Zhang and Harry Timmermans

Abstract This chapter investigates household time use behavior by especially focusing on timing decisions on interdependent daily activities. Timing decisions on various life choices have been unsatisfactorily presented in literature. At best, such timing decisions have been presented based on survival analysis, which has various attractive statistical features, however, ignores decision-making mechanisms. This chapter argues that the utility of activity participation and trip-making behavior changes over time, and timing decisions within a given period of time interact across activities/trips and across household members. This study derives the optimal timing functions for both nonshared and shared activities/trips by different household members, where interdependencies among activities/trips over time and household's coupling constraints are endogenously represented. The applicability of the developed model is empirically examined. Behavioral implications of analysis results are finally discussed.

Keywords Time use · Timing utility · Coupling constraints · Intrahousehold interaction · Interdependencies among activities/trips · Shared activities/trips · Sequential correlation · Sequencing constraints

15.1 Introduction

Time use surveys usually include activities such as work, school, travel to/from work/school, housework, eating, shopping, childcare, reading, sleeping, sports, entertaining friends, hobbies, religious activities, and social activities at various

J. Zhang (✉)
Hiroshima University, Higashi-Hiroshima, Japan
e-mail: zjy@hiroshima-u.ac.jp; junyizh24@gmail.com

H. Timmermans
Eindhoven University of Technology, Eindhoven, The Netherlands

J. Zhang (ed.), *Life-Oriented Behavioral Research for Urban Policy*,
DOI 10.1007/978-4-431-56472-0_15

locations (e.g., home, workplace, school, restaurants, and hotels: but without geocoding) throughout a period of one or several days. For example, 41 activities[1] are coded in the Multinational Time Use Study (Gauthier et al. 2006). With the support of various data,[2] time use has been studied in various disciplines[3] to analyze topics such as economic activities, labor, gender, quality of life, leisure, and travel behavior (Michelson 2006; Pentland et al. 2013; Kimberly 2015).

Decision-making processes in daily activities (including relevant trips) involve the planning, execution, and adaptation of a number of interrelated choices across space and over time. Such choices include what to do (generation of activities) and when and how long to do it (time use, including timing), where to do it (destination), with whom (companion), and how to reach a destination (choice of travel mode and/or travel route). Understanding these choices over time and across space is essential for decisions on policies related to transportation, such as flexible or staggered working hours, transportation network planning, road pricing, and travel information provision. A good understanding of the above decisions is also crucial to provide a logical measurement of the value of time (VOT), which is extremely important in evaluating various urban policies. Time is limited and therefore valuable. As a result, the meaning (i.e., the value) of time in a certain time period may be different from that in other periods, even though the same activity is performed. People may choose to participate in a certain activity because of time (timing) constraints, or purposely choose the timing of a particular activity, even taking into account the influence of biological responses (e.g., sleeping habit and tiredness). In either case, it seems that logically quantifying the value of time in consideration of the above decision-making mechanisms and phenomena is needed.

When time use decisions are quantified, transportation researchers have done a better job within the framework of the activity-based approach, which argues that travel is derived from activity participation (e.g., Hensher and Stopper 1979; Jones 1990; Gerike et al. 2015). The activity-based approach has played an extremely important role in understanding why people travel, and has also provided various useful insights into decisions on transportation policies since its birth in the 1980s. In fact, most transportation studies seek to devise ways to reduce traffic congestion during peak hours. In line with such considerations, understanding why people travel at a specific time, i.e., timing decisions, is crucial. However,

[1]The 41 activities are: paid work; paid work at home; paid work, doing a second job; attending school; attending classes; traveling to/from work; cooking; washing up; doing housework; doing odd jobs; gardening; shopping; childcare; domestic travel; dressing/toilet; receiving personal services; eating meals and snacks; sleeping; traveling for leisure; going on excursions; actively participating in sports; passively participating in sports; walking; doing religious activities; doing civic duties; attending cinema or theatre; going to dances or parties; visiting social clubs, pubs, or restaurants; visiting friends; listening to the radio; watching the television or video; listening to records, tapes, or CDs; studying; reading books; reading papers or magazines; relaxing; conversing; entertaining friends; knitting; sewing; or other hobbies, pastimes, or activities.

[2]http://timeuse-2009.nsms.ox.ac.uk/information/studies/ (accessed January 25, 2016).

[3]http://www.eijtur.org/ (accessed January 25, 2016).

existing insights are extremely limited. Since the 2000s, some relevant studies have emerged about the development of activity–travel scheduling models, which examine the underlying behavioral mechanisms that give rise to activity sequencing over a period of time (e.g., Garling et al. 1998; Arentze and Timmermans 2000, 2005; Ettema and Timmermans 2003; Joh et al. 2003; Zhang et al. 2005a). In addition, recent changes in policy and forecasting needs have led to the development of an emerging class of activity–trip scheduling process surveys (Doherty 2004; Doherty and Papinski 2004). In essence, activity–trip scheduling behavior concerns the organization of an activity agenda in space and over time, and thus involves decisions regarding destinations, timing, and duration. Destination choices have been widely studied, and nested choice models [e.g., the nested logit and generalized nested logit models (Koppelman and Wen 2000), the nested paired combinatorial logit model (Fujiwara and Zhang 2005)] have dominated the literature. With respect to duration of activity, two research streams have emerged: one applying proportional or accelerated hazard models (see Lee and Timmermans (2007) for a review of recent studies), and another that is mainly based on Becker's (1965) time allocation model [e.g., the individual-based model by Kitamura and Fujii (1998), the household-based model by Zhang et al. (2002, 2005b), and Zhang and Fujiwara (2006)]. In addition, the introduction of temporal constraints makes it possible to simultaneously represent durations of various activities across the course of a given time period (e.g., a day). More recently, more appealing models and theories have been proposed (e.g., Joh et al. 2002, 2006).

Compared with destination choice and duration, research on timing decisions remains scarce. For activity–travel scheduling behavior, timing decisions are problematic because decision-makers must make various interdependent timing decisions (i.e., multidimensional decisions) in a given time period. If the focus of analysis shifts from an individual to a multiperson household, the problem becomes even more complicated because some timing decisions are influenced by intrahousehold interactions. Therefore, ideally, interdependencies must be systematically incorporated not only into timing decisions across activities but also when factoring household members into modeling timing decisions.

In household decision-making, different members may need to adjust their schedules to meet various household needs, especially when participation in allocated or shared activities is required. An allocated activity such as daily shopping is an activity performed by one or more household members, and it involves a household task. Because the "products" of participation in allocated activities are usually consumed later, timing constraints may occur with respect to the end time. For example, to prepare a dinner with fresh vegetables, a household member may need to buy these vegetables and this trip needs to be completed before preparation of dinner starts. In contrast to allocated activities, participation in shared activities usually involves a negotiation process, because different members need to agree about the start and end times. Such coupling constraints reflect the fact that one has to be with particular people at the same location at (approximately) the same time. As a result, decisions about the timing of shared activities are more complicated than those of other activities.

Existing models have at best treated coupling constraints exogenously. In contrast, this study attempts to develop a multidimensional timing decision model of household activity–travel behavior with endogenous coupling constraints. The model is developed according to the principle of random utility maximization, which assumes that a household tries to maximize its utility. Household utility is defined as an additive-type function, which is the sum of the household members' utilities. The utility of a member is further specified using a similar additive-type function, which is the sum of utilities of activities/trips. In turn, the utility of an activity/trip is defined as an integral of its timing utility, i.e., the utility of performing the activity/trip at a specific point of time. From the concept of timing utility, the influence of timing constraints and sequential correlation can easily be incorporated. *Multidimensional timing* is emphasized to take into account the interdependencies of timing decisions related to different activities/trips over the course of a day. The proposed model can also be applied to represent the sequence of activity–travel behavior endogenously. Representing timing endogenously makes it possible to clarify when and why an activity/trip is conducted during a calendar unit of time, and derives a meaningful value for time.

This chapter is organized as follows. Section 15.2 discusses some conceptual issues related to household scheduling behavior, especially from the perspective of timing decisions. Section 15.3 derives a multidimensional household timing decision model. Section 15.4 first describes the data used in this study, and then explains the model estimation, which is followed by a discussion of the implications of the estimation results. Finally, this case study concludes with a discussion of important future research issues.

15.2 Conceptual Issues

15.2.1 Definition of Scheduling Behavior

Scheduling decisions usually involve the following four major choice facets: (1) schedule content, (2) time, (3) space, and (4) agent. "Content" describes what the decision is about. In this study, content refers to all possible activities and trips. Time is concerned with when the content is executed. This is the central concern of this study. "Space" refers to where the activity is executed. Spatial concerns are especially important from the perspective of urban/regional and transportation planning. However, a study of spatial choices is beyond this study. "Agent" refers to the person(s) and/or organization(s) involved in a scheduling decision. An agent can be an independent individual, or several interdependent group members (e.g., household members, colleagues in the same office, a businessperson and his/her clients, friends, or organizations). This study examines scheduling behavior, focusing on an endogenous representation of multidimensional timing in the context of multiperson households.

15.2.2 Group Behavior, Activity Classification, and Sequence

Existing research has shown that decisions made by different members of a household are not independent, suggesting the existence of intrahousehold interaction (Timmermans et al. 1992; Borgers and Timmermans 1993; Molin et al. 1997; Vovsha et al. 2004; Zhang et al. 2005b). The nature of such intrahousehold interaction is strongly influenced by the nature of the activity. Studies of family decision-making show that the involvement of household members varies with decision type (Davis 1976). This is also true for activity–travel behavior. A compulsory activity is by definition constrained to a particular household member, and is often also constrained by time, location, and duration. This means that such activities are likely to be given a high priority and leave the household member less flexibility to perform them. In turn, this may affect the allocation of other activities. However, allocated activities will also be influenced by role patterns within the household.

Activity scheduling involves interdependent choices of what activities to conduct, where and when to conduct them, coupled with mode and route choices. Although individuals and households may decide on these various choice facets in a variety of ways, existing models have typically assumed that decisions concerning activity type, the people involved, location, timing, and travel are made in a fixed sequence in an attempt to reduce the complexity of the problem.

15.2.3 Timing: Multidimensional Considerations

Some activities and trips may be performed by an individual at any time. For others, start and/or end times may be designated a priori. In such cases, individual decisions about timing are constrained. For example, a businessperson has to be on time for a meeting with his/her clients at a designated time and place. Airline passengers face strict departure times for flights. In this sense, timing decisions vary according to types of activities/trips and may be influenced by timing constraints. Participation in an activity reduces the available remaining time and consequently places time pressure on performing other activities scheduled later that day. The existence of such time constraints forces individuals to decide how to make effective use of their limited available time. For example, the more time they spend on one activity, the less they can spend on another; the later they leave a place, the later they start performing another activity. In this sense, it seems unrealistic to assume that activity timing can be determined independently. Decisions about various duration/timing episodes interact. Needless to say, utility of activity participation may depend on when the activity is performed. Traditional unidimensional timing models, such as hazard models, cannot reflect such interdependent timing behavior in a satisfactory manner. Multispell competing risk models (e.g., Popkowski Leszczyc and Timmermans 2002) can be used to represent multidimensional timing decisions from a statistical perspective. In contrast, simultaneous representations of timing decisions based on utility theory may be a better alternative from a behavioral perspective.

15.3 Model Development

15.3.1 Specification of Timing Utility

Previous studies have suggested that the utility of activity participation or travel is dependent upon its timing (Arentze and Timmermans 2000; Ashiru et al. 2003; Zhang et al. 2005a). The concept of timing utility is useful in the study of timing decisions. Because decision-makers may exhibit heterogeneous timing preferences, it is necessary to adopt some general utility functions with operational forms. In theory, a timing function could have either a continuous or a discrete form. These two forms have both advantages and disadvantages. By assuming the discrete form of timing utility, one can adopt the widely applied discrete choice modeling approaches to represent timing decisions (e.g., Zhang et al. 2004); however, categorizing continuous time into the appropriate number of time slots is problematic. For example, Fujiwara et al. (2001) attempted to solve such problems partially by using a paired combinatorial logit (PCL) model; however, such a categorization inevitably involves arbitrary and subjective judgments. Too many categories could result in a nonoperational model specification. To avoid such arbitrariness in model specification, the continuous form is adopted for the timing utility function in this study. Two major timing utility functions seem worthy of further investigation. One is the gamma probability density (GPD) function [Eq. (15.1)], the effectiveness of which has been examined by Zhang et al. (2005a). Another is the bell-shaped function proposed by Joh et al. (2003). Because the bell-shaped function has a much more complex form with more unknown parameters than the GPD function, this study adopts the following GPD function.

$$u_{ni}(t) = \frac{\beta_{ni}^{\alpha_{ni}} t^{\alpha_{ni}-1}}{\Gamma(\alpha_{ni})} \cdot \exp(-\beta_{ni} t) \tag{15.1}$$

$$\Gamma(\alpha_{ni}) = \int_0^{\infty} y^{\alpha_{ni}-1} e^{-y}\, dy \tag{15.2}$$

$$\alpha_{ni} > 0,\ \beta_{ni} > 0 \tag{15.3}$$

Here, α_{ni} and β_{ni} indicate the shape and scale parameters of utility $u_{ni}(t)$ that individual n derives from performing activity or trip i, respectively, and $\Gamma(\cdot)$ is the gamma function.

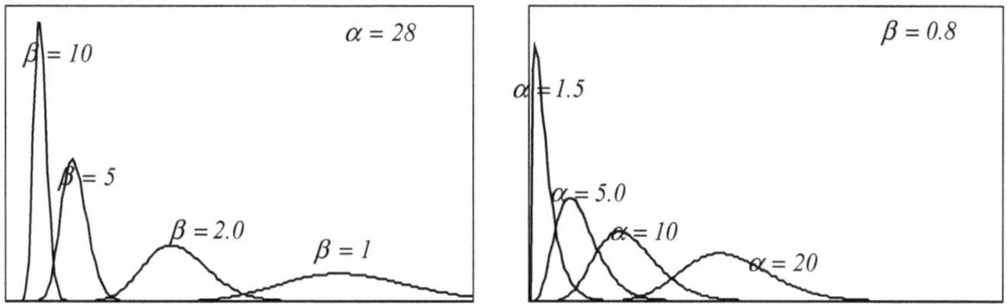

Fig. 15.1 Special cases of gamma probability density function

Different values of α_{ni} and β_{ni} result in different timing distributions, and the shape of the utility function can be either skewed or symmetric (see Fig. 15.1). As a result, the GPD function can include various forms of distribution as special cases, such as the exponential function or the normal distribution function. Adoption of the GPD function implicitly assumes that for each activity or trip, the timing utility follows a one-peak distribution, i.e., the timing utility first increases and starts to decrease after reaching a certain point in time. It should be recognized that this is also a limitation of the GPD function. In other words, if a timing distribution has two or more peaks, it is necessary to introduce additional rational logics into the model specification. This paper only examines the applicability of the GPD function to the representation of household timing decisions. Exploring other forms of timing functions is left as a future research issue.

15.3.2 Modeling Observed Interdependency: The Individual Level

Because each individual's available time is limited (here, 24 h in a day), conducting an activity for a longer period of time implies that another activity needs to be either shortened or canceled. In this sense, interdependencies among activities/trips over the course of a day need to be introduced into the model of activity participation, including timing decisions. Taking this into account, it is assumed here that utility is time-additive and time-separable, and that an individual determines the timing of an activity or a trip by maximizing his/her total utility over a given period of time. Individual n's total utility U_n is defined as the sum of utilities of all activities and trips over the target period of time [Eq. (15.4)]. Note that the start time of the ith activity or trip is also the end time of the $i-1$th activity or trip. Start and end times are the dependent variables in this study. Optimal timing can be obtained by solving the following optimization problem consisting of Eqs. (15.4) and (15.5), where Eq. (15.5) indicates the available time constraint.

Maximize

$$U_n = \sum_i U_{ni} = \sum_i \int_{t_{ni-1}}^{t_{ni}} u_{ni}(s)\, ds \tag{15.4}$$

Subject to

$$\sum_i \tau_{ni} = \sum_i (t_{ni} - t_{ni-1}) = T_n \tag{15.5}$$

where,

n, i individual and activity/trip, respectively,
U_{ni} individual n's utility from performing the ith activity/trip,
$u_{ni}(s)$ individual n's timing utility from performing the ith activity/trip at time s,
t_{ni-1} the start or departure time when individual n performs the ith activity/trip,
t_{ni} the end or arrival time when individual n performs the ith activity/trip,
τ_{ni} the duration that individual n performs the ith activity/trip, and
T_n the time available to individual n.

15.3.3 Modeling Observed Interdependency: The Household Level

In household decisions, interactions among household members with respect to multidimensional timing decisions take place because of participation in joint or shared activities and trips, which result in coupling constraints. To incorporate such coupling constraints into the model, the activities/trips should be properly classified. In this study, activities are first classified into in-home activities and out-of-home activities. The out-of-home activities are further divided into independent, allocated, and shared (joint) activities. An independent activity is an activity that does not involve a household task and is performed by a single household member. Shared activities are those activities that require the presence of all or a subset of household members. An allocated activity is usually a household task that is assigned to a specific household member. The shared activities may be synchronized or unsynchronized. In the former case, household members conduct the shared activity together from beginning to end. In the latter case, household members share parts of the activity. This study only deals with synchronized activities. The classification described above assumes that decisions on activities in each category are homogeneous. However, this may not be true in the sense that task allocation mechanisms may differ between activities. If such heterogeneity is a concern, a finer classification involving more detailed categories of activities is required.

Applying this classification, the modeling framework defined in Eqs. (15.4) and (15.5) can be rewritten for the context of household decisions as follows:

Maximize

$$U_h = \sum_n \sum_i U_{hni} = \sum_n \sum_i \int_{t_{hni-1}}^{t_{hni}} u_{hni}(s)\, ds \tag{15.6}$$

Subject to

$$\sum_i \tau_{hni} = \sum_i (t_{hni} - t_{hni-1}) = T_{hn} \tag{15.7}$$

where,

- h, n, i household, individual member, and activity/trip, respectively,
- U_{hni} the utility of individual n of household h performing the ith activity or trip,
- $u_{hni}(s)$ timing utility of individual n of household h performing the ith activity or trip at time s,
- t_{hni-1} start or departure time of individual n of household h performing the ith activity or trip (equal to the end time of $i - 1$th activity/trip),
- t_{hni} end or arrival time of individual n belonging to household h performing the ith activity or trip (equal to start time of $i + 1$th activity/trip),
- τ_{hni} duration of the ith activity or trip performed by individual n of household h, and
- T_{hn} the time available to individual n of household h.

It may be seen that household utility takes an additive type of utility function, which consists of the members' utilities. Such a specification assumes that the final decision-maker is the household rather than an individual household member. However, to reach a final decision, the household takes each member's preferences into account. Decisions about shared activities first require such a model specification because the resultant timing needs to reflect the preferences of all the members involved. Each member must take such shared activities into account to determine the timing of his/her nonshared activities. In other words, members may need to adjust the schedules of their activities/trips. Thus, the abovementioned additive type of household utility function is adopted here to incorporate the preferences of all the household members involved in the decision-making process. Of course, there are other possible household utility functions including multilinear and isoelastic types (see Zhang et al. 2005b; Zhang and Fujiwara 2006). Because introducing those types of function results in nonoperational model structures, such as the first attempt to examine household multidimensional timing decisions from the perspective of group decision-making, this paper only examines the effectiveness of the additive type of household utility function. In line with our previous research about household decisions (see Zhang et al. 2005b; Zhang and Fujiwara 2006), the principle of household utility maximization is applied.

15.3.4 Deriving the Household Timing Decision Model

In Eqs. (15.6) and (15.7), the dependent variable is timing (start time or end time) t_{hni} at which individual n belonging to household h performs activity i or makes a trip i. Maximization of Eq. (15.6) subject to Eq. (15.7) leads to the household timing decision model. To derive this model, the first derivative is calculated with respect to each timing variable t_{hni}. The timing variable of the shared activity/trip is included in all the household members' utility functions, but that of a nonshared activity/trip is only related to the member of interest. Therefore, to derive the optimal timing, it is necessary to distinguish between shared and nonshared activities/trips.

15.3.4.1 Timing Function of a Nonshared Activity/Trip

The first-order derivative for the timing of nonshared activity/trips is given below.

$$\begin{aligned}\frac{\partial U_{hn}}{\partial t_{hni}} &= \frac{\partial}{\partial t_{hni}}\left[\int\limits_{t_{hni-1}}^{t_{hni}} u_{hni}(s)\,ds + \int\limits_{t_{hni}}^{t_{hni+1}} u_{hni+1}(s)\,ds\right] \\ &= u_{hni}(t_{hni}) - u_{hni+1}(t_{hni})\end{aligned} \tag{15.8}$$

Substituting Eq. (15.1) into Eq. (15.8) and setting Eq. (15.8) to equal zero, the following equation, including the optimal timing $\hat{t}_{hni}$, can be obtained.

$$\hat{t}_{hni}^{\alpha_{hni+1}-\alpha_{hni}} \cdot \exp\{-(\beta_{hni+1} - \beta_{hni})\,\hat{t}_{hni}\} = \frac{\Gamma(\alpha_{hni})}{\Gamma(\alpha_{hni+1})} \cdot \frac{\beta_{hni+1}^{\alpha_{hni+1}}}{\beta_{hni}^{\alpha_{hni}}} \tag{15.9}$$

To obtain an explicit function of optimal timing, Eq. (15.9) is rewritten below based on a logarithm transformation.

$$(\alpha_{hni+1} - \alpha_{hni}) \ln\left(\hat{t}_{hni}\right) - (\beta_{hni+1} - \beta_{hni})\hat{t}_{hni} = \ln\left(\frac{\Gamma(\alpha_{hni})}{\Gamma(\alpha_{hni+1})} \cdot \frac{\beta_{hni+1}^{\alpha_{hni+1}}}{\beta_{hni}^{\alpha_{hni}}}\right) \tag{15.10}$$

Further transformation of Eq. (15.10) results in the following timing function for nonshared activities/trips.

$$\hat{t}_{hni} = \frac{(\alpha_{hni+1} - \alpha_{hni}) \ln\left(\hat{t}_{hni}\right) - \ln\left(\frac{\Gamma(\alpha_{hni+1})}{\Gamma(\alpha_{hni})}\frac{\beta_{hni}^{\alpha_{hni}}}{\beta_{hni+1}^{\alpha_{hni+1}}}\right)}{(\beta_{hni+1} - \beta_{hni})} \tag{15.11}$$

15.3.4.2 Timing Function of a Shared Activity/Trip

Similarly, the first-order derivative condition for the timing of shared activities/trips can be derived as below.

$$\frac{\partial U_h}{\partial t_{hni}^j} = \sum_n \frac{\partial U_{hni}}{\partial t_{hni}^j} = \sum_n \frac{\partial}{\partial t_{hni}^j} \left\{ \int_{t_{hni-1}}^{t_{hni}^j} u_{hni}(s)\, ds + \int_{t_{hni}^j}^{t_{hni+1}} u_{hni+1}(s)\, ds \right\}$$
$$= \sum_n \left(u_{hni}\left(t_{hni}^j\right) - u_{hni+1}\left(t_{hni}^j\right) \right) = 0 \tag{15.12}$$

where $\hat{t}_{hni}^j$ is the jth timing variable of household h's shared activity/trip, but the ith timing variable of individual n's activity/trip.

As a result, transformation of Eq. (15.12) leads to the following optimal timing function $\hat{t}_{hni}^j$ for the shared activity/trip.

$$t_{hni}^j = \frac{\sum_n \left(\frac{\beta_{hni+1}^{\alpha\, hni+1} (t_{hni}^j)^{\alpha_{hni+1}}}{\Gamma(\alpha_{hni+1})} \cdot \exp\left(-\beta_{hni+1} t_{hni}^j\right) \right)}{\sum_n \left(\frac{\beta_{hni}^{\alpha\, hni} (t_{hni}^j)^{\alpha_{hni}-1}}{\Gamma(\alpha_{hni})} \cdot \exp\left(-\beta_{hni} t_{hni}^j\right) \right)} \tag{15.13}$$

15.3.5 Simplifying Household Timing Decision Model Structure

Observing Fig. 15.1, it is obvious that as the value of positive shape parameter α_{ni} increases, both mean and variance of timing distribution increase, resulting in a flatter timing distribution and change in the shape of the distribution from left skewed toward the normal distribution. In contrast, the scale parameter β_{ni} shows the opposite trend. In other words, if the explanatory variable for α_{ni} and β_{ni} has different signs for shape and scale parameters, the timing distribution changes in a consistent way. Otherwise, the timing distribution varies with the values of the same explanatory variable for scale/shape parameters. On the other hand, allowing the coexistence of activity/trip-specific shape and scale parameters not only makes the estimation of Eqs. (15.11) and (15.13) very complicated, but also makes the parameter interpretations very confusing, especially from a policy perspective. Therefore, this study attempts to simplify the model structure without loss of generality by assuming that the shape parameter differs across individual household members, but is invariant across activities/trips. Based on this assumption, Eqs. (15.11) and (15.13) can be rewritten as below.

$$t_{hni} = \frac{\alpha_{hn}(\ln(\beta_{hni+1}) - \ln(\beta_{hni}))}{(\beta_{hni+1} - \beta_{hni})} \tag{15.14}$$

$$\hat{t}_{hni}^j = \frac{\sum_n \left(\frac{\beta_{hni+1}^{\alpha\, hn} (\hat{t}_{hni}^j)^{\alpha\, hn}}{\Gamma(\alpha_{hn})} \cdot \exp\left(-\beta_{hni+1} \hat{t}_{hni}^j\right) \right)}{\sum_n \left(\frac{\beta_{hni}^{\alpha_{hn}} (\hat{t}_{hni}^j)^{\alpha\, hn-1}}{\Gamma(\alpha_{hn})} \cdot \exp\left(-\beta_{hni} \hat{t}_{hni}^j\right) \right)} \tag{15.15}$$

15.3.6 Behavioral Implications of Timing Functions

As described above, the timing function for each activity/trip is derived based on the principle of household random utility maximization. This assumption is made because it is expected that the proposed model could be useful for economic evaluations of transportation policies. Moreover, because of the differing levels of involvement of household members, different forms of timing functions are derived with respect to shared and nonshared activities/trips. It is obvious that there is no structural difference in the timing functions for an activity and a trip in the same position in the schedule, or within each type of activity/trip. To capture the differences between activity and trip, activity-specific and trip-specific attributes could be introduced into the timing function. This will be explained below. If the homogeneity of each type of activity/trip were a problem, one could simply make a finer classification of activities and trips. Some major behavioral features of the derived timing functions are summarized below.

15.3.6.1 Modeling Interdependencies Among Activities/Trips

Endogenous representation of observed interdependencies

As shown in Eqs. (15.11) and (15.13), each timing variable is derived as a function not only of its own shape and scale parameters, but also of the parameters of the next activity or trip. In this sense, the derived timing functions can represent such observed interdependencies among activities and/or trips over the course of a day endogenously. Because the timing decision of an activity or a trip is influenced by that of the subsequent one, it is first-order interdependence that is incorporated into the model. As described below, the scale and shape parameters are defined as a function of the attributes of the household and its members, so the observed heterogeneity existing in the aforementioned interdependencies may be properly captured.

Endogenous representation of unobserved interdependencies

In addition to observed interdependencies among activities/trips, interdependencies may also be caused by the influence of unobserved factors. Because the parameters α_{hn} and β_{hni} are both positive, we propose to meet these two conditions and incorporate heterogeneity into timing decisions by defining these two parameters using the following functions.

$$\alpha_{hn} = \exp\left(\Delta_{hn} + e_{hn}^{\alpha}\right) \tag{15.16}$$

$$\beta_{hni} = \exp\left(\Delta_{hni} + e_{hni}^{\beta}\right) \tag{15.17}$$

where, Δ_{hn}, Δ_{hni} are deterministic terms consisting of the observed factors influencing the shape parameter α_{hn} and the scale parameter β_{hni}, respectively, and e^{α}_{hn}, e^{β}_{hni} are stochastic terms reflecting the influence of unobserved factors on α_{hn} and β_{hni}.

15.3.6.2 Representation of Activity/Trip Sequence in an Indirect Manner

It is not difficult to observe that to derive the timing function, it is only necessary to know where the relevant activity or trip is located in the overall schedule for a given time period. It is not necessary to identify the content of the activity/trip beforehand. In other words, index i in Eqs. (15.11) and (15.13) refers to the ith event in the overall schedule, and it can be either an activity or a trip. Note that Δ_{hn}, Δ_{hni} in Eqs. (15.16) and (15.17) can include any kind of observed factors that influence the shape and scale parameters. If a dummy variable about activity type or trip type is introduced as one of the influential factors, then one can obtain all the timing utilities with respect to both activities and trips corresponding to each optimal timing variable. In other words, as long as the number of activities and trips performed in a day is given, it is possible to calculate the timing utilities for both activity and trip at each ordered location of the schedule over the course of a day. For example, it is expected that a household member may decide whether to participate in an activity or to make a trip by comparing the utilities of the activity and the trip. Thus, the calculated timing utilities could be used to represent the activity/trip sequence indirectly in theory.

15.3.6.3 Endogenous Representation of Coupling Constraints

A coupling constraint means that two or more people have to be together in a specific time period and at a specific place. Such coupling can involve either an activity or a trip. In this paper, a synchronized shared activity/trip is classified to represent such coupling constraints in household scheduling behavior. The presence of coupling constraints may force household members to adjust their schedules. It can also be expected that each member's timing decisions concerning the nonshared activities/trips may influence the timing when household members undertake them. Thus, the timings of shared and nonshared activities/trips interact, and it is difficult to assume that either a one-way or a two-way influence is more realistic. Therefore, instead of making such an assumption, this paper proposes to derive each timing function by defining each member's utility as a function of the utilities obtained from performing all the possible activities/trips in a choice set. As a result, the timing functions for both shared and nonshared activities/trips are derived simultaneously in an endogenous way. The influence of coupling constraints is explicitly incorporated into the relevant timing function(s), as shown in Eqs. (15.14) and (15.15).

15.3.7 Model Estimation Method

As Eqs. (15.18) and (15.19) show, each timing variable is derived as a function not only of its own information, but also of information from the next activity/trip. This means that the derived optimal timing variables interact and may both be influenced by the same set of unobserved attributes of the household and its members, suggesting that it is necessary to represent the statistical correlation in the model. Because of the error terms $e^{\alpha}_{hn}, e^{\beta}_{hni}$ in Eqs. (15.16) and (15.17), it is quite difficult to estimate the timing functions shown in Eqs. (15.14) and (15.15) directly. To estimate the timing functions based on an operational method, it is assumed that Eqs. (15.14) and (15.15) can be transformed as follows:

$$\hat{t}_{hni} = v_{hni} + \varepsilon_{hni} = \frac{\tilde{\alpha}_{hn}\left(\ln\left(\tilde{\beta}_{hni+1}\right) - \ln\left(\tilde{\beta}_{hni}\right)\right)}{\left(\tilde{\beta}_{hni+1} - \tilde{\beta}_{hni}\right)} + \varepsilon_{hni} \tag{15.18}$$

$$\hat{t}^{j}_{hni} = v^{j}_{hni} + \varepsilon^{j}_{hni} = \frac{\sum_{n}\left(\frac{\tilde{\beta}^{\tilde{\alpha}_{hn}}_{hni+1}(\hat{t}^{j}_{hni})^{\tilde{\alpha}_{hn}}}{\Gamma(\tilde{\alpha}_{hn})}\cdot\exp\left(-\tilde{\beta}_{hni+1}\hat{t}^{j}_{hni}\right)\right)}{\sum_{n}\left(\frac{\tilde{\beta}^{\tilde{\alpha}_{hn}}_{hni}(\hat{t}^{j}_{hni})^{\tilde{\alpha}_{hn}-1}}{\Gamma(\tilde{\alpha}_{hn})}\cdot\exp\left(-\tilde{\beta}_{hni}\hat{t}^{j}_{hni}\right)\right)} + \varepsilon^{j}_{hni} \tag{15.19}$$

$$\tilde{\alpha}_{hn} = \exp(\Delta_{hn}) \tag{15.20}$$

$$\tilde{\beta}_{hni} = \exp(\Delta_{hni}) \tag{15.21}$$

where $\varepsilon_{hni}, \varepsilon^{j}_{hni}$ are the transformed error terms.

15.3.7.1 Introduction of the First-Order Sequential Correlation

The above transformation has some positive features for representing timing decisions. First, the unobserved interdependencies among activities/trips can be incorporated into the model by assuming that the error terms $\varepsilon_{hni}, \varepsilon^{j}_{hni}$ are correlated. One can define such correlations in various ways. The multivariate normal distribution may be the most desirable in the sense that it can flexibly represent the correlations between error terms. However, one of the difficulties in applying the multivariate normal distribution is the calculation of the multidimensional integral. Even though some advanced methods have recently been proposed to overcome such calculation issues, the calculation itself is still very complicated and time consuming. In this study, to overcome this computational problem and make the estimation of the timing function more practical, a concept of first-order sequential correlation is introduced. The sequential correlation is defined as the correlation between error terms of neighboring activities/trips (i.e., ε_{ni} and ε_{ni+1}). It is further assumed that these two error terms follow a bivariate normal distribution.

$$f(\varepsilon_{ni}, \varepsilon_{ni+1}) = \frac{1}{2\pi\sigma_i\sigma_{i+1}\sqrt{1-\rho^2}} \exp\left\{ -\frac{\left[\left(\frac{\varepsilon_{ni}}{\sigma_i}\right)^2 - 2\rho\frac{\varepsilon_{ni}}{\sigma_i}\frac{\varepsilon_{ni+1}}{\sigma_{i+1}} + \left(\frac{\varepsilon_{ni+1}}{\sigma_{i+1}}\right)^2\right]}{2(1-\rho^2)} \right\} \tag{15.22}$$

where ρ is correlation between error terms ε_{ni} and ε_{ni+1}, and σ_i, σ_{i+1} are the corresponding standard deviations.

15.3.7.2 Representing Nonnegative Timing and Sequencing Constraints

In this study, the timing of each activity or trip is defined as the length of time from a predefined reference time (referred to as 0:00 here). Therefore, the derived optimal timing variable should first meet this nonnegative condition. In addition, because of activity/trip sequences, the timing (start time in this study) of the *i*th activity/trip should occur before the timing of the $i+1$th activity/trip (i.e., sequencing constraint). Such conditions are described in the following Eqs. (15.23)–(15.25).

$$\hat{t}_{ni} > 0,\ \hat{t}_{ni+1} > \hat{t}_{ni} \tag{15.23}$$

$$\hat{t}_{ni} > 0 \quad \Rightarrow \quad \hat{t}_{ni} = v_{ni} + \varepsilon_{ni} > 0 \quad \Rightarrow \quad \varepsilon_{ni} > -v_{ni} \tag{15.24}$$

$$\hat{t}_{ni+1} > \hat{t}_{ni} \quad \Rightarrow \quad \hat{t}_{ni+1} = v_{ni+1} + \varepsilon_{ni+1} > \hat{t}_{ni} \quad \Rightarrow \quad \varepsilon_{ni+1} > \hat{t}_{ni} - v_{ni+1} \tag{15.25}$$

As a result, the probability that describes the nonnegativity and sequencing constraints is given below.

$$\begin{aligned}\text{Prob}\left(\hat{t}_{ni} > 0, \hat{t}_{ni+1} > \hat{t}_{ni}\right) &= \text{Prob}\left(\varepsilon_{ni} > -v_{ni}, \varepsilon_{ni+1} > \hat{t}_i - v_{ni+1}\right) \\ &= \int_{-v_i}^{\infty}\int_{\hat{t}_i - v_{i+1}}^{\infty} f(\varepsilon_{ni}, \varepsilon_{ni+1}) d\varepsilon_{ni}\, d\varepsilon_{ni+1}\end{aligned} \tag{15.26}$$

Equation (15.26), with a double integral, can be further transformed into the following equation with a single integral based on coordinate rotation (Zhang et al. 2004).

$$\text{Prob}\left(\hat{t}_{ni} > 0, \hat{t}_{ni+1} > \hat{t}_{ni}\right) = \left\{1 - \Phi\left(\frac{\hat{t}_{ni} - v_{ni+1}}{\sigma_{i+1}\sqrt{1-\rho^2}}\right)\right\}\left\{1 - \Phi\left(\frac{v_{ni}}{\sigma_i\sqrt{1-\rho^2}}\right)\right\} \tag{15.27}$$

Equation (15.27) represents the nonshared activity/trip. In the case of a shared activity/trip, because its timing may influence all members' timing decisions about consecutive activities/trips, Eq. (15.27) needs to be revised to reflect intrahousehold decision-making mechanisms. Instead of $\hat{t}_{ni}$ in Eq. (15.23), the shared activity/trip timing $\hat{t}^{j}_{hni}$ is introduced. Then the following conditions need to be met with respect to each household member.

$$\hat{t}^{j}_{hni} > 0, \quad \hat{t}_{hni+1} > \hat{t}^{j}_{hni} \tag{15.28}$$

For each member, the relevant probability related to Eq. (15.28) can be written as follows:

$$\mathrm{Prob}\left(\hat{t}^{j}_{hni} > 0, \hat{t}_{ni+1} > \hat{t}^{j}_{hni}\right) = \left\{1 - \Phi\left(\frac{\hat{t}^{j}_{hni} - v_{hni+1}}{\sigma_{i+1}\sqrt{1-\rho^2}}\right)\right\}\left\{1 - \Phi\left(\frac{v^{j}_{hni}}{\sigma_i\sqrt{1-}}\right.\right. \tag{15.29}$$

Because the shared activity timing $\hat{t}^{j}_{hni}$ is included in Eq. (15.29) for each member, it is necessary to estimate these equations simultaneously. Note that $\hat{t}_{hni+1}$ may also be the timing of a shared activity/trip.

Needless to say, timing decisions may be influenced by timing constraints (e.g., the designated time of a meeting and departure time of a flight). In addition, because an activity–travel survey is usually conducted within a predesignated time period, it cannot be expected that each respondent started the first activity/trip precisely at the beginning of the time period, and/or ended the last one at the end of the survey period. Therefore, it is necessary to represent this censored timing properly in the model. Zhang et al. (2005a) discussed such issues in the context of individual decision-making. However, their approach can be directly applied to the context of household decision-making, which is the main focus of this study. Because this case study does not deal with these issues, detailed model specifications will not be shown here, and readers are recommended to refer to Zhang et al. (2005a).

15.3.7.3 Applying a Maximum Likelihood Method for Model Estimation

Because only nonnegative timing and activity/trip sequencing constraints are relevant in this case study, the resultant household activity–travel timing decision model can be specified by Eqs. (15.30)–(15.33). The model can be estimated using the conventional maximum likelihood method.

$$\log \mathrm{L} = \sum_{h=1}^{H}\sum_{n=1}^{N}\sum_{i=1}^{I} \ln(\mathrm{p_{hni}}) \tag{15.30}$$

$$p_{hni} = \left\{1 - \Phi\left(\frac{\Theta_{hni+1}}{\sigma_{i+1}\sqrt{1-\rho^2}}\right)\right\}\left\{1 - \Phi\left(\frac{\Theta_{hni}}{\sigma_{i}\sqrt{1-\rho^2}}\right)\right\} \quad (15.31)$$

$$\Theta_{hni} = \delta^{j}_{hni}v^{j}_{hni} + \delta_{hni}v_{hni} \quad (15.32)$$

$$\Theta_{hni+1} = (\delta^{j}_{hni}\hat{t}^{j}_{hni} + \delta_{hni}\hat{t}_{hni}) - (\delta_{hni+1}v_{hni+1} + \delta^{j+1}_{hni+1}v^{j+1}_{hni+1}) \quad (15.33)$$

where p_{hni} indicates the probability with respect to the ith (nonshared or shared) activity/trip performed by individual n, belonging to household h, and δ is a dummy variable to indicate whether an activity/trip is shared (1: Yes, 0: No).

15.4 Model Estimation Results

15.4.1 Data

The proposed model was estimated using the activity diary data originally collected for the Albatross model (Arentze and Timmermans 2005), which was developed to explore the potential of a new generation of rule-based transport demand models. Albatross predicts the schedule of a maximum of two adult members of a given household on a given day. Because this study attempts to represent household activity–travel timing decision behavior, data from single-member households and the households with missing attributes were excluded from this study. To simplify the discussion of the proposed household timing decision model, the original 48 types of activities were first recategorized into two major types: shared and nonshared activities. Shared activities are distinguished only for out-of-home activities. To avoid inconsistencies in the reported timing data, activities here are considered to be shared if both the husband and wife have the same start and end times. The nonshared activities are further classified into in-home activities and out-of-home independent and allocated activities, even though they have the same form of timing function.

In total, 3075 households provided their activity data. Figures 15.2, 15.3 and 15.4 show the distribution of the numbers of nonshared and shared activities. It is clear that females perform more activities than their spouses (on average, 16 activities/day versus 14 activities/day) both on weekdays and weekends (t values of tests of the differences between husband and wife are 14.30 for activities overall, 13.64 on weekdays and 4.39 on weekends). Irrespective of whether it is a weekday or weekends, each household performs about one shared activity on average. There are significant differences between weekdays and weekends with respect to females' activities and shared activities (t values of tests of the differences between weekdays and weekends are 4.43 for the female's activities and 5.74 for the shared

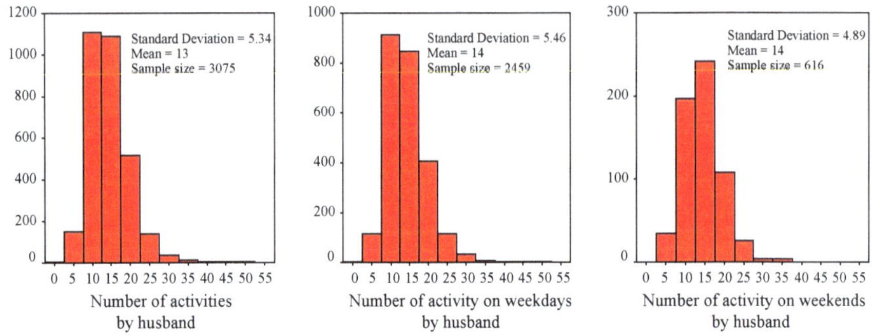

Fig. 15.2 Distribution of number of activities performed by husband

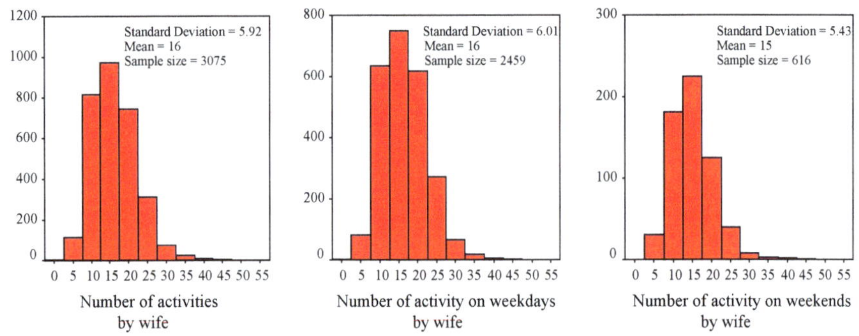

Fig. 15.3 Distribution of number of activities performed by wife

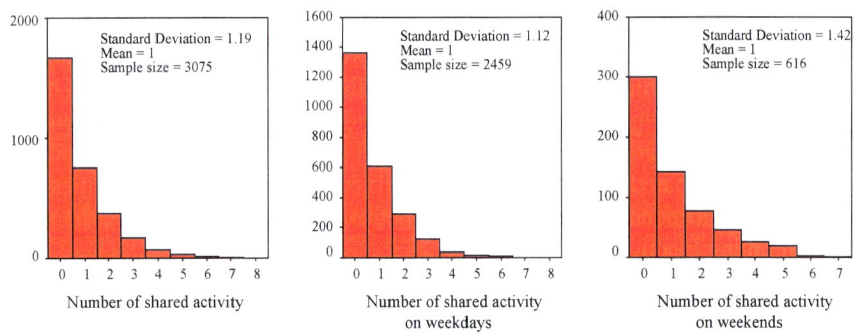

Fig. 15.4 Distribution of number of shared activities by husband and wife

activities), but no difference is observed concerning the husband's activities (the relevant t value is just 0.09).

Even though each member conducts many activities every day, because it is the first attempt to apply the proposed household timing decision model, this paper deals with only two successive activities (the fifth and sixth activities in the day of the survey) on weekdays. In other words, trip-making behavior is excluded from this case study. The resulting sample includes 593 households. The timing distributions related to the fifth and sixth activities are shown in Fig. 15.5. A trial using the full data set is left for future research.

15.4.2 Explanatory Variables

Factors influencing household timing decision behavior are introduced into the model via the scale and shape parameters of the derived timing utility functions. For that purpose, Δ_{hn}, Δ_{hni} in Eqs. (15.17) and (15.18) are rewritten as follows:

$$\Delta_{hn} = \pi_n^{\alpha} + \theta_n^{\alpha}\,\Omega_h + \mu_n^{\alpha}\,\Psi_{hn} \tag{15.34}$$

$$\Delta_{hni} = \pi_{ni}^{\beta} + \theta_{ni}^{\beta}\,\Omega_h + \mu_{ni}^{\beta}\,\Psi_{hn} + \sum\nolimits_k \gamma_k X_{hnik} \tag{15.35}$$

$$\Omega_h = \sum_p \rho_p Z_{hp} \tag{15.36}$$

$$\Psi_{hn} = \sum_q \kappa_q Y_{hnq} \tag{15.37}$$

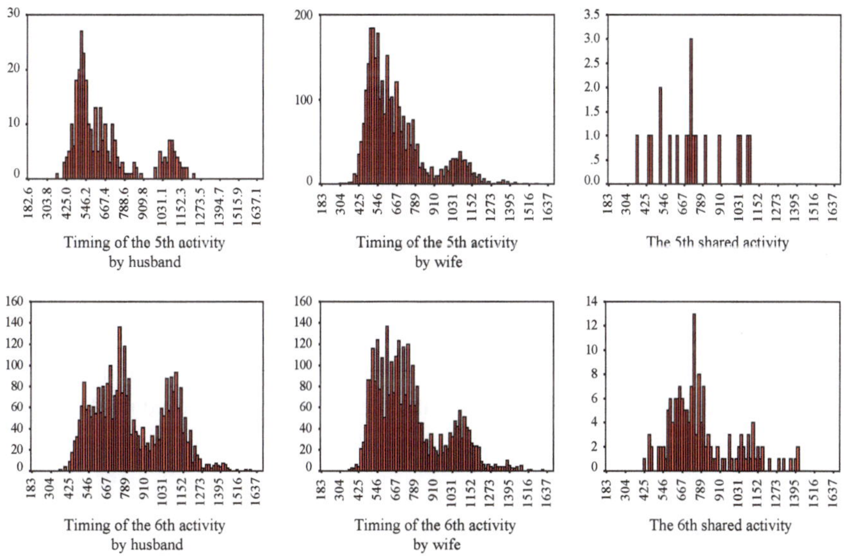

Fig. 15.5 Timing distributions of nonshared and shared activities (*upper part*: husband, *middle part*: wife, *lower part*: shared activity)

where the variables are as follows:

X_{hnik} the kth activity-specific variable used to explain scale parameter β_{hni},

Y_{hnq} the qth individual attribute used to explain both α_{hn} and β_{hni}, Z_{hp} the pth household attribute used to explain both α_{hn} and β_{hni},

θ_n^α the influence of household attributes on shape parameter α_{hn}; the parameter for one household member needs to be fixed at unity,

θ_{ni}^β the influence of household attributes on scale parameter β_{hni} of the ith activity; one activity parameter needs to be fixed at unity for each member,

μ_n^α the influence of individual attributes on shape parameter α_{hn}; the parameter for one household member needs to be fixed at unity,

μ_{ni}^β the influence of individual attributes on scale parameter β_{hni} of the ith activity; one activity parameter needs to be fixed at unity for each member,

$\gamma_k, \rho_p, \kappa_q$ the parameters of relevant variables, and

$\pi_n^\alpha, \pi_{ni}^\beta$ constant terms.

Individual and household attributes may have different influences on a decision about the timing of each activity. Because these two types of attributes are common to all activities, their direct introduction to each timing function will considerably reduce the degree of freedom in the model estimation. To overcome this problem, as shown in the above equations, individual attributes are combined into one composite variable, and household attributes into another. These are then introduced into Eqs. (15.34) and (15.35). Table 15.1 shows household and individual attributes, and activity-specific attributes.

15.4.3 Model Estimation

15.4.3.1 Effectiveness of the Proposed Model

Estimation results are shown in Table 15.2. MacFadden's Rho-squared is 0.4952. Most of the explanatory variables are statistically significant at the 99 % level, suggesting observed heterogeneity in household timing decisions. Most of the correlations and standard deviations related to sequential correlation are statistically significant. This supports the adoption of the bivariate normal distribution to represent sequential correlations. All these results suggest that the proposed model is good enough to represent household activity timing decision behavior in this case study.

15.4.3.2 Effect of the Shape Parameter on Timing Utility

Because the gamma probability density function is adopted as the timing utility function, an increase in the value of the shape parameter results in an increasing mean and variance of the timing distribution, and consequently the left-skewed

Table 15.1 Explanatory variables

Household attributes	(1) Socio-economic class 1: minimum 2: low 3: medium 4: high (2) Age of oldest member 1: 25 years old or younger 2: 26–45 years old 3: 46–65 years old 4: older than 65 years old (3) Household type 1: single, no work 2: single, work 3: double, one work 4: double, two work 5: double, no work (4) Number of cars (5) Number of bikes
Individual attributes	(1) Working hours (2) Car availability (3) Bike availability
Activity-specific attributes	(1) Type of activity – In-home activity – Out-of-home independent activity – Out-of-home allocated activity – Out-of-home shared activities (2) Travel party 1: Alone 2: Travel with household member 3: Travel with other outside household 4: Travel with household member and other outside household

timing distribution becomes flatter and moves toward the right-hand side of the time axis. In contrast, the scale parameter shows the opposite trend. In other words, if an explanatory variable has different signs for the shape and scale parameters, the timing distribution changes in a consistent way. If the signs of these parameters differ, the timing distribution varies with the difference in the scale/shape parameters of the same explanatory variable. Therefore, by interpreting the signs of the shape and scale parameters, the influences of various factors on timing distribution can be captured. Because the influences of the scale and shape parameters on timing distribution go in different directions, the meaning of each variable under study must be interpreted carefully. Note that the shape parameter is assumed to vary with household and member, but to be invariant across activities. The explanatory variables for the shape parameter are simply each member's attributes, including car availability, bicycle availability, and official work hours per week. All these variables are statistically significant and have positive parameters. This means that when the scale parameter is fixed, the high availability

Table 15.2 Model estimation results[a]

Explanatory variable		Estimated parameter	t-score	
<u>Constant term</u> ($\pi_n^{\alpha}, \pi_{ni}^{\beta}$)				
Shape parameter: wife's timing utility function		−1.2318	−8.381	**
Scale parameter: the 2nd Nonshared activity				
(1) Husband's timing utility function		−10.9348	−10.670	**
(2) Wife's timing utility function		21.6476	12.267	**
Scale parameter: the 2nd shared activity				
(1) Husband's timing utility function		−3.2945	−6.165	**
(2) Wife's timing utility function		4.6698	7.828	**
<u>Household attribute</u> ($\Omega_h = \sum_p \rho_p Z_{hp}$)				
Household type	- Single member with job	−1.5420	−1.530	
	- Two-member with one job	9.4992	9.037	**
	- Two-member with two jobs	2.5906	3.600	**
	- Two-member with no job	19.1237	10.539	**
Socio-economic class		−0.3987	−1.667	*
Age of the oldest member		2.5525	6.662	**
Number of cars		0.1672	0.409	
Number of bikes		−0.2196	−2.622	**
<u>Individual attribute</u> ($\Psi_{hn} = \sum_q \kappa_q Y_{hnq}$)				
Car availability (1: Yes, 0: No)		0.2212	3.376	**
Bike availability (1: Yes, 0: No)		0.8594	9.166	**
Official work hours per week		0.1982	6.887	**
<u>Activity-specific attribute</u> ($\sum_k \gamma_k X_{hnik}$)				
In-home activity (1: Yes, 0: No)		−11.9426	−18.151	**
Out-of-home independent activity (1: Yes, 0: No)		−2.0864	−3.172	**
Out-of-home allocated activity (1: Yes, 0: No)		3.7604	3.453	**
<u>Influence of household composite attribute on shape parameter of each member's timing utility function: Nonshared activity</u> (θ_n^{α})				
(1) Influence on husband's timing utility function				
The 1st activity		2.5865	18.253	**
The 2nd activity		−0.5901	−5.324	**
(2) Influence on wife's timing utility function				
The 1st activity		0.6000	2.664	**
The 2nd activity		−5.6987	−13.296	**
<u>Influence of individual composite attribute on scale parameter of timing utility function: Nonshared activity</u> (μ_{ni}^{β})				
(1) Husband	The 1st activity	4.4449	9.176	**
	The 2nd activity	−1.4351	−2.708	**
(2) Wife	The 1st activity	12.0598	11.519	**
	The 2nd activity	−16.3063	−10.760	**

(continued)

Table 15.2 (continued)

Explanatory variable		Estimated parameter	t-score	
Influence of individual composite attribute on scale parameter of timing utility function: Shared activity (μ_{ni}^{β})				
(1) Husband	The 1st activity	8.2242	8.188	**
	The 2nd activity	0.6979	1.760	*
(2) Wife	The 1st activity	1.3205	14.844	**
	The 2nd activity	−3.5896	−10.115	**
Influence of subsequent missing activity on scale parameter ($\tilde{\beta}_{hni} : i > \mathrm{I}$)				
(1) Nonshared activity	Husband's timing utility function	3.9896	27.487	**
	Wife's timing utility function	3.2843	15.143	**
(2) Shared activity	Husband's timing utility function	2.4435	17.503	**
	Wife's timing utility function	0.3171	5.557	**
Influence of subsequent missing activity on activity timing ($v_{hni} : i > \mathrm{I}$)				
Husband's timing: Nonshared activity		44.5896	32.573	**
Wife's timing: Nonshared activity		70.7712	32.011	**
Timing of shared activity		29.7925	18.727	**
Parameter related to sequential correlation				
(1) Husband	Standard deviation of the 5th activity (σ_5)	75.9615	21.006	**
	Standard deviation of the 6th activity (σ_6)	0.0403	0.992	
	Correlation (ρ)	0.0219	0.321	
(2) Wife	Standard deviation of the 5th activity (σ_5)	95.2358	20.895	**
	Standard deviation of the 6th activity (σ_6)	0.3702	4.269	**
	Correlation (ρ)	−0.6199	−24.484	**
Initial logarithm likelihood[b]		−3342.20		
Converged logarithm likelihood		−1687.17		
McFadden's Rho-squared		0.4952		
Sample size		593		

[a]Timing is calculated as the time difference (in minute) from the midnight (0:00). It is further divided by 1000 in order to guarantee the model estimation, because of the software requirement
[b]Initial logarithm likelihood is calculated by setting the constant terms and standard deviations to the estimated values
*Significant at 90 % level; **Significant at 99 % level

of cars or bicycles and longer working hours result in a left-skewed timing utility function tending toward the right-hand side of the time axis. In other words, households with a high availability of cars or bicycles and longer working hours prefer to start activities later. On the other hand, the constant term for the scale parameter of the female timing utility function is significantly negative, implying that women prefer an early start to each activity.

15.4.3.3 Influential Factors of Coupling Constraints

This study derives the timing utility function for shared activities. This includes information on all the household members involved. Focusing on synchronized shared activities allows the endogenous representation of coupling constraints in the model. The influence of coupling constraints on each member's activity timing decision is incorporated into the model with the aid of sequential correlations. In this case study, percentages of the shared activities are 3 and 3.5 % of the total sample for the fifth and sixth activities. Of course, such a small sample is insufficient to reveal the general decision-making mechanisms related to the timing of shared activities, but it is still useful to explore the influential factors of such decision-making mechanisms. The variables introduced to explain the shared activity timing decisions are simply each member's attributes, because it is assumed that each member has a different preference for shared activities. The scale parameter is assumed to vary across household members.

The parameter (β_{hni}), representing the influence of individual attributes on the scale parameter, shows positive values except for the wife's sixth activity. This means that households with a greater availability of cars or bicycles and longer working hours prefer an earlier start for each activity. Because the shape and scale parameters play contrary roles in determining the timing utility, in general the actual preferences of each household can be only calculated by comparing shape and scale parameters. However, in this case, the wife's sixth activity timing shows a consistent direction of variation for both parameters.

15.4.3.4 Influential Factors of Timing Decisions About the Nonshared Activity

Activity-specific attributes are activity types: in-home activities, out-of-home independent activities, and out-of-home allocated activities. The model estimates negative parameters for the first two types of activities, and positive parameters for the last activity. Negative scale parameters mean that household members prefer a later start for in-home activities and out-of-home independent activities. In contrast, a positive parameter pulls the timing distribution curve back from the right- to the left-hand side along the time axis.

Household attributes

Household attributes show a similar influence on the timing of both the husband and the wife: a positive parameter for the fifth activity and a negative parameter for the sixth activity. Because the parameters for single members with jobs, socioeconomic class and number of bicycles are negative, and the other parameters are all positive, these results show that households with a single employed member, higher socioeconomic class, and more bicycles tend to start the fifth activity later and the sixth activity earlier than do others. The degree of influence is stronger for the fifth activity of the husband, and for the sixth activity of the wife. Other attributes show the opposite influence.

Individual attributes

The estimated parameters of husband and wife attributes are positive for the fifth activity and negative for the sixth activity. Because all individual attributes, including car and bicycle availability and official work hours have positive parameters, households with greater availability of cars and bicycles and longer working hours tend to start the fifth activity earlier and the sixth activity later.

15.5 Conclusions and Future Research Issues

The utility of performing an activity or making a trip changes over time. When an individual makes decisions about the timings of activities/trips, he/she usually faces various constraints, for example, the existence of designated start (departure) and/or end (arrival) times (i.e., authority constraints). Timing decisions within a given period of time (e.g., a day) also interact across activities/trips. These mechanisms become much more complicated in the context of household decisions, where household members usually share a certain period of time to conduct some activities jointly and/or take trips together, and/or some members must take responsibility for household maintenance tasks such as shopping, and picking up and dropping off children. Coupling constraints are especially problematic in modeling household timing decisions because it is necessary to incorporate the preferences of all the members involved in decisions. Conventional modeling approaches have typically incorporated such coupling constraints exogenously, i.e., by treating the constraints as explanatory variables for decision-making. From the behavioral perspective, timing not only constrains other decision(s), but also involves decisions, just as other choices do. Therefore, it is necessary to represent the abovementioned mechanisms related to timing endogenously.

As a case study focusing on daily time use, this study first adopts a gamma probability density function to represent timing utility. Two types of timing functions are successfully derived: one for nonshared activities/trips and the other for shared activities/trips. The function for a nonshared activity/trip performed by a household member only includes information about a member, while that for a shared activity/trip includes information of all the household members involved. To incorporate interdependencies among activities/trips over a day, this study further introduces the concept of the first-order sequential correlation between error terms of timing functions of neighboring activities/trips based on a bivariate normal distribution. In theory, all the nonnegative conditions of timing variables, activity/trip sequencing, timing constraints, and censored timings can be endogenously represented based on the same bivariate normal distribution. Timing functions for shared activities/trips are used to represent a household's coupling constraints endogenously by using sequential correlations related to all relevant members. The resulting household timing decision model can be estimated using the conventional maximum likelihood method.

The estimation results of the household timing model show that husbands and wives do not have homogeneous preferences for timing decisions. The factors explaining the shape and scale parameters of the gamma distribution reveal inconsistent influences of coupling constraints on the timing distribution. This not only reflects the complexities of household timing decisions, but also raises the question of how to justify the derived influences. However, it is not sufficient to justify this conclusion based on the data/model adopted in this study (i.e., internal validity). External validity is also required. In other words, the justification should also be based on external information.

Because the results obtained from this study are based on a limited sample size with only two successive activities on weekdays, future research must first estimate the model by collecting data from more people. Second, it is necessary to investigate how to select more suitable variables to explain timing decisions. In this study, we adopted a very limited set of variables including household and individual attributes and activity attributes. The explanatory power is insufficient. Selection of explanatory variables should be based on theoretical reasoning, rather than the availability of data. Third, different people may prefer to participate in different activities at different points in time, so a finer classification of activities may be helpful. A change in preferences may be also caused by space–time settings, such as a wish to avoid congestion on roads or at activity locations. Incorporating factors related to space–time settings seems important. There may exist various types of timing distributions. Even though the gamma probability density function has a general form of distribution, to reflect the actual timing distributions more properly it may be necessary to explore the possibility of applying other types of distributions such as the bell-shaped function (Joh et al. 2003). Because representing various timing constraints is one good feature of the derived household timing model, this should be examined in the future. This study adopted an additive-type utility function to represent timing decisions without weighting any activities/trips. In reality, people attach different levels of importance to each activity/trip, suggesting the necessity of introducing such weight parameters into the model. This study assumes one form of timing distribution. Depending on the types of activities/trips and their spatial–temporal constraints, the timing distributions may yield curves that are considerably different. The simultaneous representation of different timing distributions in the same modeling framework clearly generates new difficulties for model estimation. Therefore, a methodological breakthrough is expected to overcome the tradeoff between model complexity and operationalization. Finally, incorporating budget constraints could contribute to the improved measurement of the value of time over time, which is very important in the evaluation of transportation policy.

References

Ashiru O, Polak JW, Noland RB (2003) The utility of schedules: a model of departure time and activity time allocation. In: Paper presented at the 10th international conference on travel behaviour research, Lucerne, 10–15 Aug

Arentze T, Timmermans HJP (2000) Albatross: a learning based transportation oriented simulation system. European Institute of Retailing and Services Studies, Eindhoven

Arentze T, Timmermans HJP (2005) Albatross version 2: a learning-based transportation oriented simulation system. European Institute of Retailing and Services Studies, Eindhoven

Becker GS (1965) A theory of the allocation of time. Econ J 75:493–517

Borgers A, Timmermans HJP (1993) Transport facilities and residential choice behaviour: a model of multi-person choice processes. Papers Reg Sci 72(1):45–61

Davis HL (1976) Decision making within the household. J Consum Res 2:241–260

Doherty ST (2004) Rules for assessing activity scheduling survey respondents data quality. In: Compendium of papers CD-ROM, the 83rd annual meeting of the transportation research board, Washington D.C., 11–15 Jan

Doherty ST, Papinski D (2004) Is it possible to automatically trace activity scheduling? In: Paper presented at the EIRASS conference on progress in activity-based analysis, Maastricht, The Netherlands, 28–31 May

Ettema D, Timmermans HJP (2003) Modelling departure time choice in the context of activity scheduling behavior. In: Compendium of papers CD-ROM, the 83rd annual meeting of the transportation research board, Washington D.C., 12–16 Jan

Fujiwara A, Zhang J (2005) Development of car tourists' scheduling model for 1-day tour. Transp Res Rec 1921:100–111

Fujiwara A, Kanda Y, Sugie Y, Okamura T (2001) The effectiveness of non-IIA models on time choice behavior analysis. J East Asia Soc Transp Stud 4(2):305–318

Garling T, Kalen T, Romanus J, Selart M, Vilhelmson B (1998) Computer simulation of household activity scheduling. Environ Plan A 30:665–679

Gauthier AH, Gershuny J, Fisher K (2006) Multinational time use study: user's guide and documentation. Version 2. The United Nations Economic Commission for Europe (UNECE). Available at http://www.unece.org/fileadmin/DAM/stats/gender/timeuse/Downloads/MTUS_Users'Guide.pdf. Accessed 29 May 2016

Gerike R, Gehlert T, Leisch F (2015) Time use in travel surveys and time use surveys—Two sides of the same coin? Transp Res Part A 76:4–24

Hensher DA, Stopher PR (1979) Behavioral travel demand modelling. Croom Helm, London

Joh CH, Arentze T, Timmermans HJP (2002) Modeling individuals' activity-travel rescheduling heuristics: theory and numerical experiments. Transp Res Rec 1807:16–25

Joh CH, Arentze T, Timmermans HJP (2003) A theory and simulation model of activity-travel rescheduling behavior. In: Selected proceedings of the 9th world conference on transportation research (CD–ROM)

Joh C-H, Arentze T, Timmermans HJP (2006) Characterisation and comparison of gender-specific utility functions of shopping duration episodes. J Retail Consum Serv 13:249–259

Jones P (1990) Development in dynamic and activity-based approaches to travel analysis. Gower, Aldcrshot

Kimberly F (2015) Metadata of time use studies. Last updated 31 December 2014. Centre for Time Use Research, University of Oxford, United Kingdom. http://www.timeuse.org/information/studies/

Kitamura R, Fujii S (1998) Two computational process models of activity-travel choice. In: Garling T, Laitila T, Westin K (eds) Theoretical foundations of travel choice modeling. Elsevier, Oxford, pp 251–279

Koppelman FS, Wen CH (2000) The paired combinatorial logit model: properties, estimation and application. Transp Res Part B 34:75–89

Lee B, Timmermans HJP (2007) A latent class accelerated hazard model of activity episode durations. Transp Res Part B 41(4):426–447

Michelson WH (2006) Time use: expanding explanation in the social sciences. Routledge, New York

Molin EJE, Oppewal H, Timmermans HJP (1997) Modeling group preferences using a decompositional preference approach. Group Decis Negot 6:339–350

Pentland WE, Harvey AS, Lawton MP, McColl MA (2013) Time use research in the social sciences. Kluwer Academic Publishers, New York

Popkowski Leszczyc PTL, Timmermans HJP (2002) Unconditional and conditional competing risk models of activity duration and activity sequencing decisions: an empirical comparison. J Geogr Syst 4:157–170

Timmermans HJP, Borgers A, van Dijk J, Oppewal H (1992) Residential choice behaviour of dual-earner households: a decompositional joint choice model. Environ Plan A 24:517–533

Vovsha P, Gliebe J, Petersen E, Koppelman F (2004) Sequential and simultaneous choice structures for modeling intra-household interactions in regional travel models. In: Timmermans HJP (ed) Progress in activity-based analysis. Elsevier, Amsterdam, pp 223–257

Zhang J, d Fujiwara A (2006) Representing household time allocation behavior by endogenously incorporating diverse intra-household interactions: a case study in the context of elderly couples. Transp Res Part B 40(1):54–74

Zhang J, Timmermans HJP, Borgers A (2002) A utility-maximizing model of household time use for independent, shared and allocated activities incorporating group decision mechanisms. Transp Res Rec 1807:1–8

Zhang J, Sugie Y, Fujiwara A, Suto K (2004) A dynamic bi-ordered-probit model system to evaluate the effects of introducing flexible working hour system. In: Selected proceedings of the 10th world conference on transport research, Istanbul, Turkey, 4–8 July (CD-ROM)

Zhang J, Fujiwara A, Ishikawa N (2005a) Developing a new activity-trip scheduling model based on utility of timing incorporating timing constraints, censored timing and sequential correlation. In: Paper presented at the 84th annual meeting of the transportation research board, Washington D.C., 9–13 Jan

Zhang J, Timmermans HJP, Borgers A (2005b) A model of household task allocation and time use. Transp Res Part B 39:81–95

Chapter 16
Models of Behavioral Change and Adaptation

Soora Rasouli and Harry Timmermans

Abstract This chapter explains and summarizes models of behavioral change and adaptation, which have received less application in the life choice analysis associated with urban policy. Related to various life choices, life trajectory events are major decisions with a relatively long-lasting impact, such as demographic events, job change and purchase of major resources such as a house and a car. These life trajectory events may co-vary over time and lead to dynamic changes in activity-travel repertoires. Such decision problems have hitherto been predominantly modeled in urban and transportation science using classic discrete choice models. However, because such decisions differ from daily choices, other modeling approaches may be more beneficial. The authors present discrete choice models with lifetime utility and social dynamics, attitudinal models, technology acceptance model, norm activation model, and value belief norm theory for modeling lifecycle decisions and/or lifecycle driven behavioral change.

Keywords Life trajectories · Theory of innovation diffusion · Lifetime utility · Social dynamics · Attitudinal model · Technology acceptance model · Norm activation model · Value belief norm theory

16.1 Introduction

Life trajectories describe the evolution of an individual throughout the individual's lifecycle through sequential stages of life domain careers. The identification and demarcation of careers depends on the field of study, but may include a demographic career, a housing career, a job career, an education career, a vehicle

S. Rasouli · H. Timmermans (✉)
Eindhoven University of Technology, Eindhoven, The Netherlands
e-mail: J.P.Timmermans@tue.nl

J. Zhang (ed.), *Life-Oriented Behavioral Research for Urban Policy*,
DOI 10.1007/978-4-431-56472-0_16

ownership career, etc. Generally, careers refer to personal states of an individual or of particular resources.

Recently, in parallel with the shift in interest from cross-sectional to dynamic activity-based analysis, researchers in travel behavior, geography and urban planning have evidenced increasing interest in life trajectories as important factors influencing the dynamics of travel-related decisions (e.g., Verhoeven 2005a, b, 2006, 2007; Beige and Axhausen 2008, 2012; Oakil et al. 2011a, b). The modeling of these life trajectory decisions relates to careers such as demographics, housing and job choice. Modeling these long-term decisions is critically important because they define the action spaces within which daily activity-travel behavior takes places. In addition, they concern mobility tools such as vehicle holdings and public transit passes. Thus, it is assumed that changes in these careers may prompt individuals and households to reconsider their current activity-travel behavior and adapt to the new circumstances or to the shifting needs by changing one or more facets of their current activity-travel patterns and adapt their current repertoire.

Transitions in careers reflect changes in outcomes of underlying choices. The need for change may be endogenously or exogenously triggered. Endogenous change reflects changing needs and desires or weakening constraints, allowing an individual to realize existing needs that hitherto were impossible to realize. Exogenous change induces individuals to reconsider current choices and adapt to changing circumstances. Transitions may also signify gradual moves forward to achieving particular ambitions and goals.

Most life trajectory transitions are the result of explicit choices or decisions. It is no surprise therefore that researchers, almost without exception, have rather uncritically applied their discrete choice apparatus, which they have been applying routinely to predict transport mode, destination and route choice behavior, to model housing choice, job choice, etc. These choices differ, however, in several respects from daily decisions. First, they involve a longer time perspective and create commitments. Few people will start a personal relationship with the a priori mind set or expectation to end it soon. Buying a new house is more than having shelter, but signifies building a home and often involves a considerable investment decision. Most jobs involve a contract that spans a longer period of time. Choosing an educational program is meant to develop the knowledge and skills deemed required to attain certain jobs. Because these programs demand a substantial investment in time and last over a longer time span, they require a certain commitment. Starting a personal or a business relationship is based on trust and a mutual understanding of long-term commitment. Thus, although transitions in life trajectories presume the right opportunities occurring in time (and space), which may last for just a split second, the actual decision typically involves a longer time perspective.

Second, because of this longer time perspective and the commitments involved, the consequences of decisions may have major ramifications if the wrong decision is made. Breaking up a relationship tends to be painful for at least one party; ending school or closing a business may be seen as failure and a waste of the time, money and other resources spent on the education, or the development of the business; a house is not instantaneously consumed, but the benefits and disadvantages are rather experienced over a longer period of time.

Third, although the right opportunities that lead to transitions may occur just in a split second, careers are often embedded in specific plans. These plans set targets across the life course in some chronological order. Certain states may only be accessible if certain conditions in the same or in other careers are satisfied. These conditions may not be sufficient to attain the desired states, but are necessary. For example, completion of a postdoc project may be a necessary albeit not sufficient condition to become an assistant professor; a certain job with an appropriate income may be needed to buy a house of a desired profile. Life trajectories represent different paths in the (partial) realization of these plans. If certain stages turn out to be unattainable, plans need to be adjusted.

Finally, in the context of urban and travel behavior research, lifecycle trajectories define the larger space-time context within which mid-term and short-term activity-travel decisions are or have to be made. Home and job locations define the pegs of the action space of individuals within which feasible daily activity-travel patterns may emerge. The repository of vehicles limits the available choice options, and in turn these options influence action spaces. In addition to constraints, life trajectory stages influence the needs and desires of individuals and households, influencing activity-generating processes. Lifecycle transitions may induce reconsidering current activity-travel scripts and trigger adaptations.

What is the relevance of this attempt to identify the fundamental properties of lifecycle events and transitions? We will argue, to stimulate the discussion, that dominant choice models in urban and transportation science and their underlying theories at best only partially capture these life trajectory processes or may even fail to validly formalize the quintessence of the decision problem. Consequently, we should either elaborate current choice models to better represent the very nature of these choice processes or explore the applicability of alternate models that have not yet been extensively studied in urban and travel behavior research.

In this chapter, we will endeavor both avenues. First, in the next section, we will critically reflect on dominant choice models and underlying theories in urban and travel behavior research and identify shortcomings and caveats in the ways these models are applied from a life trajectory perspective. This section is meant to stimulate discussion and identify issues for future research. Second, in Sect. 16.3, we will outline some alternate modeling approaches that have found less application in urban and travel behavior research compared to discrete choice models, but that may offer a valuable approach to model particular processes of change and adaptation. To the extent that life trajectory decisions involve behavioral change and adaptation, these theories and models may be inspirational for formulating life trajectory travel-oriented models of behavioral change. From the outset, we wish to stipulate that we do not claim to provide a comprehensive overview of the potentially relevant literature.

16.2 Life Trajectories and Choice Models

Over the years, a plethora of different models has been developed to describe and predict travel-related choice behavior. Table 16.1 gives a crude overview, differentiating between models of riskless and risky behavior as one dimension, and between utility-maximizing (rational) choice models, and models of bounded rational behavior. The cells give examples of different modeling approaches for combinations of these dimensions. The overwhelming share of studies in urban and transportation science dealing with the choice of particular facets of activity-travel behavior has conceptualized choice under certain conditions and assumed rational choice behavior. Most comprehensive activity-based models of travel demand have adopted a similar modeling approach (Rasouli and Timmermans 2014a). The most widely applied model belonging to this category is the multinomial logit model (Ben Akiva and Lerman 1985; Train 2003).

Although the mathematical specification of the MNL model can be derived from multiple, even competing theories of choice behavior, the most common foundation of the MNL model is random utility theory (McFadden 1978), assuming a stochastic utility function and the principle of utility-maximizing behavior. More advanced discrete choice models have relaxed the strict assumptions underlying the MNL model by allowing for varying variance terms and co-variances between error terms, but these advances did not affect the general modeling approach nor the principle of utility-maximizing behavior. Arguably, in applying choice models, urban and transportation researchers seem to have been more fascinated and driven by the application of a particular model rather than the desire to develop new or adjusted models that do sufficient justice to the specific characteristics of the decision problem at hand. For example, the multinomial logit model has not only been applied to model short-term decisions such as destination, route and transport mode choice, but also to long-term life trajectory decisions such as vehicle holdings and housing choice, mostly based on cross-sectional data.

While the notions of an instantaneous utility function and utility maximizing behavior may be defendable for destination and transport mode choice, this representation does not fully capture or is even too simplistic to do justice to the complexity and repercussions of life trajectory events such as buying a house, which is often the most expensive choice people make during their life. Housing choice has a number of unique features that are not incorporated in the modeling process. While destination, transport mode and route choice reflect the outcomes of a learning process in which travelers can explore different options over time, experience

Table 16.1 Classification of different types of choice models

	Rational choice models	Models of bounded rationality
Riskless choice	Utility-maximizing models	Decision heuristics
Risky choice	Expected utility Maximizing models	Prospect theoretical models Regret minimizing models

the consequences of their choice, and either reinforce or adjust their behavior, housing choice decisions are made only a few times during a lifetime.

Moreover, the set of possible choices may be huge and is not fixed. Thus, in light of the lack of experience and information and the flux in the market, the housing decision process often evolves across different stages. In the first phase, individuals will explore some available options, collect information using different media, perhaps assisted by experts, to frame their decision. Next, they often contact a real estate agent to site visit a limited set of properties. Because further search involves time, effort and money, typically the best of the limited set of inspected properties is judged against needs and desires and affordability, implications are assessed against the current and desired new lifestyle of the household and a decision is made to buy the house, extend the search process or end it to wait for new opportunities in the future.

Buying a new house does not only satisfy particular housing needs. Depending on the distance of relocation, the complete configuration of a household's job and activity locations and the social networks of its members may change, affecting commuter travel times, travel times for other activities, the feasibility of activity agendas, possible activity duration, etc. Assuming that buying a new house involves extra expenditure, expenditures on other daily activities and products may need to be reduced; opportunity costs need to be considered. Thus, the housing decision process likely has repercussions across different domains of a household lifestyle.

Because often people live in the same house for many years, the attributes of the house, its physical and social neighborhood and accessibility to a multitude of activity locations are not only judged against current needs but also against anticipated future needs that may be induced by life trajectory events. Even if decision-making would be myopic, housing generates a lifetime utility or a utility across a longer time horizon.

Random utility models constitute a meager representation of this process and largely fail to mimic its essence. The typical two-step procedure of first identifying the choice set and then predicting the choice of a particular house from the choice set is nothing but a technical way to reduce the complexity of the modeling process, but has little to do with the actual decision process. Potential housing buyers do not truly have a choice set; they may have a consideration set but only in its original process meaning. The principle of utility maximization and simultaneously choice does not seem valid for many housing choice decisions. Often the housing market clearing process is conceptualized as an auction, but in many countries in the world housing markets regulations and consumer protection in fact are antagonistic to the very notion of an auction. Moreover, the number of attributes included in housing choice models, particularly those developed in transportation research, is often very limited with a focus on transport-related attributes. Acknowledging that simple models may have an advantage, including very few attributes make these models overly simplistic to be of any use. Models developed in the housing choice literature tend to be better in this regard, but still the different lifestyle domains are rarely depicted in a balanced way.

If choice set generation would be given a behavioral interpretation, it could be viewed as evidence of bounded rationality in the sense that individual try to simplify the decision problem (Rasouli and Timmermans 2015). Other models of bounded rationality have substituted the notion of systematic, full information comparison of alternatives against a set of decision criteria for a set of simple decisions heuristics. Arguably, models of bounded rationality better mimic the actual decision making process in the sense that they represent a way of how individuals cope with the potentially large set of attributes affecting the housing choice decision. However, these models of bounded rationality share with the dominant utility-maximizing models the limitations that the larger decision process is ill-represented and that the decision problem is confined to only particular aspects of a household's lifestyle.

Another general class of choice models is based on decision-making under risk and uncertainty (see Rasouli and Timmermans 2014b for a recent overview). Risk means that the uncertain conditions are known and defined, whereas uncertainty means that the decision-maker has to attain and assess the degree of uncertainty. Some models are the equivalent of rational choice models under conditions of uncertainty. They predict that individuals will choose the alternative with the highest payoff or utility, which is defined as the expected value of the outcomes of the decisions. However, as limited empirical support has been found for this model in many fields of application, several alternate models of bounded rationality under uncertainty have been formulated. Prospect theoretic (Kahneman and Tversky 1979) and regret-based models have become most popular in travel behavior analysis (Avineri 2009; Chorus et al. 2008; Chorus 2011), although it should be noted that the number of studies involving modeling choice and decision-making under conditions of uncertainty is still surprisingly small.

Because buying a house or vehicle has a long lasting effect, one would suspect that individuals do have to consider various sources of uncertainty. The future value of the property, the ability of reselling the house if needed, the future evolution of mortgage rates, changing population distribution in the neighborhood are just of few examples of uncertain factors that may affect the utility or value of a house. Yet, we are not aware of any study in urban and transportation research where such uncertainty has been taken into account when life trajectory decisions are modeled.

Thus, in completing this section of our chapter, we argue that the travel behavior community has by and large uncritically applied modeling approaches commonly used for day-to-day activity-travel decisions to long-term life trajectory decisions. It suggests that either current modeling approaches should be elaborated to better capture the quintessence of long-term life trajectory decisions or that yet other modeling approaches should be explored and judged for their applicability in urban and transportation research.

In this chapter, without trying to be comprehensive, we discuss some alternative theories and approaches that may be useful to model certain kinds of life trajectory decisions. Some of these approaches have found limited application in urban and travel behavior research, whereas to the best of our knowledge others have not been applied in urban and transportation research yet. Where relevant, we will refer to existing applications in urban and travel behavior research.

16.3 Selected Alternate Models

Urban and transportation research has mostly relied on applied physics and economics in borrowing (choice) modeling frameworks and elaborating or applying these to choice and decision-making processes relevant for these disciplines. However, particularly social psychology has put forward many alternative theories and models of decision making, while other applied disciplines such as marketing research and environmental research also have developed models that may be relevant for urban and transportation research in general and the modeling of life trajectory decisions in particular.

Life trajectory decisions concern a transition in the status of lifecycle careers, manifested in life trajectory events that have long-lasting implications. The actual decision, representing the end of the decision process, is driven by a motivation to change the career. Motivations may also relate to the desire to change current behavior, which in some cases requires dramatic change in long-term drivers of day-to-day behavior. In this section, we will describe some modeling approaches that have been developed to model behavioral change and assess their potential for modeling life trajectory decisions that are relevant for transportation. The different approaches will be divided into aggregate and individual models.

The focus of attention of aggregate models is concerned with the aggregated outcomes of individual decisions. In contrast, individual level models aim at predicting behavioral intentions and choices of individuals. Although these outcomes are typically aggregated, the difference between the two streams of work concern the data input to the models and the definition of their explanatory variables. Aggregate models are based on aggregated data, whereas individual-level models are based on individual-level data.

16.3.1 Aggregate Modeling Approaches

16.3.1.1 Statistical Models of Temporal Interdependencies

Most research on the relationship between life trajectory events and activity-travel behavior has attempted to find evidence of significant effects of life trajectory events on behavior. It is based on the contention that life trajectory decisions trigger individuals and households to reconsider their habitual behavior that reflects s state of equilibrium (e.g., Waerden et al. 2003a, b; Klöckner 2004). Life trajectory events may involve substantial changes in available resources and choice options, and may also induce changes in activity agendas in reaction to or in anticipation of such events. Both qualitative and quantitative studies have been conducted to explore these dynamics.

Stanbridge et al. (2004—see also Stanbridge and Lyons 2006) conducted a qualitative study on the effects of residential relocation on travel behaviour. They concluded that relocation decisions are partly influenced by travel considerations. Relocation forces or prompts households to reappraise their current travel options once post-relocation travel is experienced. Similar evidence has been found in other qualitative studies (e.g., Krizek 2003; Prillwitz and Lanzendorf 2006, 2007; Rocci 2006; Hannes et al. 2007). Other lifecycle events may have a similar impact as, for example, illustrated in Lanzendorf (2010), who examined the impact of the birth of a child and found evidence of changes in transport mode.

Quantitative studies seem to have followed two modeling approaches: hazard and competing risk models, and Bayesian belief networks. Hazard and competing risk models examine the effects of a set of explanatory variables on continuous interval times between successive implementations of single activity-travel facets or on state changes. In contrast, Bayesian belief networks focus on the conditional choice probabilities of discretionized or inherently categorical variables in a network. Consequently, they require the researcher to define a time window to calculate these conditional choice probabilities. The advantage of the Bayesian approach is the richness in the specification of the relationships between the variables of interests; the disadvantage, however, is that the results are dependent on the selected time window.

Chen and Chen (2006) applied hazard models to the Puget Sound panel data and concluded that a change in residential location affected time allocation and travel patterns of individuals. Using the same data set, Rasouli et al. (2015) found that job changes (transitions between being employed and unemployed and vice versa) led to a change in shopping-travel patterns. Beige and Axhausen (2006) investigated the interrelationships between lifecycle events, such as residential choice, education, employment duration, car availability, driver's license and season's tickets using hazard/competing risk models. Their data showed that people with a driver's licence or public transport season ticket are more likely to move house.

Verhoeven et al. (2005a, b, 2006) and Xie et al. (2006) used a Bayesian network to represent the interdependencies between life trajectory events, resources and activity-travel patterns. The network included life trajectory events such as change in residential location, change in household composition, change in work location, change in study location, and other events such as change in car possession and availability, change in public transport pass and change in (household) income. The learned network, using data of 710 respondents, indicated that structural lifecycle events influence each other. Significant effects were found in within-events dependencies across time periods; between one event and another event during the same time period and across time periods, and between one event and personal characteristics. Vanhunsel et al. (2007a), elaborating Janssens (2005) and Janssens et al. (2006) applied the Q-learning algorithm for the same purpose, and showed (Vanhunsel et al. 2007b) that a regression tree used to generalize the Q-table leads to faster results.

16.3.1.2 Theory of Innovation Diffusion

Some life trajectory decisions are concerned with major expenditures such as buying a house, a boat or a car. A potentially relevant framework for investigating such decisions at the aggregate level is the theory of innovation diffusion. Various phenomena show a high degree of similarity in their particular evolution over time and sometimes space. The theory of innovation diffusion (Rogers 1962) has been formulated to describe how a new idea or product becomes popular, spreads through a population and ultimately reaches some level of saturation. The theory describes particular regularities at an aggregate level; it is not a theory of individual choice.

Underlying the typical S-shape diffusion curve that defines the theory of innovation diffusion is the idea that individuals exhibit a different attitude to innovations and change, and differ in their willingness to try different new products. The theory identifies five different adopter categories. First, innovators representing a relatively small fraction of the population are those individuals who wish to be among the very first trying the innovation. Second, a slightly larger fraction of the population shows interest in the new innovation and belongs to the category of Early Adopters. If the innovation still has more followers, the third category called Early Majority represents a larger share of the population who adopts only after they receive evidence that the innovation works or of its popularity. Next is the Late Majority – a more or less equal share of people, who are more skeptical of change, and less sensitive to innovations, and only adopt after a large share of the population has embraced the innovation before them. Finally, there is the category of Laggards, a group of conservative individuals, who are very skeptical of change and the last to adopt an innovation, if they adopt at all.

Mathematically, the well-known S-shaped logistic function is used to describe the diffusion process. That is:

$$p = \frac{S}{1 + e^{(\alpha - \beta T)}} \tag{16.1}$$

where,

p	the proportion of the population adopting an innovation,
S	the satiation level, $S \leq 1$,
T	time,
α, β	parameters to be estimated, respectively representing the proportion at $T = 0$, and the rate at which this proportion changes with increasing time

If the whole population ultimately uses an innovation, S is equal to 1. In most cases, however, the proportion of people adopting a certain new product is much smaller. For example, the market share of electric cars may only be a few per cent. If α is large, the proportion at time zero is very small. With increasing T, $(\alpha - \beta T)$ becomes increasingly smaller, implying that the proportion of the population adopting the innovation increases at an increasing rate. Once $(\alpha - \beta T)$ becomes negative, the rate of change systematically decreases until the e-term goes to zero and the diffusion and adoption process converges to the satiation level.

Some simple algebra shows that the above logistic function can be estimated using linear regression analysis:

$$S = p(1 + e^{(\alpha - \beta T)}) \tag{16.2}$$

$$S = p + pe^{(\alpha - \beta T)} \tag{16.3}$$

$$S - p = pe^{(\alpha - \beta T)} \tag{16.4}$$

$$\frac{S - p}{p} = e^{(\alpha - \beta T)} \tag{16.5}$$

$$\ln(\frac{S - p}{p}) = \alpha - \beta T \tag{16.6}$$

In case of spatial diffusion processes, in which the rate of adoption is some function of the distance from the center of origin, parameters α and β can be made a polynomial function of distance to capture spatially diverging diffusion processes. The model can be simply expanded to include different socio-demographic variables and different environmental variables assumed to influence the diffusion and adoption process. However, if we wishes to relax the symmetric nature of the diffusion process, implied by Eq. (16.6), more elaborated functions that capture non-symmetric forms are required.

Although innovation diffusion models address the issue of change, their aggregate nature makes them difficult to link to life trajectory events. Hence, in that sense their direct relevance for lifecycle studies is limited. However, these models may be useful, for instance, for modeling the adoption of electric cars. The adoption can be made a function of socio-demographic variables.

16.3.2 Individual-Level Modeling Approaches

16.3.2.1 Discrete Choice Models

The literature in travel behavior research that has explicitly taken a life trajectory perspective has tried to find relationships in the data, relying on statistical concepts. Their choice theoretical basis is weak, or has not really been articulated. In this section, we discuss two approaches that can be viewed as extensions of classic choice theory. The first approach is based on the concept of lifetime utility and thus better captures the idea that housing and job choice generate utility for a longer period of time. The second approach is based on the contention that individual choice behavior depends on social dynamics and thus offers a potentially relevant approach for those life trajectory decisions that may be influenced by social dynamics.

Lifetime Utility

Golounov et al. (2007) offer a relevant example of a model of lifetime utility. Their domain of application concerns car sharing, which may be difficult to view as a life trajectory decision, but a similar approach can be developed for the typical choices considered in this stream of literature. In line with such life trajectory decisions, the choice involves a substantial financial investment, which should be traded-off against other major investment decisions such as a house, children's education, and other expensive consumer durables. Moreover, the choice implies a loan or the spending of savings, implying that the decision-maker needs to decide whether the choice is affordable. Most importantly, consumption of the product is not immediate, but rather stretches out across a much longer period of time, implying that time-dependent utilities should be taken into account. Thus, life trajectory decisions can be seen as dynamic choice problems and these dynamics should be incorporated into the model.

The core of the model concerns the trade-off of spending money on the decision under investigation (leasing a new car), or spending the money on other goods, subject to budget constraints. The authors model change in intertemporal consumer utility as a result of possible car lease. To account for lifetime utility, the dynamic decision problem is conceptualized in terms of a vector of payments, and a vector of remaining car values. The disutility of spendings and the utility of remaining car value, and therefore the total utility change from choosing a choice option depend on the discount rate. The dynamic decision problem is solved by assuming that consumers will choose the option that maximizes total utility across time.

Let the random utility for option j of individual n be written as:

$$U_{nj} + \varepsilon_{nj} \tag{16.7}$$

where U_{nj} is the utility of alternative j for individual n, the ε_{nj}-s are independently and identically Gumbel distributed errors. Because individuals may make more than one choice, let m be an index for observation m out of M observed choices (observations) per individual (1, …, m, … M). Thus, if an individual is observed to have made M consecutive choices from a set of alternatives J_m, with $j_{nm} \in J_m$, the utility of choice option j in choice situation m, U_{njm}, is given by:

$$\begin{aligned} U_{njm}(\boldsymbol{\beta}_\mathbf{n}) &= \sum_{t=t_0}^{T} [(1+\beta_{1n})^{-t}(\beta_{2n}S_{jmt} + \beta_{3n}V_{jmt})], if \quad j \neq 0 \\ U_{n0m}(\boldsymbol{\beta}_\mathbf{n}) &= \beta_{0n} \end{aligned} \tag{16.8}$$

where each option j is represented by a vector of payments S_{jmt}, and vector of remaining car values V_{mtj}. To describe the random coefficients in the model, $\boldsymbol{\beta}_\mathbf{n}$ defines a vector (β_{0n}, β_{1n}, β_{2n}, β_{3n}) in which the parameters are unobserved for each n. These parameters vary across individuals with vector density function $f\boldsymbol{\beta}_\mathbf{n}|\boldsymbol{\theta}, x_n)$, where x_n is a set of observed characteristics of individual n, and $\boldsymbol{\theta}$ is a parameter vector. Assuming that the error terms are independently and identically Gumbel distributed within and across choices, and are independent of $\boldsymbol{\beta}_\mathbf{n}$, S_{jmt} and V_{jmt}, the probability that person n chooses alternative j in choice m is equal to:

$$p_{njm} = \frac{\exp(U_{njm}(\boldsymbol{\beta}_\mathbf{n}))}{\sum_{j'=1}^{J_m} \exp(U_{nj'm}(\boldsymbol{\beta}_\mathbf{n}))} \tag{16.9}$$

The unconditional probability is the integral of the conditional probability over all possible values of $\boldsymbol{\beta}_\mathbf{n}$ which depend on their density function $f\boldsymbol{\beta}_\mathbf{n}|\boldsymbol{\theta}, x_n)$:

$$Q_{njm}(\boldsymbol{\theta}) = \int L_{njm}(\boldsymbol{\beta}_\mathbf{n})f(\boldsymbol{\beta}_\mathbf{n}|\boldsymbol{\theta},x_n)d\boldsymbol{\beta}_\mathbf{n} \tag{16.10}$$

Denote $j(n\ ,m)$ as the alternative j that individual n chooses in choice m. Then, conditional on $\boldsymbol{\beta}_\mathbf{n}$, the probability of the observed sequence of choices $j(n,\ 1)$, …, $j(n,\ m)$, … , $j(n,\ M)$ for individual n is a standard multinominal logit probability:

$$H_n(\boldsymbol{\beta}_\mathbf{n}) = \prod_m L_{nj(n,m)m}(\boldsymbol{\beta}_\mathbf{n}) \tag{16.11}$$

The unconditional probability is the integral of the conditional probability over all possible values of $\boldsymbol{\beta}_\mathbf{n}$, which depends on the density function $f\boldsymbol{\beta}_\mathbf{n}|\boldsymbol{\theta}, x_n)$:

$$P_n(\boldsymbol{\theta}) = \int H_n(\boldsymbol{\beta}_\mathbf{n})f(\boldsymbol{\beta}_\mathbf{n}|\boldsymbol{\theta},x_n)d\boldsymbol{\beta}_\mathbf{n} \tag{16.12}$$

This mixed logit approach allows $\boldsymbol{\beta}_\mathbf{n}$ to vary randomly across individuals. We assume that the true values of $\boldsymbol{\beta}_\mathbf{n}$ are not known, but we can estimate their distribution in the population. More advanced models can be estimated by assuming dependencies in the error terms.

Discrete Choice Model of Social Dynamics

Some life trajectory decisions such as residential choice and vehicle choice may be induced by a multitude of endogenous and exogenous drivers of change. One of these drivers is social influence. Individuals may be triggered to consider particular options because these have become more popular or mainstream in (parts of) their social network. Because in certain decision contexts, some people may exhibit a tendency to mimic or copy the behavior of others because they like to belong to the same group or gain the respect of some people, including such mechanisms into choice models would be beneficial. It should be noted that other people show exactly the opposite tendency: to differentiate oneself from a particular group exactly the opposite or at least different behavior is exhibited.

Blume and Durlauf (2003) developed a discrete choice theoretic approach to examine dynamical aspects of social interaction. Their model assumes that individual choice behavior is influenced by the accumulated choices of all other members of a social network or population. Brock and Durlauf (2001) derive results for the equilibrium state of this system. The model can be expressed as follows. They assume that individual choices are based not only the private utility derived from a particular choice, but also from the social utility associated with the choice. They consider a binary choice, where each of the binary choices is coded into y_n. The realization of the binary choice is coded as $y_n = \{-1, 1\}$. The space of all possible binary actions of the population is N-tuple $\mathbf{y} = (y_1, y_2, \ldots, y_N)$. The utility of individual n of choosing action j is assumed to consist of:

$$U_{nj} = V_{nj} + S_{nj}(\rho_n^e(\mathbf{y}_{-n})) + \varepsilon(y_n) \tag{16.13}$$

where,

U_{nj}	the utility of individual n with respect to choice j,
V_{nj}	the private utility of individual n with respect to choice j,
$S_{nj}(\rho_n^e(\mathbf{y}_{-n}))$	the social utility caused by influence of the social interactions on the utility of individual n with respect to choice j,
$\rho_n^e(\mathbf{y}_{-n})$	the conditional probability measure individual n places on the choices of others at the time of making his own decision, and
$\mathbf{y}_{-n}$	the vector of choices of all individuals other than n

Two different models were derived from this basic concept. The first model is based on the assumption of a constant degree of dependence across individuals. If it is assumed that

$$S_{nj}(\rho_n^e(\mathbf{y}_{-n})) = S_{ni}(\bar{m}_n^e) = \theta\, \mathbf{y}\, \bar{m}_n^e \tag{16.14}$$

where, $\bar{m}_n^e$ is the average of the subjective expected value from the perspective of individual n of individual n' choice ($\bar{m}_n^e = (N-1)^{-1} \sum_{n' \neq n} m_{n',n}^e$), and $\theta > 0$.

Theoretically, this specification assumes that individual choice behavior is based on an expectation of the mean choice level, which is independent of the error terms. The latter means that individuals do not communicate or coordinate their decisions. Assuming an extreme value distribution for the error terms, the probability than individual n will choose option j is then equal to:

$$p_{ni} = \frac{\exp(\beta(V_{ni} + \theta\, \mathbf{y}_n\, \bar{m}_n^e))}{\sum_{y_{ni'}} \exp(\beta(V_{ni'} + \theta\, \mathbf{y}_{ni'} \bar{m}_n^e))} \tag{16.15}$$

The second specification captures conformity by assuming that

$$S_{ni}(\bar{m}_n^e) = -\theta/2(\mathbf{y}_n - \bar{m}_n^e)^2 \tag{16.16}$$

This model assumes that social utility decreases with increasing deviance from the mean. Dugundji and Walker (2005) and Dugundji (2013) expanded this model from the binary case to the trinomial case and derived the equilibrium conditions for this model.

16.3.2.2 Attitudinal Models

Choice models in urban planning and transportation research express the relationship between attributes of the choice alternatives and choice probabilities. This focus is understandable in that these disciplines, by their very nature, try to change these attributes to achieve particular goals, and therefore have a need to predict consumer response to changing attributes. However, behavioral change may also come about without changing any of the attributes of the choice alternatives but rather as a change in attitudes that people hold. For example, the policy objective to reduce environmental emission by increasing the market share of electric cars may be achieved by changing attributes of electric cars; it may also be achieved by campaigns to increase environmental awareness of particular groups to change their attitudes. It means that some life trajectory decisions such as vehicle choice may also be influenced by the attitudes that people have about particular topics, such as environmental policies, that may affect their choice and decision-making regarding these life trajectory decisions. Classic random utility models lack the variables and mechanisms to successfully predict choice behavior that is primarily driven by attitudes.

Relative to random utility theory, attitudinal theories have found less application in urban and travel behavior research. However, these theories and associated models have dominated related fields such as marketing and environmental psychology. The best-known attitudinal theories are the theory of reasoned action and its successor the theory of planned behavior. Originally, attitude theories were concerned with general behavioral dispositions of individuals with respect to organizations and institutions, social groups and societal issues. These general dispositions were, however, found to be poor predictors of behavior. One possible reason for this lack of predictive success may be that the effects of multiple other factors unique to the specific choice context are ignored. Fishbein and Azjen (1975) argued that general dispositions only indirectly influence choices in specific contexts by impacting factors that are more closely linked to the behavior of interest. They, therefore, formulated the theory of reasoned action (Fishbein and Azjen 1975; Azjen and Fishbein 1980), which was later extended to the theory of planned behavior (Azjen 1985, 1991).

Random utility theory implicitly assumes that changes in choice sets and their attributes will induce behavioral change conform the estimated parameters of the choice model that capture the marginal effects of attribute changes on choice probabilities. These models thus rely on the estimated relationships between attribute levels and choice probabilities. However, these models lack the actual mechanisms that induce such change. Where random utility models emphasize the input-output relations in choice behavior, keeping the actual process as a black box, in contrast, models based on the theory of reasoned action and planned behavior explicitly identify the concept of intention to reflect the strength of underlying motivations to engage in particular behaviors. In general, the stronger intentions, the more likely an individual will engage in the behavior of interest. However, an individual can only transform intentions into actual behavior if he/she can be engaged in that behavior at free will. The theory uses the concept of behavioral control to signify the extent that the individual has access to the required choice options and resources. Thus, the concept is quite similar to the notion of space-time and budget constraints often used in activity-based approaches to travel demand (Rasouli and Timmermans 2014a).

A commonly made assumption is that intentions and behavioral control interact in their effects on actual behavior. Intentions are assumed to positively influence performance to the extent that the individual has behavioral control, and behavioral control is assumed to be positively related to performance to the extent that the individual is motivated to become engaged in the behavior of interest. In the theory of planned action, the concept of actual behavior control was replaced with the concept of perceived behavioral control. It defines an individual's perception of the ease or difficulty of performing the behavior of interest. It is assumed that individual behavior is strongly influenced by the confidence an individual has in his/her ability to perform. Perceived behavioral control, jointly with behavioral intention, directly influence behavioral achievement. The theory of planned behavior postulates three conceptually independent determinants of intention: (i) attitude towards the behavior of interest; (ii) subjective norms, and (iii) degree of perceived behavioral control. Attitude toward the behavior of interest defines the degree to which an individual is positively or negatively disposed to the behavior in question. An example might be concerns about the environment may co-vary with a positive disposition to buy hybrid or electric cars. Subjective norms relate to the perceived social pressure to perform or not to perform the behavior of interest. One can imagine that the probability of buying a speedy car with high fuel consumption may be different if all friends of an individual own the same type of cars, or that all friends are users of public transport or all drive electric cars. The degree of perceived behavioral control refers to the perceived ease or difficulty of performing the behavior in question. Here again, the decision to buy or not to buy an electric car may depend on an individual's perception to what extent his/her routine activity travel behavior would be impacted by the more frequent charging activities and the extra time each charging episode takes. The more positive the attitude and subjective norms, and the greater the perceived behavioral control, the stronger an individual's intention to perform the behavior in question. The relative importance of these concepts in predicting behavioral intention varies across context. Figure 16.1 summarizes the theory.

As to attitudes, a cognitive approach to attitude formation is adopted, typically based on Fishbein and Ajzen's (1975) expectancy-value model of attitudes. This model assumes that attitudes develop from the beliefs people hold about the choice alternative of interest by associating an object or behavior to certain

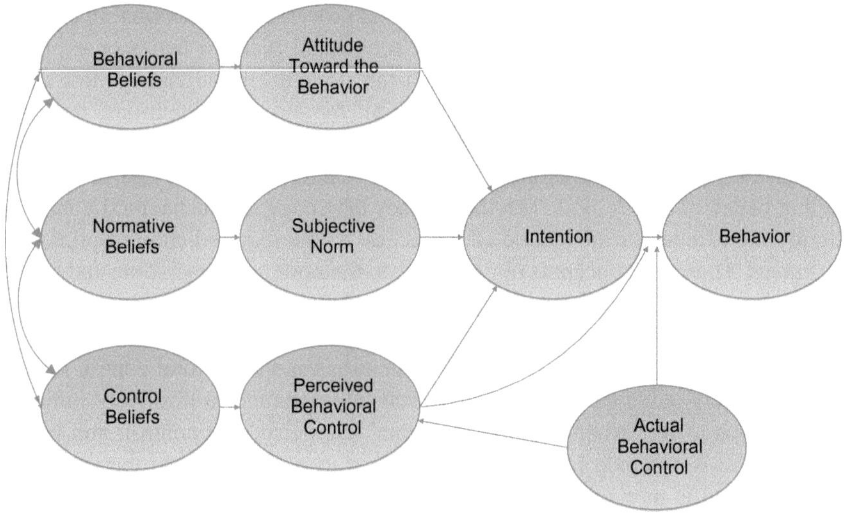

Fig. 16.1 The theory of planned action

outcomes. Mathematically, the outcome's subjective value is assumed to contribute to the attitude in direct proportion to the strength of the belief,

$$A_{nj} = \sum_{k=1}^{K} b_{nk} e_{njk} \tag{16.15}$$

where,

A_{nj} is the attitude of individual n with respect to object or behavior j;
e_{njk} is the subjective evaluation of individual n of salient belief k about choice alternative j;
b_{nk} is individual nth strength of salient belief k defined as the subjective probability that a given behavior will generate a certain outcome

Note that mathematically this function strongly resembles a linear utility function. The main difference is that in this case all terms on the right hand side of the equation are separately and explicitly measured. In most applications of the theory of planned behavior, belief strength is assessed by means of a 7-point graphic scale (e.g., likely-unlikely) and evaluation by means of a 7-point evaluative scale (e.g., good-bad). Alternatively, one can find the optimal scaling. The belief and evaluation scales can be rescaled by adding constants θandϑ respectively (Holbrook 1977). Then, the model becomes

$$A_{nj} = \sum_{k=1}^{K} (b_{nk} + \theta)(e_{njk} + \vartheta) \tag{16.16}$$

$$A_{nj} = \sum_{k=1}^{K} (b_{nk}e_{njk} + b_{nk}\vartheta + \theta e_{njk} + \theta\vartheta) \tag{16.17}$$

$$A_{nj} = \sum_{k=1}^{K} b_{nk}e_{njk} + \vartheta \sum_{k=1}^{K} b_{nk} + \theta \sum_{k=1}^{K} e_{njk} + \theta\vartheta) \tag{16.18}$$

To estimate the rescaling parameters ϑ and θ, we regress the attitude measure on $\sum_{k=1}^{K} b_{nk}e_{njk}, \sum_{k=1}^{K} b_{nk}$ and $\sum_{k=1}^{K} e_{njk}$ and divide the unstandardized regression coefficients $\sum_{k=1}^{K} b_{nk}$ and $\sum_{k=1}^{K} e_{njk}$ by the coefficient obtained for $\sum_{k=1}^{K} e_{njk}$. The resulting values provide least-squares estimates of belief strength and evaluation.

For subjective norms, a similar equation is used

$$N_{nj} = \sum_{k=1}^{K} m_{njk}s_{jk} \tag{16.19}$$

where,

N_{nj} is the subjective norm of individual n with respect to object or behavior j;
s_{jk} is the strength of social norm k about choice alternative j;
m_{njk} is individual nth motivation to comply with social norm k about choice alternative j;

Finally, perceived control is assumed to be equal to

$$C_{nj} = \sum_{k=1}^{K} p_{njk}c_{njk} \tag{16.20}$$

where,

C_{nj} is the perceived control of individual n with respect to object or behavior j;
p_{njk} is the perceived power of individual n of belief k about choice alternative j;
c_{njk} is individual nth control belief of belief k about choice alternative j;

Social norm in this context is defined as the perceived social pressure to engage in a certain type of behavior.

Over the years, the level of sophistication in measuring these concepts and estimating their relationships has dramatically increased. Nowadays, the standard is to use multiple indicators for each concept and estimate a structural equation model to identify the direct and indirect relationships identified by the model.

It should be evident that these attitudinal models are models of behavioral change and are not per se directly linked to life trajectories. However, it is possible to examine whether particular attitudes are related to different lifecycle stages and in that sense a link between life trajectories and attitudes may be established. Although the number of applications of this model in urban and travel behaviour research is still relatively limited, the potential usefulness of this approach to study behavioural change in travel behaviour has been advocated by, for example, Gärling (2005), Gärling et al. (1998, 2001, 2002), Fujii and Gärling (2003, 2005), and Gärling and Fujii (2006). Although the following examples do not concern life trajectory events, they do illustrate the contention that for some choice problems attitudes may be more important than utilities. For example, Fujii and Kitamura (2003) investigated the effects of a one-month free bus pass on travel behaviour, and found an increase in positive attitudes towards the bus, and intensified use of the bus at the expanse of decreased car travel. Similarly, Bamberg et al. (2003a, b) found that the provision of a free pass to students led to changing attitudes, subjective norms and perceptions of behavioural control. Other examples of this kind of work include Bamberg and Schmidt (2003), Chatterjee and Ma (2006), Fujii et al. (2001), Fujii and Gärling (2005, 2006), Fujii and Taniguchi (2005, 2007), and Loukopoulos et al. (2004, 2005, 2006).

Compared to random utility and discrete choice theory, the Theory of Planned Behavior has some limitations. Perhaps the most important of these is fact that it ignores economic factors influencing choices. Although, as the above examples illustrate, it is not difficult to imagine choice problems in which attitudes play a dominant role, it is difficult to imagine that these attitudes will not be traded-off against the utility derived from the choice alternatives, costs, etc. Moreover, although to some extent this also applies to stated choice models, constraints are not explicitly taken into account and the time frame between the intention and actual choice is not addressed. Another criticism raised against original attitudinal theory was the lack of rigor in measurement and parameter estimation. Developments with respect to structural equation models have, however, put that criticism to rest. In fact, structural models allow for much more complexity than commonly used random utility models. Yet, for urban transportation planners, the fact that attributes of the choice alternatives are ignored limits the applicability of these models.

In that sense, the further development of elaborated hybrid choice models may be beneficial. Hybrid models have been introduced in transportation research to include attitudinal and psychological constructs in choice models. However, this has typically been done in rather restrictive ways by assuming that both socio-economic variables and latent attitudes directly influence the utility of choice alternatives according to a linear model, and therefore choice probabilities. Forecasting with such models remains relatively difficult. Attitudes are assumed related to socio-economic variables, but often such relationships are weak and may not hold over time.

16.3.2.3 Technology Acceptance Model

Particularly, life trajectory decisions related to mobility resources such as electric cars, can be viewed in terms of consumer interest in new technology. The intention to buy new technology and the ultimate buying decision are strongly influenced by people's attitudes towards such new technology. The technology acceptance model, introduced by Davis (1985), represents an attempt to identify the motivations underlying acceptance of new technology. As will be discussed, this theory shares concepts with the theory of planned behavior, and adds components specifically related to technology.

Building on earlier work about motivations (e.g., Schultz and Slevin 1975; Bandura 1982), Davis (1985, 1989) argued that motivations underlying the acceptance of technology are influenced by (i) perceived usefulness, (ii) perceived ease of use, and (iii) attitude towards using the system. Perceived usefulness relates to the degree an individual believes that the use of a new technology would enhance particular objectives, such as for example reduction of energy. Perceived ease of use is defined as the degree to which an individual believes the use of a new technology is free of physical or mental effort. Attitudes are assumed influenced by perceived usefulness and perceived ease of use. In that sense, the technology acceptance model can be viewed as a special case of the theory of reasoned action. Figure 16.2 gives a summary of this original framework.

Later, Davis et al. (1993) hypothesized that perceived usefulness may also have a direct and not only an indirect effect on behavior. Venkatesh and Davis (1996) subsequently deleted the component of attitudes and assumed that perceived ease of use may influence perceived usefulness and that both these concepts influence behavioral intention.

In later work (Venkatesch and Davis 2000), the authors identified a set of factors influencing perceived usefulness. In particular, the mentioned image, subjective norm, job relevance, quality and result demonstrability. Experience and voluntariness were added as factors influencing behavioral intention, while experiences also moderate the relationship between subjective norm and perceived usefulness (Fig. 16.3). Venkatesh (2000) identified further factors influencing perceived ease of use. More specifically, he argued that perceived ease of use is influenced by self-efficacy, perceptions of external control, anxiety, playfulness, enjoyment and usability.

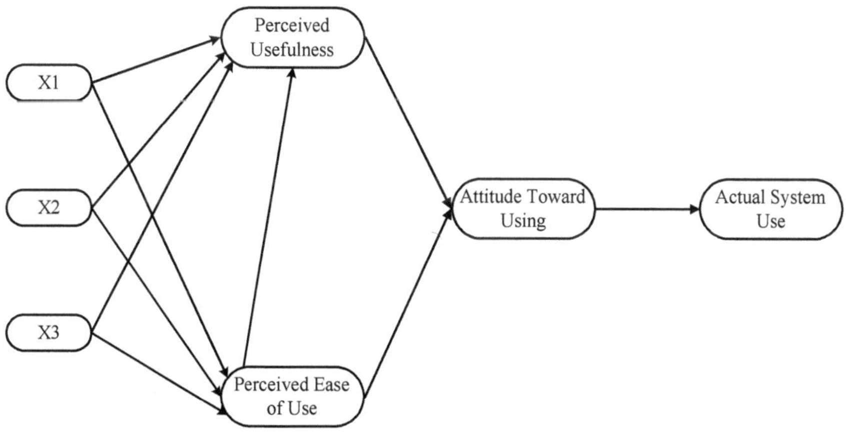

Fig. 16.2 The original technology acceptance model

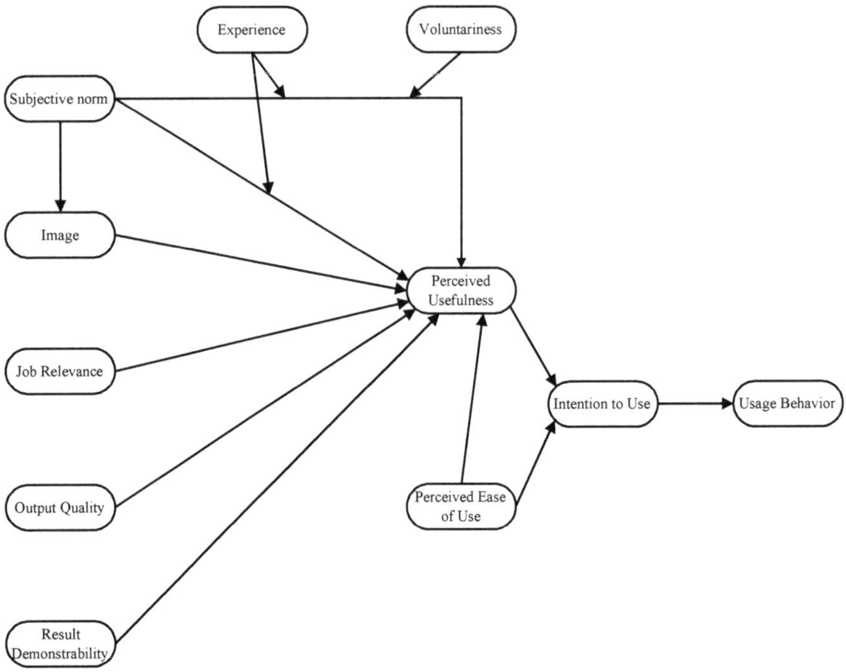

Fig. 16.3 Venkatesch (2000) technology acceptance model

It will be evident that not all these constructs are equally relevant or important for the kind of choice problems of interest to transportation researchers. Specific operationalisations will be required if one would apply this modeling approach to a problem related to life trajectory decisions.

16.3.2.4 Norm Activation Model

While the technology acceptance model focused on the acceptance of new technology as an example of behavioral change, other attitudinal models have been advocated and formulated in environmental sciences to address changing attitudes and behavior with regard to environmental issues. These models also are concerned with behavioral change, and in case with shifts in dispositions towards pro-environmental attitudes and behavior. To the extent that life trajectory decisions involve behavioral change, these theories and models may be inspirational for formulating life trajectory travel-oriented models of behavioral change.

Schwartz (1977) formulated the norm activation model to study pro-environmental behavior/intentions of individuals. The model identifies three types of antecedents to predict pro-environmental behavior: awareness of consequences, ascription of responsibility, and personal norms. Awareness of consequences addresses the question whether the individual is aware of the harmful consequences of his actions. Ascription of responsibility is concerned with the question whether the individual feels responsible for the negative consequences of not acting pro-socially or pro-environmentally. The personal norm dictates whether an individual should perform a particular action that prevents negative outcomes.

The norm activation model has been given two different interpretations, differing in terms of the relationships between the key core concepts of the model (Steg and De Groot 2010). First, it has been interpreted as a sequential model, emphasizing that problem awareness influences a personal norm that directly affects pro-environmental intention/behavior via ascription of responsibility. The second interpretation is that both problem awareness and ascription of responsibility directly influence a personal norm, which acts as an immediate predictor of pro-environmental intention/behavior (Steg and De Groot 2010).

More recently, the basic model has been expanded. It has been argued that pro-social and pro-environmental behavior reflects a combination of pro-social motives and self-interest (Bamberg and Moser 2007; Onwezen et al. 2013; Han 2015). Consequently, attitude toward the behavior and social/subjective norm have been added to the basic model, bringing this revised model closer to the original attitudinal models. Other authors (e.g., Perugini and Conner 2000; Bagozzi et al. 2003) argued that individuals assess the consequences of attaining and not attaining their goals. These assessments then result in corresponding (anticipated) favorable or unfavorable emotions from engaging in particular behavior. In particular, pride and guilt have been added to the model (e.g., Harth et al. 2013). Feelings of pride trigger compliance with the personal norm, while anticipated guilt induces violating the personal norm. Similarly, it has been argued that an individual's attitude toward engaging in ecofriendly behavior and perceived social pressure play an important role (e.g., Klockner 2013; Matthies et al. 2012). Attitudes are assumed to depend on the awareness of any negative consequences of behavior and affect behavioral intention.

16.3.2.5 Value Belief Norm Theory

The VBN theory, developed by Stern et al. (1999), can be viewed as an elaboration of norm activation theory. It adds the concepts of values and ecological worldview to the model. VBN theory assumes that an individual's eco-friendly intentions and behavior are determined by pro-environmental personal norms, which in turn are activated by the sequential process of values-ecological worldview-awareness of adverse consequences, and ascribed responsibility. Value orientations such as biospheric, altruistic, and egoistic values are directly related to the ecological worldview (Stern 2000).

Although the model may not be directly relevant for transportation and urban research, the norm activation framework, which states that individuals' awareness of conceivably harmful consequences of their behavior, together with a feeling of responsibility for these possibly detrimental consequences of not behaving

Chatterjee K, Ma K (2006) Behavioural responses to a new transport option—a dynamic analysis using a six-month panel survey. In: Proceedings of the 11th international conference on travel behaviour research, Kyoto, August 16–20 (CD-ROM)
Chen C, Chen X (2006) What it takes for people to change? A time question. In: Proceedings of the 11th international conference on travel behaviour research, Kyoto, August 16–20 (CD-ROM)
Chorus CG (2011) A new model of random regret minimization. Eur J Transp Infrastruct Res 10:181–196
Chorus CG, Arentze TA, Timmermans HJP (2008) A random regret-minimization model of travel choice. Transp Res Part B 42:1–18
Davis F (1985) A technology acceptance model for empirically testing new end-user information systems. MIT Sloan School of Management, Cambridge, MA
Davis F (1989) Perceived usefulness, perceived ease of use, and user acceptance of new technology. MIS Q 13:319–340
Davis F (1993) User acceptance of computer technology: system characteristics, user perceptions. Int J Man Mach Stud 38:475–487
Dugundji E (2013) Socio-dynamic discrete choice: theory and application. Doctoral dissertation, University of Amsterdam
Dugundji E, Walker J (2005) Discrete choice with social and spatial network interdependencies. Transp Res Rec 1921:70–78
Fishbein M, Azjen I (1975) Belief, attitude, intention and behavior. Addison-Wesley, Reading, MA
Fujii S, Gärling T (2003) Application of attitude theory for improved predictive accuracy of stated preference methods in travel demand analysis. Transp Res Part A 37:389–402
Fujii S, Gärling T (2005) Temporary structural change: a strategy to break car-use habit and promote public transport. In: Underwood G (ed) Traffic and transport psychology. Elsevier, Amsterdam, pp 585–592
Fujii S, Gärling T (2006) Role and acquisition of car-use habit. In: Gärling T, Steg L (eds) Threats to the quality of urban life from car traffic: problems, causes, and solutions. Elsevier, Amsterdam, pp 235–250
Fujii S, Kitamura R (2003) What does a one-month free bus ticket do to habitual drivers? An experimental analysis of habit and attitude change. Transportation 30:81–95
Fujii S, Taniguchi A (2005) Reducing family car use by providing travel advice or requesting behavioural plans: an experimental analysis of travel feedback programs. Transp Res Part D 10:385–393
Fujii S, Taniguchi A (2007) Determinants of the effectiveness of travel feedback programs: a review of communicative mobility management measures for changing travel behavior in Japan. Transp Policy 13:339–348
Fujii S, Gärling T, Kitamura R (2001) Changes in drivers' perceptions and use of public transport during a freeway closure: effects of temporary structural change on cooperation in a real-life social dilemma. Environ Behav 33:796–808
Gärling T (2005) Changes in private car use in response to travel demand management. In: Underwood G (ed) Traffic and transport psychology. Elsevier, Amsterdam, pp 551–571
Garling T, Fujii S (2006) Travel behavior modification: theories, methods, and programs. Proceedings of the 11th international conference on travel behaviour research, Kyoto, August 16–20 (CD-ROM)
Gärling T, Gillholm R, Gärling A (1998) Reintroducing attitude theory in travel behavior research: the validity of an interactive interview procedure to predict car use. Transportation 25:129–146
Gärling T, Fujii S, Boe O (2001) Empirical tests of a model of determinants of script-based driving choice. Transp Res Part F 4:89–102
Gärling T, Eek D, Loukopoulos P, Fujii S, Johansson-Stenman O, Kitamura R, Pendyala R, Vilhelmson B (2002) A conceptual analysis of the impact of travel demand management on private car use. Transp Policy 9:59–70

Golounov V, Dellaert B, van Soest F, Timmermans HJP (2007) Mixed-Logit heterogeneous intertemporal lifetime utility model of car-leasing behavior using conjoint choice data. In: Compendium of papers CD-ROM, the 86th annual meeting of the transportation research board, Washington D.C., January 21–25

Han H (2015) Travelers' pro-environmental behavior in a green lodging context: converging value-belief-norm theory and the theory of planned behavior. Tour Manag 47:164–177

Hannes E, Janssens D, Wets G (2007) The use of choice heuristics in daily activity travel behaviour: an expert system. In: Paper presented at the CUPUM 2007 conference, Iguassa Falls

Harth N, Leach CW, Kessler Th (2013) Guilt, anger, and pride about in-group environmental behaviour: different emotions predict distinct intentions. J Environ Psychol 34:18–26

Holbrook MB (1977) Comparing multiattribute attitude models by optimal scaling. J Consum Res 4:165–171

Janssens D (2005) Calibrating unsupervised machine learning algorithms for the prediction of activity-travel patterns. Doctoral dissertation, Hasselt University, Faculty of Applied Economics, Belgium

Janssens D, Lan Y, Wets G, Chen G (2006) Allocating time and location information to activity-travel patterns through reinforcement learning. Knowl-Based Syst 20(5):466–477

Kahneman D, Tversky A (1979) Prospect theory: an analysis of decisions under risk. Econometrica 47:263–291

Kim J, Rasouli S, Timmermans HJP (2014a) Expanding the scope of hybrid choice models allowing for mixture of social influences and latent attitudes: application to intended purchase of electric cars. Transp Res Part A 69:71–85

Kim J, Rasouli S, Timmermans HJP (2014b) Hybrid choice models: original formulation and recent progress incorporating social influence and nonlinear utility functions. Procedia Environ Sci 22:20–34

Klöckner C (2004) How single events change travel mode choice a life span perspective. In: Paper presented at the 3rd international conference of traffic and transport psychology, Nottingham, UK, September 5–9

Klöckner C (2013) A comprehensive model of the psychology of environmental behavior: a meta-analysis. Glob Environ Change 23:1028–1038

Krizek K (2003) Residential relocation and changes in urban travel. J Am Plann Assoc 69:265–281

Lanzendorf M (2010) Key events and their effect on mobility biographies: the case of child birth. Int J Sustain Transp 4(5):272–292

Loukopoulos P, Jakobsson C, Gärling T, Schneider CM, Fujii S (2004) Car user responses to travel demand management measures: goal setting and choice of adaptation alternatives. Transp Res Part D 9:263–280

Loukopoulos P, Gärling T, Jakobsson C, Meland S, Fujii S (2005) Choices of activity- and travel change options for reduced car use. In: Timmermans HJP (ed) Progress in activity-based analysis. Elsevier, Amsterdam, pp 489–501

Loukopoulos P, Jakobsson C, Gärling T, Meland S, Fujii S (2006) Understanding the process of adaptation to car-use reduction goals. Transp Res Part F 9:115–127

Matthies E, Selge S, Klöckner CA (2012) The role of parental behaviour for the development of behaviour specific environmental norms: the example of recycling and re-use behavior. J Environ Psychol 32:277–284

McFadden D (1978) Modelling the choice of residential location. In: Karlqvist A, Snickars F, Weibull J (eds) Spatial interaction theory and planning models, North Holland, pp 75–96

Oakil ATM, Ettema DF, Arentze TA, Timmermans HJP (2011a) Longitudinal model of longer-term mobility decisions: framework and first empirical tests. J Urban Plann Dev 137:220–229

Oakil ATM, Ettema DF, Arentze TA, Timmermans HJP (2011b) Dynamics in car ownership and life cycle events: a longitudinal analysis. In: Compendium of papers CD-ROM, the 90th annual meeting of the transportation research board, Washington, D.C., January 23–27

Onwezen MC, Antonides G, Bartels J (2013) The norm activation model: an exploration of the functions of anticipated pride and guilt in pro-environmental behavior. J Econ Psychol 39:141–153

Perugini M, Conner M (2000) Predicting and understanding behavioral volitions: the interplay between goals and behaviors. Eur J Soc Psychol 30:705–731

Prillwitz J, Lanzendorf M (2006) Impact of life course events on car ownership. In: Compendium of papers CD-ROM, the 85th annual meeting of the transportation research board, Washington D.C., January 22–26

Prillwitz J, Lanzendorf M (2007) Interactions among residential relocations, life course events and daily commute distances. In: Compendium of papers CD-ROM, the 86th annual meeting of the transportation research board, Washington, D.C., January 21–25

Rasouli S, Timmermans HJP (2014a) Activity-based models of travel demand: promises, progress and prospects. Int J Urban Sci 18:31–60

Rasouli S, Timmermans HJP (2014b) Applications of theories and models of choice and decision-making under conditions of uncertainty in travel behaviour research. Travel Behav Soc 1:79–90

Rasouli S, Timmermans HJP (2015) Models of bounded rationality under certainty. In: Rasouli S, Timmermans HJP (eds) Bounded rational choice behavior: applications in transport. Emerald Publishers

Rasouli S, Timmermans HJP, van der Waerden PJHJ (2015) Employment status transitions and shifts in daily activity-travel behavior with special focus on shopping duration. Transportation 42(6):919–931

Rocci A (2006) Why don't we change our mobility behaviours? Acceptance and hindrance to a change: the case study of the Greater Paris Region as compared to Nagoya. In: Proceedings of the 11th international conference on travel behaviour research, Kyoto, August 16–20 (CD-ROM)

Rogers EM (1962) Diffusion of innovations. Free Press, Glencoe

Schultz RL, Slevin DP (1975) A program for research in implementation. In: Schultz RL, Slevin DP (eds) Implementing operations research/management science. American Elsevier, New York

Schwarz SH (1977) Normative influences on altruism. Adv Exp Soc Psychol 10:221–279

Stanbridge K, Lyons G (2006) Travel behaviour considerations during the process of residential relocation. In: Proceedings of the 11th international conference on travel behaviour research, Kyoto, August 16–20 (CD-ROM)

Stanbridge K, Lyons G, Farthing S (2004) Travel behaviour change and residential relocation. In: Paper presented at the 3rd international conference of traffic and transport psychology, Nottingham, UK

Steg L, De Groot J (2010) Explaining prosocial intentions: testing causal relationships in the norm activation model. Br J Soc Psychol 49:725–743

Stern PC (2000) Toward a coherent theory of environmentally significant behavior. J Soc Issues 56:407–424

Stern PC, Dietz T, Abel T, Guagnano GA, Kalof L (1999) A value-belief-norm theory of support for social movements: the case of environmentalism. Res Human Ecol 6:81–97

Train K (2003) Discrete choice methods with simulations. Cambridge University Press, Cambridge

Venkatesh V (2000) Determinants of perceived ease of use: integrating control, intrinsic motivation, and emotion into the technology acceptance model. Inf Syst Res 11:342–365

Venkatesh V, Davis F (1996) A model of the antecedents of perceived ease of use: development and test. Decis Sci 27:451–481

Venkatesh V, Davis F (2000) A theoretical extension of the technology acceptance model: four longitudinal case studies. Manage Sci 46:186–204

Verhoeven M, Arentze TA, Timmermans HJP, van der Waerden PJHJ (2005a) Modeling impact of key events on long-term transport mode choice decisions: decision network approach using event history data. Transp Res Rec 1926:106–114

Verhoeven M, Arentze TA, Timmermans HJP, van der Waerden PJHJ (2005b) Examining temporal effects of lifecycle events on transport mode choice decisions. In: Proceedings of the computers in urban planning and urban management conference, London (CD-ROM: 15)

Verhoeven M, Arentze TA, Timmermans HJP, van der Waerden PJHJ (2006) Modeling the influence of structural lifecycle events on transport mode choice decisions using a structure learning algorithm. In: Proceedings of the 11th international conference on travel behaviour research, Kyoto, August 16–20 (CD-ROM)

Verhoeven M, Arentze TA, Timmermans HJP, van der Waerden PJHJ (2007) Simulating the influence of life trajectory events on transport mode behavior in an agent based system. In: Proceedings of the 10th IEEE conference on intelligent transportation systems. IEEE, New York, NY, pp 107–112

Vanhunsel M, Janssens D, Wets G (2007a) Calibrating a new reinforcement learning mechanism for modeling dynamic activity-travel behavior and key events. In: Compendium of papers CD-ROM, the 86th annual meeting of the transportation research board, Washington, D.C., January 21–25

Vanhulsel M, Janssens D, Wets, G (2007b) Use of a relational reinforcement learning algorithm to generate dynamic activity-travel patterns. In: Paper presented at TRISTAN VI, Phuket Island, Thailand

Waerden PJHJ van der, Borgers AWJ, Timmermans HJP (2003a) Key events and critical incidents influencing transport mode choice switching behavior: an exploratory study. In: Compendium of papers CD-ROM, the 82nd annual meeting of transportation research board, Washington, D.C., January 12–16

Waerden PJHJ van der, Borgers AWJ, Timmermans HJP (2003b) The influence of key events and critical incidents on transport mode choice switching behaviour: a descriptive analysis. In: Proceedings of the 10th international conference on travel behaviour research, Lucerne, August 10–15 (CD-ROM)

Xie C, Wang H, Nozick LK (2006) Modeling travel mode choice behavior by a Bayesian network. In: Compendium of papers CD-ROM, the 85th annual meeting of the transportation research board, Washington D.C., January 22–26

Chapter 17
Behavioral Changes in Migration Associated with Jobs, Residences, and Family Life

Junyi Zhang, Yubing Xiong, Ying Jiang, Nobuhito Tanaka, Nobuaki Ohmori and Ayako Taniguchi

Abstract This chapter first explores migration-related urban issues and then illustrates migration dynamics. It further points out the limitations of existing migration theories. To overcome the shortcomings of existing theories, this chapter presents a new analysis framework for migration, where multiple life choices, including migration, are simultaneously incorporated by expanding the theory of planned behavior. To empirically confirm the applicability of the new framework, a web-based questionnaire survey about migration associated with employment, dwellings and child rearing was implemented in Japan in 2015. This is the first study to reveal such interrelated behavioral changes in multiple life domains from the perspective of decision-making process. Such a theoretical reformulation could provide more scientific insights into cross-sectoral policies of migration than existing theories.

Keywords Migration dynamics · Microlevel theory · Life course · Mobility biographies · Behavioral changes · Behavioral interdependencies · Theory of planned behavior · Japan

---

J. Zhang (✉) · Y. Xiong · Y. Jiang · N. Tanaka
Hiroshima University, Higashi-Hiroshima, Japan
e-mail: zjy@hiroshima-u.ac.jp; junyizh24@gmail.com

N. Ohmori
Utsunomiya University, Utsunomiya, Japan

A. Taniguchi
University of Tsukuba, Tsukuba, Japan

J. Zhang (ed.), *Life-Oriented Behavioral Research for Urban Policy*,
DOI 10.1007/978-4-431-56472-0_17

17.1 Migration-Related Urban Issues

Migration has always been a fundamental component of human history (Lee 1966; Kniveton et al. 2011) and has been studied in various disciplines such as regional economics, demography, sociology, and geography (Chi and Voss 2005). People migrate for various reasons (e.g., work, study, and marriage) from village to village, from village to city, from city to city, and from country to country, while the outcomes of migration may be either prosperity or misery for people and/or for society. An examination of global urban development practices suggests that cities with various population sizes can be economically prosperous. However, cities of different sizes may need to achieve sustainable development in different ways, and migration is clearly a major factor in determining city size. In reality, various optimal/ideal city sizes may be possible depending on how the notion of "optimal" or "ideal" is defined. This book describes people's life choices at the individual/household level. Migration that is optimal or ideal for an individual or a houschold is not necessarily so for society. As stated in Chi and Voss (2005), "migration is a large concern for policy makers because flows of population can significantly affect local political, social, economic, and ecological structures for both sending and receiving areas (p. 11)."

According to Globalization101.org (2013), flows of goods and capital across countries have driven globalization, which has stimulated international migration. Currently, international migrants account for about 3 % of the world's population and would form a country with the world's fifth largest population if they all lived in the same place. The main motivation for international migration is economic factors, and other motivations come from civil strife, war, and political and religious persecution as well as environmental problems (e.g., natural disasters). At the national level, overconcentration of populations in many megacities across the world (e.g., Tokyo, Jakarta, Manila, Seoul, Shanghai, Karachi, Beijing, New York, Mexico City, Mumbai, and New Delhi) has caused various urban development and social issues. In Japan, as an Asian model of a prosperous country, the majority of young people have continued to migrate for work and residence from small cities to the three metropolitan areas (Tokyo, Osaka and Nagoya regions), where around half of the nation's population is now concentrated. As a result, many small cities in Japan now face serious population issues, for example, an ever-increasing proportion of elderly people, difficulties in ensuring mobility for elderly people, and insufficient support for child rearing and women's labor participation. It is predicted that many of these small cities will disappear in future if their current situations cannot be improved.

Similar issues to those caused by migration in Japan can be observed in other developed countries. Smith and Sage (2014) found that the long-distance movement of young adults is a leading cause of demographic and population changes in England and Wales. Muilu and Rusanen (2003) showed empirically that without the support of the young population, small areas, especially remote rural areas, cannot remain viable or maintain their economic functions in the long term. Thissen et al. (2010) argued that "together with the ageing of the European population, youth migration related to the transition from secondary to higher education is increasingly responsible for the declining numbers of young people in rural areas (p. 435)." Using 1970–2000 US Census data, Chen and Rosenthal (2008) revealed that young and highly educated households, especially highly educated couples, are more likely to move to cities with higher quality business environments. Thissen et al. (2010) found that local attachments appear to be the most important factor explaining youths' migration intentions. Other factors include their social background, migration history, and perceptions of employment opportunities, even though there are obvious regional differences caused by the structure, culture, and landscape of the regions. Ek et al. (2008) reported that if living conditions (educational and vocational opportunities) could not be improved and psychosocial resources (lack of social support, passive coping strategies, and greater pessimism) of young adults in rural and remote areas of Northern Finland could not be enhanced, young adults would continue to out-migrate to cities. Interestingly, Vilhelmson and Thulin (2013) found that most young adults in Sweden have integrated the Internet into their migration decision-making processes—from the formation of vague plans and thoughts, to more active plans and actual moves. The Internet reinforces many recent movers' migration motives and intentions, and facilitates their decisions to move and choices of destinations. On the other hand, the counter-urbanization phenomenon has been observed in some European countries. Bijker et al. (2012) found that people in the north of the Netherlands who migrated to less popular rural areas were mainly young; many of them were employed and highly educated, most of them had simply returned to their original rural areas, and only a small percentage had moved from urban areas. Bijker et al. concluded that the migrants in their study were most similar to the migrants to the fringe areas of Denmark.

Out-migration by young people to cities is also common in developing countries. Childs et al. (2014) revealed that communities that had thrived for centuries in Nepal's rugged mountain environments are facing rapid population declines caused by the out-migration of youth, and this posed a potential long-term threat to agricultural production, the family-based care system for the elderly, socioeconomic inequalities, and human capital. In China, the total number of young adults moving from rural to urban areas reached 153 million in 2010, and accounted for about 30 % of total rural labor.[1] Furthermore, the accelerated rural depopulation driven by the vast and increasing out-migration of young labor has imposed huge obstacles to improving land use efficiency and coordinating urban–rural development in China, such as low efficiency in rural residential land use, and the lateral expansion of rural dwellings at the expense of farmland loss, decrease in the ability of rural development, and deterioration of rural residential environments (Liu and Liu 2010; Li et al. 2014). Jiang et al. (2015) found that under China's Urbanization Plan 2014–2020,

[1]Ministry of Human Resources and Social Security (2011) Human Resources and Social Security Undertakings Statistical Bulletin of 2010 (in Chinese; http://w1.mohrss.gov.cn/gb/zwxx/2011-05/24/content_391125.htm).

under which the uniquely Chinese household registration (*hukou*[2]) system will be gradually abolished, about 40 % of rural migrant workers stated that they would choose to live in a city. If this were the case, a dramatic increase in energy consumption by rural migrants could be expected, especially if their social security and housing issues could be properly resolved through the *hukou* reforms. About 60 % of the respondents in the study by Jiang et al. were young workers from rural areas, and more focused insights into those young workers could be derived from that study. Crivello (2015) examined young Peruvians' aspirations and the role of migration in their imagined futures and concluded that aspirations are about much more than abstract "futures;" aspirations determine young Peruvians' actions in the present and to a large extent can explain their current realities. Nugin (2014) argued that young people's out-migration from the rural areas in Estonia should be depicted as moving "forward" rather than "away;" however, this does not necessarily mean that they would never go back home, considering the constantly changing rural context in post-socialist Estonia. Nugin concluded that one of the additional options for rural areas to survive is to attract young people from other areas with the appeal of change and self-realization in a small community.

17.2 Migration Dynamics

17.2.1 General Descriptions

Various theories have been proposed for and applied to migration in various disciplines, including macrolevel, mesolevel, and microlevel theories. As summarized well by Hagen-Zanker (2008), major macrolevel theories include neoclassical macromigration theory, dual labor market theory, and world systems theory. Mesolevel theories include social capital theory, institutional theory, network theory, and the new economics of labor migration. Microlevel theories include Lee's push–pull theory, neoclassical micromigration theory, behavioral models, and the theory of social systems. Macrolevel theories emphasize the role of macrolevel economic and social factors in migration (e.g., Massey et al. 1993; Groenewold et al. 2012). As long as a behavior changes over time, it is desirable to understand it in a dynamic fashion. Migration is not invariant over time (Kennan and Walker 2013). For example, at the macrolevel, Castles (2010) proposed to capture migration within the wider phenomena of social change and social transformation, arguing that migration is also part of national and global social change. However, previous studies revealed that economic and social factors cannot fully explain why

[2]The traditional *hukou* system means that city residents' rights to public services depend on whether or not they have a *hukou*. As most rural migrants do not have a city *hukou*, they receive unequal access to urban public services, consequently discouraging them from permanently residing in cities.

people migrate, and they have consequently emphasized the importance of considering microlevel factors such as individual expectations, values, beliefs, and personality traits (e.g., Boneva and Frieze 2001; Tabor and Milfont 2011; Van Dalen and Henkens 2012, 2013). Kennan and Walker (2013) formulated a dynamic programming-based migration behavior model, which represents decisions of migration locations over time by defining transition probabilities from one location to another. They estimated a model using the National Longitudinal Study of Youth in the USA, and found that expected income and home location are important determinants of migration decisions. Mesolevel theories are developed to incorporate the influence of collectives and social networks on migration at the household or community level. Related to this, another dynamic feature of migration is reflected in the phenomenon of chain migration, which consists of three stages: (1) pioneer migration, (2) labor migration, and (3) family migration (MacDonald and MacDonald 1964). As stated by Haug (2012), pioneer migration usually involves quick decisions on the migration destination and job hunting, with exceptionally high costs and risks. Once pioneer migrants have settled, more workers from home may be attracted because of the transfer of social capital (i.e., labor migration). After that, family reunification becomes feasible in the third stage. Such chain migration can be modeled as a diffusion process (i.e., an S-shaped curve) and it is maintained on the basis of social networks. As for the connections across the three levels, Haug (2012) on the basis of a literature review stated that "the migration decision-making of individual actors (microlevel) is embedded in social contexts (mesolevel) and is based on underlying macro-structural conditions."

As argued by King (2012), "migration is not always, by any means, a one-off event which ends in settlement, but an ongoing process that is reevaluated several times over the life-course." Thus, even though a life course perspective is crucial for migration decisions, limited studies of young adults' decisions can be found in the literature. Chatterjee and Scheiner (2015) presented an excellent review of the application of life-course approaches to travel behavior (often labelled "mobility biographies"), including migration in general. Scheiner's research group conducted a retrospective survey about residential biographies, travel behavior, and holiday trips, and employment biographies with respect to students (954 people) of TU Dortmund University, and their parents (1787 people) and grandparents (1294 people) (Albrecht et al. 2015; Doering et al. 2015). The survey was conducted every term from 2007 to 2012. Albrecht et al. (2015) and Doering et al. (2015) made an initial attempt to reveal intergenerational socialization effects with respect to migration and work trip mobility.

17.2.2 A Case Study Based on the Life-Course Approach

Using data from a life history survey (1400 people) conducted in Japan in 2010 (Zhang et al. 2014), as explained in Chap. 2 of this book, we extracted 1770 samples from young adults (number of people * times migrated) for this case study.

"Young adults" in Japan refers to the population aged from 15 to 34 years old.[3] There were 393, 671, and 706 young adults in the 1980s, 1990s, and 2000s, respectively, who moved from their original places of residence to new ones. It is found[4] that while the proportion of total migrants going to large cities in Japan rose from 28 % in the 1980s to 32 % in 2000s, migration to medium-sized cities remained almost unchanged; however, migration into small cities dropped from 35 % in the 1980s to 30 % in the 2000s.

Based on the above 1770 samples, Xiong et al. (2016) revealed more complicated migration patterns.

As for the overall sample, there were more young adult females who migrated to small cities: 5.99 % from large cities (males: 4.49 %), 5.88 % from medium-sized cities (males: 2.99 %), and 26.53 % from small cities (males: 22.21 %). As for adult males, more migration within large cities (22.90 %) and within medium-sized cities (24.97 %) was observed. It is further shown that 10.65 % of females moved from small to large cities, which is about four percentage points higher than the figure for adult males. In total, more adult males preferred relocation to medium or large cities (4.03 % points higher in large cities and 4.69 % points higher in medium-sized cities than the figure for females), but more females moved to small cities (about 8.71 % points more than males).

The 1990s generation preferred relocation within small cities (26.68 %), but not relocation within medium-sized cities (19.82 %), compared with the 1980s and 2000s generations. Relocation to large cities grew over time (27.47 % in the 1980s, 29.21 % in the 1990s, and 32.01 % in the 2000s). In contrast, relocation to small cities saw a peak in the 1990s (35.36 % in the 1980s, 37.71 % in the 1990s, and 30.03 % in the 2000s), but the drop from the 1990s to the 2000s was much more remarkable than the increase from the 1980s to the 1990s. Conversely, we observed a dip of relocation to medium-sized cities in the 1990s, but this recovered almost to the same level as the 1980s.

Furthermore, young adults' residential relocation choices differ in response to life events such as changes in household structure, workplace, and car ownership within the previous five-year period, or in anticipation of such events in the subsequent five-year period. Specifically, this occurs if household structure changes during the previous or subsequent five years are associated with a preference among older young adults to live in large cities instead of medium-sized and small cities. When they had changed their place of employment within the previous five years or planned to do so in the subsequent five years, younger adults relocated to large cities. However, if they changed their car ownership status within that period, they had a lower probability of relocating to large cities.

[3]Statistics Bureau of Japan: http://www.stat.go.jp/english/data/nenkan/1431-02.htm.

[4]Here, Tokyo, Yokohama, Osaka, and Nagoya are treated as large cities (each has a population of more than 2.0 million). Sapporo, Sendai, Saitama, Kawasaki, Kyoto, Kobe, Hiroshima, and Fukuoka cities are grouped into medium-sized cities (each has a population of over 1.0 million). The remaining cities (170 cities were included in the survey) are classified as small cities.

By incorporating the effects of life events, changes in quality of life-oriented living environment (including residential environment) characteristics at the city level, as well as household attributes and sociodemographics of young adults in Japan, Xiong et al. (2016) estimated a residential relocation choice model without the property of independence of irrelevant alternatives. Their model confirmed that there were clear differences in relocation decisions across generations of young male and female adults, diverse influences of a variety of living environment attributes, and varied influences of state dependence and future expectations of different types of cities. Choice of residential location and/or workplace is a matter for an individual and/or a household. It may be associated with factors such as marriage and child rearing, or use of free time. It is true that having a job is to make a living. However, without a better environment in which to enjoy life, policies that focus only on employment will eventually fail. With such considerations, the above migration behavior analysis should be improved by incorporating the influence of other aspects of life.

17.3 Behavioral Changes Across Life Domains: A New Way of Thinking

Most of the above migration theories and models deal with migration decisions by referring to behavioral outcomes that supposedly reveal people's preferences; however, the internal processes underlying behavioral outcomes are ignored. For this purpose, methodologies that examine behavioral changes are useful, including behavioral change stage models (Prochaska and DiClemente 1983; Prochaska and Velicer 1997), the theory of planned behavior (TIB) (Triandis 1977). Prochaska and DiClemente (1983) and Prochaska and Velicer (1997) argue that health behavior change involves progress through six stages of change: (1) precontemplation (no intention to take action within the next six months), (2) contemplation (the intention to take action within the next six months), (3) preparation (intention to take action within the next 30 days, and some behavioral steps have been taken in this direction), (4) action (changed overt behavior for less than six months), (5) maintenance (changed overt behavior for six months or more), and (6) termination (no temptation to relapse and 100 % confidence). Both the theory of planned behavior and the theory of interpersonal behavior emphasize the importance of attitudes, social norms, and intentions, while the latter further argues that habits cannot be ignored. Studies based on the above theories/models have been conducted to investigate various forms of behavior, such as energy consumption (e.g., Nachreiner et al. 2015; Chen 2016), environmental behavior (e.g., Botetzagias et al. 2015; De Leeuw et al. 2015), travel (e.g., Bamberg 2013; Rowe et al. 2016), purchase of green products (e.g., Yazdanpanah and Forouzani 2015; Paul et al. 2016), behavior concerning fertility (e.g., Mencarini et al. 2015), child rearing (e.g., Guo et al. 2016), and tourism (e.g., Han 2015).

17.3.1 Limitations of Existing Theories

As described in Sect. 17.2.1, previous studies have developed various methodologies to examine migration at the macro-, meso-, and microlevels, in which various factors are assumed to affect migration decisions. The factors assumed to exist in these theories may all work to explain migration decisions; however, we argue that migration decisions are, after all, a matter for an individual or a household. Especially in policymaking, it is necessary to understand not only the results of migration (e.g., where people actually moved), but also the process of migration decisions. For example, in Japan, the central government has sought to encourage more people to migrate into local cities from the three megacities (Tokyo, Nagoya, and Osaka) by adopting various policies. However, the resistance to migrating to local cities is remarkable. Therefore, it is important to understand how to encourage people's behavioral changes in migration.

In line with the above considerations, Hoppe and Fujishiro (2015) applied the theory of planned behavior to predict migration decisions by making use of potential migrants' expectations and attitudes toward migration and careers (i.e., the anticipated job benefits of migration, and career aspirations) as well as beliefs. The decision-making was conceptualized as having three phases: the predecisional, preactional, and actional phases. The predecisional phase corresponds with intentions, the preactional phase starts with exploring options for migrating by gathering information, and the actional phase involves definite actions for the move (e.g., making logistical arrangements). Such phases follow the basic idea of Prochaska and DiClemente (1983), Prochaska and Velicer (1997). Hoppe and Fujishiro (2015) found that respondents are motivated to migrate, not only by the expectation of finding a job, but also by the opportunity to advance their careers. However, they could not find any interaction between the anticipated job benefits (of migration) and career aspirations. The study by Hoppe and Fujishiro (2015) concluded that it is necessary to combine the theory of planned behavior with the behavioral change stage model for a better understanding of migration. Using the National Longitudinal Study of Youth in the USA, Liu et al. (2010), based on a dynamic econometric model with self-selection, found that children's educational outcomes are affected by migration and maternal employment after controlling for the possible endogeneity of relevant decisions. In the context of international migration, Groenewold et al. (2012) revealed a significant influence of perceptions (threat to living conditions, benefits of and barriers to migration), cues to action, and self-efficacy on migration intentions. Interestingly, Kniveton et al. (2011) integrated the insights of the theory of planned behavior into an agent-based model to quantify the numbers of migrants generated by changes in climate. Such efforts of cleverly utilizing agent-based models created a new way to apply the theory of planned behavior in practice.

As for theories of behavioral changes, we point out that there are serious drawbacks, considering the fact that all existing studies, to the best of our knowledge, have focused on only a single form of behavior, such as environmental behavior, travel, or fertility behavior. If a change in a behavior is constrained by other behaviors, how can existing theories of behavioral changes be applied? For example, environmental attitudes and relevant social norms may not only influence the intention to change from commuting by car to using mass transit systems, but may also affect intentions to introduce energy-saving electronic appliances at home. If people enjoy the use of a car and various domestic electronic appliances as part of a comfortable modern lifestyle, then the habits of driving and using appliances cannot be treated separately. Because car use and other life choices may be interrelated, whether and how many old habits could be broken partially depends on how strongly the two behaviors are interrelated. In addition, the timing and duration of change also differ according to life choices. Applying similar sociopsychological approaches may not work well to unfreeze the two habits at the same time. A delay in reforming one form of behavior may lead to a failure to change another, and as a result, neither of the two types of behaviors may eventually change. The above arguments are probably equally applicable to intentions.

In summary, it seems that existing theories of behavioral change need to be modified to reflect the potential interdependencies across life choices. In the following case study, we provide empirical evidence based on data collected in Japan in 2015.

17.3.2 A Survey in Japan

We conducted an Internet questionnaire survey with the working population of the Tokyo Capital Area, including the Tokyo Metropolitan Area, Kanagawa, Chiba, Saitama, Ibaragi, Tochigi, Gunma, and Yamanashi Prefectures in December 2015. The survey includes items about migration, employment, child rearing, and dwellings, focusing especially on young people. Specific items mainly concern (1) migration history and reasons for previous migration as well as the influences of other people; (2) type of current job, location of workplace, duration of tenure, and mode of commuting; (3) current residential location, current and ideal residential environment (in terms of distance to daily facilities), and car ownership; (4) household structure (including the presence of children, members' residential location, and their coresidence with a parent); (5) items based on the theory of planned behavior (mainly attitudes, social norms, and intentions) with respect to migration, jobs, child rearing, and dwellings; (6) intended migration destinations in future and the conditions for future migration; and (7) information about discretional activities in daily life. The purpose of the above survey is to clarify the extent to which the working population of the Tokyo Capital Area would like to migrate to local cities and to encourage more people to work/live there. We conducted the survey with the assistance of a major Internet survey company in Japan, and collected valid data from 1000 workers aged 20–40 (Table 17.1), which is a representative sample of the working population in the Tokyo Capital Area.

Table 17.1 Distributions of age and gender of the working respondents by prefecture

Attribute	Prefecture								
	Tokyo (23 wards) (%)	Kanagawa (%)	Chiba (%)	Saitama (%)	Ibaragi (%)	Tochigi (%)	Gunma (%)	Yamanashi (%)	Subtotal (%)
Male: 20 s	1.6	3.6	2.4	2.8	1.4	1.0	1.0	0.4	14.2
Male: 30 s	2.4	5.8	3.4	4.4	2.2	1.6	1.6	0.6	22.0
Male: 40 s	2.4	5.6	3.2	4.0	2.0	1.4	1.4	0.6	20.6
Female: 20 s	1.4	3.0	2.0	2.2	1.0	1.0	0.8	0.4	11.8
Female: 30 s	1.8	3.8	2.6	3.0	1.4	1.0	1.0	0.4	15.0
Female: 40 s	1.8	4.2	2.8	3.4	1.6	1.0	1.2	0.4	16.4
Subtotal	11.4	26.0	16.4	19.8	9.6	7.0	7.0	2.8	100.0

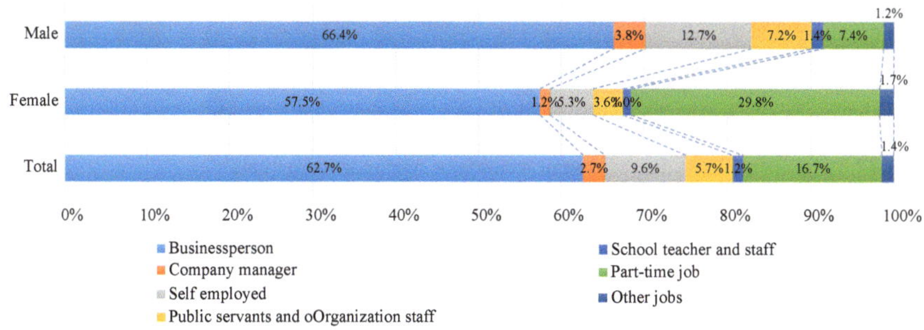

Fig. 17.1 Distribution of jobs by type

Table 17.2 Life stages by workplace

Workplace	Life stages					
	Single (%)	Married without child (%)	Married with one child (%)	Married with two or more children (%)	Single parent (%)	Total (%)
Tokyo: 23 wards	54.4	16.3	12.8	14.9	1.7	100.0
Other areas of Tokyo	49.4	14.2	13.7	19.4	3.3	100.0

As for types of jobs (Fig. 17.1), more than 60 % of the working respondents are businesspeople, and about 30 % of the female respondents are part-time workers, a proportion that is more than four times higher than that of male respondents. There are more single people and married couples without children in the 23 wards of Tokyo than respondents in other life stages, compared with other areas (Table 17.2). As Fig. 17.2 shows, the parents of 66.4 % of the respondents were living in the Kanto region (which has a large overlap with the Tokyo Capital Area).

In the survey, respondents reported their migration histories (the maximum was five times) and reasons for each migration (see Fig. 17.3: note that each respondent can provide one or more reasons). The average number of migrations reported is 2.4. The most common reason was for employment (32.9 %) (job change: 13.1 %; (voluntarily: 9.8 %); to find a job: 13.0 %; job relocation: 6.2 %; inheritance of family business: 0.6 %). This finding is consistent with traditional migration theories, which emphasize the role of economic factors (e.g., Massey et al. 1993; Groenewold et al. 2012), and other previous studies (e.g., Fahr and Sunde 2006; Kennan and Walker 2010; Huinink et al. 2014). It is also consistent with the observations by the Central Government of Japan.[5] In our previous study using a

[5]http://www.mlit.go.jp/hakusyo/mlit/h26/hakusho/h27/html/n1211000.html (accessed January 30, 2016).

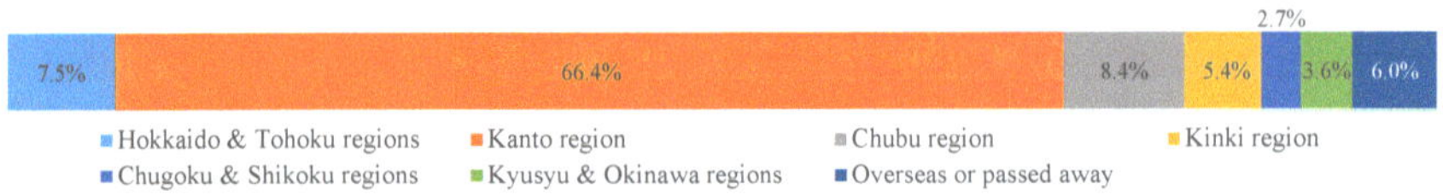

Fig. 17.2 Distribution of the residential location of respondents' parents

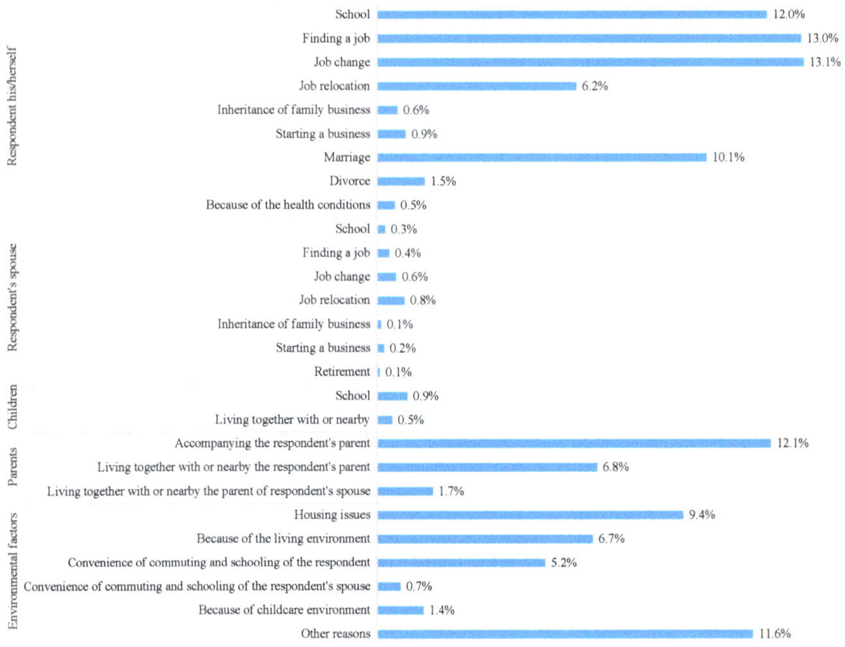

Fig. 17.3 Reasons of migration in the past

life history survey conducted with residents in various Japanese cities in 2010 (Zhang et al. 2014), the peak ages for both job mobility and residential relocation were observed to be between 25 and 30 years old. This also supports the above findings. Interestingly, more than 20 % of respondents reported that their migration was to accompany their parents (the respondent's parent: 12.1 %; the parent of the respondent's spouse: 6.8 %). There are some studies in the literature on the effects of parental migration on their children's lives (e.g., Clifton-Sprigg 2015; Graham et al. 2015); however, no study has clarified how parents affect their children's migration. In this sense, this finding is new. As shown in Fig. 17.2, 66.4 % of respondents live close to their parents (within the same region: Kanto). This suggests that the distance to a parent's residence is also critical in migration decisions. This may be a particular characteristic of Japan and some Asian countries with a strong tradition of caring for parents. It is worth conducting an international comparison to clarify this point. Other strong reasons for migration are going to

Table 17.3 Shares of behavioral change stages with respect to migration from Tokyo, Japan

Age groups	20 s	30 s	40 s	Total
Sample size (persons)	259	380	361	1000
Behavioral change stages				
(1) Migration was already decided, but not because of respondents' own will	7.7 %	4.2 %	3.9 %	5.0 %
(2) Be willing to live in the current residence city	32.8 %	47.6 %	42.9 %	42.1 %
(3) Have not even considered future residence	23.6 %	17.4 %	23.8 %	21.3 %
(4) Have considered future residence, but have hesitated to decide	18.9 %	18.9 %	14.1 %	17.2 %
(5) Intend to move to other places in Japan	9.3 %	7.9 %	9.1 %	8.7 %
(6) Already started to prepare for future migration based on respondent's own will	1.5 %	0.8 %	1.7 %	1.3 %
(7) Already decided to move to other places in Japan	3.1 %	1.1 %	1.1 %	1.6 %
(8) Considering to move to overseas, or preparing for overseas migration, or already decided to move to overseas	3.1 %	2.1 %	3.3 %	2.8 %
Total	100.0 %	100.0 %	100.0 %	100.0 %

school (12.0 %) and getting married (10.1 %), which is consistent with our intuitions. Furthermore, environmental factors cannot be ignored: there are housing issues (9.4 %), the living environment (6.7 %), and the convenience of commuting and schooling of the respondent (5.2 %).

17.3.3 Evidence of Interrelated Behavioral Changes Across Life Domains

As shown in Table 17.3, among all the respondents, 42.1 % are willing to reside in the current city, 21.3 % have not even considered their future residence, 5.0 % of respondents have already decided to migrate, but not voluntarily, and 2.8 % of responses are related to overseas migration. In other words, 71.2 % of these respondents may have ruled out voluntary relocation to other places in Japan. The strongest resistance to migration is expressed by those in their 30s: 47.6 % reported that they were willing to live in the current city of residence. This willingness to remain shows the largest variation across the three age groups (32.8 %–47.6 %). In contrast, variations across age groups with respect to other behavioral changes are unremarkable. In relation to migration to other places in Japan, 17.2 % of respondents have considered their future residence—however, they hesitated to decide; 8.7 % intended to move to other places in Japan; 1.3 % had already begun preparation for future voluntary migration, and just 1.6 % had already decided to move to other places in Japan. The above 28.8 %

of respondents (i.e., 288 people) were asked to report their potential migration places, with the assumption that they had already decided to migrate. As a result, 166 people reported that they would migrate to one of the three megacity regions (Tokyo, Nagoya, or Osaka), i.e., 16.6 % in total. A total of 122 people [30 people aged in their 20s (3.0 % of the total), 44 people aged in their 30s (4.4 %), and 48 people aged in their 40s (4.8 %)] reported that they would migrate to local cities (103 people: 10.3 %) and rural areas (19 people: 1.9 %), i.e., 12.2 % in total. These results are consistent with our intuition; that is to say, most people do not want to move from the Tokyo Capital Area once they have settled there. This suggests a difficulty in resolving the fundamental issues caused by the overconcentration of the Japanese population. Since 2014 in particular, the Japanese government has actively implemented various policies to encourage more people to move to places beyond the three megacity regions, to revitalize local cities and rural areas. However, it remains questionable how large the influence of these percentages—3.0 % in their 20s, 4.4 % in their 30s, 4.8 % in their 40s, and 12.2 % overall—is on the revitalization of local cities and rural areas. A comparison of the three age groups reveals that those in their 20s have the lowest percentage of people who are willing to live in the current city of residence, while this is highest for those in their 30s. The proportions of those intending to move to other places in Japan are similar among the three age groups. The proportion of those in their 20s and 30s that hesitate to move is higher (by 4.8 % points) than those in their 40 s. The proportion of those in their 20s who have already decided to move to other places in Japan is highest (3.1 %); however, the proportions moving to other places in Japan are similar in the three age groups.

Next, the concurrence of behavioral changes in terms of migration and of job, child rearing, and residence are shown in Tables 17.4, 17.5, 17.6. We conducted a χ^2 test to examine whether the behavioral changes between each of the above three pairs of life domains are independent, and rejected the hypotheses of independence in all cases on statistical grounds (as shown at the bottom of each table). Given this interdependence across life domains, even though some young people may intend to migrate to local cities, they may not do so, because behavioral changes in other domains do not support such a change.

Among those who intend to move to other places in Japan (8.7 %), those who either intend to change jobs (35.6 %), those preparing for a voluntary job change (9.2 %), or those who have already decided on a voluntary job change in future (1.1 %) only account for about 46 %. For the remainder, 24.1 % hesitate to decide whether to continue their current job or change it, and 29.9 % are willing to continue their current job. As for changes of dwelling, those who intend to change to another residence in future (70.1 %), who are already preparing to move (5.7 %), or who have decided to change residence in the near future (3.4 %) account for about 80 %. Concerning change in the child rearing domain, those who either intend to have children or to have more children in future (33.3 %), who are currently planning to have children (4.6 %), or who have decided to do so in the near future (2.3 %) only account for about 40 %. Thus, the intention to migrate in future is much more consistent with potential changes in residence than with changes in jobs or child rearing.

Table 17.4 Joint occurrence of behavioral changes between migration and job

Migration	Job					
	Future job was decided, but not because of own will (%)	Willing to continue the current job (%)	Have hesitated about whether to continue the current job or not (%)	Intend to have a change in job (%)	Already started to prepare for a job change based on own will (%)	Already decided to have a change in job based on own will (%)
	(2.5)	(49.5)	(25.2)	(16.3)	(3.9)	(2.6)
(1) Migration was decided, but not because of respondents' own will	24.0	42.0	22.0	8.0	0.0	4.0
(2) Be willing to live in the current residence city	1.4	63.2	18.8	13.1	1.9	1.7
(3) Have not even considered future residence	1.9	47.4	33.8	13.6	1.9	1.4
(4) Have considered future residence, but have hesitated	1.2	36.6	33.7	22.1	5.2	1.2
(5) Intend to move to other places in Japan	0.0	**29.9**	**24.1**	***35.6***	***9.2***	***1.1***
(6) Already started to prepare for future based on own will	0.0	**38.5**	**15.4**	*7.7*	***30.8***	*7.7*
(7) Already decided to move to other places	6.3	**18.8**	**25.0**	***25.0***	***12.5***	***12.5***

(continued)

Table 17.4 (continued)

Migration	Job					
	Future job was decided, but not because of own will (%)	Willing to continue the current job (%)	Have hesitated about whether to continue the current job or not (%)	Intend to have a change in job (%)	Already started to prepare for a job change based on own will (%)	Already decided to have a change in job based on own will (%)
(8) Considering to move to overseas, or preparing for, or already decided to move to overseas	0.0	35.7	17.9	3.6	14.3	28.6

Independence test for all categories: CHISQ = 321.9 (DF = 35, $p = 0.000$); Independence test for categories excluding items (1) and (8) of migration: CHISQ = 132.1 (DF = 20, $p = 0.000$)

Table 17.5 Joint occurrence of behavioral changes between migration and residence

Migration	Dwelling				
	Satisfied with current dwelling and no need to change (%)	Have not considered whether to change the dwelling or not in future (%)	Have hesitated about whether to change the dwelling in future or not (%)	Intend to change the dwelling in future (%)	Already started to prepare for changing the dwelling (%)	Already decided to change the dwelling (%)
	(28.1)	(18.2)	(9.2)	(36.4)	(4.4)	(3.7)
(1) Migration was decided, but not because of respondents' own will	24.0	14.0	14.0	28.0	4.0	16.0
(2) Be willing to live in the current residence city	47.7	15.4	6.4	26.1	2.4	1.9
(3) Have not even considered future residence	18.3	35.7	8.0	34.7	1.4	1.9
(4) Have considered future residence, but have hesitated	9.3	13.4	19.8	48.3	7.6	1.7
(5) Intend to move to other places in Japan	**8.0**	**9.2**	**3.4**	***70.1***	***5.7***	***3.4***
(6) Already started to prepare for future based on own will	0.0	0.0	0.0	***30.8***	***61.5***	***7.7***

(continued)

Table 17.5 (continued)

Migration	Dwelling					
	Satisfied with current dwelling and no need to change (%)	Have not considered whether to change the dwelling or not in future (%)	Have hesitated about whether to change the dwelling in future or not (%)	Intend to change the dwelling in future (%)	Already started to prepare for changing the dwelling (%)	Already decided to change the dwelling (%)
(7) Already decided to move to other places	**6.3**	**6.3**	**12.5**	***31.3***	***6.3***	***37.5***
(8) Considering to move to overseas, or preparing for, or already decided to move to overseas	17.9	7.1	7.1	46.4	7.1	14.3

Independence test for all categories: CHISQ = 431.2 (DF = 35, $p = 0.000$); Independence test for categories excluding items (1) and (8) of migration: CHISQ = 411.0 (DF = 25, $p = 0.000$)

Table 17.6 Joint occurrence of behavioral changes between migration and child rearing

Migration	Child rearing						
	No intention to marry or to have a child (%)	The current number of children is ideal and no intention to have more children (%)	Have not considered whether to marry and have any child or not, or whether to have more children or not (%)	Have hesitated about whether to marry and have any child or not, or whether to have more children or not (%)	Intend to have a child or to have more children (%)	Have started to prepare for having a child or having more children (%)	Already decided to have a child or to have more children (%)
	(16.7)	(21.7)	(18.1)	(9.0)	(26.8)	(4.5)	(3.2)
(1) Migration was decided, but not because of respondents' own will	10.0	28.0	14.0	8.0	26.0	8.0	6.0
(2) Be willing to live in the current residence city	17.1	28.7	16.2	7.6	23.0	4.5	2.9
(3) Have not even considered future residence	18.3	16.4	28.2	10.3	24.4	0.9	1.4
(4) Have considered future residence, but have hesitated	14.5	16.3	15.1	9.3	34.9	7.6	2.3
(5) Intend to move to other places in Japan	20.7	12.6	16.1	10.3	**33.3**	***4.6***	**2.3**

(continued)

Table 17.6 (continued)

Migration	Child rearing						
	No intention to marry or to have a child (%)	The current number of children is ideal and no intention to have more children (%)	Have not considered whether to marry and have any child or not, or whether to have more children or not (%)	Have hesitated about whether to marry and have any child or not, or whether to have more children or not (%)	Intend to have a child or to have more children (%)	Have started to prepare for having a child or having more children (%)	Already decided to have a child or to have more children (%)
(6) Already started to prepare for future based on own will	7.7	23.1	15.4	7.7	***38.5***	***0.0***	***7.7***
(7) Already decided to move to other places	18.8	0.0	6.3	6.3	***43.8***	***18.8***	***6.3***
(8) Considering to move to overseas, or preparing for, or already decided to move to overseas	14.3	17.9	10.7	17.9	17.9	0.0	21.4

Independence test for all categories: CHISQ = 113.0 (DF = 42, $p = 0.000$); Independence test for categories excluding items (1) and (8) of migration: CHISQ = 71.8, (DF = 30, $p = 0.000$)

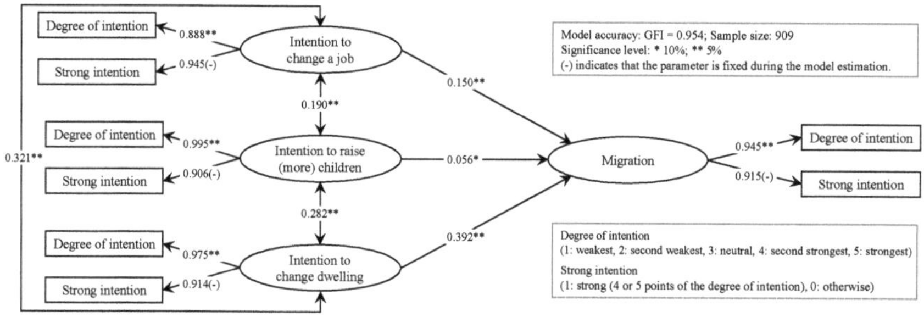

Fig. 17.4 Correlations of intentions across life domains: migration, job, dwelling, and child rearing

Keeping the above interdependencies across life domains in mind, we estimated a structural equation model, focusing only on intentions in different life domains, to test whether intention to migrate is affected by intentions to change job, dwelling, or child rearing. The model estimation reflects correlations among the latter three items. Figure 17.4 illustrates the estimation results. The goodness of fit (GFI) value is 0.954, suggesting that the model fit is sufficient to support the above hypothesis. Obviously, intentions with respect to jobs, dwellings, and child rearing all have a statistically significant effect on intention to migrate. Significant correlations of intentions are also confirmed with respect to jobs, dwellings, and child rearing. The intention to change dwelling has the strongest influence on the intention to migrate, where its effect size (i.e., the direct effect: 0.392) is more than twice as high as that of employment (0.150) and seven times higher than that of child rearing (0.056). Concerning intentions to change jobs, dwellings, or child rearing, the correlation between jobs and dwellings is highest (0.321) and the lowest correlation is observed between jobs and child rearing. To the best of our knowledge, this is the first study to reveal such interrelated behavioral changes in multiple life domains. The above findings suggest that it is necessary to reformulate traditional theories of behavioral changes by properly reflecting interdependency across life domains. It is also expected that such reformulation of theories of behavior could provide further sound insights into cross-sectoral policies to support migration.

17.4 Conclusions

Urban policies are intended not only to regulate people's behavior using various laws, institutional rules, and economic measures (but consensus building is required), but also to encourage voluntary changes in people's behavior in desirable directions through efficient communication. In particular, voluntary behavioral changes are essential for sustainable urban development, which requires close collaboration between various stakeholders over a considerable period. In the context of migration, such collaboration largely determines the population size and structure of a city/region, which is the most important input for almost all urban policies. On the other hand, no city/region could survive without connections to other parts of a nation or the world. Migration also determines and reflects the development patterns of a nation, which in turn affect the development of cities/regions. Thus, understanding migration behavior is essential for being able to make decisions on urban policies.

The population size of a city/region is important for its development, but the quality of its population is much more important (Romer 1990). Florida (2002a, b) and Zachary (2000) argued that regional innovation and economic growth are strongly associated with the creativity and diversity of a region, and it is especially important to attract talented individuals or those with high levels of human capital, because the presence of such human capital in turn attracts and generates innovative, technology-based industries. In fact, the importance of such high-quality human capital in urban and region development has been long recognized (Ullman 1958; Jacobs 1961). More empirical evidence is provided by Mathur (1999). To attract such human capital successfully, there is no doubt that economic incentives (salaries or relative deprivation elsewhere) are important; however, the roles of factors such as amenities, recreation, and lifestyles are crucial (Gottlieb 1995; Kotkin 2000; Glaeser et al. 2001; Lloyd and Clark 2001; Florida 2002a, 2002b). According to Yigitcanlar et al. (2007), knowledge workers prefer to live in a city that not only has affordable housing, but also high-quality urban services/facilities (e.g., child rearing, school education, and health care), a rich retail environment, and an attractive entertainment environment (professional sports, music, arts, and historical sites), and also offers a rich life in retirement. Frenkel et al. (2013), emphasizing that knowledge workers play three roles: household members, workers, and leisure consumers, further revealed that land uses related to culture, education, and lifestyle influence knowledge workers' residential behavior, in addition to the socioeconomic level of the city, the affordability of its housing, commuting time, and travel time to the city center. Households with culture-oriented lifestyles prefer to live in a city center, and households with home-oriented lifestyles prefer a suburban residence.

Based on an extensive literature review about various macro-, meso-, and microlevel studies, Hagen-Zanker (2008) concluded that migration decisions should be considered at a household level, where social networks, migration institutions (e.g., rules and norms governing the network that reduce transaction and migration costs), and relative deprivation (relative income, levels of inequality in a community) are emphasized. This argument is in line with our viewpoint about the intrahousehold and social interactions seen in studies of residential behavior (e.g., Zhang and Fujiwara 2009), car ownership (Zhang et al. 2009; Kuwano et al. 2011), time use (Zhang et al. 2002; Zhang and Fujiwara 2006), energy consumption (Yu et al. 2012), and tourist behavior (Wu et al. 2013). Additionally, we would like to argue for the importance of analysis of other life choices in migration studies, a view supported by the above review and empirical evidence of the interdependency across life domains revealed in Chap. 2 of this book. Human behavior, including migration behavior, changes over time.

As shown in the review in Sects. 17.2 and 17.3, there exist various dynamic behavior models in the literature; however, most previous studies have strongly focused on behavioral outcomes, rather than the process underlying them. This is true for not only migration behavior, but also for other life choices. With the above arguments in mind, it seems that the framework shown in Fig. 17.5 is necessary to address both behavioral changes related to the decision-making process and temporal dynamics related to behavioral outcomes (i.e., decision results) simultaneously by incorporating various interdependencies. In relation to behavioral changes, intentions are not only affected by attributes and norms, but also by experience and expectation. The influence of experience is called "state dependence" (Heckman 1981). Previous studies have widely represented state dependence by directly linking behavioral outcomes (choice results) over time (e.g., Kitamura 1990; Hunt 2008; De Jong et al. 2012; Carro and Traferri 2014; Zhang et al. 2014; Plum and Ayllon 2015), and have also shown that many human decisions are forward-looking (e.g., Manski 1999; Chan and Stevens 2004; Khan and Dhar 2007; Van der Klaauw and Wolpin 2008; Van der Klaauw 2012; Zhang et al. 2014; Tran et al. 2015). However, considering the importance of behavioral changes related to the decision-making process, it seems more logical to represent state dependence

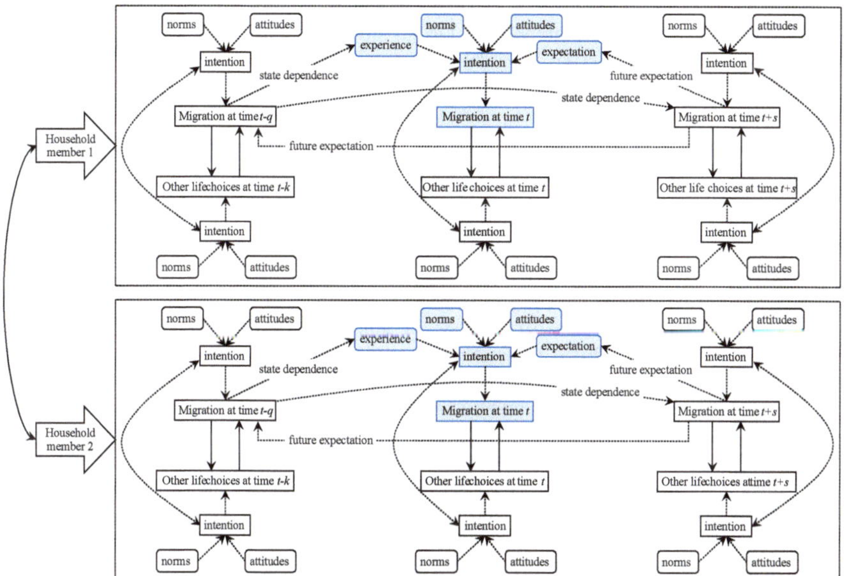

(Note: Influences of experience and expectation life are applicable not only to migration at time t, but also to migration at other time points as well as to other life choices. For the sake of simplicity, only the influences on migration at time t are illustrated)

Fig. 17.5 A conceptual framework of behavioral changes and temporal dynamics across life domains

and future expectations via intentions. The correlations revealed in Fig. 17.4 should also be reflected. There are various challenges (such as surveys, modeling, and policy applications) to realizing this comprehensive but complicated framework. In surveys, it is not an easy task to collect data, especially about items of behavioral change over time using methods such as panel surveys, considering the burden these place on respondents. Innovative survey methods (including retrospective surveys) should be developed. As for modeling, both utility-based approaches with attractive features for economic evaluations of policies (e.g., Yu et al. 2012), but also agent-based approaches with flexibility in managing various complex aspects (e.g., Kniveton et al. 2011) should be further improved to deal with large sets of life choices.

References

Ajzen I (1988) Attitudes, personality, and behavior. Dorsey, Chicago
Ajzen I (1991) The theory of planned behavior. Organ Behav Hum Decis Process 50:179–211
Albrecht J, Doering L, Holz-Rau C, Scheiner J (2015) The relevance of the place of childhood and adolescence for residential choice in later life: a life-course and intergenerational approach. In: Compendium of papers CD-ROM, the 94th annual meeting of transportation research board, Washington, D.C., 11–15 Jan
Bamberg S (2013) Changing environmentally harmful behaviors: a stage model of self-regulated behavioral change. J Environ Psychol 34:151–159
Bijker RA, Haartsen T, Strijker D (2012) Migration to less-popular rural areas in the Netherlands: exploring the motivations. J Rural Stud 28(4):490–498
Boneva BS, Frieze IH (2001) Toward a concept of a migrant personality. J Soc Issues 57(3):477–491
Botetzagias I, Dima A-F, Malesios C (2015) Extending the theory of planned behavior in the context of recycling: the role of moral norms and of demographic predictors. Resour Conserv Recycl 95:58–67
Carro JM, Traferri A (2014) State dependence and heterogeneity in health using a bias-corrected fixed-effects estimator. J Appl Econom 29(2):181–207
Castles S (2010) Understanding global migration: a social transformation perspective. J Ethnic Migr Stud 36(10):1565–1586
Chan S, Stevens AH (2004) Do changes in pension incentives affect retirement? A longitudinal study of subjective retirement expectations. J Public Econ 88(7–8):1307–1333
Chatterjee K, Scheiner J (2015) Understanding changing travel behavior over the life course: contributions from biographical research. In: A Resource paper for the workshop "Life-Oriented Approach for Transportation Studies" at the 14th international conference on travel behaviour research, Windsor, UK, 19–23 July
Chen M-F (2016) Extending the theory of planned behavior model to explain people's energy savings and carbon reduction behavioral intentions to mitigate climate change in Taiwan–moral obligation matters. J Clean Prod 112(2):1746–1753
Chen Y, Rosenthal SS (2008) Local amenities and life-cycle migration: do people move for jobs or fun? J Urban Econ 64:519–537
Chi G, Voss P (2005) Migration decision-making: a hierarchical regression approach. J Reg Anal Policy 35(2):11–22
Childs G, Craig S, Beall CM, Basnyat B (2014) Depopulating the Himalayan highlands: education and outmigration from ethnically Tibetan communities of Nepal. Mt Res Dev 34(2):85–94

Clifton-Sprigg J (2015) Educational spillovers and parental migration. Labour Econ 34:64–75
Crivello G (2015) 'There's no future here': the time and place of children's migration aspirations in Peru. Geoforum 62:38–46
De Jong MG, Lehmann DR, Netzer O (2012) State-dependence effects in surveys. Mark Sci 31(5):838–854
De Leeuw A, Valois P, Ajzen I, Schmidt P (2015) Using the theory of planned behavior to identify key beliefs underlying pro-environmental behavior in high-school students: implications for educational interventions. J Environ Psychol 42:128–138
Doering L, Albrecht J, Scheiner J, Holz-Rau C (2015) Mobility socialization in work trip biographies: work trips over the life course of two generations. In: Compendium of papers CD-ROM, the 94th annual meeting of transportation research board, Washington, D.C., 11–15 Jan
Ek E, Koiranen M, Raatikka V-P, Jarvelin M-R, Taanila A (2008) Psychosocial factors as mediators between migration and subjective well-being among young Finnish adults. Soc Sci Med 66:1545–1556
Fahr R, Sunde U (2006) Spatial mobility and competition for jobs: some theory and evidence for Western Germany. Reg Sci Urban Econ 36(6):803–825
Florida R (2002a) Bohemia and economic geography. J Econ Geogr 2:55–71
Florida R (2002b) The economic geography of talent. Ann Assoc Am Geogr 92:743–755
Frenkel A, Bendit E, Kaplan S (2013) Residential location choice of knowledge-workers: the role of amenities, workplace and lifestyle. Cities 35:33–41
Glaeser EL, Kolko J, Saiz A (2001) Consumer city. J Econ Geogr 1:27–50
Globalization101.org (2013) Migration and Globalization (http://www.globalization101.org/uploads/File/Migration/migration.pdf. Accessed 28 Jan 2016)
Graham E, Jordan LP, Yeoh BSA (2015) Parental migration and the mental health of those who stay behind to care for children in South-East Asia. Soc Sci Med 132:225–235
Groenewold G, de Bruijn B, Bilsborrow R (2012) Psychosocial factors of migration: adaptation and application of the health belief model. Int Migr 50(6):211–231
Gottlieb PD (1995) Residential amenities, firm location and economic development. Urban Stud 32:1413–1436
Guo JL, Wang TF, Liao JY, Huang CM (2016) Efficacy of the theory of planned behavior in predicting breastfeeding: meta-analysis and structural equation modeling. Appl Nurs Res 29:37–42
Hagen-Zanker J (2008) Why do people migrate? A review of the theoretical literature. Maastricht University, Maastricht Graduate School of Governance, Working Paper MGSoG/2008/WP002. Downloadable from http://papers.ssrn.com/sol3/papers.cfm?abstract_id=1105657. Accessed 29 Jan 2016
Han H (2015) Travelers' pro-environmental behavior in a green lodging context: converging value-belief-norm theory and the theory of planned behavior. Tour Manag 47:164–177
Haug S (2012) Migration and return migration: the cause of Italian migrants in Germany. Kakanien Revisited 1–11. http://www.kakanien-revisited.at/beitr/labourmigration/SHaug1.pdf. Accessed 29 Jan 2016
Heckman JJ (1981) Heterogeneity and state dependence. In: Rosen S (ed), Studies in labor markets. University of Chicago Press, Chicago
Hoppe A, Fujishiro K (2015) Anticipated job benefits, career aspiration, and generalized self-efficacy as predictors for migration decision-making. Int J Intercult Relat 47:13–27
Huinink J, Vidal S, Kley S (2014) Individuals' openness to migrate and job mobility. Soc Sci Res 44:1–14
Hunt LM (2008) Examining state dependence and place attachment within a recreational fishing site choice model. J Leisure Res 40(1):110–127
Jacobs J (1961) The death and life of great American cities. Random House, New York
Jiang Y, Zhang J, Jin X, Ando R, Chen L, Shen Z, Ying JQ, Fang Q, Sun Z (2015) Rural migrant workers' residential, commuting, and energy consumption preferences in the changing context of urban China. Transp Res Part D (under review)

Kennan J, Walker JR (2010) Wages, welfare benefits and migration. J Econom 156(1):229–238
Kennan J, Walker JR (2013) Modeling individual migration decisions. In: Constant AF, Zimmermann KF (eds), International handbook on the economics of migration. Edward Elgar Publishing, Cheltenham, UK (Chapter 2)
Khan U, Dhar R (2007) Where there is a way, is there a will? The effect of future choices on self-control. J Exp Psychol Gen 136(2):277–288
Kitamura R (1990) Panel analysis in transportation planning: an overview. Transp Res Part A Gen 24(6):401–415
King R (2012) Theories and typologies of migration: an overview and a primer. In: Willy Brandt series of working papers in international migration and ethnic relations 3/12, Malmö Institute for Studies of Migration, Diversity and Welfare, Malmö University, Sweden
Kniveton D, Smith C, Wood S (2011) Agent-based model simulations of future changes in migration flows for Burkina Faso. Glob Environ Change 21:S34–S40
Kotkin J (2000) The new geography. Random House, New York
Kuwano M, Zhang J, Fujiwara A (2011) A dynamic discrete choice model with multi-dimensional social interactions. Transp Res Rec 2231:68–75
Lee E (1966) A theory of migration. Demography 3:47–57
Li Y, Liu Y, Long H, Cui W (2014) Community-based rural residential land consolidation and allocation can help to revitalize hollowed villages in traditional agricultural areas of China: evidence from dancheng county, Henan Province. Land Use Policy 39:188–198
Liu YS, Liu Y (2010) Progress and prospect on the study of rural hollowing in China. Geogr Res 29(1):35–42
Liu H, Mrozb TA, van der Klaauw W (2010) Maternal employment, migration, and child development. J Econom 156:212–228
Lloyd R, Clark TN (2001) The city as entertainment machine. In: Gatham KF (ed) Research in urban sociology, vol 6. Critical Perspectives on Urban Redevelopment, Oxford, JAI/Elsevier, pp 357–378
MacDonald JS, MacDonald LD (1964) Chain migration, ethnic neighbourhood formation and social networks. Milbank Meml Fund Q 42(1):82–97
Manski CF (1999) Analysis of choice expectations in incomplete scenarios. J Risk Uncertain 19(1–3):49–65
Massey DS, Arango J, Hugo G, Kouaouci A, Pellegrino A, Taylor JE (1993) Theories of international migration: a review and appraisal. Popul Dev Rev 19(3):431–466
Mathur VK (1999) Human capital-based strategy for regional economic development. Econ Dev Q 13(3):203–216
Mencarini L, Vignoli D, Gottard A (2015) Fertility intentions and outcomes: implementing the theory of planned behavior with graphical models. Adv Life Course Res 23:14–28
Muilu T, Rusanen J (2003) Rural young people in regional development—the case of Finland in 1970–2000. J Rural Stud 19(3):295–307
Nachreiner M, Mack B, Matthies E, Tampe-Mai K (2015) An analysis of smart metering information systems: a psychological model of self-regulated behavioural change. Energy Res Soc Sci 9:85–97
Nugin R (2014) "I think that they should go. Let them see something": the context of rural youth's out-migration in post-socialist Estonia. J Rural Stud 34:51–64
Paul J, Modi A, Patel J (2016) Predicting green product consumption using theory of planned behavior and reasoned action. J Retail Consum Serv 29:123–134
Plum A, Ayllon S (2015) Heterogeneity in unemployment state dependence. Econ Lett 136:85–87
Prochaska JO, DiClemente CC (1983) Stages and processes of self-change of smoking: toward an integrative model of change. J Consult Clin Psychol 51(3):390–395
Prochaska JO, Velicer WF (1997) The transtheoretical model of health behavior change. Am J Health Promot 12(1):38–48
Romer PM (1990) Endogenous technological change. J Polit Econ 98(5):S71–S102

Rowe R, Andrews E, Harris PR, Armitage CJ, McKenna FP, Norman P (2016) Identifying beliefs underlying pre-drivers' intentions to take risks: an application of the theory of planned behaviour. Accid Anal Prev 89:49–56
Smith DP, Sage J (2014) The regional migration of young adults in England and Wales (2002–2008): a 'conveyor-belt' of population redistribution? Child Geogr 12(1):102–117
Tabor AS, Milfont TL (2011) Migration change model: exploring the process of migration on a psychological level. Int J Intercult Relat 35(6):818–832
Thissen F, Fortuijn JD, Strijker D, Haartsen T (2010) Migration intentions of rural youth in the Westhoek, Flanders, Belgium and the Veenkoloniën, The Netherlands. J Rural Stud 26(4):428–436
Triandis H (1977) Interpersonal behaviour. Brookds/Cole, Monterey CA
Tran MT, Zhang J, Fujiwara A (2015) Interdependences between current choices and future expectations in the context of Hanoians' residential location choices. Transp B: Transp Dyn, 1–8
Ullman EL (1958) Regional development and the geography of concentration. Papers Reg Sci 4(1):179–198
Van Dalen HP, Henkens K (2012) Explaining low international labour mobility: the role of networks, personality, and perceived labour market opportunities. Popul Space Place 18(1):31–44
Van Dalen HP, Henkens K (2013) Explaining emigration intentions and behaviour in the Netherlands, 2005–10. Popul Stud 67(2):225–241
Van der Klaauw W (2012) On the use of expectations data in estimating structural dynamic choice models. J Labor Econ 30(3):521–554
Van der Klaauw W, Wolpin KI (2008) Social security and the retirement and savings behavior of low income households. J Econom 145(1–2):21–42
Vilhelmson B, Thulin E (2013) Does the internet encourage people to move? Investigating Swedish young adults' internal migration experiences and plans. Geoforum 47:209–216
Wu L, Zhang J, Fujiwara A (2013) Representing the influence of multiple social interactions on monthly tourism participation behavior. Tour Manag 36:480–489
Xiong Y, Zhang J, Kayama Y (2016) Disentangling the young adults' residential relocation choices in Japan. Asian Transp Stud 4(1):78–95
Yazdanpanah M, Forouzani M (2015) Application of the theory of planned behaviour to predict Iranian students' intention to purchase organic food. J Clean Prod 107:342–352
Yigitcanlar T, Baum S, Horton S (2007) Attracting and retaining knowledge workers in knowledge cities. J Knowl Manag 11:6–17
Yu B, Zhang J, Fujiwara A (2012) A household time use and energy consumption model with multiple behavioral interactions and zero-consumption. Environ Plan B 40(2):330–349
Zachary PG (2000) The global me: new cosmopolitans and the competitive edge—picking globalism's winners and losers. Perseus Books, New York
Zhang J, Fujiwara A (2006) Representing household time allocation behavior by endogenously incorporating diverse intra-household interactions: a case study in the context of elderly couples. Transp Res Part B 40:54–74
Zhang J, Fujiwara A (2009) Intrahousehold interaction in transit-oriented residential choice behavior represented in stated preference approach. Transp Res Rec 2134:73–81
Zhang J, Timmermans HJP, Borgers A (2002) A utility-maximizing model of household time use for independent, shared and allocated activities incorporating group decision mechanisms. Transp Res Rec 1807:1–8
Zhang J, Kuwano M, Lee BJ, Fujiwara A (2009) Modeling household discrete choice behavior incorporating heterogeneous group decision-making mechanisms. Transp Res Part B 43:230–250
Zhang J, Yu B, Chikaraishi M (2014) Interdependences between household residential and car ownership behavior: a life history analysis. J Transp Geogr 34:165–174

Chapter 18
Future Perspectives of the Life-Oriented Approach

Junyi Zhang

Abstract This book has attempted to provide a general picture about the life-oriented approach by focusing on major life choices. In reality, there are so many types of life choices and it is therefore impossible to cover all of them in a single book. Here, first, this chapter makes brief discussions on research issues related to several life choices excluded from the previous chapters. Second, relevance of the life-oriented approach to cross-sectoral planning and policy as well as general public services is described. Third, future research from the perspective of making use of Big Data is illustrated. Fourth, it is discussed how to put the life-oriented approach into practice. Finally, this chapter describes future perspectives of the life-oriented approach in general, as a truly scientific system.

Keywords Interdependencies · Life-oriented behavior analysis system · Cross-sectoral policy · Public services · Big data & open government data · Citizen participation · Non-reductionism

18.1 Additional Remarks on Life Choice Studies

The previous chapters have provided rich insights into analyses of various life choices; however, there are still more life choices that need to be explored within the life-oriented approach. Here, I provide additional discussions on the following life choices that are also important to urban policy: residential behavior, time use, expenditure, habitual life choices, social network, and general travel behavior.

First, residential behavior involves long-term decisions (e.g., where to reside, whether to purchase a house or rent, and how long to reside), that may have

J. Zhang (✉)
Hiroshima University, Higashi-Hiroshima, Japan
e-mail: zjy@hiroshima-u.ac.jp; junyizh24@gmail.com

J. Zhang (ed.), *Life-Oriented Behavioral Research for Urban Policy*,
DOI 10.1007/978-4-431-56472-0_18

long-lasting impacts on many other life choices. Residential behavior has been widely studied together with travel behavior, where residential self-selection is a core behavioral phenomenon. A dominating argument is that residential self-selection comes from two sources: attitudes and sociodemographic traits. This argument would be true if decisions were made only on residential choice and travel behavior (Zhang 2014). In reality, residential and travel behavior are a part of people's life choices. Accordingly, omission of information about other life choices may also result in the existence of residential self-selection and it is therefore necessary to extend the decision boundary of residential and travel behavior research. In line with such consideration, Zhang (2014) proposed a new framework to analyze residential and travel behavior research considering the influence of residential self-selection issues by treating other life choices as the third source of the self-selection, based on the life-oriented approach. Zhang (2014) further presented several promising methodologies how to represent the residential self-selection under this new framework from static and dynamic perspectives, including multiple discrete-continuous choice modeling, modeling of future expectation and other behavioral dynamics, and choice models with flexible error structures.

Second, even though everybody has the same amount of time per day (24 h), per week (7 days), and per year (365 days), income levels of individuals with the same attributes are not the same. This means that the economic productivity of time use differs between individuals. Time is a kind of tradable resource in the market (e.g., housekeeping and chauffeur services). It is worth investigating what such features of time use mean for urban policy research, considering the interdependencies between activities and their connections with monetary expenditure. Unfortunately, little has been done with respect to joint analysis of time use and expenditure behavior (Zhang 2009). Because money and time are resources for decisions on many other life choices, it is not unrealistic to assume that decisions on monetary expenditure and time use are associated with other life choices. There are two types of monetary expenditure: utilitarian and hedonic expenditure. Utilitarian expenditure is for problem solving and hedonic expenditure for obtaining better affective experience (or enjoyment of life). It is expected that the more expensive a purchase, the higher its dependence on other life choices. On the other hand, spending time at a certain place usually involves energy consumption. Due to limited time, people have to trade off not only between in-home activities and out-of-home activities, but also between different in-home activities. In this sense, examining household energy consumption needs to treat in-home and out-of-home activities within the same analysis framework (see Yu and Zhang 2016), and types of in-home activities should be distinguished for the analysis of energy consumption. In line with such considerations, interestingly, a new type of energy-saving system has just been developed in Japan.[1] This system can automatically control lights and air conditioners in response to the resident's activity patterns at home,

[1]http://www.shimztechnonews.com/topics/t091007.html (in Japanese; Accessed May 14, 2015).

which are automatically detected based on the use of various electronic appliances via the in-home network. Considering that rebound effects cannot be ignored during the deployment of such new technology (Yu and Zhang 2016), it is worth clarifying whether such a new energy-saving system can actually reduce the overall household energy consumption. People usually spend one-third of a day sleeping, mainly at home. As sleeping time is a core indicator of a healthy lifestyle, health behavior and energy consumption behavior might be interrelated as a consequence of time use. Furthermore, there is a so-called solitude issue related to those young people who dislike face-to-face communication with others.[2] In recent years, people have been able to communicate with others via social media such as Facebook and LINE, without leaving home. This trend is especially prevalent among young people. Positively speaking, social media have dramatically improved people's lives. However, the above solitude issue is surely a serious social issue, which needs more research.

Third, in reality, some daily activities are habitual (e.g., Gärling and Axhausen 2003; Wood and Neal 2009). People may perform different habitual behaviors over a different length of time. For example, employed persons usually commute daily on weekdays; people may go shopping mainly on weekends; tourists may repeat their overseas travel annually or over several years. It is necessary to clarify how to represent time-use behavior involving habits. If two or more habits are behaviorally connected, their representation will become even more challenging. For this purpose, the time window for their representation should be clarified, because once the time window is extended, some habitual behaviors may be no longer habitual. A habitual activity may constrain participation in other daily activities. Once the living environment is changed, the habitual activity may become nonhabitual, consequently resulting in a changing interdependence structure among activities. In line with such considerations, long-term observation of various life choices is required. There are some time use related policies; for example, flexible working hours, flexible work contracts, and telework. Changes in time use patterns may have various impacts on people's daily life, not just the time spent on other activities. For example, in the case of telework, it may also lead to the reconsideration of residential functions and even the location of residence. Furthermore, people may participate in some activities more frequently in specific seasons. For example, people may enjoy more physical activities during spring and fall than during summer and winter. During spring and fall, more people may like to take a bicycle than during summer and winter. These seasonal activities may affect people's time use patterns in different ways.

Fourth, people live in a networked society. People's social networks are formed with a reflection of interpersonal bonds (e.g., Easterbrook and Vignoles 2013), needs in life (e.g., Lin et al. 2014; Tetreault et al. 2014), personality and

[2]http://ec.europa.eu/eurostat/statistics-explained/index.php/Being_young_in_Europe_today_-_digital_world (Accessed May 14, 2015).

attachment styles (e.g., Yaakobi and Goldenberg 2014), etc. Various studies on social networks have been done in link with subjective well-being (e.g., Pinquart and Sorensen 2000; Cheng et al. 2009; Huxhold et al. 2013), lifestyles (e.g., Baghaei et al. 2011; Sandra et al. 2011), residential choice (e.g., Magdol 2000; Viry 2012; Oishi et al. 2013), travel behavior (e.g., Schönfelder and Axhausen 2003; Larsen et al. 2006; Kowald et al. 2013), health (e.g., Li and Zhang 2015; Mohnen et al. 2015; Rook 2015), time use (e.g., Moore et al. 2013; Chang and Hsiao 2014), tourism (e.g., Larsen et al. 2007; Kim and Tussyadiah 2013) and so on. For example, in case of travel behavior research, one fundamental question is how to understand the associations between social networks, interrelated life choices, and daily activity-travel behavior. Social networks may mold various life choices and the resulting daily activity-travel behavior on one hand, while participating in various life activities allows people to get to know new members living in different locations on the other. Additionally, better accessibility supported by transport network and services may help people to form new social networks, which may provide them with more opportunities and enlarge their choice sets for enjoying a better life. However, such an effect may not appear soon and should be therefore captured over a longer period. In recent years, social networking via the Internet has become much more popular than ever before, which brings in more complexities. Better understanding of social networks needs more detailed information about people's social connections; however, such survey effort inevitably causes serious privacy issues. To avoid privacy issues, Big Data of social networking should be cleverly utilized based on innovative data fusion techniques. Furthermore, it might be worth exploring joint optimization of urban service networks and social networks, considering the social dimension of sustainable urban development.

Last but not the least, travel behavior should be reexamined from the viewpoint of life considerations. For this, trip-making behavior can be classified into two types: one is made reluctantly and the other willingly. In the former case, a trip maker has to be patient with the trip (e.g., commuting) and sometimes he/she may do something (e.g., reading, listening to music, and surfing the Internet) to relieve boredom (i.e., multitasking during travel). In the latter case, the trip maker may feel excited at the thought of participating in the subsequent activities (e.g., leisure and/or tourism activities) or may feel the travel is helpful because he/she can make use of the travel time to prepare for the subsequent activity (e.g., a business meeting). The willingness of trip making may also result from the liking of travel. The utility of trip making in the former case should be at least nonpositive and in the latter case at least nonnegative. In summary, positive utility derived from travel may result from three sources: travel liking, multitasking during travel, and expectation of activity participation after travel. Recently, studies of subjective well-being in the context of trip making have been attracting ever-increasing attention from travel behavior researchers. In particular, considering that the ideal travel time of many people is not zero (e.g., Redmond and Mokhtarian 2001), the preferred distance from home to each type of daily facility has been under-researched. More studies are required, especially for specifying the proper size of a city and further realizing the transformation to sustainable urban forms. Life choices affect travel mode choices while on the other, there are more travel mode choice variables influencing other life choices. The activity-based approach is a powerful tool for understanding travel behavior, but the effects of daily travel behavior on life choices are greatly under-researched. Thus, the accumulative effects of daily travel behavior on various life choices from a long-term perspective should be examined, considering the long-term nature of transportation planning. Furthermore, more life choice variables should be introduced to the travel behavior research framework. However, the paradigm shift from the activity-based approach to the life-oriented approach does not simply suggest extending the decision boundary. Rather, it suggests a new way of thinking about transportation planning and policy with better consensus building. The availability of transport access to various facilities and locations is essential to people's life. In line with this consideration, it is important to promote further the study of social exclusion (e.g., Stanley and Vella-Brodrick 2009; Stanley et al. 2011) in the context of transportation. For this purpose, the life-oriented approach could provide a new type of "compass" to guide social exclusion studies by paying more attention to various life domains with respect to different population groups in various contexts (e.g., aging society, depopulated areas, and natural disasters).

18.2 Relevance to Cross-sectoral Policymaking

The life-oriented approach may serve well for integrated planning and policies. For example, integrated land use and transportation planning needs a better understanding of people's decisions on activity participation at different locations and the resulting travel behavior. Healthy city planning should focus on improving not only people's lifestyle habits, but also their living environment that can facilitate their participation in more outdoor physical activities and social contacts with others. Low-carbon urban planning highly relies on how much people will live a low-carbon life in terms of transit-oriented and non-motorized travel behavior, residential behavior, energy consumption behavior, and eating behavior, etc. Inclusive transport policy needs to eliminate various exclusions, such as physical exclusion, geographical exclusion, economic exclusion, time-based exclusion, fear-based exclusion, and space exclusion (Church et al. 2000), which may prevent some people's access to various services for supporting their daily lives. Incorporating various interdependencies in life choices may not only allow the above examples of integrated planning and policies to be made in a more accurate way, but also enhance their effectiveness to improve people's quality of life in a better way, than ignoring the interdependences as done in independent planning and policies. In case of transportation planning, the activity-based approach (e.g., Axhausen and Gärling 1992; Algers et al. 2005), arguing that travel is a derived demand from activity participation, has been proved to be superior to the traditional trip-based approach. Barton (2009) stated that modern planning was invented in response to inhumane living conditions in the 19th century cities; however, in the last century the connection was lost and argued that land use planning should aim to the improvement of health and well-being. In line with this argument, Barton (2009) concluded, based on extensive literature review, that health and well-being is affected by physical activity, active travel, recreational activity, and diet, which may be further influenced by land use planning at the neighborhood level. Barton further concluded that health is closely tied with economic sustainability (in terms of jobs and income), social sustainability (in terms of the reduction of inequality, building inclusive and supportive communities), and environmental sustainability.

Considering the complexity of various interdependent life choices and the importance of reflecting them into urban policymaking, it may be worth developing a kind of life-oriented behavior analysis system (e.g., Fig. 18.1). Conceptually, the system may consist of (1) database of life choices, (2) behavioral modeling modules, and (3) policy modules. The life-oriented approach requires more data than existing single discipline. Innovative survey methods should be developed by trading off between respondents' answering burdens and rich information that is required to represent various interdependencies across life choices. In this regard, it is necessary to package various life choices and conduct each packaged survey separately. Meanwhile, existing data (especially Big Data) related to various life choices should be cleverly applied to supplement the use of the surveys required by the life-oriented approach. The above database (1) contain various life choices surveys conducted at the individual and household level, Big Data, and supply-side data of various urban services. The modeling modules cover behavioral models with respect to various life choices by explicitly incorporating the cause-effect

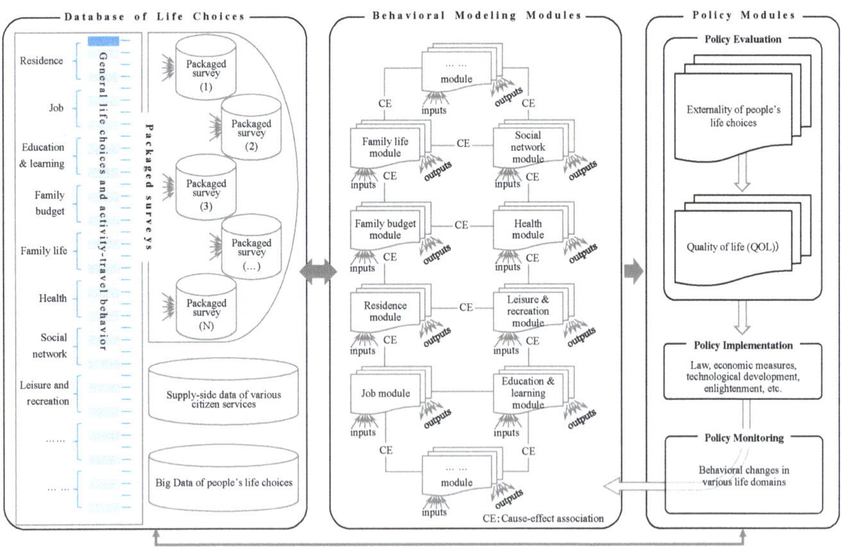

Fig. 18.1 A conceptual illustration of the life-oriented behavior analysis system

associations connected by various inputs and outputs. The policy module includes policy evaluation, implementation, and monitoring. The evaluation should focus on not only QOL but also various externalities caused by people's life choices (the externalities may also influence QOL), the implementation covers laws, economic measures, technological development, and enlightenment and so on, and the monitoring should pay more attention to behavioral changes in various life domains.

18.3 Relevance to General Public Services

Globally, people are continuing to migrate to cities. Governments, firms and other organizations provide various services to them. All these stakeholders usually claim that they aim to improve people's quality of life (QOL); however, their claims often hold within their own territories, reflecting their own interests and benefits. In many cases, different stakeholders understand people's QOL and its associations with various life choices differently. Governments have taken up many responsibilities, such as insuring public safety, guaranteeing essential infrastructures, promoting economic development, protecting the environment, and providing services to each individual citizen with respect to various life domains (e.g., residence, job, education, health, leisure and recreation, and travel). Different public services are usually accessible at different departments, partially because of specialty and efficiency of service provision. A particular public service may be associated with two or more life choices, while a particular life choice may need supports from two or more public services. In this sense, integration of and collaboration among public services are not a choice, but a "must" from a citizen's point of view. In other words, public services must be citizen-centered. This argument is consistent with that of the life-oriented approach, which aims to support various policy decisions involving interdependent life choices.

For example, *One-Stop-Government*, the integration of public services from a citizen's point of view, is a solution to realize citizen-centered public service provision (e.g., Wimmer 2002; Kunstelj and Vintar 2010). Under the one-stop paradigm, all of a citizen's business can be completed in a single contact, either face to face or via other means (e.g., phone, fax, Internet). To make the one-stop scheme possible, Tambouris and Spanos (2002) proposed an architecture for integrated public service delivery based on life events in the context of e-government, where service is handled by front-office, mid-office, and back-office in a sequential way. They discussed how such an architecture could service for one-stop government not only within one public authority, but also across all public authorities. They further identified three areas that need technical innovations: central portal (a central access point to information and services), service integration (for creating and invoking composite services), and service coordination (to locate all essential information for service provision). Composite service refers to the workflow, inputs, and outputs of all elementary and basic services that are required to fulfil one life event.

Consumer's point of view is indispensable to the provision of any service. Even though studies on services can be traced back to the era of Adam Smith, service science, formally advocated by Innovate America in 2004, attaches the most importance to the value co-creation between consumers and service providers (Maglio et al. 2010). Service science argues the necessity of paradigm shift from goods-dominant logic to service-dominant logic, where the former looks at economic exchange in terms of the production and distribution of units of output, while the latter suggests that market exchange is the process of parties using their specialized knowledge for mutual service provision benefits, i.e., value co-creation. Service science also claims that it aims to improve people's QOL and consumer modeling is at its core. In this sense, the life-oriented approach is consistent with the idea of service science. Different from private services, public services need to pay more attention to social welfare of the whole society. Therefore, future research should figure out how to make use of the life-oriented approach to realize various value co-creations during the process of public services provision.

18.4 More General Perspectives

The life-oriented approach deals with behavioral research for urban policy. Considering behavioral complexities involved in the life-oriented approach, it is necessary to conduct more studies by directly focusing on various urban issues, rather than just treating behaviors themselves. To understand life choices for urban policy, clearly, it is not a wise idea to focus on a specific discipline, for example, economics, psychology, or sociology. It is not a realistic choice, either, to develop a unified theory that can accommodate various interrelated life choices within the same modeling framework. Nevertheless, theoretical studies should be further promoted for scientifically guiding our understanding about various life choices. Society is sometimes too complex for models. For this reason, more qualitative research is required to derive some useful theories. Meanwhile, it is still worth applying various statistical approaches and simulation models to capture the complicated interdependencies involved in various life choices. More studies on the life-oriented approach should be implemented by exploring how to cultivate it as a new major behavioral research stream for supporting more general public policy decisions. Dialogue among researchers from various disciplines should be further promoted.

18.4.1 Use of Open Government Data

Data collection is a troublesome task in promoting studies on the life-oriented approach, because it needs respondents to answer many questions about their life choices, some of which may be sensitive to privacy issues. To understand why people make a particular choice in their life, questionnaire surveys are still a powerful tool. As stated by Alexopoulos et al. (2014), governments are one of the largest producers and collectors of data in many different domains. Recently, a number of open government data movements sprung up around the world, with transparency, data reuse, and participatory governance as three major reasons (Ubaldi 2013; Attard et al. 2015). Examples[3] of open government data include education, employment, industrial information, health, housing, transport and infrastructure, energy and environment, meteorological/weather information, geospatial information, crime and justice, government accountability and democracy, governmental budget, and public administration, etc. Currently, there are more than 30 countries with open data portal sites.[4] Research on how to make use of open government data based on the idea of the life-oriented approach should not be neglected.

18.4.2 Relevance to Understanding of Citizen Participation

Democratic public policymaking requires citizen participation (or public involvement), which ideally needs to represent the whole population. However, there are various constraints to citizen participation. Tonn and Petrich (1998) summarized five constraints in the United States: work-related, consumerisms, social capital, personal, and built environment constraints. Work places major constraints on the amount and quality of people's discretionary time and attention. Consumerism as a lifestyle (e.g. time spent watching television, shopping, and engaging in entertainment activities) takes time away from community pursuits and also requires time and effort to produce sufficient income to maintain the lifestyle. Social capital is a prerequisite for citizenship; however, population mobility, time pressure, lack of leadership, and economic stratification lead to decline in social capital. Many people fear public speaking because of enormous pressures to conform, threat of psychological harm, and their intuitive feeling about social tendencies towards intolerance. Built environment refer to land use, building designs, and transportation systems. The loss of great good places and the retreat of people to their homes only exacerbates difficulties in building social capital. Car-rather than people-oriented land uses may discourage people to participate in community activities because of longer travel time. Constraints related to work, lifestyle, and built environment are closely related to individual time use of both activity and travel, and social networking. To overcome any constraint may require a concerted effort to simultaneously overcome several constraints. Coglianese (2006) further revealed that the more significant barriers to citizen participation are cognitive and motivational, even with more sustained efforts to create user-friendly tools for

[3]https://www.gov.uk/government/publications/open-data-charter/g8-open-data-charter-and-technical-annex.

[4]http://www.soumu.go.jp/johotsusintokei/whitepaper/ja/h25/html/nc121240.html.

participation. Ravensbergen and VanderPlaat (2009) argued that poverty is a serious barrier to citizen participation of low-income people, and Irvin and Stansbury (2004) stated that one ideal condition for enhanced citizen participation is that citizens have enough income to attend meetings without harming their ability to provide for their families. The life-oriented approach has potential to contribute to a better understanding of citizen participation for value co-creation between public service providers and citizens. Relevant studies should be promoted in the future. If citizens can voluntarily engage in citizen participation, achieve a sustainable society will not be a dream.

18.4.3 Toward a Truly Scientific System

There are many disciplines dealing with human behavior. As argued by Kuhn (1962), any discipline may face a crisis of paradigm shift when abnormal events that it cannot address come to accumulate. Such a crisis has motivated the proposal of the life-oriented approach. As argued by the famous psychologist Kantor (1958), scientific systems must aspire toward validity, significance, and comprehensiveness (Fryling and Hayes 2010). Validity refers to internal consistency or lack of contradiction. Significance describes the relationship of an individual scientific system to others. When an individual scientific system shares the meta-assumptions of others, it is considered significant. Validity is a prerequisite for significant interactions with other scientific systems, but validity itself does not assure significance. Comprehensiveness means an adequate account of all of the events that fall within the scope of the scientific system. Importantly, comprehensiveness is only valued when it is construed within a system that is both valid and significant. From the validity viewpoint, the authors of this book have shown that there are complicated and diverse "chicken-and-egg" interdependencies across life choices, suggesting the necessity of treating multiple life choices within a unified analysis framework. The life-oriented approach can serve as such a unified framework. Considering interdependencies across life choices meets the requirements of significance and comprehensiveness. Reductionism has been widely adopted in various scientific research treating complex systems. Life choices are such a complex system. Reductionism decomposes a complex system into elements and assumes that as long as characteristics of each element can be revealed, the whole system can be understood (e.g., Sawyer 2002). However, because of interdependencies across life choices, it is not desirable to treat different life choices separately. In other words, reductionism has its serious limitations in representing interdependent life choices. Therefore, it is necessary to promote studies on the life-oriented approach based on the idea of non-reductionism (e.g., Sawyer 2002) that treats interdependent decisions as one cohesive unit of analysis. Studies based on non-reductionism may contribute to develop the life-oriented approach as a truly scientific system.

References

Alexopoulos C, Zuiderwijk A, Charalabidis Y, Loukis E, Janssen M (2014) Designing a second generation of open data platforms: Integrating open data and social media. In: Janssen M, Scholl HJ, Wimmer MA, Bannister F (eds), Electronic Government, Lecture Notes in Computer Science. Springer Berlin Heidelberg, 230–241

Algers S, Eliasson J, Mattsson LG (2005) Is it time to use activity-based urban transport models? A discussion of planning needs and modelling possibilities. Ann Reg Sci 39(4):767–789

Attard J, Orlandi F, Scerri S, Auer S (2015) A systematic review of open government data initiatives. Gov Inf Q 32:399–418

Axhausen KW, Gärling T (1992) Activity-based approaches to travel analysis: conceptual frameworks, models, and research problems. Transp Rev 12(4):323–341

Baghaei N, Kimani S, Freyne J, Brindal E, Berkovsky S, Smith G (2011) Engaging families in lifestyle changes through social networking. Int J Hum Comput Interact 27(10):971–990

Barton H (2009) Land use planning and health and well-being. Land Use Policy 26(Supplement 1):S115–S123

Chang T-S, Hsiao W-H (2014) Time spent on social networking sites: understanding user behavior and social capital. Syst Res Behav Sci 31(1):102–114

Cheng S-T, Lee CKL, Chan ACM, Leung EMF, Lee J-J (2009) Social network types and subjective well-being in chinese older adults. J Gerontol Ser B 64(6):713–722

Church A, Frost M, Sullivan K (2000) Transport and social exclusion in london. Transp Policy 7:195–205

Coglianese C (2006) Citizen participation in rulemaking: past, present, and future. Duke Law J 55(5):943–968

Easterbrook M, Vignoles VL (2013) What does it mean to belong? Interpersonal bonds and intragroup similarities as predictors of felt belonging in different types of groups. Eur J Soc Psychol 43(6):455–462

Fryling MJ, Hayes LJ (2010) An interbehavioral analysis of memory. Eur J Behav Anal 11:53–68

Gärling T, Axhausen KW (2003) Introduction: habitual travel choice. Transp 30(1):1–11

Huxhold O, Fiori KL, Windsor TD (2013) The dynamic interplay of social network characteristics, subjective well-being, and health: the costs and benefits of socio-emotional selectivity. Psychol Aging 28(1):3–16

Irvin RA, Stansbury J (2004) Citizen participation in decision making: is it worth the effort? Public Adm Rev 64(1):55–65

Kantor JR (1958) Interbehavioral psychology. The Principia Press, Chicago

Kim J, Tussyadiah IP (2013) Social networking and social support in tourism experience: the moderating role of online self-presentation strategies. J Travel Tourism Mark 30(1–2):78–92

Kowald M, Van den Berg P, Frei A, Carrasco JA, Arentze T, Axhausen KW, Mok D, Timmermans HJP, Wellman B (2013) Distance patterns of personal networks in four countries: a comparative study. J Transp Geogr 31:236–248

Kuhn TS (1962) The structure of scientific revolutions. The University of Chicago Press, Chicago

Kunstelj M, Vintar M (2010) One-stop government: critical analysis of the concept and its implementation in the selected countries. In: Nemec J, Peters BG (eds) State and administration in a changing world. NISPAcee Press, Slovak Republic, pp 131–156

Larsen J, Urry J, Axhausen KW (2006) Mobilities, networks and geographies. Ashgate, Aldershot

Larsen J, Urry J, Axhausen KW (2007) Networks and tourism—mobile social life. Ann Tourism Res 34(1):244–262

Li T, Zhang Y (2015) Social network types and the health of older adults: exploring reciprocal associations. Soc Sci Med 130:59–68

Lin H, Tov W, Qiu L (2014) Emotional disclosure on social networking sites: the role of network structure and psychological needs. Comput Hum Behav 41:342–350

Magdol L (2000) The people you know: the impact of residential mobility on mothers' social network ties. J Soc Pers Relatsh 17(2):183–204

Maglio PP, Kieliszewski CA, Spohrer JC (2010) Handbook of service science. Springer, New York

Mohnen SM, Volker B, Flap H, Subramanian SV, Groenewegen PP (2015) The influence of social capital on individual health: is it the neighbourhood or the network? Soc Indic Res 121(1):195–214

Moore J, Carrasco JA, Tudela A (2013) Exploring the links between personal networks, time use, and the spatial distribution of social contacts. Transportation 40(4):773–788

Oishi S, Kesebir S, Miao FF, Talhelm T, Endo Y, Uchida Y, Shibanai Y, Norasakkunkit V (2013) Residential mobility increases motivation to expand social network: but why? J Exp Soc Psychol 49:217–223

Pinquart M, Sorensen S (2000) Influences of socioeconomic status, social network, and competence on subjective well-being in later life: a meta-analysis. Psychol Aging 15(2):187–224

Ravensbergen F, VanderPlaat M (2009) Barriers to citizen participation: the missing voices of people living with low income. Community Dev J 45(4):389–403

Redmond LS, Mokhtarian PL (2001) The positive utility of the commute: modeling ideal commute time and relative desired commute amount. Transportation 28:179–205

Rook KS (2015) Social networks in later life: weighing positive and negative effects on health and well-being. Curr Dir Psychol Sci 24(1):45–51

Sandra B, Jeroen L, Lise K, Jacqueline D, Nijpels G (2011) Association between social network characteristics and lifestyle behaviour. Psychol Health 26:94

Sawyer RK (2002) Emergence in psychology: lessons from the history of non-reductionist science. Hum Dev 45:2–28

Schönfelder S, Axhausen KW (2003) Activity spaces: measures of social exclusion? Transp Policy 10(4):273–286

Stanley JR, Vella-Brodrick D (2009) The usefulness of social exclusion to inform social policy in transport. Transp Policy 16(3):90–96

Stanley JK, Hensher DA, Stanley JR, Vella-Brodrick D (2011) Mobility, social exclusion and well-being: exploring the links. Transp Res Part A 45(8):789–801

Tambouris E, Spanos E (2002) An architecture for integrated public service delivery based on life-events. Electron Markets 12(4):281–288

Tetreault S, Freeman A, Carriere M, Beaupre P, Gascon H, Deschenes PM (2014) Understanding the parents of children with special needs: collaboration between health, social and education networks. Child Care Health Dev 40(6):825–832

Tonn BE, Petrich C (1998) Everyday life's constraints on citizenship in the united states. Futures 30(8):783–813

Ubaldi B (2013) Open government data: towards empirical analysis of open government data initiatives. In: OECD working papers on public governance, No. 22, OECD Publishing, Paris. doi:10.1787/5k46bj4f03s7-en

Viry G (2012) Residential mobility and the spatial dispersion of personal networks: effects on social support. Soc Netw 34(1):59–72

Wimmer MA (2002) A European perspective towards online one-stop government: the eGOV project. Electron Commer Res Appl 1(1):92–103

Wood W, Neal DT (2009) The habitual consumer. J Consum Psychol 19(4):579–592

Yaakobi E, Goldenberg J (2014) Social relationships and information dissemination in virtual social network systems: an attachment theory perspective. Comput Hum Behav 38:127–135

Yu B, Zhang J (2016) Household energy consumption behavior. In: Zhang J (ed) Life-oriented behavioral research for urban policy. Springer, Berlin. (Chapter 5)

Zhang J (2009) A model of pedestrian time and monetary consumption behavior at city center. In: Timmermans HJP (ed) Pedestrian behaviour: models data collection and applications. Emerald, West Yorkshire, pp 157–193

Zhang J (2014) Revisiting the residential self-selection issues: a life-oriented approach. J Land Use Transp 7(3):29–45

MIX
Papier aus verantwortungsvollen Quellen
Paper from responsible sources
FSC® C105338

If you have any concerns about our products,
you can contact us on
ProductSafety@springernature.com

In case Publisher is established outside the EU,
the EU authorized representative is:
Springer Nature Customer Service Center GmbH
Europaplatz 3, 69115 Heidelberg, Germany

Printed by Libri Plureos GmbH
in Hamburg, Germany